Modules for BASIC NURSING SKILLS FIFTH EDITION

Volume II

Modules for BASIC NURSING SKILLS

Volume II

FIFTH EDITION

Janice Rider Ellis, R.N., Ph.D.

Elizabeth Ann Nowlis, R.N., Ed.D.

Patricia M. Bentz, R.N., M.S.N.

Shoreline Community College
Seattle, Washington

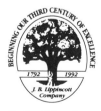

J. B. Lippincott Company Philadelphia

New York London Hagerstown

Sponsoring Editor: Donna L. Hilton, RN, BSN
Developmental Editor: Marian Bellus
Coordinating Editorial Assistant: Susan Perry
Project Editor: Amy P. Jirsa
Indexer: Anne Cope
Design Coordinator: Kathy Kelley-Luedtke
Designer: Susan Blaker
Cover Design: Larry Pezzato
Production Manager: Helen Ewan
Production Coordinator: Nannette Winski
Compositor: Tapsco, Inc.
Printer/Binder: Courier Companies, Inc.

5th Edition

1 3 5 6 4 2

Library of Congress Cataloging-in-Publication Data
(Revised for vol. 2)

Ellis, Janice Rider.
  Modules for basic nursing skills.

  Includes bibliographical references and index.
  1. Nursing—Outlines, syllabi, etc. 2. Nursing—
Problems, exercises, etc. I. Nowlis, Elizabeth Ann.
  II. Bentz, Patricia M. III. Title. [DNLM: 1. Nursing—
programmed instruction.   WY 18 E47m]
RT52.E44 1992   610.73'076   91-21752
ISBN 0-397-54908-3 (v. 1)
ISBN 0-397-54909-1 (v. 2)

Contents

v

Unit 10
SPECIAL THERAPEUTIC AND SUPPORTIVE PROCEDURES

Unit 11
PROVIDING MEDICATION AND INTRAVENOUS THERAPY

List of Skills

The following skills are included in this volume. For easy reference, a module number and a page number are provided for each skill.

Skill	Module	Page
Albumin administration	57	538
Bladder irrigation	48	295
Blood and blood products administration		
Albumin	57	538
Autologous transfusion	57	526
Cryoprecipitate	57	539
Platelets	57	535
Whole blood and packed red cells	57	530
Catheter irrigation	48	295
Catheterization		
Caring for a patient with a catheter	39	111
Inserting a urinary drainage catheter	39	114
Intermittent self-catheterization	39	113
Removing a Foley catheter	39	113
Chest tubes		
Assisting with insertion	44	207
Assisting with removal	44	214
Care of the patient with chest tubes	44	210
Stripping or milking	44	208
Colostomy/ileostomy care		
Changing a dressing	38	84
Changing a pouch	38	84
Irrigating a colostomy	38	86
Obtaining specimens	38	84
Coughing	41	151
Cryoprecipitate administration	57	539
Deep breathing	41	149
Dressings, sterile, changing	37	60
Ear irrigation	48	297
Epidural catheter care	59	573

To the Instructor

The fifth edition of *Modules for Basic Nursing Skills* continues to provide a resource for students to learn basic skills and procedures. We have used the same nursing-process-oriented, self-instructional approach that has proven valuable in previous editions.

As we prepared this edition, we have tried to look at our instructions and directions from a student's standpoint. We have tried to clarify this new language of health care that students are learning at the same time they are mastering skills. We recognize that the formal, official terms used for equipment and skills are not always the same as the "shorthand" that students will hear in a clinical setting. Therefore, we have provided both sets of terms in many instances.

As more students enter the college setting with varied educational backgrounds, language and reading levels become ever more important. In a skills text, perhaps more than anywhere else, the focus must be on clear, straightforward language. We are grateful for the responses of our students in helping us with this task.

COMPREHENSIVE SKILLS COVERAGE

There are now 59 modules in two volumes. Volume 1 contains the most basic skills and is appropriate by itself for some courses enrolling LPN/LVN students, as well as for courses for nursing aides and nursing assistants. Volumes 1 and 2 together are most useful in programs for RN students. Because programs vary considerably from state to state and from institution to institution, we have tried to make the two volumes as adaptable as possible to many different programs by offering comprehensive coverage of nursing skills.

ORGANIZATION

The modules are organized into units that reflect broad concepts of nursing care. This structured presentation will help the student understand how individual skills relate to particular human needs and to the nursing process. The first unit focuses on skills that students must master in order to deal safely and effectively with patients. As in the previous edition, throughout the two volumes skills are arranged in a progression from simple to complex, but each module is self-contained so that skills can be omitted or reordered according to the needs of particular programs.

SELF-INSTRUCTIONAL FORMAT

By consistently emphasizing the nursing process and appropriately highlighting rationale, the format of the modules focuses on the student's practice and mastery of skills and procedures. The elaborate program of features is designed to encourage understanding, independent learning, and self-instruction.

Module Contents

An outline of the module contents helps the student identify the information and specific skills that are included in the module.

Prerequisites

The list of prerequisites lets the student know what other modules and significant material are essential to successful completion of the particular module. This information is especially helpful when the order of modules is adjusted to meet the needs of individual nursing programs. It can also be used advantageously by the student who wishes to prepare for a particular patient-care situation.

Overall Objective

A general statement of the overall objective concisely describes what the student can expect to learn in the module.

xi

Specific Learning Objectives

Arranged in tabular form, the outline of learning objectives previews the important steps in the skill and indicates what basic knowledge and application of knowledge are required in addition to psychomotor skills.

Learning Activities

The learning activities provide additional guidance to the student about what steps to take in order to accomplish the desired objectives.

Vocabulary

A list of key terms for each skill is provided. These terms are defined in the Glossary at the back of each volume.

MODULE CORE

The discussion of each procedure includes necessary background information and step-by-step instructions, with carefully chosen photographs and technically precise illustrations.

Instructions are presented in a nursing process format when the skill is one that is used with patients and when the nursing process is appropriate to the skill. The steps in the process—Assessment, Planning, Implementation, and Evaluation—are clearly delineated by headings. This emphasis reinforces for students the fact that nursing process is relevant to practice. Nursing diagnoses are not included in the procedure itself. Where appropriate, the nursing diagnoses for which the particular skill might be used are presented in a separate section.

Documentation is included with every skill. The increasing emphasis on documentation for both evaluative and legal reasons makes the learning of correct documentation essential. Our premise is that although systems differ in *how* documentation is done, *what* needs to be documented is fairly standard. We have included specific examples of flow sheets and progress notes (in both narrative and SOAP formats) to help students make the transition to the record system they will be asked to use.

Rationale for the use of each skill is explained at the beginning of every module. Rationale for the specific actions that are part of the procedure are highlighted throughout the discussion by the use of italic type.

Because the approach to many skills is the same, whenever possible a general procedure for a group of specific procedures has been identified. The purpose of this is to facilitate the student's ability to transfer basic principles from one situation to another. We have tried to do this in a way that does not create confusion and that can be followed when practicing the skill.

Illustrations were carefully chosen to help the students as they work through the module independently. We have expanded the examples of charting and have placed the examples of nursing progress notes on chart facsimiles to help the student transfer knowledge to the actual clinical setting.

References

The references given are to research data regarding the skill or the recommendations of an authoritative agency such as the Centers For Disease Control (CDC). The most recent research is cited. In the case of skills, this research is may be older than expected. For example, the many excellent studies on the procedure and timing used for taking temperatures were done 10 years ago, but remain the basis for current recommendations. The CDC change their recommendations only when their decision-making bodies determine that the data warrant a change. You will note that the most recent recommendations from the CDC are from 1988.

Unfortunately, there is little research data to support many of the nursing techniques used. Therefore, you will also note an emphasis within the modules on consulting policy and procedure manuals in institutions. These are generally established by groups of nurses working together with legal as well as health care goals in mind. Learning to use the official policy and procedure manual will be an asset both to the student and to the practicing nurse.

Performance Checklist

The performance checklist follows the nursing process approach and can be used for quick review and for evaluation of the student's performance in terms of psychomotor skills. To facilitate review and evaluation, all steps of each procedure, including those which are first presented as part of a general procedure, are outlined in the performance checklist.

Quiz

A self-test is provided at the end of each module to allow students to test their mastery of the material in the module. The quizzes may also be used by instructors for evaluation purposes.

Glossary

The terms in the vocabulary lists are defined in the glossary at the back of each volume. The glossaries are a convenient reference source for students.

Answers to Quizzes

Answers to the quizzes are given at the end of each volume.

Index

An index is provided at the back of each volume.

CONVENIENT PACKAGING

The pages of both volumes are three-hole punched and perforated, so students can either tear them out and hand them in or keep them in notebooks.

TESTING SUPPLEMENT

A test bank accompanying Volumes 1 and 2 includes multiple-choice questions for all the skills that are covered.

Modules for Basic Nursing Skills, Volumes 1 and 2, Fifth Edition, can be used in conjunction with the text by Ellis and Nowlis, *Nursing: A Human Needs Approach,* Fourth Edition, which treats the theory behind nursing practice. However, the two volumes of modules are designed to stand alone and can be used by themselves in a course addressing nursing skills. *Mod-*

ules for Basic Nursing Skills can also be used in conjunction with any other text covering nursing theory or fundamentals.

We would like to thank Carole C. Wonsiewicz and the following individuals for their reviews of the manuscript at various stages and for their many useful suggestions:

Betty Sue Ashby, RN, PhD
Level I Coordinator
Southside Regional Medical Center
School of Nursing
Petersburg, VA

Marylee Evans, BSN, MSN
University of Rhode Island
Kingston, RI

Maryanne Ludy, RN, MSN
Professor of Nursing
Valencia Community College
Orlando, FL

Ann Carignan, RN, MSN
Professor of Nursing
Valencia Community College
Orlando, FL

We are especially grateful to our students and colleagues who used the modules as they were originally written, worked through the changes made for the first four editions, and assisted in the planning of this revision. Their constant feedback has been essential to us.

J.R.E.
E.A.N.
P.M.B.

To the Student

The modules in these two volumes are designed to enable you to learn the procedures that are basic to your role as a health care provider. Each module contains the following parts, unless they are not applicable to a particular skill:

Module Contents

The outline of the module contents provides you with an overview of all the information and specific skills contained in the module. Often a module contains several skills, and these will all be listed in the contents.

Prerequisites

The list of prerequisites describes the specific skills or abilities needed to master the new skill and indicates other modules that contain information necessary to an understanding of the skill.

Overall Objective

A general statement of the overall objective describes the basic skill that is taught in the module.

Specific Learning Objectives

A table of specific learning objectives breaks down the basic skill you are studying into specific subskills on which you can test yourself after completing the module.

Learning Activities

The learning activities are designed to help you progress safely and gradually into performing the new skill. Practice, in whatever setting is available, is essential to skillful performance. The amount of practice needed by each student will differ, depending on manual dexterity and previous experience. If your school provides audiovisual aids to use with the mod-

ule, view them after reading the module but before actually practicing the skill. Do not hesitate to contact your instructor if you encounter difficulties.

Vocabulary

The vocabulary list gives key terms used in the module. A glossary at the back of each volume gives the definitions of these terms, though some are best understood in the context of the module itself.

Module Core

The discussion of each procedure includes necessary background information and step-by-step instructions, with carefully chosen photographs and technically precise illustrations.

Instructions are presented in a nursing process format when the skill is one that is used with patients and when the nursing process is appropriate to the skill. The steps in the process—Assessment, Planning, Implementation, and Evaluation—are clearly delineated by headings. This emphasis reinforces for students the fact that nursing process is relevant to practice. Nursing diagnoses are not included in the procedure itself. Where appropriate, the nursing diagnoses for which the particular skill might be used are presented in a separate section.

Documentation is included with every skill. The increasing emphasis on documentation for both evaluative and legal reasons makes the learning of correct documentation essential. Our premise is that although systems differ in *how* documentation is done, *what* needs to be documented is fairly standard. We have included specific examples of flow sheets and progress notes (in both narrative and SOAP formats) to help students make the transition to the record system they will be asked to use.

Rationale for the use of each skill is explained at the beginning of every module. Rationale for the specific actions that are part of the procedure are

xv

highlighted throughout the discussion by the use of italic type.

Because the approach to many skills is the same, whenever possible a general procedure for a group of specific procedures has been identified. The purpose of this is to facilitate the student's ability to transfer basic principles from one situation to another. We have tried to do this in a way that does not create confusion and that can be followed when practicing the skill.

An increasing number of people are being cared for at home who were previously cared for in the acute care hospital. Therefore, we have added a discussion of how you would integrate the information on a particular skill into your planning for home care. Another area of increasing importance in health care is long-term care. In long-term care, adaptations of procedures and techniques may also be needed. We have added references to these changes and adaptations where appropriate.

References

The references given are to research data regarding the skill or the recommendations of an authoritative agency such as the Centers For Disease Control (CDC). The most recent research is cited. In the case of skills, this research is may be older than expected. For example, the many excellent studies on the procedures and timing used for taking temperatures were done 10 years ago, but remain the basis for current recommendations. The CDC change their recommendations only when their decision-making bodies determine that the data warrant a change. You will note the most recent recommendations from the CDC are from 1988.

Unfortunately, there is little research data to support many of the nursing techniques used. There-

fore, you will also note an emphasis within the modules on consulting policy and procedure manuals in institutions. These are generally established by groups of nurses working together with legal as well as health care goals in mind. Learning to use the official policy and procedure manual will be an asset both to the student and to the practicing nurse.

Performance Checklist

The performance checklist is used as a guide for practicing the skill and judging your performance of it.

Quiz

The quiz is a brief review for self-testing.

Glossary

The glossary at the back of each volume provides definitions for the key vocabulary terms.

Answers to Quizzes

The answer key at the end of each volume allows you to score yourself on the quizzes.

Index

An index is provided at the back of each volume.

We hope you will find gaining these essential skills to be a satisfying endeavor, and we wish you our best as you begin your studies.

J.R.E.
E.A.N.
P.M.B.

Modules for
BASIC
NURSING
SKILLS FIFTH EDITION

Volume II

Unit 7

COMPLEX INFECTION CONTROL

MODULE 34
Isolation Technique

MODULE 35
Sterile Technique

MODULE 36
Surgical Asepsis: Scrubbing, Gowning, and Gloving

MODULE 37
Wound Care

1

Module 34
Isolation Technique

Module Contents

Rationale for the Use of This Skill
Nursing Diagnoses
Resources for Isolation Procedures
Creating Barriers to Microorganisms
Disease-Specific Isolation Precautions
Category-Specific Isolation Precautions
   Strict Isolation
   Respiratory Isolation
   Wound and Skin Precautions
   Enteric Precautions
   Blood/Body Fluid Precautions
   Protective Isolation
   Compromised Host
Specific Isolation Procedures
   Preparing the Room
   Entering the Room

   Double-Bagging
   Caring for Linen
   Caring for Dishes and Food Trays
   Leaving the Room
   Transporting the Patient in Isolation
General Procedure for Isolation
   Assessment
   Planning
   Implementation
   Evaluation
   Documentation
Patient, Family, and Staff Cooperation
Combating Sensory Deprivation
Home Care

Prerequisites

Successful completion of the following modules:

VOLUME 1

Module 1   An Approach to Nursing Skills
Module 2   Basic Infection Control
Module 3   Safety
Module 6   Documentation

3

Overall Objective

To carry out correct isolation technique, placing emphasis on safety for patients, visitors, staff, and self.

Specific Learning Objectives

	Know Facts and Principles	Apply Facts and Principles	Demonstrate Ability	Evaluate Performance

1. *Purpose*
  a. To protect patient
  b. To protect environment
	Know two major purposes of isolation.	Given a patient situation, identify which of two major purposes of isolation should be utilized.	In the clinical setting, identify purposes for isolation in use.	Evaluate with instructor.

2. *Types*
  a. Rationale
  b. Disease-specific
  c. Category-specific
    (1) Strict
    (2) Respiratory
    (3) Wound and skin
    (4) Enteric
    (5) Blood/body fluid
    (6) Protective
    (7) Compromised host
	Discuss various types of isolation and rationale for use of each.	Given a patient situation, identify type of isolation procedure appropriate.	In the clinical setting, choose appropriate type of isolation for patient.	Evaluate own performance with instructor.

3. *Procedures*
  a. Preparing the room
  b. Entering the room (gown, mask, gloves)
  c. Double-bagging
  d. Caring for linen
  e. Leaving the room
  f. Transporting the patient in isolation
  g. General procedure
	Describe various procedures necessary for patient isolation.	Given a patient situation, state which procedure would be appropriate to carry out.	Carry out various types of isolation procedures correctly.	Evaluate own performance with instructor using Performance Checklist.

4. *Teaching*	List important facts to teach patient, family, and auxiliary staff.	Given a patient situation, plan teaching appropriate for type of isolation.	Instruct patient, family, and auxiliary staff on isolation procedure.	Evaluate own performance with patient, family, staff, and instructor.
5. *Sensory deprivation*	State causes and effects of sensory deprivation. List techniques that can be used to prevent or decrease effects of sensory deprivation.	Given a patient situation, identify possible effects of sensory deprivation and list nursing techniques that could be used to decrease them.	Recognize potential and real effects of sensory deprivation and use nursing techniques to intervene.	Evaluate own performance by sharing experience with instructor and classmate.

Learning Activities

1. Review the Specific Learning Objectives.
2. Read the section on isolation in the chapter on infection in Ellis and Nowlis, *Nursing: A Human Needs Approach,* or comparable material in another textbook.
3. Look up the module vocabulary terms in the Glossary.
4. Read through the module and mentally practice the techniques.
5. In the practice setting:
   a. With a partner, practice preparing to enter and leave the various types of isolation rooms: strict, respiratory, wound and skin, enteric, blood/body fluid, protective, and compromised host. Evaluate each other's performance using the Performance Checklist.
   b. With a partner, practice double-bagging, alternating so that each of you has a turn being inside the room and outside the room. After you have done the procedure the first time, evaluate yourselves, using the Performance Checklist. Then switch roles and repeat the procedure. Again, evaluate yourselves and repeat the procedure as necessary.
   c. When you are satisfied that you can carry out the procedure, have your instructor evaluate your performances.
6. In the clinical setting:
   a. Consult your clinical instructor for an opportunity to carry out isolation procedure.

Vocabulary

AIDS
compromised host
isolation
microorganisms
sensory
   deprivation

Isolation Technique

Rationale for the Use of This Skill

The isolation of an institutionalized patient may become necessary for various reasons. Whatever the reason, the nurse must understand the rationale and be able to carry out the procedure correctly. This is true not only to perform correctly, but so that explanations can be given to the patient, the patient's family, and the auxiliary staff regarding the procedures and the reasons for them.

Two main systems are used for placing the patient in isolation: disease-specific isolation precautions and category-specific isolation precautions. Because both approaches are accepted by the Centers for Disease Control (CDC) and facilities may choose to implement either type, nurses should be familiar with both. In this module we will discuss the preparation of the room for isolation and the correct method for entering and leaving the room. We will also consider sensory deprivation as a potential problem for the isolated patient.[1]

▶ *Nursing Diagnoses*

> The following nursing diagnoses are problems commonly experienced by patients in isolation:
>
> Social Isolation: Related to confinement imposed by isolation regimen
> Knowledge Deficit: Related to lack of experience with infection control measures
> Diversional Activity Deficit: Boredom related to confinement imposed by isolation
> High Risk for Infection: Related to suppressed immune system

RESOURCES FOR ISOLATION PROCEDURES

To meet the hospital accreditation standards, each facility must have an infection control officer. This officer might be a nurse or someone on the laboratory staff. In large medical centers, the infection control officer is sometimes a physician epidemiologist. This person monitors infections and helps establish policy regarding isolation within the facility.

[1] You will note that rationale for action is emphasized throughout the module by the use of italics.

The procedure manual of a facility outlines the specific method its staff should use. Review this resource *for clarification* regarding isolation if you are unsure of how to proceed in an individual situation.

CREATING BARRIERS TO MICROORGANISMS

The principle behind isolation technique is to create a physical barrier that prevents the transfer of microorganisms. To do this, you have to know how the organisms are transmitted and take measures to prevent that transmission. For example, if an organism is airborne, it is reasonable to start wearing masks and keep the door of the patient's room closed. If, however, the organisms are only transferred by contact with drainage or secretions on linen and items used in care, masks are unnecessary, and only direct contact with the patient is hazardous.

In other words, the barriers created for effective isolation should be appropriate to the goal—preventing the spread of select microorganisms from the patient to the environment or from the environment to the patient.

In 1983 the Centers for Disease Control altered long-standing guidelines and introduced a new system, Disease-Specific Isolation Precautions, which set up appropriate isolation measures for the various infectious diseases. However, many facilities continue to use the older Category-Specific Isolation Precautions. Each system has its advantages and disadvantages, and both are used in various health care agencies.

Since the widespread use of body substance precautions, many facilities use a specific isolation designation only rarely because all patients are being treated as if they have infections that can be transferred by blood, body fluids, or any other body substance (see Module 2, Basic Infection Control). A specific isolation designation may be reserved for infections transmitted via the respiratory tract or certain extremely virulent infections. Be sure to check the policy in any facility where you work. An infection control manual may be available for your use and you may also consult the infection control specialist to make the best decision regarding an individual patient situation.

DISEASE-SPECIFIC ISOLATION PRECAUTIONS

Under Disease-Specific Isolation Precautions, each infectious disease is considered separately, and guidelines that use only those procedures considered necessary to attain the goal are then set up (Table 34–1). An advantage of this system is that it is adaptable to individualized care plans (Moree & Garner, 1984). This approach has also been termed more logical *because it minimizes unnecessary precautions and equipment use* (Veterans Administration). After consulting a list of diseases with recommendations for isolation, nurses can fill out a single card that lists the appropriate precautions to take for a specific disease (Figure 34–1).

CATEGORY-SPECIFIC ISOLATION PRECAUTIONS

Many hospitals continue to use the system known as category-specific isolation *to protect people from pathogens infecting a given patient*. This approach has separate cards and instructions for diseases fitting into various categories, which are determined by how the organisms are transmitted. The five types of isolation generally used in this system are strict isolation, respiratory isolation, wound and skin precautions, enteric precautions, and blood/body fluid (universal) precautions. In view of the current concern about diseases transmitted by body fluids, blood and body fluid precautions are used more frequently than enteric precautions, which are limited to vomitus and feces.

Under this system, patients who have a suppressed immune system are designated either *protective isolation* or, more frequently, *compromised host*. It has been proven that the most effective measure for infection control is handwashing (Centers for Disease Control, 1985).

Strict Isolation

Strict isolation is used if the identified pathogens are transmitted through the air and by contact. Precautions to be taken include placing the patient in a private room with the door closed; wearing a gown, mask, and gloves when entering the room; washing hands on entering and leaving the room; and double-bagging (for decontamination) linens and other articles used in the care of the patient (Figure 34–2).

Respiratory Isolation

If the pathogens involved are airborne, respiratory isolation is carried out. It is desirable to place the patient in a private room with the door closed. Masks must be worn, but gowns and gloves are not necessary unless there is direct contact with linens or secretions. Hands should be washed on entering and leaving the room. Any article contaminated with secretions from the patient must be disinfected or double-bagged for disposal or decontamination (Figure 34–3).

Wound and Skin Precautions

For the patient with a wound infected with microorganisms that can be spread by contact, wound and skin precautions are observed. Isolation of the patient is not required, but a private room is desirable. Gowns must be worn when in direct contact with the patient, and gloves should be used when in direct contact with the infected area. Masks are necessary only during dressing changes. Hands are washed on entering and leaving the room. Instruments, dressings, and linens must be double-bagged for decontamination or disposal (Figure 34–4).

Enteric Precautions

Enteric precautions are used when the pathogens involved are transmitted by direct contact with the gastrointestinal system. A private room is necessary for the pediatric patient. Gowns must be worn when in direct contact with the patient and gloves when in direct contact with the patient or with contaminated material. Masks are not necessary. Hands are washed on entering and leaving the room. Linen should be double-bagged. Urine, feces, and vomitus should be discarded in an adjoining private bathroom, and any articles contaminated with them must be discarded or disinfected. (Urine is included *because of the proximity of the urinary and intestinal tracts.*)(Figure 34–5).

Blood/Body Fluid Precautions

Masks are not needed, since organisms are not airborne. Gowns and gloves are necessary only for direct contact with the patient or with soiled linen or equipment. Meticulous handwashing is essential, and a special needle and syringe disposal box should be used. The double-bagging of linen and the disposal of diet trays depends on the type of disease and organism. Blood specimens collected from patients on blood precautions should be prominently labeled so all persons handling the specimens can take necessary precautions (Figure 34–6).

Table 34–1 Disease-Specific Isolation Precautions

Disease	Precautions Indicated				Infective Material	Apply Precautions How Long?	Comments
	Private Room?	Masks?	Gowns?	Gloves?			
Decubitus ulcer, infected							
Draining, major	Yes	No	Yes, if soiling is likely	Yes, for touching infective material	Pus	Duration of illness	Major = draining and not covered by dressing or dressing does not adequately contain the pus.
Draining, minor	No	No	Yes, if soiling is likely	Yes, for touching infective material	Pus	Duration of illness	Minor or limited = dressing covers and adequately contains the pus, or infected area is very small.
Diarrhea, acute– infective etiology suspected (see gastroenteritis)	Yes, if patient hygiene is poor	No	Yes, if soiling is likely	Yes, for touching infective material	Feces	Duration of illness	
Diphtheria Cutaneous	Yes	No	Yes, if soiling is likely	Yes, for touching infective material	Lesion secretions	Until 2 cultures from skin lesions, taken at least 24 h apart after cessation of antimicrobial therapy, are negative for *Coryne-bacterium diphtheriae*	
Pharyngeal	Yes	Yes	Yes, if soiling is likely	Yes, for touching infective material	Respiratory secretions	Until 2 cultures from both nose and throat taken at least 24 h apart after cessation of antimicrobial therapy	
Meningococcemia (meningococcal sepsis)	Yes	Yes, for those close to patient	No	No	Respiratory secretions	For 24 h after start of effective therapy	See CDC Guideline for Infection Control in Hospital Personnel for recommendations for prophylaxis after exposure.
Gastrointestinal	Yes	No	Yes, if soiling is likely	Yes, for touching infective material	Feces	Until off antimicrobials and culture-negative	In outbreaks, cohorting of infected and colonized patients may be indicated if private rooms are not available. *(continued)*

© 1992 by J.B. Lippincott Company

Table 34–1 (*Continued*)

Disease	Precautions Indicated				Infective Material	Apply Precautions How Long?	Comments
	Private Room?	Masks?	Gowns?	Gloves?			
Respiratory General	Yes	Yes, for those close to patient	Yes, if soiling is likely	Yes, for touching infective material	Respiratory secretions and possibly feces	Until off antimicrobials and culture-negative	In outbreaks, cohorting of infected and colonized patients may be indicated if private rooms are not available.
Tuberculosis (new, active case)	Yes	Yes, if patient coughing	Yes, if soiling with respiratory secretions likely	Yes, for touching infective material, such as tissues used for cough	Respiratory secretions	For 2 weeks after antituberculosis therapy initiated	Use of ultraviolet lights or filtered air systems recommended.
Skin, wound or burn	Yes	No	Yes, if soiling is likely	Yes, for touching infective material	Pus and possibly feces	Until off antimicrobials and culture-negative	In outbreaks, cohorting of infected and colonized patients may be indicated if private rooms are not available.
Urinary	Yes	No	No	Yes, for touching infective material	Urine and possibly feces	Until off antimicrobials and culture-negative	Urine and urine-measuring devices are sources of infections, especially if the patient (or any nearby patients) has indwelling urinary catheter. In outbreaks, cohorting of infected and colonized patients may be indicated if private rooms are not available.

Protective Isolation

The patient who is particularly susceptible to infection is placed in protective, also called reverse, isolation to provide protection from the pathogens in the environment. A private room with the door closed is required. Gowns and masks must be worn by all who enter the room. Gloves need to be worn only by those having direct contact with the patient. Hands are washed on entering and leaving the room. All items

taken into the room should be individually evaluated for their potential to contaminate and harm the patient. *Because the room and its contents are considered clean,* no special measures are taken when removing articles and linens (Figure 34–7).

Compromised Host

The designation *compromised host* usually means that the patient has a suppressed immune system and is

(Front of Card)

Visitors—Report to Nurses' Station Before Entering Room

1. Private room indicated?   _____ No
                              _____ Yes
2. Masks indicated?   _____ No
                              _____ Yes for those close to patient
                              _____ Yes for all persons entering room
3. Gowns indicated?   _____ No
                              _____ Yes if soiling is likely
                              _____ Yes for all persons entering room
4. Gloves indicated?   _____ No
                              _____ Yes for touching infective material
                              _____ Yes for all persons entering room
5. Special precautions   _____ No
   indicated for handling blood? _____ Yes
6. Hands must be washed after touching the patient or potentially contaminated articles and before taking care of another patient.
7. Articles contaminated with _____ should be
                                          infective material(s)
   discarded or bagged and labeled before being sent for decontamination and reprocessing.

(Back of Card)

Instructions

1. On Table B, Disease-Specific Precautions, locate the disease for which isolation precautions are indicated.
2. Write disease in blank space here: _____
3. Determine if a private room is indicated. In general, patients infected with the same organism may share a room. For some diseases or conditions, a private room is indicated if patient hygiene is poor. A patient with poor hygiene does not wash hands after touching infective material (feces, purulent drainage, or secretions), contaminates the environment with infective material, or shares contaminated articles with other patients.
4. Place a check mark beside the indicated precautions on front of card.
5. Cross through precautions that are *not* indicated.
6. Write infective material in blank space in item 7 on front of card.

Figure 34–1. Sample instruction card for disease-specific isolation precautions.

therefore *less capable of self-protection against pathogens.* Many facilities are now using the procedure for compromised host more often than that for protective isolation, *since it is thought to be as effective.* The procedure is less stringent and may not include use of mask and gown. More often it includes meticulous handwashing and the requirement that persons who have a cold or other infection do not enter the room

or come close to the patient. Some facilities also prohibit live plants in the environment, *because soil can be a growth medium for pathogens.*

SPECIFIC ISOLATION PROCEDURES

A variety of specific procedures are used as part of isolation. To begin you must know how to enter and
(*text continues on page 14*)

Strict Isolation
Visitors-Report to Nurses' Station Before Entering Room

1. **Private Room**—*necessary;* door must be kept closed.

2. **Gowns**—must be worn by all persons entering room.

3. **Masks**—must be worn by all persons entering room.

4. **Hands**—must be washed on entering and leaving room.

5. **Gloves**—must be worn by all persons entering room.

6. **Articles**—must be discarded, or wrapped before being sent to Central Supply for disinfection or sterilization.

Figure 34–2. Strict isolation sign.
(*Courtesy Shamrock, Inc., Bellwood, Illinois*)

Respiratory Isolation
Visitors-Report to Nurses' Station Before Entering Room

1. **Private Room**—*necessary;* door must be kept closed.

2. **Gowns**—not necessary.

3. **Masks**—must be worn by all persons entering room if susceptible to disease.

4. **Hands**—must be washed on entering and leaving room.

5. **Gloves**—not necessary.

6. **Articles**—those contaminated with secretions must be disinfected.

7. **Caution**—all persons susceptible to the specific disease should be excluded from patient area; if contact is necessary, susceptibles must wear masks.

Figure 34–3. Respiratory isolation sign.
(*Courtesy Shamrock, Inc., Bellwood, Illinois*)

Wound & Skin Precautions
Visitors—Report to Nurses' Station Before Entering Room

1. **Private Room**—desirable.

2. **Gowns**—must be worn by all persons having direct contact with patient.

3. **Masks**—not necessary except during dressing changes.

4. **Hands**—must be washed on entering and leaving room.

5. **Gloves**—must be worn by all persons having direct contact with infected area.

6. **Articles**—special precautions necessary for instruments, dressings, and linen.

NOTE: *See* Manual for Special Dressing Techniques to be used when changing dressings.

Figure 34–4. Wound and skin precautions sign.
(*Courtesy Shamrock, Inc., Bellwood, Illinois*)

Enteric Precautions
Visitors-Report to Nurses' Station Before Entering Room

1. **Private Room**—Necessary for children only.

2. **Gowns**—must be worn by all persons having direct contact with patient.

3. **Masks**—not necessary.

4. **Hands**—must be washed on entering and leaving room.

5. **Gloves**—must be worn by all persons having direct contact with patient or with articles contaminated with fecal material.

6. **Articles**—special precautions necessary for articles contaminated with urine and feces. Articles must be disinfected or discarded.

Figure 34–5. Enteric precautions sign.
(*Courtesy Shamrock, Inc., Bellwood, Illinois*)

Blood/Body Fluid Precautions

Private room: See Back

Masks: Not Indicated

Gowns: Indicated if soiling with blood or body fluids is likely

Gloves: Indicated for touching blood or body fluids

Handwashing: HANDS MUST BE WASHED after touching the patient or potentially contaminated articles

Goggles: To be worn if contamination of eyes with secretions is likely

Articles: Articles contaminated with infected material should be discarded (double bagging only necessary if soaking through is likely) or bagged and labeled and sent to Central Supply

Special note: Patient must have own needle disposal box. Report all needle-stick injuries to Employee Health or Emergency Room.

VISITORS REPORT TO NURSES STATION BEFORE ENTERING ROOM

Figure 34–6. Blood/body fluid precautions sign.

Protective Isolation
Visitors—Report to Nurses' Station Before Entering Room

1. Private Room—*necessary;* door must be kept closed.

2. Gowns—must be worn by all persons entering room.

3. Masks—must be worn by all persons entering room.

4. Hands—must be washed on entering and leaving room.

5. Gloves—must be worn by all persons having direct contact with patient.

6. Articles—*see* manual text.

Figure 34–7. Protective isolation sign.
(*Courtesy Shamrock, Inc., Bellwood, Illinois*)

leave the room correctly. These procedures are discussed first. Additional procedures are required to care for equipment and supplies in the isolation room. These are presented next. Then, on occasion the patient in the isolation room must be transported to another department for a procedure or a test. This procedure is provided last. Then we present a General Procedure for approaching all isolation situations in which you will choose which of the specific procedures you need in the care of the individual patient.

Preparing the Room

Preparation of a room for isolation procedure varies, depending on the type of isolation required. In some instances, such as strict isolation, it is appropriate to remove unnecessary furniture and equipment from the room. In other cases the room does not need to be changed in any way. If good handwashing technique is followed, patients under wound and skin precautions and blood and body fluid precautions can share a room with another patient, according to CDC guidelines. We recommend that you review the policy at your facility, but generally you will need:

1. A private room with running water
2. A sign on the outside of the door indicating what preparation is needed before entering the room and which type of isolation is being carried out (Figures 34–2 through 34–7)
3. A stand of some sort (often a bedside stand is used) placed just outside the door to hold isolation laundry bags, gowns, masks, gloves, and other items specific to the care of an individual patient. In some hospitals these stands are prepared and kept in the central supply department and requisitioned when needed.
4. A laundry hamper for inside the room
5. A wastebasket (preferably large) lined with plastic
6. A thermometer and blood pressure equipment, including stethoscope, which should be left in the room
7. Special containers as needed for used needles, syringes, and instruments.

In facilities that have areas especially designed for use with isolation patients, necessary items are stored in the anteroom outside the patient's room. Such special areas are also equipped with sinks with knee controls.

Entering the Room

One component of care that will prove helpful as you prepare to enter an isolation room is *organization*. Make sure you have all the equipment you need before you are gowned and in the room. *To stand helpless in the room, waiting for someone to bring you forgotten items, is frustrating and time-consuming for you and other workers, not to mention the patient.*

You may need to wear a gown, a mask, and gloves, depending on the specific situation. Determine which items you need to wear. Follow the specific directions below for those items.

1. Obtain needed equipment.
2. Wash hands for infection control.
3. Put watch in plastic bag.
4. Put on gown, gloves, mask as needed.

Gown

An isolation gown is used to protect the care provider's clothing from microorganisms that can be spread on clothing. Gowns are usually worn for strict and respiratory isolation and when providing direct care to patients who have drainage or secretions that may contain infectious organisms. Isolation gowns may be made of washable cotton cloth or disposable paper.

1. Wash your hands (see Module 2, Basic Infection Control). Take off any rings, *because the regular handwashing procedure may not remove microorganisms lodged beneath them.*
2. If the room does not have a wall clock and you need a watch to perform some aspect of care, remove your watch and place it in a plastic bag, *so that it is protected but visible.*
3. Put on gown, making sure that all parts of your uniform are covered and that the ties are fastened securely.

Masks

Masks may be made of washable cloth or disposable material. *Masks protect against airborne microorganisms and droplet nuclei on which they are carried.* To do this effectively, all inhaled air must pass through the mask material before reaching the mouth and nose. *As masks are worn they become moist from the wearer's breath and can therefore wick microorganisms through from the surface to the wearer.* Therefore, masks should be changed as soon as moisture is detected on the surface. In addition, *masks collect microorganisms on the outside surface, concentrating them in that location.* For this reason do not hang a mask around your neck and reuse it. *This increases the chance of contaminating your hands with organisms from the mask and of transferring organisms from your hands to the mask that will be over your mouth and nose.*

1. Place clean mask over nose and mouth.
2. Fasten both sets of ties securely.
3. Bottom edge should be tucked under chin and the top edge should fit snugly across the bridge of nose. If you wear glasses, tuck the mask under the lower edge of your glasses *to prevent your glasses from steaming up from your breath.* Some masks have a metal strip that can be molded to fit snugly over the bridge of your nose and under your eyes.

Gloves

Gloves are always used in isolation in the same way as they are used for other patients. Gloves should be kept inside of the room so that they can be put on and changed as needed when providing care. In addition, clean gloves may be worn for all care in a strict isolation situation. In these situations, gloves must be kept outside of the room and donned before entering. If you will need to change gloves while in the room, you may wish to double-glove (that is, put one pair over the other) to keep your hands covered when you are changing gloves. If gloves are to be donned outside of the room, use the following steps.

1. Put on both gloves.
2. Tuck the sleeves of the gown securely inside the cuffs of the gloves.

When removing soiled gloves, it is wise to turn them inside out as you pull them off. This encloses the contaminated surface inside of the glove. Small items to be disposed of may be encased in a soiled glove by turning the glove inside out over the item. This provides a compact, moisture-proof cover *to decrease the number of microorganisms being released into the room and to prevent contamination of your hands.*

3. Remove soiled gloves by turning them inside out as you pull gloves off.
   a. Peel first glove off touching only the outside with other gloved hand.
   b. Hold first glove in second hand.
   c. Slide ungloved fingers inside of second glove and turn glove inside out over first glove while removing it.

Double-Bagging

You may use a double-bagging technique for contaminated items removed from an isolation room (except a protective isolation room). One nurse inside of the room and one nurse outside carry out this procedure. This procedure may be used for wet linen or for items that are being sent to another department.

1. If you are the inside nurse, place used items in appropriate containers: linen in the linen hamper, glass bottles and jars in a brown paper bag, paper garbage in a plastic-lined wastebasket. Take care not to fill the bags too full, *because full bags are difficult to double-bag without breaking technique.* Carefully close and secure the bag.
2. If you are the outside nurse, form a cuff on another bag, spreading it to receive the bag from the nurse on the inside. *The cuff protects your hands from contact with the contaminated items inside the bag.*
3. If you are the inside nurse, place the bag holding contaminated items directly into the bag being held by the outside nurse. Be careful to touch only the inside of the bag (Figure 34–8).

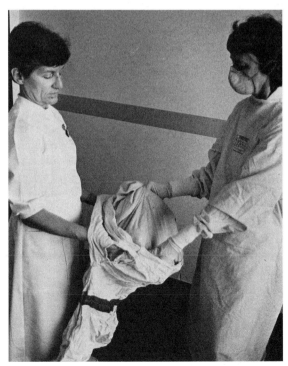

Figure 34–8. Double-bagging wet linens from a strict isolation room.
(*Courtesy Ivan Ellis*)

4. If you are the outside nurse, fold over and carefully secure the top of the outside bag.
5. Mark the bag in the manner prescribed by the facility. Most isolation linen bags are red (as opposed to another color for regular linen) or have a red stripe sewn on them. Brightly colored plastic tape can be used to mark paper or plastic bags. A felt-tipped marking pen is often used to indicate the contents of the bag, *so that proper sterilization or destruction processes can be carried out.*
6. Dispose of the bag in the proper place. Check the procedure book at your facility for any special procedures related to the care of nondisposable equipment.

As an alternative to having two nurses, an open laundry hamper may be set up outside of the isolation room. The inside nurse can then place the soiled laundry bag into the clean bag. Other items are more difficult to double-bag without a second nurse. Paper bags set on a stand outside of the isolation room tend to fall over or close, making it difficult to put an item in the bag.

Note: Do not put lids or caps on glass jars or bottles being sent to be sterilized or incinerated. *A jar or bottle with a lid or cap in place will explode in an autoclave or incinerator, possibly causing injury to hospital staff.*

Caring for Linen

Care should be taken to touch only the inside of the laundry bag with the soiled linen or contaminated hands. This maintains the outside as clean as is possible. The clean dry bag of soiled linen may be handled just as any soiled linen bag is handled because all are considered contaminated.

Double-bagging technique is recommended by the CDC whenever linen is contaminated with moisture that might leak through to those handling the bag at any point. This provides extra protection to hospital workers. In some facilities all soiled linen from isolation rooms is handled by double-bagging as an extra precaution.

Caring for Dishes and Food Trays

Whether food trays are cleaned or disposed of depends on whether or not the disease can be transmitted by oral secretions such as saliva. For example, the trays of patients with AIDS can be removed from the room and placed on the unit's cart for used diet trays, since the hot soapy water used in the hospital kitchen removes the weak organisms of this disease (Lusby & Schietinger, 1985). In contrast, the diets for patients with tuberculosis or hepatitis A may be served on disposable dishes with disposable utensils. If disposables are not available, the trays are placed in marked plastic bags before they are put on the unit's cart for used diet trays.

Leaving the Room

This procedure assumes you are wearing a gown, mask, and gloves. It can be modified if you are not using all three.

1. Complete your work in the room.
2. Remove your gloves and dispose of them as described previously.
3. Untie waist ties.
4. Wash your hands.
5. Untie neckline ties, dropping the gown over your shoulders. Do not touch the outside of the gown.
6. Pull off the gown, touching the inside only and turning the gown inside out as you take it off. Fold it with all outside surfaces toward the center and place it in the laundry hamper (Figure 34–9).
7. Touching the ties only, untie your mask and discard it in a wastebasket or, if it is a cloth mask, in a laundry hamper.
8. Wash your hands.
9. Using a paper towel as a barrier on the doorknob, open the door. Discard the paper towel inside the room.
10. Wash your hands outside the room.

Note: The reuse technique for gowns is seldom used, except perhaps in protective isolation situations. If it is used in your facility, check the procedure book *to be certain you are following the exact procedure.*

Transporting the Patient in Isolation

Sometimes a patient in isolation must be transported to another area. This should be done only when absolutely necessary. Precautions vary according to the type of isolation in use. Generally, it is essential to keep in mind *who* you are protecting and from *what*. *A patient in protective isolation must be protected from all those with whom he or she comes in contact.* Therefore, all who care for the patient in another department must wear gowns and masks. During transport a patient in respiratory isolation must wear a mask, a pa-

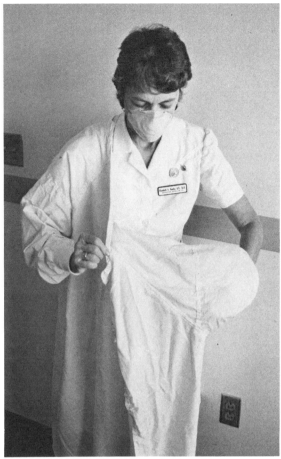

Figure 34–9. Removing an isolation gown by touching only the neck and inside surfaces.
(*Courtesy Ivan Ellis*)

tient in wound isolation should wear a gown, and a patient in strict isolation must wear a gown and mask and should be covered by a sheet or bath blanket. All items that are touched by the patient must be disinfected. Consult your facility procedure book for specific instructions.

GENERAL PROCEDURE FOR ISOLATION

Assessment
1. Check the type of isolation ordered for the patient *in order to plan for care*.

2. Identify the type of infection or the reason for protective precautions.
3. Check the equipment on the stand outside the door or in the anteroom and inside the room *to be sure you have everything you need* for the procedure you intend to perform.

Planning
4. Wash your hands *for infection control*.
5. Gather any equipment you need that is not outside or inside the room.

Implementation
6. Identify the patient *to be sure you are performing the procedure for the correct patient*. Explain to the patient what you are doing. This may be unnecessary if the patient has been in isolation for an extended period of time.
7. Carry out the aspects of isolation technique necessary for the type of isolation ordered when entering the room and giving patient care.
8. Give care as planned.
9. Carry out the aspects of isolation technique necessary for the type of isolation ordered when leaving the room.

Evaluation
10. Evaluate, using the following criteria:
   a. All necessary equipment readily available.
   b. All aspects of the particular isolation procedure correctly carried out.
   c. Patient cared for safely and made comfortable.

Documentation
11. Record care given appropriately. There may be a place to check (✓) that isolation procedure was carried out.

PATIENT, FAMILY, AND STAFF COOPERATION

One of your responsibilities with regard to isolation procedure is making sure the patient and the patient's family understand the reasons for the type of isolation

Example of Progress Notes Using Narrative Format

DATE/TIME	
3/12/94 1620	Pt placed in respiratory isolation per order after report on sputum specimen. Weak but comfortable. States, "I just want to rest." ———————————— S. Danton, RN

DATE/TIME	
3/14/94	Psychosocial status:
1800	S "I feel so bored. I wish more of my friends would visit me."
	O Appears sad and restless. Pacing room for long periods of time this PM.
	A Diversional deficit.
	P Consult with family regarding visits from friends and possible diversional activities.
	S. Danton, RN

Example of Progress Notes Using SOAP Format

being carried out and that they respond to this knowledge with appropriate actions. This responsibility extends to the hospital staff and the physician as well. Remember that the chain will only be as strong as its weakest link.

No one likes isolation procedures, perhaps the patient least of all. For this reason, emphasize the do's rather than the don'ts. *A positive approach may yield more in terms of observable results.*

COMBATING SENSORY DEPRIVATION

Closely related to the idea that isolation procedure is extra work that no one really likes to do is the idea that patients in isolation feel that no one really wants to take care of them. This feeling may be prompted by the fact that they are always the last to be cared for (and cold meals communicate a lot!), by careless remarks made outside doors but within hearing, and by countless nonverbal exchanges. In addition, those who do come to visit isolated patients (family, friends, staff) are often covered from head to toe, making normal communication impossible. Isolation rooms are usually stripped of pictures, plants, and other decorative items, making the total setting rather dismal. The variety of stimulation isolated patients receive is less, and it can be less meaningful too. Usually these patients have limited interaction with others. As a result, patients in isolation can develop any one or a combination of the following problems: decreased alertness and motivation, increased complaints, loneliness, depression, and anger.

You can intervene positively in this process by giving care to an isolated patient first, by answering the call light promptly, and by stopping in the doorway to wave. Provide the patient with puzzles, paperback books, and other paper items that can be burned. Often the family can provide such items.

Home Care

When individuals with infectious diseases are being cared for at home, the patient, the family, and caregivers are taught how to protect themselves from infection. Isolation techniques are not used because they are unwieldy in that environment. The general instructions for basic infection control given in Module 2, Basic Infection Control, are given to the family. It is most critical to teach the patient about how to avoid spreading infection. Especially in the case of respiratory illness, the patient through careful attention to covering coughs, disposing of tissues in a paper bag, and washing hands plays a crucial role in protecting others. In addition, when a respiratory illness is present, those not needed for care are instructed to avoid entering the patient's room. This is especially true for children who are often more susceptible to infection than are adults.

When the patient has tuberculosis, you should be sure that your teaching conforms to the latest information on the transmission of that disease. When a child has a communicable disease such as chickenpox, the family may be concerned about when the child may return to school or day care. Consult your local health department for the most current recommendations regarding these communicable diseases.

References

Centers for Disease Control. (1979). *Guideline for hospital environment control.* U. S. Department of Health and Human Services.

Centers for Disease Control. (1983). *Guidelines for isolation precautions in hospitals.* U. S. Department of Health and Human Services.

Centers for Disease Control. (1985). *Guideline for handwashing and hospital environmental control.* U. S. Department of Health and Human Services.

Centers for Disease Control. (1987). Recommendations for prevention of HIV transmission in health-care settings. *MMWR, 36*(25), 1–16.

Centers for Disease Control. (1988). Update: Universal precautions for prevention of transmission of human immunodeficiency virus, hepatitis B virus, and other blood borne pathogens in health-care settings. *MMWR, 37*(24), 377–382, 387–388.

Lusby, G., & Schietinger, H. (1985). Infection precautions for people with A.I.D.S. living in the community. *Infection control.* San Francisco General Hospital.

Moree, N. A., & Garner, J. S. (1984). CDC's revised protocols keep you current with the latest epidemiological information. *American Journal of Nursing, 84,* 210.

Veterans Administration Medical Center, Seattle. Unpublished Infection Control Manual (C-3).

Performance Checklist

Preparing the Room	Unsat	Needs More Practice	Sat	Comments
1. Be sure patient will be in a private room with running water.				
2. Post sign outside indicating type of isolation.				
3. Be sure a stand is outside with appropriate supplies (disposal bags, gowns, masks, gloves as needed).				
4. Have laundry hamper for inside room.				
5. Be sure a wastebasket with plastic liner is inside of room.				
6. Be sure a thermometer, blood pressure cuff, and stethoscope are inside of room.				
7. Make certain a special container for used needles and instruments is readily available.				

Entering the Room

1. Obtain all needed equipment.				
2. Wash hands for infection control.				
3. Put watch in plastic bag.				
4. Put on gown, gloves, mask as needed.				

Gowning

1. Wash hands for infection control.				
2. Put on gown, making sure uniform is covered.				

Mask

1. Place mask over nose and mouth.				
2. Fasten both sets of ties securely.				
3. Tuck bottom edge under chin and fit the top edge snugly across the bridge of nose.				

Gloves

1. Put on clean gloves.				
2. Tuck sleeves of gown securely inside of gloves.				

	Unsat	Needs More Practice	Sat	Comments
Gloves *(Continued)*				
3. Remove soiled gloves by turning inside out as you pull gloves off. a. Peel first glove off touching only the outside with other gloved hand.				
b. Hold first glove in second hand.				
c. Slide ungloved fingers inside of second glove and turn glove inside out over first glove while removing it.				
Caring for Dishes and Food Trays				
1. Use disposables if organisms transmitted on eating utensils.				
2. Treat as other trays if organisms not transmitted on eating utensils.				
Double-Bagging				
1. Inside nurse: Place used items in appropriate containers or bags. Carefully close and secure each bag.				
2. Outside nurse: Form a cuff on outer bag and hold with hands underneath for protection.				
3. Inside nurse: Place the bag holding contaminated items directly into the bag being held by the outside nurse, being careful to touch only the inside of that bag.				
4. Outside nurse: Fold over and carefully secure top of bag.				
5. Mark bag in manner prescribed by facility.				
6. Dispose of bag in proper place.				
Caring for Linen				
1. Handle soiled linen with gloved hands.				
2. Touch only inside of laundry bag when placing soiled linen into bag.				
3. Double-bag wet linen.				

Leaving the Room	Unsat	Needs More Practice	Sat	Comments
1. Complete your work in the room.				
2. Remove gloves, touching bare hands to inside surfaces only.				
3. Untie waist ties.				
4. Wash your hands.				
5. Untie neck ties, dropping gown over shoulders.				
6. Pull off gown, touching only inside, and place in laundry hamper.				
7. Untie mask ties and discard mask carefully, touching ties only.				
8. Wash your hands.				
9. Open door, using paper towel as barrier.				
10. Wash your hands outside room.				

General Procedure for Isolation Technique

Assessment

	Unsat	Needs More Practice	Sat	Comments
1. Check type of isolation ordered.				
2. Identify reason for isolation.				
3. Check equipment outside and inside the patient's room to make sure you have everything you need.				

Planning

4. Wash your hands.				
5. Gather necessary equipment not outside or inside the patient's room.				

Implementation

6. Identify the patient. Explain what you are doing.				
7. Carry out techniques necessary to enter room.				
8. Give care as planned.				
9. Carry out techniques necessary to leave room.				

General Procedure for Isolation Technique
(Continued)

	Unsat	Needs More Practice	Sat	Comments
Evaluation				
10. Evaluate, using the following criteria: 　a. Necessary equipment readily available.				
b. Isolation procedure correctly carried out.				
c. Patient left comfortable and safe.				
Documentation				
11. Record appropriately.				

Quiz

Short-Answer Questions

1. What are the two major purposes of isolation?

   a. _____

   b. _____

2. The organism that is causing Mr. Paulson's illness can be transmitted either by air or by contact. What type of isolation would be appropriate for him? _____

3. Mrs. Raymond is a postop patient whose care has been complicated by the presence of a pathogen transmitted by direct contact, the mode of transmission being the gastrointestinal system. What type of isolation would be appropriate for her? _____

4. List three items required in the preparation of a room for isolation procedure.

   a. _____

   b. _____

   c. _____

5. How are items removed from a protective isolation room? _____
   _____

6. If you are the outside nurse double-bagging an isolation room and the inside bag touches your hand, what should you do? _____
   _____

7. A patient with severe leukemia has been ordered placed in isolation. What is the purpose of isolation for this patient? _____
   _____

   Situation: Mrs. Rogers has been in isolation for 10 days. She seems irritable and shows no interest in eating or in the activities ordered by the physician.

8. What could be the source of her problem? _____

9. List at least three nursing actions that might help Mrs. Rogers.

   a. _____

   b. _____

   c. _____

Module 35
Sterile Technique

Module Contents

Rationale for the Use of This Skill
Nursing Diagnoses
Procedures Requiring Sterile Technique
Methods of Sterilization
    Boiling Water
    Steam
    Sporicidal Chemicals
    Ethylene Oxide Gas
    Ultrasonic Sterilization
    Irradiation

Indicators of Sterility
General Principles
Sterile Procedures
    Opening a Sterile Pack
    Adding Items to a Sterile Field
        Objects
        Liquids
    Putting on Sterile Gloves
Home Care

Prerequisites

Successful completion of the following modules:

VOLUME 1
Module 1   An Approach to Nursing Skills
Module 2   Basic Infection Control
Module 3   Safety
Module 5   General Assessment Overview

25

© 1992 by J.B. Lippincott Company

Overall Objective

To identify situations in which sterile technique is needed and to recognize breaks in technique when they occur. To open a sterile pack, set up a sterile field, add sterile items or fluid to a sterile area, and put on sterile gloves.

Specific Learning Objectives

	Know Facts and Principles	Apply Facts and Principles	Demonstrate Ability	Evaluate Performance
1. *Situations requiring sterile technique*	List common situations in which sterile technique is indicated.	Given a patient situation, identify which procedures require sterile technique.	In the clinical setting, decide correctly when to use sterile technique.	Evaluate decision with instructor.
2. *Methods of sterilization*	Define *sterile.* List four methods of sterilization and give an example of when each is used. State common ways to identify sterility.	Given a situation in which sterilization is needed, identify appropriate process.	Identify whether a package is sterile.	Evaluate own performance using Performance Checklist.
3. *Movement of microorganisms*	State six ways microorganisms move from one area to another. Identify methods used to maintain sterile field.	Given a situation in which a sterile field is used, identify any actions that would potentially contaminate it.	Open sterile pack correctly. Add sterile objects to sterile field without contaminating them. Pour liquid into sterile container. Put on sterile gloves.	Evaluate own performance using Performance Checklist.

Learning Activities

1. Review the Specific Learning Objectives.
2. Read the chapter on nursing procedures and the chapter on infections in Ellis and Nowlis, *Nursing: A Human Needs Approach,* or comparable chapters in another textbook.
3. Look up the module vocabulary terms in the Glossary.
4. Read through the module and mentally practice specific procedures.
5. Review the Performance Checklist.
6. In the practice setting:
   a. Open sterile packs.
   b. Add items to a sterile field.
   c. Pour liquids into sterile containers.
   d. Put on sterile gloves. Use the Performance Checklist as a guide.
7. When you can perform these tasks correctly, select a partner.

   a. Have your partner observe your performance and evaluate you, using the Performance Checklist.
   b. Observe and evaluate your partner, using the Checklist.
   Repeat this exercise until you have mastered the skill. Arrange with your instructor for a time to have your technique checked.
8. In the clinical setting:
   a. Arrange a visit to the central supply department for your clinical group and observe the methods of sterilization used in your facility.
   b. Identify situations in which sterile technique is needed.
   c. Participate in a discussion with other students about situations requiring sterile technique.

Vocabulary

antiseptic	microorganism	sterile technique
autoclave	pathogen	sterilize
contaminated	spore	surgical asepsis
disinfect	sterile	transfer forceps
disinfectant		

Sterile Technique

Rationale for the Use of This Skill

Strict sterile technique, or surgical asepsis, is frequently necessary in nursing. It is used most extensively in operating and delivery rooms, but it is also essential when performing such nursing procedures as injections, catheterizations, dressing changes, and intravenous therapy.

The purpose of sterile technique is to eliminate all microorganisms as well as vegetative states such as spores from objects that come into contact with the tissues of the body. Sterile technique is also used to protect patients from possible infection when the normal body defenses are not intact. The nurse is responsible for identifying situations in which sterile technique is needed and for carrying out sterile procedures precisely.[1]

▶ *Nursing Diagnoses*

The most common nursing diagnoses relating to the need for sterile technique are:

High Risk for Infection: Related to interruption of skin integrity by presence of surgical incision

High Risk for Infection: Urinary related to presence of indwelling urinary catheter

PROCEDURES REQUIRING STERILE TECHNIQUE

Healthy, intact skin and mucous membranes provide an effective barrier to microorganisms, but underlying tissues provide an excellent medium for their growth. Therefore, when underlying tissues are exposed (through a wound or surgical incision), they must be protected against the entry of microorganisms by sterile technique.

Some internal body areas, such as the urinary bladder and the lungs, are normally sterile. To maintain this status, sterile technique is used whenever such an area must be entered. Although the eyes are not normally sterile, sterile technique is used in all procedures relating to them, *because the eyes are susceptible to infection and the consequences of even a minor infection in the eye can be serious.*

Common situations in which sterile technique is

used are during catheterizations, changing surgical dressings, and preparing and administering injections.

METHODS OF STERILIZATION

The ideal method of sterilization should not only render an item free of all microorganisms (including spores and vegetative forms) but should also not damage the item being sterilized, be relatively simple to use, inexpensive, and safe to those in the work place. Unfortunately, no single method of sterilization meets all these criteria for all items that must be sterilized.

Some items used in the modern hospital arrive from manufacturers in presterilized packages. However, sterilization of many items is still done in the central supply department.

As a general staff nurse, you may be involved in sending items to the central supply department for sterilization. *Because it is your responsibility to wrap or label these items correctly,* you need some familiarity with the types of sterilization processes available. If you were employed at a facility where you needed to carry out sterilization procedures, you would need more extensive education.

Any items to be sterilized must first be completely clean, no matter which method of sterilization is used. Among other reasons, *protein,* which is a part of all body secretions and excrement, *often coagulates, providing a protective barrier for microorganisms that helps them survive even the most careful sterilization procedure.*

Boiling Water

Boiling items in water is an old sterilization method but is still valuable in certain situations such as in the home. This method is no longer used in hospitals.

To use this method, completely cover the items so that all surface areas are exposed to the water. Start timing only after a rolling boil has begun. Boil for a minimum of 15 minutes. *The temperature kills microbes.* Because it is difficult to maintain sterility when removing items from boiling water and drying them, this method is most often used for items that need sterilization between uses but do not need to be sterile during use, such as bedpans and emesis basins. Some spore forms are not destroyed by boiling water.

Steam

Using steam under pressure is called *autoclaving.* It is the most commonly used sterilization procedure in health care facilities today. To kill microorganisms,

---

[1] You will note that rationale for action is emphasized throughout the module by the use of italics.

the temperatures reach as high as 250°F under 15–20 lbs pressure for approximately 30 minutes.

The high-pressure system enables the steam to reach a much higher temperature than is otherwise possible, and it is the temperature—not the pressure—that destroys microorganisms.

Some items are not appropriate for autoclaving. Rubber and plastics *may soften or melt and delicate electronic devices may be damaged by the moisture and high temperatures.* These items are sterilized using other methods.

With items that are autoclaved, the steam penetrates *the cloth wrapper and soaks into nooks and crannies, providing complete contact and sterilization.* Items should be left in an autoclave until they are cool and dry, *so that the exterior of a wrapped package can be handled, maintaining the sterility of the contents. Remember, moisture enhances the movement of microorganisms.*

Sporicidal Chemicals

The items we have mentioned that are not appropriate for autoclaving *due to potential damage* can be sterilized by soaking in a sporicidal chemical solution. An advantage is that this method is inexpensive, but a disadvantage is that items have to be soaked for long periods of time, i.e., 12–24 hours. Some surgical instruments are manually scrubbed and immersed in a chemical solution before they are rinsed and autoclaved *for extra safety.* Many respiratory therapy departments use chemical solutions to sterilize partly plastic or rubber equipment. For use in the home, a simple household bleach solution can be used to disinfect surfaces and items in use. This means that it can kill weak viruses and bacteria but not all microorganisms. It must be made clear that this procedure only disinfects and does not sterilize items the solution contacts.

Ethylene Oxide Gas

In most hospital central supply departments, the use of ethylene oxide gas has increased as a method for sterilization. One reason is that more equipment with plastic or electronic components has come into use. Another reason is that gas has become less expensive to use and the sterilizing units are better ventilated to protect workers from the toxic effects of exposure to this gas. State and federal guidelines have been mandated in regard to safety. *Because ethylene oxide gas is toxic,* all gas-sterilized items must be subjected to a waiting period before they can be used. Consult the manufacturer's recommendations for this information.

Ultrasonic Sterilization

Ultrasonic sterilization uses the principle of bombarding the item to be sterilized with countless numbers of ultrasonic waves. All particles including microorganisms are loosened and separated from the equipment. The procedure may damage electronic equipment but can readily be used on instruments and items made of rubber or plastic. This method has several advantages; it requires no waiting time after processing, is effective in removing microorganisms, and is safe for the worker.

Irradiation

A less common method of sterilization is exposure to cobalt 60 irradiation. This method can be used for all objects but is costly.

INDICATORS OF STERILITY

Indicators that react to autoclaving or gas when exposed to it for a prolonged period are used to show whether an item is sterile. They are frequently seen on packs in the form of special tape. Dark lines appear on the tape after a package has been exposed to a temperature for sufficient time to sterilize the item. Small glass-tubing indicators that contain a substance sensitive to heat are sometimes placed inside large packs to indicate sterility. The sterility of bottles of liquids is usually identified by the presence of a vacuum seal.

Every commercial product has some indicator of sterility. It is your responsibility to check the manufacturer's literature for this information, so you can ascertain the sterility of an item before using it.

Wrapped packages retain their sterility for various lengths of time depending on the type of wrapping material, the conditions of storage, and the integrity of the package. An expiration date should appear on the sterile package. Do not use the contents after that date until the item or items inside have been resterilized.

GENERAL PRINCIPLES

Microorganisms move through space on air currents. Thus, items that are exposed to the air for a prolonged period are considered contaminated. For this reason, it is important to minimize air movement or to control its direction through special ventilation to limit the movement of microorganisms. When a sterile field is open, keep doors closed, and do not shake drapes and gowns, even if they are sterile.

Microorganisms are transferred from one surface to another whenever a nonsterile object touches another object. Keep sterile objects at a distance from nonsterile ones to prevent the transfer of microorganisms. *Any contact, no matter how brief, renders sterile items nonsterile.* To preserve sterility, pick up sterile items with sterile gloves or with transfer forceps.

Microorganisms move from one object to another as a result of gravity when a nonsterile item is held above another item. For this reason, it is important to keep nonsterile objects, among them your own arm, from being over the sterile field.

Microorganisms travel rapidly along any moisture through a wicking action. If moisture connects a nonsterile surface to a sterile one, the sterile surface is considered contaminated.

Microorganisms move slowly along a dry surface. If one side of a dry object is touched, that side is contaminated, but the opposite side is still considered to be sterile. When someone picks up sterile forceps, the handle is immediately contaminated but the tips, which have not been touched, are sterile. Maintain a safety margin of approximately 1 inch around a contaminated portion.

Microorganisms are released into the air on droplet nuclei whenever a person breathes or speaks. In a situation where sterility is critical (for example, the operating room), personnel wear masks to stop this source of contamination. In the general setting a mask may be

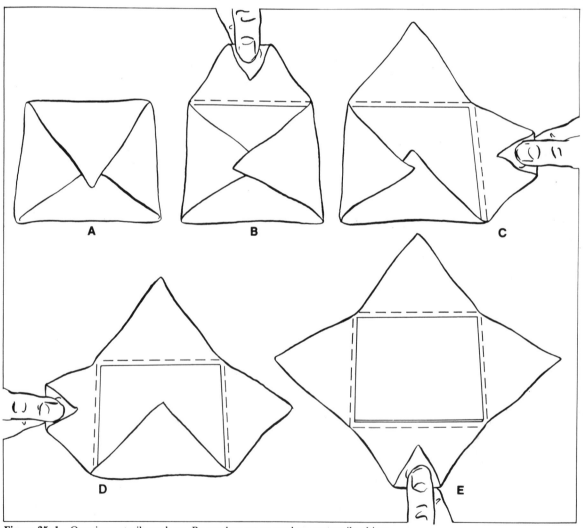

Figure 35–1. Opening a sterile package. Remember not to reach over a sterile object. **A:** Unopened package. **B:** First flap opened. **C:** Second flap opened. **D:** Third flap opened. **E:** Fourth flap opened, sterile object in center of sterile field.

omitted, but avoid talking across a sterile field, turn your head away when speaking, and speak only when necessary in a sterile environment.

Because microorganisms are in constant motion in a variety of ways, sterile areas must be protected by providing wide margins for safety. *Because you cannot guarantee what you cannot see*, it is common practice to consider anything that is out of sight to be nonsterile. A person's back is considered nonsterile, even when clothed in an originally sterile gown. Therefore, two persons in sterile gowns should always pass face to face or back to back, so there is no danger of the sterile front touching the nonsterile back. Keep gloved hands in front of you, in your line of vision. Remember that all items below your waist or below table level are considered nonsterile *because they are out of full view.*

The edge of any sterile field is potentially contaminated by microorganisms moving in from the outside. Therefore, keep sterile objects away from the edge of the field. Again, 1 inch is considered a minimum safety margin.

If you must set up a sterile field ahead of time or leave it during use, cover it with a sterile drape of some type *to prevent contamination*. Use a single thickness of paper drape or a double thickness of cloth drapes.

STERILE PROCEDURES

Opening a Sterile Pack

Before sterilization, objects are wrapped *so that they can be opened without contaminating the contents*. The wrapper, when opened, provides a sterile field. Choose a flat, hard, dry surface to prepare a sterile field. Clear a sufficient area, *so you have plenty of room to work*. As a beginner, you will find you need at least a 12-inch-square field.

When you open a sterile package, remember not to reach over a sterile object. Grasp only the outside edge of the wrapper. To accomplish this, open the far flap first, then the side flaps, and finally the flap closest to you. The item can also be turned, or you can walk around it. In some instances you may reach around the object, but it is difficult to do this without contaminating the item.

Figure 35–1 shows the proper sequence for opening a sterile package.

Adding Items to a Sterile Field

Objects. When you add additional sterile items to a sterile field, you must take care that contami-

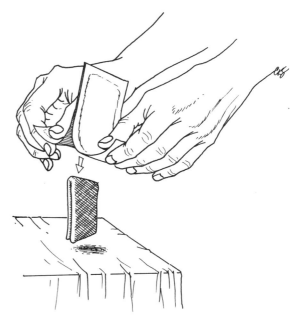

Figure 35–2. The nurse holds the package by touching only the outside and dropping the sterile contents onto the sterile field.

nation does not occur. Unwrap the item as for any sterile package. Pick it up by sliding your hand underneath the sterile covering. Gather the ends of the covering back around your wrist, forming a sterile cover for your hand, and keep the ends from dragging.

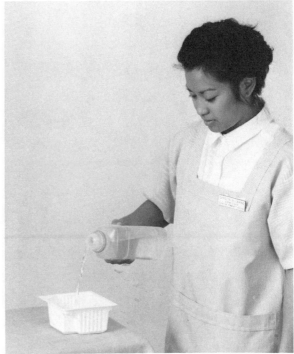

Figure 35–3. The nurse pours into a container on the sterile field by not reaching over the field and not pouring from a height that could cause splashing.

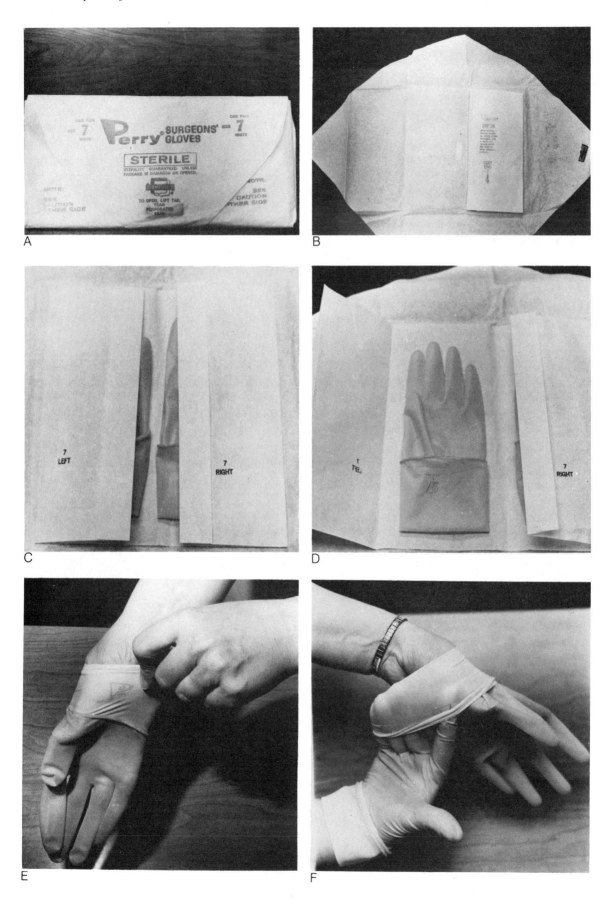

Commercially packaged sterile dressings usually come in packages that peel open. Remember that *the ends you have grasped to peel back are contaminated* and should not touch the dressing, nor should they be held over the sterile field. If one peeled-back side is folded under, it is possible to slide the dressing off over the sterile folded edge.

Place items well within the sterile field. Small items, such as gauze dressings, may be dropped from above the sterile field (Figure 35–2); large items should be put down carefully. You can use sterile forceps to remove an item from a package and place it in the sterile field.

Liquids. To pour a liquid into a container in the sterile field, pour it from 6–8 inches above the receiving container, *to avoid the possibility of the two containers touching* (Figure 35–3). Always pour a small amount of a nonsterile solution (e.g., Betadine) into a waste receptacle (*to clean the lip of the container*) before you pour the contents into the sterile receptacle. Pour slowly *to prevent splashing.*

If liquid is spilled onto the sterile field, the spot is considered contaminated if the moisture can soak through to the nonsterile table beneath. Remember that *microorganisms move rapidly through moisture.* If the drape is impervious to fluid (many disposable drapes have a plastic layer) and the sterile liquid pools up on the surface, the area is still sterile. Usually, however, this area is covered with a dry drape because moisture may attract microorganisms in the air.

Putting on Sterile Gloves

Remove rings and wash your hands before putting on sterile gloves. *Gloves may have small imperfections or may tear, and bacteria can multiply rapidly on the skin of gloved hands. A ring can also tear the glove and can harbor microorganisms.* Module 2, Basic Infection Control, outlines general handwashing procedure. Module 36, Surgical Asepsis; Scrubbing, Gowning, and Gloving, gives the procedure for a surgical scrub, required in operating and delivery rooms and before some invasive procedures. For sterile procedures such as urinary catheterizations and dressing changes, repeating the handwashing procedure described in Module 2, Basic Infection Control, twice is generally

considered adequate preparation for putting on gloves.

You should put on sterile gloves without touching the outside of the gloves, *so contamination does not occur.* Gloves are packaged uniformly *to facilitate this procedure.*

Sterile gloves are sealed in a sterile package. Open the package in the same way you would open any other sterile package, unless it is a commercially prepared paper package. In that instance, instructions for opening are printed on the outside of the package.

Inside the sterile package is a folder containing the gloves. A small, folded-back margin is provided over each glove, *so you can open the folder without touching the gloves.* The gloves in the package are arranged palm upward, with the left glove on the left side and the right glove on the right side. A cuff of 2–4 inches is folded down over each glove. Figure 35–4 shows the correct sequence for opening and putting on sterile gloves.

Open one side of the folder, either left or right, touching only the center lower corner. Pick up the exposed glove with your opposite hand (the left glove with the right hand or the right glove with the left

Home Care

Patients needing sterile dressings are often discharged home. Some of these adult and pediatric patients have central lines in place that may *require regular sterile dressing changes.* The materials and equipment are available from commercial companies. As a nurse in the hospital or as a nurse in home health care, you may be involved in performing the procedure yourself or teaching sterile technique to the care provider. Demonstrating the principles outlined in this module and having the family person return the demonstration under your supervision are helpful in maintaining a technique that will prevent infection.

Figure 35–4. Putting on sterile gloves. **A:** Obtain a sealed package of gloves. **B:** Open the outer wrapper, following the directions on the package. **C and D:** Open the inner folder at the corner without touching the gloves. **E:** Pick up the right glove with your left hand, touching only the folded cuff and put it on. **F:** Grasp the left glove under the cuff and put it on.
(*Courtesy Ivan Ellis*)

hand). Be careful to touch only the folded cuff. Then insert your free hand into the glove without touching skin to the outside of the glove. (The rhyme "sk*in* side to *in*side" may help you remember this.) Be sure you hold the glove well away from your body and from the table or package as you work. A common error is to brush the tips of the glove fingers against a nonsterile surface while manipulating, thus contaminating the gloves.

Open the second side of the folder with your bare hand, exposing the second glove. Pick up the glove with your gloved hand from under the cuff, which is the outside surface. Be sure to keep the thumb of the gloved hand rigidly extended outward or folded against the palm, *so you are not tempted to use it to grasp the other glove.* Hold the glove under its cuff by your four gloved fingers. *The cuff on the second glove protects the gloved hand from contamination by touching and also from microorganisms moving by gravity.* Carefully maneuver the second hand into the glove. When both gloves are on, turn the cuffs up by flipping them, taking care not to roll the outside of the gloves onto your skin. You may then make any necessary adjustments so the gloves fit smoothly.

Performance Checklist

Arranging a Sterile Field	Unsat	Needs More Practice	Sat	Comments
1. Wash your hands.				
2. Choose a flat, hard, dry surface.				
3. Open sterile pack, using wrapper for sterile field.				
4. Add additional sterile items, placing them well within edge of sterile field.				

Opening a Sterile Pack or Set				
1. Wash your hands.				
2. Do not cross your hand or arm over sterile area.				
3. Touch wrapper on outside only.				
4. Do not allow anything nonsterile to touch contents of pack.				

Adding Objects to Sterile Field				
1. Wash your hands.				
2. Open package away from sterile field.				
3. Drop sterile item onto sterile field, keeping hands as far from field as possible.				
4. Avoid reaching over field with arm as much as possible.				

Adding Liquid to Sterile Field				
1. Wash your hands.				
2. If the liquid is nonsterile, pour small amount over lip of bottle first, into waste receptacle.				
3. Pour from 6–8 inches above sterile container.				
4. Do not touch lip of bottle to container.				
5. Pour slowly.				
6. Keep arm as far as possible from sterile field. Avoid reaching over field if possible.				

Putting on Sterile Gloves	Unsat	Needs More Practice	Sat	Comments
1. Remove rings and wash your hands.				
2. Open wrapper so that areas touched do not touch gloves.				
3. Pick up first glove, touching only inside surface (cuff).				
4. Put on first glove without allowing outside to touch anything.				
5. Pick up second glove from under cuff with fingers (only) of gloved hand.				
6. Put on second glove, touching only inside of second glove with bare hand.				
7. Turn up cuffs, touching gloved hand only to outside of other glove. Do not let outside of glove touch your skin.				

Quiz

Multiple-Choice Questions

_____ 1. The definition of *sterile* is

    a. the absence of all germs.
    b. the absence of disease-producing microorganisms.
    c. the absence of disease-producing microorganisms and their spores.
    d. the absence of all forms of life.

_____ 2. A precision instrument for measuring pressure must be sterilized. Which of the following methods would be suitable? (1) boiling water; (2) steam under pressure; (3) ethylene oxide gas; (4) sporicidal chemicals

    a. 1 and 3   **c.** 1 and 2
    b. 2 and 4   **d.** 3 and 4

_____ 3. A metal emesis basin must be sterilized. Which of the following techniques would be appropriate? (1) boiling water; (2) steam under pressure; (3) ethylene oxide gas; (4) sporicidal chemicals

    a. 1, 2, and 3   **c.** 1 and 2 only
    b. 2, 3, and 4   **d.** All of the above

_____ 4. Which of the following is the most common sterilization process used in hospitals?

    a. boiling water   **c.** ethylene oxide gas
    b. steam under pressure   **d.** sporicidal chemicals

_____ 5. A plastic tubing to an instrument must be sterilized. The best method to use would be

    a. boiling water.   **c.** ethylene oxide gas.
    b. steam under pressure.   **d.** sporicidal chemicals.

_____ 6. In which of the following situations is sterile technique needed? (1) changing a dressing over a surgical wound; (2) changing a warm pack over an inflamed joint; (3) changing a dressing over an open decubitus ulcer; (4) changing a colostomy bag

    a. 1 and 2   **c.** 1 and 3
    b. 2 and 3   **d.** 3 and 4

_____ 7. We say the rhyme "skin side to inside" when we put on sterile gloves. From your knowledge of the basic rationale of sterile technique, this statement is

    a. correct.   **c.** partially correct.
    b. incorrect.   **d.** not relevant.

_____ 8. When adding objects to a sterile field, your arm should be

    a. anywhere convenient.
    b. as far from the sterile field as possible—at least 24 inches away.
    c. anywhere at least 12 inches above the table.
    d. kept to the side of the table, so as not to be above the sterile field.

True-False Questions

_____ 9. When a solution soaks through a sterile drape to a nonsterile table beneath, the sterile drape is considered contaminated.

_____ **10.** Persons in sterile gowns can pass one another in any way because all surfaces of their gowns are sterile.

_____ **11.** Articles dropped out of sight are considered contaminated.

_____ **12.** It is permissible to reach over a sterile object with a bare arm as long as you do not touch it.

_____ **13.** Sterile objects can be placed anywhere on the sterile field as long as they do not extend over the edge and contact a nonsterile object.

Short-Answer Question

14. Give two examples of ways in which sterility can be determined.

a. _____

b. _____

Module 36
Surgical Asepsis: Scrubbing, Gowning, and Gloving

Module Contents

Rationale for the Use of This Skill
Scrubbing
  Equipment
  Types of Scrubs
    Counted Brush-Stroke Method

Timed Method
  Procedure for Scrubbing
Gowning and Gloving
Guidelines for Working in Sterile Attire

Prerequisites

Successful completion of the following modules:

VOLUME 1
Module 1   An Approach to Nursing Skills
Module 2   Basic Infection Control
Module 3   Safety

VOLUME 2
Module 35 Sterile Technique

39

Overall Objectives

To scrub the hands and arms in a thorough manner in order to decrease the bacterial count preparatory to participating in procedures that require surgical technique. To don and function appropriately in sterile attire, identifying contamination if it occurs and taking corrective action.

Specific Learning Objectives

	Know Facts and Principles	Apply Facts and Principles	Demonstrate Ability	Evaluate Performance
1. Purposes	State three purposes of surgical scrub.	Identify which persons in a specific situation must perform surgical scrubs.		
2. Scrubbing				
a. Equipment	List equipment needed for surgical scrub and rationale for use.		Obtain and set up needed equipment for surgical scrub.	Check module to be sure all equipment is ready.
b. Types of scrub	State two major bases for planning scrub procedure.	Given a specific scrub procedure, identify major basis for planning procedure.		
c. Procedure	List steps in scrubbing procedure.	Explain rationale for each step in scrubbing procedure.	Scrub, using procedure outlined in module.	Evaluate own performance using Performance Checklist. Verify procedure with observer.
3. Gowning and gloving	List steps for putting on sterile gown. List steps of closed-glove technique. Identify part of gown considered sterile.	Identify situations in which gowning and gloving are necessary. Explain rationale for wearing gowns. Explain rationale for closed-glove technique.	Put on gown correctly. Put on sterile gloves correctly, using closed-glove technique.	Evaluate own performance using Performance Checklist. Verify with observer that contamination did not occur.
4. Guidelines for functioning in sterile attire	List six guidelines for functioning in sterile garb.	Identify reasons for guidelines.	Preserve sterility of own garb. Identify contamination if it occurs and take immediate corrective action.	Evaluate own performance. Validate with observer.

Learning Activities

1. Review the Specific Learning Objectives.
2. Look up the module vocabulary terms in the Glossary.
3. Read through the module and mentally practice the procedure.
4. Read the scrub procedures of the facility where you practice, if available.
5. With a partner, in the practice setting:
   a. Look at the scrub equipment available.
   b. Compare it with what is suggested in the module.
   c. Adapt the equipment as needed. For example, if sink foot controls are not available, arrange for someone else to turn off the water.
   d. Prepare the equipment, including a gown and gloves.
   e. Scrub your hands and arms, using the Performance Checklist (or your facility's procedure) as a guide.
   f. Have your partner observe and evaluate your performance.
   g. Put on the sterile gown and gloves, using the Performance Checklist as a guide.
   h. Have your partner observe and evaluate your performance.
   i. Reverse roles and repeat steps d–h.
   j. Repeat practice until you have mastered these skills.
   k. Ask your instructor to check your performance.
6. Ask your instructor for an opportunity to observe in an area where scrubbing, gowning, and gloving are carried out.
7. In a discussion with the instructor, compare the procedure you learned with the one you observed. Identify strengths and weaknesses.
8. Ask your instructor for an opportunity to scrub in an appropriate area where you are prepared to undertake other activities.

Vocabulary

antimicrobial	disinfectant	normal flora
antiseptic	lateral	sterile
axilla	medial	subungual
culture	microorganism	surgical asepsis

Surgical Asepsis: Scrubbing, Gowning, and Gloving

Rationale for the Use of This Skill

Handwashing alone does not eliminate normal flora on the hands. This normal flora can produce infection when introduced into an open wound. During surgical procedures, deliveries, and invasive diagnostic procedures, sterile gloves are worn. However, gloves can tear in the course of a procedure, so it is important that the hands be rendered as nearly free of microorganisms as possible. A gown too can become moist, allowing microorganisms to move from the arms to the gown's surface.

Surgical scrubbing lowers the total count of microorganisms on the hands and arms. It also removes dirt and oil from the skin, decreasing the ability of remaining microorganisms to multiply. After scrubbing, a residue of antimicrobial cleansing agent remains on the skin, which further reduces the growth of microorganisms.

Gowns and gloves worn for sterile procedures must be put on in a way that ensures that nothing nonsterile touches their outer surfaces. To maintain the highest standard of sterility, proper scrubbing, gowning, and gloving technique is essential.[1]

SCRUBBING

Every facility has its own routine for performing a surgical scrub. *The use of a specific routine ensures that all individuals maintain the same high standard.* You should always follow the procedure established by your facility or, if none exists, work to establish an appropriate procedure.

It is recommended that consultation with the infection control committee should take place in each practice setting regarding scrub policies and procedures (AORN, 1990). Presented here are the general principles related to surgical scrub as well as a sample procedure.

Equipment

A nail-cleaning device such as a metal nail file or plastic nail cleaner is necessary *to remove debris from the subungual area under the nail of each finger.* Wooden cleaning sticks (orange sticks) are not recommended, *because the wood can splinter and harbor microorganisms.*

The scrubbing device may be a sterilized reusable

---

[1] You will note that rationale for action is emphasized throughout the module by the use of italics.

scrub brush or a disposable sponge. Disposable products are individually packaged and are often impregnated with one of a variety of antiseptic detergent agents.

Liquid antibacterial soap or detergent, preferably in a container that can be operated by a foot pedal, is necessary *to reduce the number of microorganisms on the skin.* Many facilities provide a choice of cleansing agents, *so if a person is sensitive to one type, another type can be used.*

The scrub sink should be deep and wide enough *so you can hold both arms over it and water cannot splash out onto your scrub attire. Moisture can contaminate the sterile gown put on over scrub attire.* Knee-operated faucets (rather than hand-operated ones) are preferred *to prevent contamination of the hands after you have scrubbed them.*

Before you begin to scrub, adjust your cap and mask *because you may not touch them during or after scrubbing.* Open a pack that contains a sterile towel for drying the hands and arms after scrubbing and a sterile gown. Place them in a convenient location along with gloves of the correct size.

Types of Scrubs

Counted Brush-Stroke Method. This method dictates a specified number of strokes for each surface of the fingers, hands, and arms. *It ensures complete and thorough coverage of all areas, no matter how rapidly you scrub.*

Timed Method. With this method you scrub each surface of the fingers, hands, and arms for a specified time, using a prescribed anatomic pattern *to ensure that no area is missed. Timed scrubs ensure optimum contact with the cleansing agent.*

Some facilities use a combination of the counted brush-stroke method and the timed method. Others allow the individual to choose which method to use.

The procedure for scrubbing may differ from one facility to another, but certain principles of aseptic technique are common to both the counted brush-stroke scrub and the timed scrub. Either method, if properly done, is effective and ensures sufficient exposure of all skin surfaces to friction and the antibacterial soap or detergent.

Atkinson and Kohn (1986) recommend thinking of the fingers, hands, and arms as having four sides or surfaces. They further recommend following an anatomic pattern of scrub: "four surfaces of each finger, beginning with the thumb and moving from one finger to the next, down the outer edge of the fifth finger, over the dorsal (back) surface of the hand, the palmar (palm) surface of the hand, or vice versa, from small finger to thumb, over the wrist, and up the arm, in thirds, ending 2 inches (5 cm) above the elbow." *Since the hands are in the most direct contact with the sterile field,* you should begin the steps of a scrub procedure with the hands and end with the elbows. Also, you should keep the hands higher than the elbows during the scrub procedure, *to allow water to flow from the cleanest area (the hands) to the less clean area (the elbows) (AORN, 1990).*

Properly done, a surgical scrub usually takes about 5 minutes. Some recommend that the same procedure be used for every scrub (Gruendemann & Meeker, 1983), whereas others recommend 5 minutes for the first scrub of the day and 3 minutes for subsequent scrubs. Follow the policies and procedure established in your facility.

PROCEDURE FOR SCRUBBING

1. Prepare yourself for the scrub.
   a. Put on the proper surgical attire used in your facility. These are called "scrub" garments. Wearing surgical attire prevents bringing outside organisms into the area. The scrub shirt should be tucked into the scrub pants or the scrub dress fitted or tied at the waist *so that loose garments do not come into contact with scrubbed hands and arms or with the sterile drying towel.*
   b. Put on a cap or hood, shoe covers, and a mask *to cover common sources of contamination* (Figure 36–1). A new mask is available with an added splash guard (Figure 36–2).
   c. Examine your hands and forearms for cuts or blemishes. Do not scrub if there are any open lesions or breaks in skin integrity *because they can contaminate surgical wounds.*
   d. All watches, rings, and bracelets should be removed *because they harbor microorganisms beneath them* (Atkinson & Kohn, 1986).
   e. Any shade of nail polish, including clear, should not be worn *to avoid chips, which may harbor microorganisms.* Fingernails should be no longer than the tips of the fingers *to prevent puncturing the gloves.* The wearing of artificial fingernails should also be avoided *because studies have shown that a higher number of microorganisms have been cultured from the fingertips of nurses wearing artificial nails than from the fingertips of nurses with natural nails* (Gruendemann & Meeker, 1987).

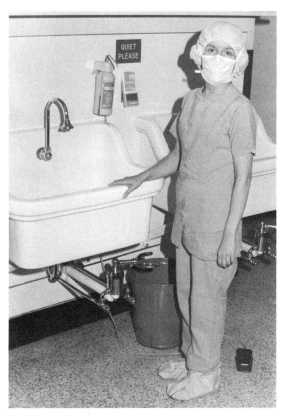

Figure 36–1. Before scrubbing, the nurse puts on surgical attire (scrub garments). Note foot pedal for liquid soap and knee-operated faucet.
(*Courtesy Ivan Ellis*)

2. Perform the prewash.
   a. Turn on the water and adjust the temperature so that it is comfortably warm. *Warm water emulsifies fats more effectively than cold water does, and hot water is hard on the skin.*
   b. Moisten your hands and arms, keeping your hands higher than your elbows *so that water will drain off your elbows, flowing from the cleanest area to the less clean area.*
   c. Using one of the liquid soaps provided, lather your hands and arms for 1 minute.
   d. Remove a brush from the dispenser and clean under each fingernail and around each cuticle with the nail cleaner included in the package. Rinse the nail cleaner after cleaning each fingernail (Figure 36–3).
   e. Rinse hands and arms thoroughly, passing them through the water *in one direction only,* from fingertips to elbow. Do not move your arms back and forth through the water.

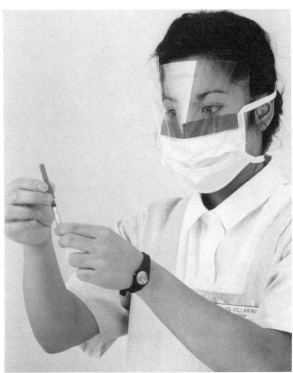

Figure 36–2. A splash guard mask protects the eyes and mucous membranes from accidental blood splashes.

3. Scrub.
   a. Counted brush-stroke method
      (1) Select a sterile brush or sponge. Apply a liquid cleanser if the brush or sponge is not impregnated with one.
      (2) Scrub the nails of the left hand 30 strokes and all skin surfaces 20 strokes, using the anatomic pattern of scrub

previously outlined (Gruendemann & Meeker, 1987).
      (a) Four surfaces of each finger, thumb to fifth finger
      (b) Over dorsal surface of hand, small finger to thumb
      (c) Over palmar surface of hand, small finger to thumb
      (d) Over the wrist
      (e) Up the arm in thirds, ending 2 inches above the elbow
      (3) Repeat step (2) for the right hand.
   b. Timed method
      (1) Select a sterile brush or sponge and apply liquid cleanser if the brush or sponge is not impregnated with one.
      (2) Scrub the nails, fingers, hand, and wrist of your left arm for 1½ minutes, using the anatomic pattern of scrub described above.
      (3) Repeat for the right nails, fingers, hand, and wrist.
      (4) Scrub from the wrist to 2 inches above the elbow, spending 1 minute on each arm (Figure 36–4).

4. Rinse.
   a. Rinse hands and arms as previously described, passing through the water in one direction from fingertips to elbow (Figure 36–5).
   b. Hands should be extended in front of you and kept at the height of your waist to avoid contamination. If a sterile towel is not available near the scrub sink, walk to the table where the towels are kept. If you must

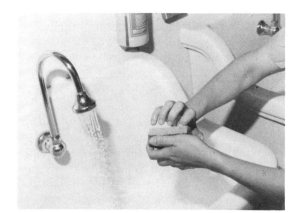

Figure 36–3. The nurse scrubs the nails briskly with a small sterile brush after the prewash has been completed. (*Courtesy Ivan Ellis*)

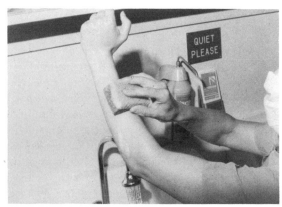

Figure 36–4. The hands and forearms are scrubbed with a sterile brush or sponge after the nails are cleaned and brushed. (*Courtesy Ivan Ellis*)

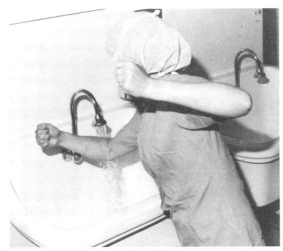

Figure 36–5. Rinse your arms, keeping the hands higher than the elbows.
(*Courtesy Ivan Ellis*)

go through closed doors, back through. Allow your arms to drip (Figure 36–6).
5. Dry your hands and arms.
   a. Pick up the sterile towel by one end.
   b. Allow the towel to unfold.
   c. Place one hand under half of the towel. Use that half to blot the opposite hand dry (Figure 36–7). Start at the fingers and move gradually up the arm.

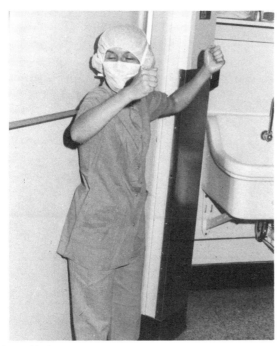

Figure 36–6. The nurse backs through a door with arms raised to prevent contamination.
(*Courtesy Ivan Ellis*)

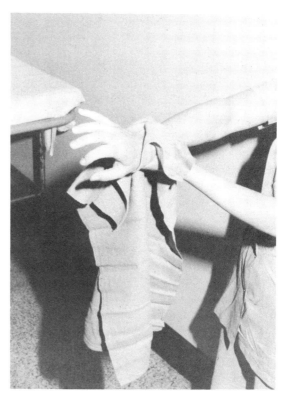

Figure 36–7. Hands and arms are dried with a sterile towel.
(*Courtesy Ivan Ellis*)

   d. Use the other half of the towel to blot the second arm dry. Again start at the fingers and move up the arm.
   e. Push the cuticles of your fingernails back with the towel as you dry your hands. *This helps to prevent ragged cuticle edges, decreasing the chance of harboring bacteria.*

You are now ready to put on a sterile gown and gloves.

GOWNING AND GLOVING

After you have scrubbed and dried your hands, you are ready to put on a sterile gown. Remember to keep your hands above your waist and higher than your elbows at all times *to make sure they do not touch anything nonsterile.*

Gowning is a two-person procedure. You will need an assistant to put on a sterile gown safely, and your assistant will need sterile forceps.

The closed-glove technique, which is described in step 7 below, is in widespread use because *it provides a way to don gloves without the possibility that they will be touched on the outside by the bare hand.* You will don the right glove first, and then the left glove.

(Open-glove technique is described in Module 35, Sterile Technique.)

1. Pick up the sterile gown carefully by its neck edge.
2. Facing the sterile field, hold the gown by the inside, top neckline in front of you and allow it to unfold (Figure 36–8).
3. Position so that you are facing the back opening.
4. Work your hands and arms carefully into the gown and into the sleeves, as far as the seam between the sleeve and the cuff. Take your time and proceed slowly. Do not push your hands out through the ends of the sleeves.
5. Turn your back to your assistant, who will now grasp the inside of the back, pull it securely onto your shoulders, and tie the neck and back waistline ties.
6. Leave the front waistline tie tied in front of you.
7. Using the closed-glove technique, put on the sterile gloves.

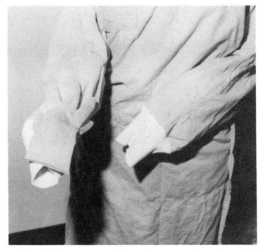

Figure 36–9. The nurse positions the sterile glove by reaching through the gown with the opposite hand. (*Courtesy Ivan Ellis*)

a. With your left hand still inside the gown, pick up the folded edge of the right glove.
b. Hold your right hand out, with the palm up, still inside the sleeve.
c. Lay the right glove on the right palm (which is still inside the sleeve). Position it with the glove fingers pointing toward the elbow and the cuff end pointing toward the fingertips. The thumb of the glove should be over the thumb of your right hand (Figure 36–9).

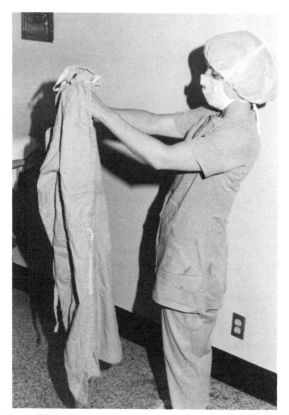

Figure 36–8. To put on a sterile gown, face the sterile field and hold the gown by the inside neck-line. Allow it to fall open and work your hands and arms carefully into the gown. (*Courtesy Ivan Ellis*)

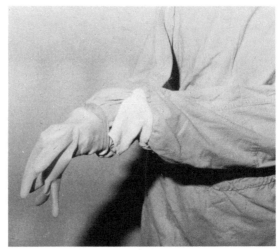

Figure 36–10. Pull up the first glove with your opposite hand still inside the gown. (*Courtesy Ivan Ellis*)

d. Use your right hand (which is still inside the gown sleeve) to grasp the bottom fold of the cuff end of the right glove. You are touching sterile gown to sterile glove.

e. With your left hand (which is still inside the gown sleeve), grasp the right glove cuff by the top fold of the cuff end, and pull the right glove cuff up and over the right gown cuff (Figure 36–10).

f. Adjust the right glove cuff over the right gown cuff as necessary, keeping the left hand inside the gown.

g. Work your right hand down into the glove. If the fingers are not in place, don't worry. You can correct them when both gloves are on.

h. Pick up the left glove with the gloved right hand.

i. Hold your left hand, palm up, inside the gown sleeve.

j. Place the left glove on the left palm (which is still inside the gown), with the glove fingers pointing toward the elbow and the cuff end pointing toward your fingertips. Position the glove thumb over the left thumb of your hand.

k. Use your left hand (which is still inside the sleeve) to grasp the bottom fold of the cuff end of the left glove.

l. Grasp the top fold of the cuff edge with the gloved right hand, and pull the glove cuff up and over the gown cuff (Figure 36–11).

m. Work your left hand down into the left glove.

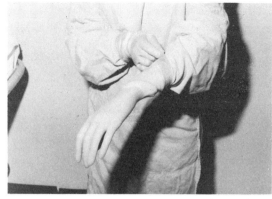

Figure 36–12. When sterile gloves are on both hands, the cuffs can be safely adjusted. (*Courtesy Ivan Ellis*)

n. Turn up and adjust the cuffs of both gloves (Figure 36–12).

o. Pull the glove fingers out at the ends to reposition your fingers if necessary.

8. With your gloved hands, untie the front waist tie of your gown.

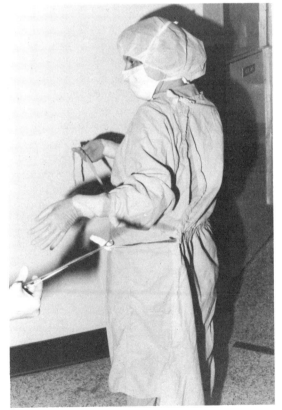

Figure 36–13. Take the tie from the forceps held by your assistant and tie the sterile gown. (*Courtesy Ivan Ellis*)

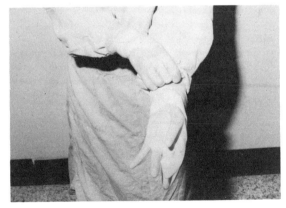

Figure 36–11. The second glove can be pulled up by the hand wearing the sterile glove. (*Courtesy Ivan Ellis*)

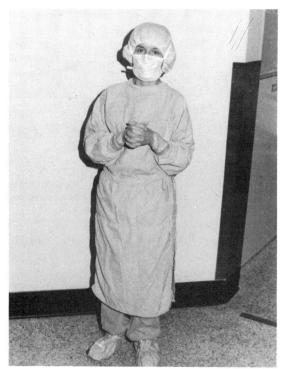

Figure 36–14.   The nurse is now properly scrubbed, gowned, and gloved.
(*Courtesy Ivan Ellis*)

9. Hold the ends carefully, keeping them above your waist.
10. Hold the shorter tie in one hand.
11. With the other hand, hold the longer tie out for your assistant to grasp with sterile forceps.
12. While your assistant is holding the tie, turn around carefully, wrapping the gown around you as you turn. This completely covers your back with the sterile gown. Be sure you are well away from all equipment when you turn.
13. Retrieve the tie from your assistant, and tie the two ties together in the front. You are now prepared to handle sterile equipment and to assist the physician performing a surgical procedure (Figure 36–13).
14. You are now in scrub attire (Figure 36–14).

GUIDELINES FOR WORKING IN STERILE ATTIRE

1. *Everything below the waist or table height is considered nonsterile.* Therefore, keep your hands above your waist and keep sterile equipment on top of the tables. When you are waiting, it is often convenient to clasp your gloved hands together in front of you to protect them.
2. *Your back is considered potentially contaminated because you cannot see what happens to it.* Do not turn your back on any sterile area. Always pass it with your face toward the sterile area.
3. Also, for the same reason, when passing another person in sterile attire, pass either face to face or back to back. If you must stand behind someone, fasten a sterile towel over that person's back.
4. *Sterility is a matter of certainty, not conjecture.* If you even suspect that a part of your attire has been contaminated, notify the appropriate person (circulating nurse, perhaps) for assistance in changing.
5. *Moisture allows microorganisms to wick quickly and easily from one area to another.* If your attire becomes wet, consider it contaminated and change it or cover it.
6. *Contamination often occurs accidentally.* To prevent this, whenever you move close to anyone, warn them verbally. Do not take it for granted that they will see you.

References

Atkinson, L. J. & Kohn, M. L. (1986). *Berry and Kohn's introduction to operating room technique* (6th ed.). New York: Mc-Graw Hill.

Gruendemann, B. J. & Meeker, M. H. (1987). *Alexander's care of the patient in surgery* (8th ed.). St. Louis: C. V. Mosby.

Standards and recommended practices for perioperative nursing. (1990). The Association for Operating Room Nurses, Inc. (AORN).

Performance Checklist

Scrubbing	Unsat	Needs More Practice	Sat	Comments
1. Prepare yourself. a. Put on surgical attire ("scrub" garments).				
b. Put on cap or hood, shoe covers, and mask.				
c. Examine hands and forearms for cuts or blemishes.				
d. Remove watches, rings, and bracelets.				
e. Remove nail polish and/or artificial nails if worn and clip nails so they are no longer in length than the fingertips.				
2. Perform the prewash. a. Turn on water and adjust temperature.				
b. Moisten hands and arms.				
c. Lather hands and arms for 1 minute.				
d. Remove brush from dispenser and clean nails, rinsing after each nail.				
e. Rinse hands and arms, keeping hands higher than elbows.				
3. Scrub. a. Counted brush-stroke method				
(1) Select sterile brush or sponge, adding liquid cleanser if necessary.				
(2) Scrub nails of left hand 30 strokes and all skin surfaces 20 strokes, using anatomic pattern outlined.				
(3) Repeat step (2) for the right hand and arm.				
b. Timed method				
(1) Select sterile brush or sponge, adding liquid cleanser if necessary.				
(2) Scrub nails, fingers, hand, and wrist of left arm for 1½ minutes, using anatomic pattern outlined.				
(a) Four surfaces of each finger, thumb to fifth finger				

Scrubbing *(Continued)*	Unsat	Needs More Practice	Sat	Comments
(b) Over dorsal surface of hand, small finger to thumb				
(c) Over palmar surface of hand, small finger to thumb				
(d) Over the wrist				
(e) Up the arm in thirds, ending 2 inches above the elbow				
(3) Repeat for right nails, fingers, hand, and wrist.				
(4) Scrub from wrist to 2 inches above elbow, spending 1 minute on each arm.				
4. Rinse. a. Rinse hands and arms, keeping hands above elbows.				
b. Keep your hands in front of you, above the waist and not higher than the axilla, and move to location of sterile towels.				
5. Dry hands and arms. a. Pick up sterile towel.				
b. Allow towel to unfold.				
c. Use half to dry first hand and arm.				
d. Use second half to dry second hand and arm.				
e. Push cuticles back as you dry.				

Gowning and Closed Gloving

	Unsat	Needs More Practice	Sat	Comments
1. Pick up gown by neck edge.				
2. Facing the sterile field, hold gown by the inside, top neckline and allow it to unfold.				
3. Position gown so that you are facing the back opening.				
4. Work hands and arms into gown to seam between gown and cuff.				
5. Turn your back to assistant for securing gown at neck and back.				
6. Leave front tie tied.				

Growning and Closed Gloving *(Continued)*	Unsat	Needs More Practice	Sat	Comments
7. Using closed-glove technique, put on sterile gloves. a. Use left hand inside gown to pick up folded edge of right glove.				
b. Hold right hand, palm up, inside gown.				
c. Position right glove on right palm.				
d. Use right hand inside gown to grasp bottom fold of cuff.				
e. Use left hand inside gown to pull right glove cuff over right gown cuff.				
f. Adjust right glove over right gown cuff.				
g. Work right hand into glove.				
h. Using gloved right hand, pick up left glove.				
i. Hold left hand, palm up, inside gown.				
j. Position left glove over left palm.				
k. Use left hand inside gown to grasp fold of glove cuff.				
l. Use gloved right hand to grasp top of fold and pull glove cuff over gown cuff.				
m. Work left hand into glove.				
n. Turn up and adjust cuffs.				
o. Reposition fingers as needed.				
8. Untie front waist tie.				
9. Hold ends above waist.				
10. Hold shorter tie in one hand.				
11. Hold longer tie out for assistant to grasp with sterile forceps.				
12. Turn around carefully, wrapping gown around you.				
13. Retrieve tie from assistant and tie two ties in front.				

Working in Sterile Attire

1. Keep your hands in front of you and above waist level, below axilla.				

Working in Sterile Attire *(Continued)*	Unsat	Needs More Practice	Sat	Comments
2. Do not turn your back on sterile field.				
3. Pass front to front or back to back with others in sterile attire.				
4. Change attire when contaminated.				
5. Change or cover attire if wet.				
6. Warn others of your movements.				

Quiz

Short-Answer Questions

1. List three purposes of a surgical scrub.

   a. _____

   b. _____

   c. _____

2. What hospital committee could you consult regarding scrub policies and procedures? _____

3. List three situations in which a nurse would be required to don a sterile gown and gloves.

   a. _____

   b. _____

   c. _____

4. Why do you remove jewelry from your hands and forearms before beginning the scrub? _____

5. Why is a wooden nail cleaner not recommended? _____

6. Why would you want a residue of antibacterial cleansing agent to remain on the skin? _____

7. Why are hands held higher than the elbows for a surgical scrub? _____

8. What is the advantage of the closed-glove technique? _____

9. When you are scrubbed, why do you always face a sterile area when you pass it? _____

10. What should you do if you suspect that one of your gloves is contaminated? _____

Module 37
Wound Care

Module Contents

Rationale for the Use of This Skill
Nursing Diagnosis
Observing and Describing the Wound
Drains
Dressing Materials
Procedure for Changing Sterile Dressings[1]
    Assessment
    Planning
    Implementation
    Evaluation
    Documentation
Shortening a Penrose Drain
Wet-to-Dry Dressings
Procedure for Removing Sutures or Skin
    Staples
    Assessment
    Planning

    Implementation
    Evaluation
    Documentation
Procedure for Emptying and Restarting a
    Wound Suction Device
    Assessment
    Planning
    Implementation
    Evaluation
    Documentation
Long-Term Care
Home Care

Prerequisites

Successful completion of the following modules:

VOLUME 1

Module 1   An Approach to Nursing Skills
Module 2   Basic Infection Control
Module 3   Safety
Module 5   General Assessment Overview
Module 6   Documentation
Module 26 Applying Bandages and Binders

VOLUME 2

Module 35 Sterile Technique

[1] For stump dressings, see Module 26, Applying Bandages and Binders. For colostomy dressings, see Module 38, Ostomy Care. For tracheostomy dressings, see Module 43, Tracheostomy Care and Suctioning. For central line dressings, see Module 55, Caring for Central Intravenous Lines.

54

© 1992 by J.B. Lippincott Company

Overall Objective

To care for wounds by changing sterile dressings and removing sutures or staples, maintaining safety and comfort for both patient and nurse.

Specific Learning Objectives

	Know Facts and Principles	Apply Facts and Principles	Demonstrate Ability	Evaluate Performance
1. *Function of dressings*	State three functions of dressings.	Given a patient situation, identify function of particular dressing.	In the clinical setting, identify function of all dressings observed.	Evaluate effectiveness of dressing in performing identified function.
2. *Drains*	State two reasons for use of wound drains. List three types of surgery in which drains are often used.	Given a patient situation, identify purpose of wound drain in use.	Shorten Penrose drain correctly under supervision.	Evaluate performance with instructor.
3. *Observations*	State observations to be made during dressing change.	Given a patient situation, describe observations accurately, using correct terminology.	Make pertinent observations during dressing change.	Evaluate own performance with instructor, using Performance Checklist.
4. *Dressing materials*	List dressing materials.	Identify various dressing materials by name. Give rationale for use of different dressing materials in various situations.	Use various types of dressing materials appropriately.	Evaluate use of dressing materials with instructor.
5. *Procedure for dressing change*	Explain how to change dressing.	Given a patient situation, identify correct ways to perform procedure. Give rationale for correct performance of procedure. Give rationale for using wet-to-dry dressing.	Change dressing correctly under supervision. Apply wet-to-dry dressing correctly under supervision.	Evaluate own performance with instructor. Evaluate own performance with instructor.
6. *Removing sutures or staples*	Describe the procedure for removing sutures or staples.		In the clinical setting, under supervision, remove sutures or staples.	Evaluate with your instructor.

(continued)

Specific Learning Objectives *(Continued)*

	Know Facts and Principles	Apply Facts and Principles	Demonstrate Ability	Evaluate Performance
7. *Emptying and restarting a wound suction device*	Describe the procedure for emptying and restarting a wound suction device.	Given a patient situation, determine whether wound suction device should be emptied and restarted.	In the clinical setting, under supervision, empty and restart a wound suction device.	Evaluate own performance with instructor.
8. *Documentation*	State items to be included on progress note regarding dressing change, removing staples or sutures, or a wound suction device.	Given a patient situation, write progress note descriptive of dressing change and wound. Give rationale for items to be included in progress note regarding dressing change and wound.	In the clinical setting, write complete and accurate progress note regarding dressing change and wound.	Provide copy to instructor for evaluation.

Learning Activities

1. Review the Specific Learning Objectives.
2. Read the chapters on procedures and infection in Ellis and Nowlis, *Nursing: A Human Needs Approach,* or comparable chapters in another textbook.
3. Look up the module vocabulary terms in the Glossary.
4. Read through the module and mentally practice the skills.
5. In the practice setting:
   a. Identify the various types of dressing materials available by name. In what kind of situation is each appropriate?
   b. Using a pillow (or other curved surface) as an abdomen, practice doing a dressing change, with the Performance Checklist as a guide. What adaptation would you make if a drain were present? If a drain were to be shortened?
   c. When you are satisfied with your performance, have another student evaluate you.
   d. Have your instructor evaluate your performance.
   e. Repeat b–d for a wet-to-dry dressing.
6. Examine a suture removal kit. Practice using the forceps to pick up a small thread and clip it with the scissors.
7. Examine a staple remover. Note how it operates.
8. Examine a wound suction device. Practice opening, draining, and re-establishing the suction.
9. In the clinical setting:
   a. Change a sterile dressing under the supervision of your instructor or a staff nurse.

Vocabulary

aseptic
contaminated
debride
excoriation

first-intention
  healing
Penrose drain
purulent
sanguineous

second-intention
  healing
serosanguineous
serous
sterile

Wound Care

Rationale for the Use of This Skill

Open wounds such as surgical wounds, decubitus ulcers, and burns require care that will promote healing and prevent further injury or deterioration of the wound. Dressings over open wounds must be sterile, and sterile technique is essential when changing dressings. Second only to the nurse's responsibility to maintain rigid sterile technique is the responsibility to observe and describe the wound carefully. A third responsibility is to choose the most appropriate dressing materials available and to apply them in the most secure and comfortable fashion possible.[2]

▶ *Nursing Diagnosis*

> The individual with the nursing diagnosis "Impaired skin integrity," specifically a surgical wound, decubitus ulcer, or burn, is in need of appropriate wound care.

OBSERVING AND DESCRIBING THE WOUND

Careful observation and accurate description of the wound are integral parts of changing a sterile dressing.

Observe the wound. Are the edges approximated? Does the wound have a smooth contour? Are inflammation and edema (swelling) present? If so, to what degree? A wound that has approximated edges and a smooth contour and that displays minimal inflammation and swelling and is healing across all layers is said to be healing by *primary (first) intention.* Scarring is minimal with this type of healing. If the wound opens or if the edges never were closely approximated, the wound heals from the inside out, and the gap fills with granulation tissue. This type of healing is called healing by *secondary intention.* It takes longer and leaves a larger scar.

Is there drainage from the surface of the wound? Drainage may be primarily *serous* (composed of serum from the body), *serosanguineous* (composed of blood and serum), or *purulent* (containing pus). The color, amount, and odor of the drainage must be identified and documented. Note the amount by stating the number of dressings saturated or stained by the drainage. Odors are best described by comparing

[2] You will note that rationale for action is emphasized throughout the module by the use of italics.

them with a familiar smell such as feces or ammonia, if that is possible. A flow sheet is frequently used to record wound assessment and treatment. Figure 37–9 is an example of a flow sheet used for monitoring a decubitus ulcer.

All types of wound drainage support the growth of microorganisms. Therefore, many measures are used to keep the wound surface clean and to move the drainage away from it. Drainage can also irritate the skin around the wound, so heavily draining wounds may need special dressing techniques to protect the skin.

DRAINS

Drains are sometimes placed during surgery *to enhance the drainage of discharge from the wound, thus promoting wound healing.* A drain may also be used *to help keep the operated area dry.* The Penrose drain is an example of such a drain (Figure 37–1).

If a considerable amount of drainage is expected postoperatively, a closed-wound drainage system is placed at surgery. This portable system consists of a drainage tube attached to a vacuum unit that gently suctions fluid from the wound. The Hemovac is an example of this type of setup (Figure 37–2). Other brands have a different shape, such as a small plastic bottle, but operate on the same principle of low suction. Commonly used after breast, hip, or perineal surgery, it helps keep the wound dry and is easily moved when the patient moves.

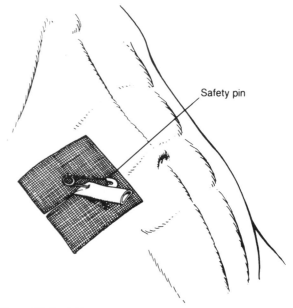

Figure 37–1. Split gauze surrounding a Penrose drain.

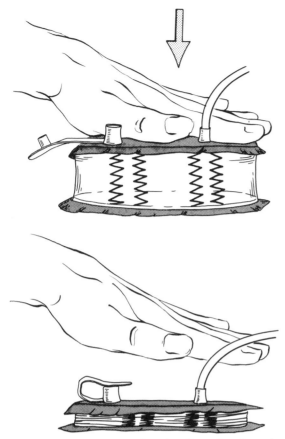

Figure 37-2. Hemovac wound suction. Open the valve and push down to reestablish suction.
(*Courtesy Zimmer, Inc., Warsaw, Indiana*)

DRESSING MATERIALS

The type of dressing materials used varies from facility to facility. Here are some of the most common types, although they may be called by different names.

1. *4 × 4s* These are sterile or nonsterile folded gauze pads, 4 inches by 4 inches in size. In most facilities 2 × 2s and 3 × 3s are also available.
2. *Fluffs* Fluffs are large pieces of sterile or nonsterile gauze that are loosely folded *to absorb drainage.* They are also used to pack wounds.
3. *ABDs (combines, combination pads)* These are large, sterile or nonsterile, absorbent pads (usually a coarse gauze covered by a finer gauze). Normally they are used over smaller dressing materials, and most are moisture-resistant on one side.
4. *Nonadherents* These are special sterile dressings that have one nonadhering surface.

Nonadherent dressings are used directly next to incisions, *to prevent injury to tissues when the dressing is removed.* They are often cut to appropriate size.

5. *Moisture-vapor-permeable* (MVP) *transparent dressings* These dressings look like a thin sheet of plastic and are often called by their brand names, such as Bioclusive, Opsite, and Tegaderm. One surface has an adhesive that adheres to dry, intact skin but not to a moist wound surface. The dressings are semipermeable and allow gases such as moisture vapor and oxygen to move through them. Larger molecules such as those found in the drainage or in bacteria, do not pass through the material. Bacteria can move from the skin surrounding the dressing to the area under it through very small crevices in the skin that are not sealed off by the dressing. MVP dressings provide a moist surface that encourages epithelialization of the wound surface (Turner, 1985). They are used primarily over small wounds and sometimes for intravenous dressings.
6. *Hydrocolloid dressings* A common brand of this type of dressing is Duoderm. It is a soft wafer than can be cut to the desired shape and size and placed over an open wound. The colloidal substance absorbs drainage at the wound surface, providing a moist environment for epithelialization and healing. The hydrocolloidal dressing is impermeable to both small and large molecules, but bacteria can move under it, as they do with MVP dressings (Turner, 1985). Hydrocolloid dressings are used over decubitus ulcers and other open skin lesions.
7. *Ostomy care materials* Materials developed to protect the skin from stool or urine after an ostomy are also valuable for protecting the skin around heavily draining wounds. They can also be used to protect skin from tape irritation—if they are placed over intact skin where tape must be removed frequently, the tape can be affixed to the skin barrier instead of the skin. One of these products, karaya, is available as a pliable wafer that can be cut to any shape and adheres to the skin. It also comes in a powder form, to be used on skin irregularities such as those caused by a scar or the umbilicus, that are near the wound. Another type, Stomadhesive, comes as a wafer or paste. A lesser degree of protection is

offered by clear liquids, such as tincture of benzoine, which dry to form a thin protective covering on the skin.

8. *Roller gauze* This is sterile gauze that comes in various widths and is used for packing as well as wrapping wounds. Roller gauze is also used to secure dressings.

9. *Tape* Tape comes in a variety of materials (adhesive, plastic, paper) and in widths from ¼ inch to 6 inches. Paper tape is generally considered hypoallergenic.

10. *Montgomery straps or ties* Commercially available, these straps are used to tie across large or bulky dressings that need frequent changing (Figure 37–3). Cut to the desired width, they include one or more eyelets. Generally, twill tape, roller gauze, or rubber bands attached with safety pins are used to secure these straps or ties. Straps may remain on the dressing until soiled, but ties are usually changed more frequently. Montgomery straps can be made from wide tape folded back, with holes cut for eyelets.

11. *Drainage bags* Disposable plastic drainage bags are sometimes used over profusely draining wounds. These bags attach to the skin with a variety of adhesives. Most have a ring that is attached to the skin and a bag that can be removed and replaced. The bags allow staff to measure drainage precisely and observe the wound. They contain odor and moisture, making the patient more comfortable (Figure 37–4).

PROCEDURE FOR CHANGING STERILE DRESSINGS

Assessment

1. Check the orders for the dressing change. In some instances the physician will want to do the first dressing change after surgery and then will write an order: "Change dressing prn." Or, you may be responsible for all dressing changes. In any case, a dressing may always be reinforced, meaning that you can apply

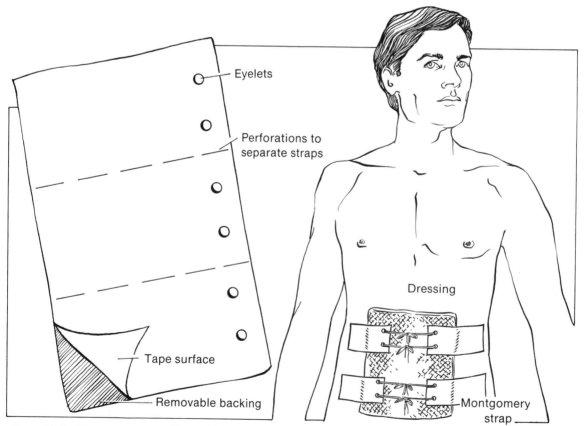

Figure 37–3. Montgomery straps allow multiple dressing changes without removing and reapplying tape each time.

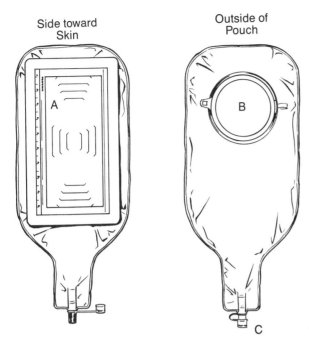

Figure 37-4. Wound or drainage collection pouch. Adhesive area, cut to fit shape of wound (A). Access opening for wound observation and care (B). Drainage port for emptying drainage (C).

additional dressings on top of dressings already in place *to absorb drainage.* Sterile dressings are used over a previous dressing *to avoid introducing organisms.* However, because they are placed on the contaminated exterior surface of the old dressing, they do not prevent the possibility of wound contamination. Keep in mind that *once drainage has penetrated to the outside of a dressing, organisms may be carried to the wound through moisture.*

2. Check the present dressing *to ascertain the type and amount of dressing materials necessary.* This information may be on the Nursing Care Plan.
3. Check the patient's unit for supplies and equipment that may already be in the room.

Planning
4. Wash your hands *for infection control.*
5. Gather the equipment. Some facilities use commercially prepared packages that include all the instruments needed. Your facility may use a partially prepared dressing tray, in which case you must add the additional sterile supplies needed. Or you may have to gather all the sterile supplies, using a sterile towel or the individual sterile packages as a sterile field. Items you may need include scissors, thumb

forceps (pickups), 4 × 4s, ABDs, tape, antiseptic solution, cotton-tipped applicators, and sterile gloves. Some facilities have special bags or paper *for the disposal of soiled dressings.* In others the bedside waste bag is used. If you follow this latter procedure, the bag should be discarded and replaced immediately after the dressing change.

Implementation
6. Identify the patient *to be sure you are performing the procedure for the correct patient,* and explain what you intend to do. Allow the patient to ask questions *to help ensure his or her cooperation.* Usually little, if any, pain is associated with a dressing change, but if some is expected, prepare the patient for it. Ask the patient to keep his or her hands away from the dressing area and to avoid talking during the procedure *to limit the number of microorganisms moving in the air.* Limit your own conversation to essential information. In some situations it may be necessary for both patient and nurse to wear masks during a dressing change.
7. Prepare the environment. Close windows and doors *to eliminate drafts that might chill the patient or carry microorganisms into the open wound.* Pull the drapes and draw the curtains around the bed *to provide privacy.* The patient should be lying flat or in low Fowler's position. Clear a working space—the overbed table serves this purpose well. Make sure your work surface is clean and dry *to prevent contamination of supplies.* Place a bag or paper *for soiled dressings* within easy reach. The bag edges can be taped to the mattress edge *for convenience.*
8. Tear strips of tape in correct lengths and place them on the edge of an easily reached surface. (If Montgomery straps are used, you will not need tape unless the straps themselves are to be changed.) Determine whether the patient has an allergy to adhesive tape, in which case you should use paper or plastic tape.
9. Expose the area to be dressed and drape the patient, if necessary, *for privacy.* A bath blanket can be used for this purpose.
10. Prepare to remove the present dressing. Loosen tapes, starting from the outside and working toward the dressing *to minimize disruption of wound healing.* If body hair makes this activity uncomfortable for the patient, you may want to shave the area before applying more tape. Some dressings are covered with an

elastic or cloth binder, in which case you must unhook or unpin the binder.

11. Put on gloves and remove the dressings. This can be done in many ways. Your facility may have a preferred procedure, so be sure to consult its procedure book. Take the outer dressings off by grasping them at the center (without applying pressure) and removing them to the side. Avoid passing dressings over any sterile area. You can use forceps or wear clean gloves to remove all dressings. *This protects you from drainage.* On rare occasions you may find that you must touch and move drains, retention sutures, and other devices in the wound to remove a soiled dressing. In such a case you should put on sterile gloves *to avoid introducing microorganisms to this area.*

Notice how many of which type of dressings are soiled *to indicate the amount of drainage when you chart.* Place the soiled dressings in the bag or on the paper designated for that use. If you used forceps or gloves, discard them.

12. Wash your hands.

13. Observe the wound, noting the approximation of the wound's edges, the presence of inflammation and edema, and the presence, appearance, and odor of drainage, if any.

14. Open all packages and arrange the sterile equipment conveniently.

15. Pour the antiseptic solution if one is being used. Use the solution of the physician's choice or the one currently in use at your facility. In some facilities the solution is available in small bottles for individual use and does not have to be poured. In any case, if you need a container for the solution, it must be sterile and you should be careful not to drip solution around the basin, especially on the cloth drapes. Also available for use in this situation are antiseptic-soaked swabsticks and small foil packages of antiseptic solution.

The most common agents used for cleansing are the iodophor compounds (Betadine, Acudyne, Povidone), which provide long-lasting antimicrobial protection. However, *they also cause skin reactions in some individuals,* and therefore you should assess the skin carefully for early signs of redness and edema when you are using them. Hibiclens is another commonly used antibacterial agent. Hydrogen peroxide is less effective as an antimicrobial, but it does clean and is less likely to provoke skin

reactions. Antimicrobials applied directly to a wound surface inhibit epithelialization.

16. Put on sterile gloves (see Module 35, Sterile Technique). In some facilities you will also be required to wear a mask.

17. Clean the skin around the wound with antiseptic solution if indicated or ordered by the physician. Using cotton balls or prepared swabs, clean around the wound. If the wound is small or is a surgical stab wound (a small puncture wound made by the surgeon) clean in ever-widening circles away from it, moving from clean to dirty (Figure 37–5). For a longer wound, you may need to use consecutive long strokes, starting each stroke at the top of the wound and moving to the bottom. Each successive stroke is farther from the wound on that side. Use another swab to clean the other side of the wound, starting at the wound edge and gradually moving out (Figure 37–6). Use each swab only once. Clean two or three times as indicated. If there are multiple wounds, such as a central incision with several drains, clean each wound separately, using fresh swabs *to avoid moving microbes from one site to another.*

18. Redress the wound, placing dressing materials carefully *so they do not slide off.* Use materials in the order they were in when the old dressing was removed, if that seemed effective. If not, redress *for greater effectiveness.*

If the wound is deep and is to be packed, place the dressings so that they contact all

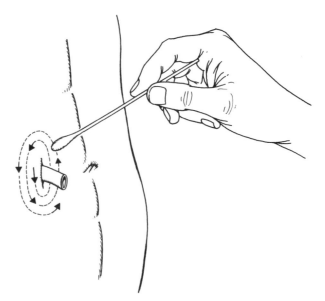

Figure 37–5. Clean around a drain by using a widening spiral starting at the drain and moving outward.

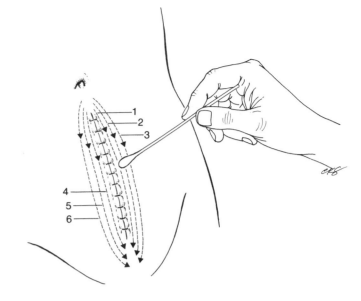

Figure 37–6. Cleaning along a large wound. Use one swab for strokes 1, 2, and 3. Use a second swab for strokes 4, 5, and 6.

surfaces of the wound. Fill the wound firmly but not so tightly that pressure is placed on its surface.

If a drain is in place, the bulk of the dressing should cover the drain area, usually in a dependent position. *To prevent excoriation of the skin around the drain site,* partially split a 4 × 4 with sterile scissors and place it snugly around the drain (see Figure 37–1). A drain site may also be dressed with two 4 × 4s. Open the 4 × 4s and fold them in half lengthwise. By folding each at right angles, each can serve as two sides of the dressing (Figure 37–7).

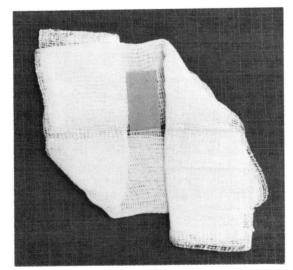

Figure 37–7. Two 4 × 4s surrounding a Penrose drain. (*Courtesy Ivan Ellis*)

Prenotched gauze squares are also available.

19. Remove your gloves and place them in the bag of soiled dressing materials.
20. Secure the dressing with tape, Montgomery straps, or a binder as indicated. Use enough tape to hold the dressing in place, but do not use more than necessary. Avoid putting tension on the tape as *this can create skin irritation and tape burns* (Figure 37–8).
21. Assist the patient to a comfortable position.
22. Care for the equipment. Remove the bag used for soiled dressings and other materials and put it in the appropriate place. Rinse any glass or metal materials used *to remove protein substances* before sending them to the central supply department.
23. Wash your hands.

Evaluation
24. Evaluate, using the following criteria:
    a. Sterile technique maintained throughout procedure.
    b. Dressing applied securely.
    c. Patient made comfortable after procedure.

Documentation
25. Record the procedure on the patient's chart, including the time the procedure was performed, observations made, dressing materials and antiseptic solution used, and any reactions of the patient. This information is sometimes entered on a flow sheet (Figure 37–9).

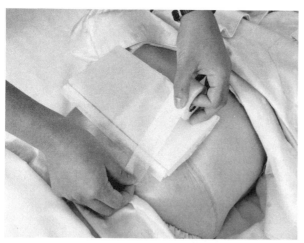

Figure 37–8. Tape should be applied to the skin without tension to prevent tape burns and skin irritation.

SHORTENING A PENROSE DRAIN

A Penrose drain is a soft, flat rubber tubing that is placed into the wound to facilitate drainage. The physician may order that a drain be shortened by a specific amount, usually *to encourage the closure of the wound from the inside out.* Therefore, the drain is pulled out of the wound the specified distance and its length inside of the wound is thus shortened. A sterile safety pin is often used to prevent the drain from slipping back inside the wound. If a drain is stapled or sutured to the skin, you must remove the staple or suture before you can shorten or remove the drain.

The drain is shortened during the dressing change. After the wound has been cleaned in step 17 complete the following:

a. Grasp the Penrose drain with a pair of forceps.
b. Gently but firmly pull the drain out the specified distance.
c. If a sterile safety pin is to be placed on the drain, you must handle it with sterile gloved hands. Remove and replace it at wound surface.
d. Using sterile scissors, clip off the excess drain, making sure that 2 inches of drain remain visible outside the wound. *This prevents the drain from sliding back into the wound where a surgical incision would be needed to remove it.*

WET-TO-DRY DRESSINGS

Wet-to-dry dressings may be used to *debride* (clean away adherent material from) the surface of the wound. Gauze that has been moistened with saline is placed in contact with the wound surface. Dressings are usually moistened by pouring the fluid from a container over the gauze, which is held in the sterile

DATE/TIME	
4/4/94	*Impairment of skin integrity: surgical wound*
0930	S *Reports minimal pain in wound area. States does not want to observe wound.*
	O *Abd drsg: 3 fluffs and 1 ABD saturated with serosanguineous drainage. Wound surface appears clean. Sterile drsg applied.*
	A *Healing progressing.*
	P *Change drsg q shift.*
	H. Gray, RN

Example of Progress Notes Using SOAP Format

DATE/TIME	
4/4/94	*Abd dressing changed. 3 fluffs and 1 ABD saturated with*
0930	*serosanguineous drainage. Edges of wound approximated with no puffiness noted and only slight redness at drain site. Patient unwilling to look at wound but offered no complaints. Resting comfortably at present.* — *H. Gray, RN*

Example of Progress Notes Using Narrative Format

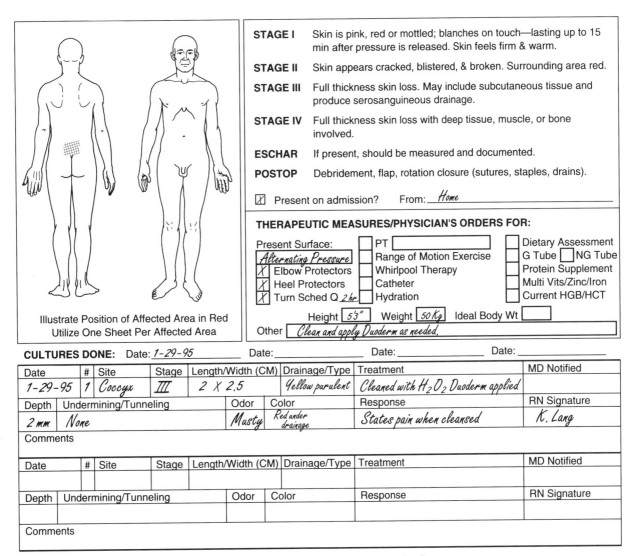

STAGE I — Skin is pink, red or mottled; blanches on touch—lasting up to 15 min after pressure is released. Skin feels firm & warm.

STAGE II — Skin appears cracked, blistered, & broken. Surrounding area red.

STAGE III — Full thickness skin loss. May include subcutaneous tissue and produce serosanguineous drainage.

STAGE IV — Full thickness skin loss with deep tissue, muscle, or bone involved.

ESCHAR — If present, should be measured and documented.

POSTOP — Debridement, flap, rotation closure (sutures, staples, drains).

☒ Present on admission?   From: *Home*

THERAPEUTIC MEASURES/PHYSICIAN'S ORDERS FOR:

Present Surface: *Alternating Pressure*
☒ Elbow Protectors
☒ Heel Protectors
☒ Turn Sched Q *2 hr*

☐ PT
☐ Range of Motion Exercise
☐ Whirlpool Therapy
☐ Catheter
☐ Hydration

☐ Dietary Assessment
☐ G Tube ☐ NG Tube
☐ Protein Supplement
☐ Multi Vits/Zinc/Iron
☐ Current HGB/HCT

Height *5'3"*   Weight *50 Kg*   Ideal Body Wt [ ]

Other: *Clean and apply Duoderm as needed.*

Illustrate Position of Affected Area in Red
Utilize One Sheet Per Affected Area

CULTURES DONE: Date: *1-29-95*   Date: _____   Date: _____   Date: _____

Date	#	Site	Stage	Length/Width (CM)	Drainage/Type	Treatment	MD Notified
1-29-95	*1*	*Coccyx*	*III*	*2 X 2.5*	*Yellow purulent*	*Cleaned with H₂O₂ Duoderm applied*	

Depth	Undermining/Tunneling	Odor	Color	Response	RN Signature
2 mm	*None*	*Musty*	*Red under drainage*	*States pain when cleansed*	*K. Lang*

Comments

Date	#	Site	Stage	Length/Width (CM)	Drainage/Type	Treatment	MD Notified

Depth	Undermining/Tunneling	Odor	Color	Response	RN Signature

Comments

Figure 37–9. Example of a wound care flow sheet. A full page would contain spaces for five entries and patient identification.

gloved hand or with sterile forceps. The hand that holds the fluid container is contaminated and cannot then be used for placing the sterile dressings (Figure 37–10).

Dry dressings are placed on top of the moist dressing. The moist surface absorbs drainage from the wound readily, and as it begins to dry it adheres to debris on the surface of the wound. When the dressing is removed, the surface debris is removed along with it. This may be uncomfortable for the patient, but moistening the dressing to prevent pulling on the surface negates the purpose of the wet-to-dry dressing. Dressings removed in this way may also disturb fresh granulation tissue, so it may be appropriate to use saline to carefully remoisten areas of the dressing that have adhered to granulating tissue rather than to debris.

Some facilities refer to any dressing that is moist at the wound surface and covered with a dry dressing as a wet-to-dry dressing. These dressings are designed to provide a moist healing environment, not to debride the wound. Be sure that you clearly understand the purpose of the dressing before proceeding.

PROCEDURE FOR REMOVING SUTURES OR SKIN STAPLES

Assessment

1. Check for an order to remove sutures or skin staples or clips.

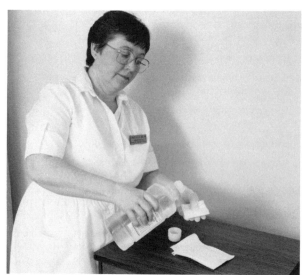

Figure 37–10. A sterile dressing can be moistened by pouring solution. The hand that holds the container is contaminated.

Planning

2. Wash your hands *for infection control.*
3. Gather the equipment you will need. The suture removal kits and staple removers used in your facility may be either disposable or nondisposable. The latter type is sterilized and packaged in the central supply department.

Implementation

4. Identify the patient *to be sure you are performing the procedure for the correct patient.*
5. Explain to the patient what you are going to do. Removal of sutures or staples may produce a pinching or pulling sensation but does not usually cause pain. If pain is anticipated, give the patient the ordered pain relief medication about 30 minutes before the procedure is to be performed.
6. If a dressing is in place, remove it as described in steps 10 and 11 of the procedure for changing sterile dressings, above.
7. If the patient's wound has been closed with sutures, gently lift each suture away from the skin with the pickup forceps. Then snip the suture close to the skin. Pull it out by pulling in line with the suture that is still inside the tissue, *in order not to traumatize tissue at the suture exit site* (Figure 37–11). *Clipping close to the skin ensures that suture material that was outside the tissue is not pulled inside, which could contaminate the wound.*

   To remove skin staples or clips, use a special instrument that is placed under the staple and pinched down to exert pressure on its center. This motion raises the ends, allowing you to remove the staple easily (Figure 37–12). Remove every other suture or staple first to determine whether the wound will hold.
8. Apply tape if ordered or if included in the procedure at your facility, *to help keep the wound edges together.* Commercially available sterile tapes (Steri-strips) are often used to approximate skin edges after suture or staple removal.

Evaluation

9. Evaluate, using the following criteria:
   a. Patient comfort
   b. Appearance of wound: approximation of wound's edges; presence of inflammation

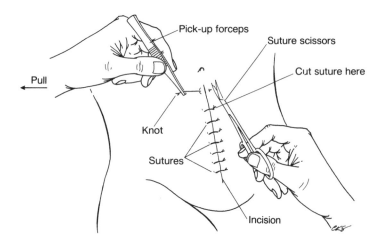

Figure 37–11. Removing sutures. Clip the suture close to the skin. Remove it by pulling in line with the stitch. Do not pull a knot into tissue.

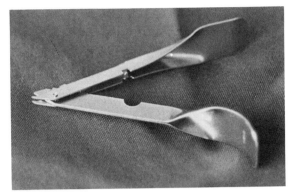

Figure 37–12. A wound staple remover.
(*Courtesy Ivan Ellis*)

and edema; presence, appearance, and odor of drainage, if any.

Documentation

10. Record the procedure on the patient's chart, including the time the procedure was performed, observations of the wound, and any reactions of the patient. Update the Nursing Care Plan as needed.

PROCEDURE FOR EMPTYING AND RESTARTING A WOUND SUCTION DEVICE

Many different brands of continuous wound suction devices are available. Three commonly used ones are the Hemovac, the Davol, and the Jackson-Pratt. These provide a much lower level of suction than do wall suctions or suction machines, and they are lightweight and allow the patient freedom of movement.

Assessment

1. Identify the type of suction device and its location.
2. Check the device to determine whether the drainage chamber contains fluid and the suction area has reexpanded.

Planning

3. Wash your hands *for infection control.*
4. Obtain a clean towel or absorbent pad to protect the bed and a container in which to measure the drainage. *Because you might contact the drainage with your hands,* it is prudent to wear clean gloves.

Implementation

5. Identify the patient *to be sure you are performing the procedure for the correct patient.*
6. Explain what you plan to do and allow the patient to ask questions.
7. Put on gloves.
8. Open the drainage port, avoiding contamination, and empty the contents into the container for measurement.
9. Clean the port with an alcohol or iodine swab.
10. Compress the suction chamber. In the Hemovac, you do this by pressing firmly down

Example of Progress Notes Using SOAP Format

DATE/TIME	
1/23/95	Impaired skin integrity: surgical wound
0830	S "Feels good to get those stitches out."
	O Skin sutures removed. Skin edges approximated without redness or puffiness.
	A Wound healing without obvious problems
	P Continue to observe.
	M. Wong, SN

Example of Progress Notes Using Narrative Format

DATE/TIME	
1/23/95	Skin sutures removed per order of Dr. Mark. Skin edges
0830	approximated. No puffiness noted. Small, reddened area at left end of incision. Patient resting comfortably. N. Sturtevant, RN

on the top of the chamber (see Figure 37–2). In the type with a bulb syringe, squeeze the bulb firmly to fill the balloon inside the suction chamber. While pressing down or squeezing firmly, reseal the drainage port. This reestablishes the vacuum and the suction.

11. Measure and empty the drainage and discard or clean the container.

12. Remove the gloves and wash your hands.

Evaluation

13. Evaluate using the following criteria:
    a. Is the container properly closed so it will not leak?
    b. Is there suction in the device?

Documentation

14. Record the amount and describe the drainage on a flow sheet if one is available. If not, you can add this information to the narrative. Also note the amount on the intake and output record, under "drainage."

LONG-TERM CARE

In the long-term care setting, the most common types of wounds are skin ulcers created by circulatory problems or through pressure. These wounds often take a long time to heal because of underlying physiologic deficits in circulation, nutrition, and oxygenation. The slow rate of healing makes progress difficult to assess. The Nursing Care Plan may specify the care techniques to be used and documentation of wound status may be done on a weekly basis rather than daily. The nurse and the physician must work collaboratively on these difficult problems. Sometimes a trial and error approach to finding the most successful care techniques is necessary.

In addition to care of the wound itself, the nurse must be even more aware of the multiple factors involved in healing and strive to support the patient through nutrition, stress reduction, positioning, activity, and oxygenation. Your fundamentals text provides more detailed information on the factors that affect wound healing.

Home Care

The patient who returns home with a surgical wound may need little more than instruction to keep the area clean and dry as healing is completed. On occasion the patient may return home with an extensive wound that requires complex management. Plans need to be made for how this is to be done at home while there is still time to teach the patient before discharge. Modifications of technique may be necessary when hospital equipment and supplies are not available at home.

For some long-term wounds, such as leg ulcers arising from poor circulation, patients may be instructed to use clean rather than sterile technique for home care. Sterile supplies are expensive and may be impossible for a person on limited income to afford. The body's own defenses may be adequate to prevent infection if the individual is in his or her own home without the assault of new and more virulent organisms to combat. Careful handwashing and the use of meticulously clean supplies may be adequate protection in this setting.

The home care nurse can teach the patient and any other caregiver and assess the progress of the wound. Some of the same concerns regarding healing may apply to the home-bound person as are found in the long-term care setting. Other physiologic problems may interfere with healing and attention to the whole person is essential.

Reference

Turner, T. D. (1985). Semiocclusive and occlusive dressings. In T. J. Rine (Ed.), *An environment for healing: The role of occlusion,* (pp. 5–14). London: Royal Society of Medicine.

Performance Checklist

Changing Sterile Dressings	Unsat	Needs More Practice	Sat	Comments
Assessment				
1. Check orders.				
2. Check the present dressing.				
3. Check the patient's unit for supplies.				
Planning				
4. Wash your hands.				
5. Gather necessary equipment.				
Implementation				
6. Identify patient and explain procedure.				
7. Prepare environment.				
8. Tear tape.				
9. Expose dressing, draping patient if necessary.				
10. Loosen tapes.				
11. Put on gloves, remove dressing and place in waste bag.				
12. Wash your hands.				
13. Observe wound.				
14. Open sterile packages and arrange equipment.				
15. Pour solution (if used).				
16. Put on sterile gloves.				
17. Clean wound with antiseptic solution if appropriate, using each swab only once. If a Penrose drain is to be shortened: a. Grasp Penrose drain with a pair of forceps.				
b. Gently but firmly pull drain out specified distance.				
c. Place sterile safety pin if needed.				
d. Clip off excess drain (leaving 2 inches).				
18. Apply dressing. a. Dry dressing—all dry components.				

Changing Sterile Dressings *(Continued)*	Unsat	Needs More Practice	Sat	Comments
b. Wet-to-dry dressing:				
(1) Moisten gauze.				
(2) Place moist gauze in contact with wound surface.				
(3) Place dry dressings over moist one.				
19. Remove gloves and place in waste bag.				
20. Secure dressing.				
21. Assist patient to position of comfort.				
22. Put on gloves and care for equipment.				
23. Wash your hands.				

Evaluation

	Unsat	Needs More Practice	Sat	Comments
24. Evaluate, using the following criteria: a. Sterile technique maintained.				
b. Dressing secure.				
c. Patient comfortable.				

Documentation

	Unsat	Needs More Practice	Sat	Comments
25. Record time, observations of wound, dressing materials and antiseptic solution used, and patient reaction.				

Removing Sutures or Staples

Assessment

	Unsat	Needs More Practice	Sat	Comments
1. Check orders.				

Planning

	Unsat	Needs More Practice	Sat	Comments
2. Wash your hands.				
3. Gather necessary equipment.				

Implementation

	Unsat	Needs More Practice	Sat	Comments
4. Identify the patient.				
5. Explain the procedure.				
6. Remove dressing, if necessary.				
7. Remove sutures or skin staples or clips.				

Removing Sutures or Staples *(Continued)*	Unsat	Needs More Practice	Sat	Comments
8. Apply tape as ordered or appropriate.				

Evaluation

	Unsat	Needs More Practice	Sat	Comments
9. Evaluate using the following criteria: a. Patient comfort.				
b. Appearance of wound: approximation of wound's edges; presence of inflammation and edema; presence, appearance, and odor of drainage, if any.				

Documentation

	Unsat	Needs More Practice	Sat	Comments
10. Record the time, observations made, and patient reaction.				

Emptying and Restarting a Wound Suction Device

Assessment

	Unsat	Needs More Practice	Sat	Comments
1. Identify type and location of suction device.				
2. Check device for drainage and suction area reexpansion.				

Planning

	Unsat	Needs More Practice	Sat	Comments
3. Wash your hands.				
4. Obtain clean towel or absorbent pad, measuring container, and clean gloves.				

Implementation

	Unsat	Needs More Practice	Sat	Comments
5. Identify patient.				
6. Explain what you plan to do.				
7. Put on gloves.				
8. Open drainage port and empty contents into container.				
9. Clean the drainage port.				
10. Compress suction chamber as appropriate and reclose drainage port while compressing.				
11. Measure and empty drainage and care for container.				
12. Remove gloves and wash your hands.				

Emptying and Restarting a Wound Suction Device (Continued)	Unsat	Needs More Practice	Sat	Comments
Evaluation				
13. Evaluate using the following criteria: a. Container is properly closed to prevent leaks.				
b. Suction is working in device.				
Documentation				
14. Record amount and description of drainage. a. On flow sheet or narrative.				
b. On intake and output record.				

Quiz
Short-Answer Questions

1. List three reasons for the application of dressings.

   a. _____

   b. _____

   c. _____

2. List three of the nurse's responsibilities with regard to dressing changes.

   a. _____

   b. _____

   c. _____

3. List four characteristics of drainage that must be noted when a dressing is changed.

   a. _____

   b. _____

   c. _____

   d. _____

4. List three characteristics of a wound that is healing by primary intention.

   a. _____

   b. _____

   c. _____

5. A special sterile dressing with a nonstick surface that is used directly next to an incision is called a _____ dressing.

6. What type of tape is generally considered to be hypoallergenic?

   _____

7. List three types of surgery in which drains are often used.

   a. _____

   b. _____

   c. _____

8. Why are ostomy supplies sometimes used for wound care? _____

9. What is the rationale underlying treatment of each wound site (drain wound, incision, etc.) separately when cleaning the wound area? _____

   _____

10. What is the purpose of a wet-to-dry dressing? _____

   _____

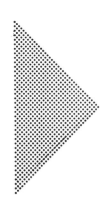

Unit 8

COMPLEX PROCEDURES RELATED TO ELIMINATION

MODULE 38
Ostomy Care

MODULE 39
Catheterization

75

Module 38
Ostomy Care

Module Contents

Rationale for the Use of This Skill
Nursing Diagnoses
Bowel Diversion Ostomies
Urinary Diversion Ostomies
Ostomy Appliances
Appearance of a Normal Stoma
Health Teaching Toward Self-Care
Obtaining Specimens From Ostomies
Home Care
Long-term Care
Procedure for Changing a Colostomy or Ileostomy Pouch or Dressing
  Assessment
  Planning
  Implementation
  Evaluation
  Documentation
Applying a Colostomy Dressing
Procedure for Irrigating a Colostomy
  Assessment
  Planning

  Implementation
  Evaluation
  Documentation
Problems
Procedure for Changing a Urinary Drainage Appliance
  Assessment
  Planning
  Implementation
  Evaluation
  Documentation
Procedure for Catheterizing an Ileoloop
  Assessment
  Planning
  Implementation
  Evaluation
  Documentation

Prerequisites

1. *Successful completion of the following modules:*

VOLUME 1

Module 1   An Approach to Nursing Skills
Module 2   Basic Infection Control
Module 3   Safety
Module 5   General Assessment Overview
Module 6   Documentation
Module 11 Hygiene
Module 18 Collecting Specimens
Module 28 Administering Enemas

VOLUME 2

Module 39 Catheterization

2. Review of the anatomy and physiology of the gastrointestinal and urinary systems

77

Overall Objective

To care for patients with an "ostomy," using correct technique while maintaining cleanliness and an environment conducive to the patient's dignity and self-respect.

Specific Learning Objectives

	Know Facts and Principles	Apply Facts and Principles	Demonstrate Ability	Evaluate Performance
1. *Types of ostomies*	Differentiate between various types of ostomies.	Explain why skin care is different for different ostomies, based on effect of urine and feces on skin.	Correctly identify type of drainage to expect when assigned patient with ostomy.	Verify identification with instructor.
2. *Appliances*	Describe various appliances available.		In the clinical setting, choose an appropriate appliance.	Evaluate with your instructor.
3. *Changing a colostomy or ileostomy pouch*	List steps in procedure for changing colostomy pouch.	Given a patient situation, decide whether pouch should be changed.	Change colostomy or ileostomy pouch correctly.	Check pouch for security, leaks, and cleanliness. Evaluate own performance using Performance Checklist.
4. *Observations*	List observations to make before, during, and after procedure.	Given a patient situation, identify observations that are significant.	Identify which observations are significant. Institute corrective action if necessary.	Evaluate own performance with clinical instructor.
5. *Documentation*	State information and observations that need to be documented.	Given a patient situation, record data as though on chart.	Document procedure and observations correctly.	Evaluate with instructor.

Learning Activities

1. Review the Specific Learning Objectives.
2. Look up the module vocabulary terms in the Glossary.
3. Read through the module and mentally practice the procedure.
4. In the practice setting:
   a. Examine the various types of appliances available.
   b. Read the instructions on any appliances and adhesives available.
   c. Examine colostomy irrigation equipment.
   d. Using a simulated ostomy on a mannequin:
      (1) Change the ostomy pouch using the Performance Checklist as a guide.
      (2) Set up a colostomy irrigation using the equipment available. Do a mock irrigation if possible, using the Performance Checklist as a guide.
      (3) When you have mastered these skills, ask your instructor to check your performance.

Vocabulary

adhesive	colostomy	excoriate	ostomate
anastomose	descending	ileoconduit	ostomy
appliance	transverse	ileobladder	skin barrier
asymmetry	double-barrel	ileoloop	stoma
cecostomy	enterostomal therapist	ileostomy	ureterostomy

Ostomy Care

Rationale for the Use of This Skill

More advanced surgical techniques have led to increasing numbers of patients with surgical diversions of fecal and urinary elimination pathways. Comprehensive care requires that the nurse understand the different types of diversions and the reasons for them. Cleanliness, skin care, and odor control are other concerns. Because a surgical diversion is a profound change in body structure and function, the nurse must also provide supportive care, helping patients to make the necessary psychosocial adjustments.

Ostomies usually drain either fecal material or urine. Rarely does the same ostomy drain both. Bowel diversion ostomies and urinary diversion ostomies, although similar in appearance and in appliances used, differ in one important element: urine drains from the sterile ureters, and any opening into the urinary system offers a pathway for infection directly to the kidneys.

The nurse must also constantly assess the condition of the surrounding skin for problems that can be caused by constant moisture on the skin as well as by urine or fecal material.[1]

▶ Nursing Diagnoses

Examples of some nursing diagnoses that may be appropriate for the patient with an ostomy include:

Impairment in Skin Integrity: High risk related to skin around stoma being exposed to urine/fecal material

Disturbance in Body Image: Actual related to presence of stoma and surgical alteration of elimination

Knowledge Deficit: Related to management of ostomy

BOWEL DIVERSION OSTOMIES

Bowel diversion ostomies may be temporary or permanent. Persons with a chronic disease of the bowel may have an ostomy *so that the diseased bowel can rest for a period of time to heal.* Others who have severe bowel injury that requires reconstructive surgery may

also have a temporary diversion *so that healing can take place.* More commonly, a permanent bowel diversion is performed for the person who has a malignancy of the rectum or lower bowel.

All bowel diversion ostomies drain fecal material. The consistency of the material depends on the portion of the bowel that remains and the length of time the ostomy has been in place.

An ileostomy empties from the end of the small intestine. Because a large part of the water in the stool in the ileum is not normally absorbed until the stool is lower in the intestinal tract, the fecal material may be very liquid. After the ileostomy has been in place for a while, the ileum often assumes a degree of this water-absorbing function, which produces a less liquid stool, although not one that is truly formed. The discharge from the stoma also *contains digestive enzymes, which increase the risk of impairment of skin integrity.* Odor is not usually a major problem.

A cecostomy empties from the first part of the large intestine. Some digestive enzymes are usually present, and the stool may be liquid. Neither the cecostomy nor the ileostomy should need to be irrigated, *since the stool is not formed and moves through the intestinal tract without stimulation.*

A person with an ileostomy or a cecostomy wears a drainage pouch, formerly referred to as a bag. A new surgical ileostomy technique, called the continent ileostomy or Kock Pouch, has been devised. During this procedure, a pouch of small intestine is formed to serve as a reservoir for feces.

A "nipple" valve is formed onto the skin and a catheter is introduced at regular intervals to drain the liquid fecal material. When not accessed, the valve closes *so that the patient does not need to wear an appliance.* Sometimes a small amount of leakage will occur. In that case, the person wears a light dressing for absorption.

A colostomy can be located anywhere along the entire length of the large intestine. The further along the bowel it is located, the more solid the stool is, because the large intestine reabsorbs water and the colon is less active than more proximal portions of the intestine. The larger the portion of intestine that remains, the less frequent the bowel movements, *because there is more space for fecal material to accumulate.*

There are several types of colostomies. A descending or sigmoid colostomy with resection removes the diseased portion of the colon and/or rectum and forms a permanent colostomy. A transverse colostomy is often done by removing a portion of the diseased transverse colon and forming a loop of bowel, which is either cauterized (matured) in the

---

[1] You will note that rationale for action is emphasized throughout the module by the use of italics.

operating room (a current procedure) or brought through the abdominal wall with a glass rod beneath the loop, to be cauterized later (an older procedure). A double-barrel colostomy procedure removes only the diseased portions of the colon and brings both ends to the surface. Two stomas are formed; the proximal delivers stool, and the distal produces mucus. The latter is sometimes referred to as a *mucus fistula.* Both loop and double-barrel colostomies may be temporary, in cases in which the distal bowel primarily needs a "resting" period. The severed bowel is anastomosed later.

As with the ileostomy and cecostomy, the longer a colostomy has been in place, the more normal the consistency of the stool is, *because remaining portions of the intestine increase water reabsorption to compensate for the lost area.*

The general location of a planned ostomy, which depends on the underlying pathology, is determined by the surgeon. However, in many large medical centers the *enterostomal therapist* (ET), usually a nurse, is consulted. Several factors regarding the placement of the stoma are taken into consideration. Patients should be able to see the stoma easily, *so that if they are caring for themselves, they can see what they are doing.* The stoma should never be placed in areas such as a body crease, near scar tissue, or by bony prominences, *since any of these could interfere with the appliance's tight fit* (Figure 38–1).

URINARY DIVERSION OSTOMIES

All urinary diversions provide drainage of urine that bypasses the bladder. *A urterostomy is an opening of a ureter directly onto the abdominal surface.* Ureterostomies can be right, left, or bilateral. In the bilateral ureterostomy each opening is covered by a separate appliance. Another variation is to anastomose one ureter into the other and bring that ureter to the skin, forming only one stoma. The opening is small— about as large in diameter as a pencil—and drains urine continuously so that an appliance must be worn.

To simplify the actual diversion, the physician may perform a more elaborate surgical procedure called *ileoloop, ileobladder, or ileoconduit.* (The prefix *ileal* is also used.) In this procedure a section of the ileum (small intestine) or some other part of the intestine, such as the cecum, is dissected from the rest of the intestine, and then the intestinal ends are reattached. (Although some surgeons use sections other than the ileum, the term *ileo* is still used.) Both ureters are attached to this separate segment of intestine and drain into it. One end of the intestinal segment is closed, and the other opens onto the abdomen as a stoma (Figure 38–2). The stoma is the size of an ileostomy (about 1½ inches in diameter) and drains urine continuously. *The advantage of this type of urinary diversion is having one stoma that is larger and more easily fitted with an appliance. This procedure reduces the risk of ascending kidney infection because the mucous membrane of the intestinal segment serves as a barrier to microorganisms.*

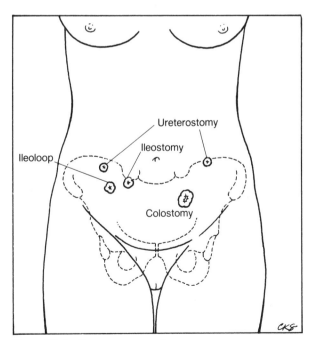

Figure 38–1. Common ostomy sites.

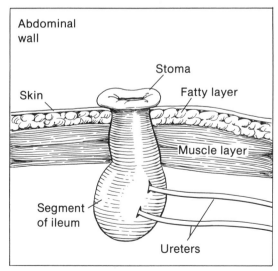

Figure 38–2. To form an ileoloop, a portion of the ileum is formed into a pouch for storing the urine.

A technique being done with increasing frequency is the continent ileoconduit. This is similar to the bowel diversion technique known as the continent ileostomy or Kock pouch. Again, a portion of the ileum is dissected and folded back on itself to form a structure for urine storage. A "nipple" valve is constructed onto the skin so that a stoma is formed and a catheter can be introduced at intervals to drain the urine. Figure 38–3 shows a catheter being used to drain a continent ileoconduit. See Module 39, Catheterization, for the procedure for draining the continent ileoconduit.

OSTOMY APPLIANCES

Ostomy appliances are manufactured by many companies. No one type of appliance is best for all patients. An enterostomal therapist is the best resource person to consult when making a selection. If no therapist is available, a salesperson at the surgical supply store may be able to explain the various types of appliances. For convenience, many facilities carry only one brand of appliance, but the patient should be made aware of all available options, *so a personal choice can be made for ongoing care.* Ostomy appliances

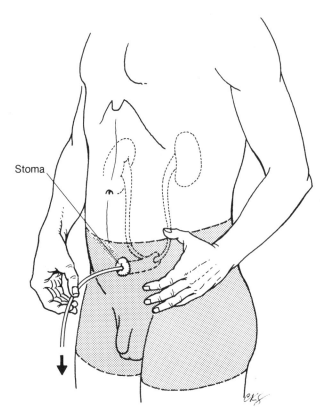

Figure 38–3. The patient uses a clean catheter to periodically drain a continent ileostomy.

Stoma

and accessories can also be ordered at most pharmacies (Table 38–1).

While in the hospital, the patient can use a temporary, disposable pouch with a peel-off adhesive square (Figure 38–4**A**). A hole the size of the stoma is cut in the square. Only the mucous membrane of the stoma is permitted to project through the hole. (*The mucus protects the membrane from irritation.*) *The skin surrounding the stoma can be irritated easily if urine or stool drains across it.* After the hole is cut, the covering is peeled from the adhesive and the pouch is applied to the skin.

It is important to use a "see-through" appliance while the patient is in the hospital with a new stoma, *so that staff can see the stoma and assess its condition.* If the pouch is partially full, it can be opened and drained from the bottom. It can then be rinsed with an asepto syringe and warm water while in place. *Removing and reapplying adhesive pouches can irritate the skin.*

Most patients use a disposable pouch, but patients who have had a colostomy for some time may be more familiar and comfortable with a permanent pouch. Permanent appliances usually have a solid ring faceplate that fits around the stoma (Figure 38–4). Faceplates come in various sizes, and the size needed by an individual patient may change over time. The pouch is fastened to the faceplate, which is held in place by a skin barrier: a karaya gum ring, a solid-pectin adhesive (such as Stomadhesive), or a liquid adhesive. A belt is usually attached to the faceplate and worn around the patient's waist (Figure 38–4**C**). *The belt is designed to support the weight of the pouch as it fills, preventing it from pulling the adhesive loose and causing leakage.* Normally, the pouch has a closure at the bottom, so it can be drained. The closure clip may be reused even if the pouch is disposable.

A person who has established good colostomy control may wear only a flat dressing over the stoma except when irrigating the colostomy.

Appliances used for urinary drainage ostomies are similar to those already described. Special adhesives that cannot be broken down by urine are used. Urinary pouches are drained from the bottom. They are replaced every 2–3 days to prevent urinary infection.

APPEARANCE OF A NORMAL STOMA

It is important that both patients with an ostomy and nurses recognize the appearance of a normal stoma *so that they can identify problems early and intervene if necessary. Since the stoma is formed from normal intestinal*

Table 38–1 Commonly Used Ostomy Products

Product	Manufacturer	Uses
Moisturizing cream	Hollister Cream (Hollister) Bard Cream (Bard) Sween Cream (Sween)	Applied to lubricate dry skin around stoma. Apply sparingly so that the skin barrier used will adhere.
Powders	Stomadhesive (ConvaTec) Karaya (many manufacturers) Baby powder (many manufacturers) Corn starch (many manufacturers)	Powders applied to irritated or moist skin enable barriers to more tightly adhere to the skin.
Skin sealers	Skin Gel (Hollister) Bard Protective Barrier (Bard) Skin Prep (United)	Can be used over powder to protect the skin from adhesive barriers.
Skin barriers	Premium Skin Barrier (Hollister) ReliaSeal (Bard) Stomahesive Barrier (ConvaTec) Comfeel (Coloplast) Various sheets, rings, and wafers (many manufacturers)	Skin barriers help protect the skin from irritation caused by the discharge from the ostomy. Most skin barriers can be applied to moist or irritated skin.
Sealing pastes	Premium Paste (Hollister) Karaya Paste (Hollister) Stomahesive Paste (ConvaTec) Comfeel Paste (Coloplast)	These pastes fill in skin cracks and crevices to ensure a tight seal.
Deodorants	UltraFresh (Mentor) Ostozyme (Shelton) Banish (United) White vinegar (household 1:3 water)	Deodorants are used in the pouch to decrease odor.

tissue, it is highly vascular, and as such it should resemble other mucous membranes of the body and be red and smooth. *Because there are no nerve endings in this tissue,* the stoma can be irritated and even necrotic without causing the patient pain. This fact mandates careful and continual assessment. Although the stoma will be edematous (swollen) at first, this will subside in 5–10 days. Any sign of a bluish color, excoriation, or asymmetry should be reported at once.

To avoid early complications, Petillo (1987) recommends assessment of the appearance of the stoma every 2 hours for the first 24 hours and then every 4 hours for the next 48–72 hours.

HEALTH TEACHING TOWARD SELF-CARE

Unless the patient is very debilitated or seriously ill, an important nursing goal is to teach the patient to perform ostomy self-care. The nurse must be both totally accepting of the appearance of the stoma and competent and knowledgeable in the care of ostomies. After the nurse has mastered the various procedures, a teaching plan should be set up and shared with the health care team.

Some hospitals have a health teaching outline for teaching the patient with a new ostomy. If the facility has an enterostomal therapist on the staff, this person may give instructions to the patient or be a useful resource to you so that you can teach the patient. At first, the patient may be reluctant to actively enter a teaching program *because of both fear and depression related to the realization that such a basic function as elimination has been surgically altered.* This is particularly true if the surgery has been done as an emergency and the patient had little time to prepare (Edwards & Krouse, 1987). If your approach is both straightforward and supportive, the patient will soon understand the goal as one of regaining independence.

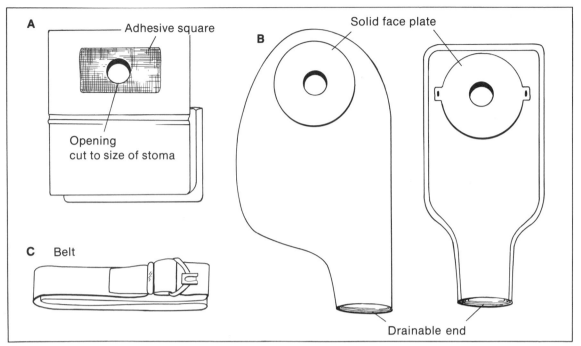

Figure 38–4. Examples of equipment used for colostomy. **A:** Temporary pouch held on skin by an adhesive square. Adhesive squares when round are called "wafers." **B:** Permanent pouches. **C:** Belt with hook on each end is to support pouch, length adjustable.

OBTAINING SPECIMENS FROM OSTOMIES

At times, a stool or urine specimen will be needed from the patient with a fecal or urinary diversion *to identify the presence of blood, glucose, bacteria, or parasites.* Even if the pouch has just been changed, it is preferable to secure the specimen directly from the stoma, *since it will not have had time to deteriorate in the pouch or to become contaminated if the pouch is not new.* A tongue blade can be used to gently collect a specimen of stool from an intestinal stoma, and a syringe without a needle can aspirate a small amount of urine from a urinary diversion. Review these procedures in Module 18, Collecting Specimens.

🏠 Home Care

Visits by the home health nurse after the person with an ostomy (these persons are referred to as "ostomates") is discharged from the hospital *make the transition much easier.* The nurse can supervise the ostomy care procedure as the patient performs what may be a new and frightening experience. Erickson (1987) states that it should be recognized that the pouch that worked well for the patient in the hospital may fail to be satisfactory when used in the home because of the resumption of normal activity. If this is the case, the home health nurse can consult with the enterostomal therapist to discover a pouch that may be more effective. Again, it is important to emphasize exercise and adequate diet and fluid intake *so that elimination, both bowel and urinary, is facilitated. To avoid excessive intestinal gas formation,* patients should be taught to avoid gas-producing foods such as cabbage and beans.

The home health nurse can also act as a resource. Self-help groups within most communities meet regularly to talk about the physical and psychologic impacts of living with an ostomy. These groups offer ways of overcoming any disruptions in life *caused by having an ostomy* and have proven invaluable for many people with a temporary or permanent elimination diversion.

LONG-TERM CARE

The nurse in the long-term care setting has an added responsibility when caring for the older resident who has had an ostomy for some period of time and may be living in the facility because of impairments other than elimination. Some of these people have been performing their own ostomy care for years but find they have gradually lost the ability to continue giving themselves ostomy care. It is important for you to understand the type of ostomy and the procedure needed for a specific client *so that you can offer what has been usual and satisfactory to the client.* It also becomes vital to maintain proper exercise and diet *to maintain adequate fecal elimination through an ostomy. To ensure adequate urinary elimination and decrease the risk of urinary tract infection,* it is essential to provide enough oral fluids for the person in your care who has a urinary diversion. With adaptations for the individual resident, you can modify certain procedures in this module for use within the long-term care setting.

PROCEDURE FOR CHANGING A COLOSTOMY OR ILEOSTOMY POUCH OR DRESSING

Assessment

1. Identify the type of ostomy the patient has and its location.
2. Check skin integrity around the stoma.
3. Note the amount of fecal material in the pouch or on the dressing.
4. Determine whether the patient is being taught self-care at this time.

Planning

5. Wash your hands *for infection control.*
6. Gather the following equipment needed to change a pouch or dressing:
   a. Cleansing supplies, including tissues (for wiping away stool), warm water, mild soap, a washcloth, and a towel. In some facilities, clean disposable cloths are used for cleaning colostomies.
   b. Clean pouch of the type currently being used.
   c. Seal or use adhesive to prevent leakage. (This may be attached to the pouch.)
   d. Clean belt. The patient usually has two— one to be worn while the other is washed and dried. The belt being worn can be used

again if it is clean. Temporary appliances may not have a belt.
   e. Dressing materials.
   f. Receptacle for the soiled pouch or dressing. A bedpan can be used initially. *For both aseptic and aesthetic reasons,* place the soiled pouch or dressing in a paper bag or wrap it in newspaper or paper towels for disposal. *This keeps the linen clean and helps contain odor.*
   g. Protective spray. The skin around the stoma may be protected by spraying with a liquid skin protector.
   h. Clean gloves.
7. Determine whether the patient is to participate in the procedure, and if so, in what way.
8. Choose the appropriate location for performing the procedure. On the one hand, *the bathroom offers the patient more privacy and is more like the setting the patient will use at home.* On the other hand, *the bedside is usually more convenient for the nurse because the stoma can be clearly seen and there is a place to put needed equipment.* At this time make your plans based on the patient's needs.

Implementation

9. Identify the patient *to be sure you are performing the procedure on the correct patient,* and explain what you are planning to do. If the patient is to participate, explain each step and the rationale behind it.
10. Take the patient to the bathroom or provide privacy by screening at the bedside.
11. Remove the soiled dressing or appliance (see specific instructions below). Wear gloves when *handling the soiled material.* At home, however, the patient may not choose to wear gloves to perform colostomy care.
12. Using warm water and a mild soap, cleanse the skin around the stoma thoroughly *to remove all fecal residue.* Inspect the skin for redness or irritation.
13. Cover the stoma with a tissue *to prevent stool from leaking onto the clean skin.* (An ileostomy may leak more than a colostomy.) Change this tissue as necessary during the procedure.
14. Dry the skin around the stoma carefully, patting gently. Do not rub, *to avoid irritating the skin.*
15. Apply a skin protective if needed. Use sparingly *because a thin coating is sufficient for protection and will not interfere with pouch attachment.*

16. Allow the skin to dry thoroughly *so the pouch will adhere firmly.* Some patients use a hair dryer on a low setting for this purpose although the risk of a burn might make this an unwise practice.
17. Remove the tissue from the stoma and apply the clean pouch or dressing as outlined below.
18. Remove your gloves and wash your hands thoroughly *for infection control.*

Evaluation
19. Evaluate using the following criteria:
    a. Pouch or dressing secure.
    b. Area clean.
    c. No odor.
    d. Patient comfortable.
20. If the patient is being taught the procedure, add:
    a. Patient able to change pouch using correct technique.
    b. Patient verbalizes understanding of key points in care.

Documentation
21. Record the following information:
    a. The amount, color and consistency of the fecal material in the pouch.
    b. The application of the clean pouch and dressing change.
    c. The knowledge and capability of the patient to participate in the procedure or ability to change the pouch independently.

APPLYING A COLOSTOMY DRESSING

Colostomy dressings are uncommon except in the case of a newly created colostomy that is nonfunctioning. Since most colostomies are functioning, the patient returns from the operating room with an appliance in place. If a colostomy dressing is used, a sterile 4 × 4 held in place with paper tape is usually sufficient.

PROCEDURE FOR IRRIGATING A COLOSTOMY

The physician determines whether a colostomy should be irrigated. Not all colostomies need to be irrigated for effective functioning, although irrigation may be done *if constipation develops.* For some people, a colostomy does not function well without irrigation. When irrigation is performed daily, a regular routine should be established *to facilitate cleanliness and odor control and to prevent embarrassing emptying of the bowel at inconvenient times and places.* To this end, set up a regular time for irrigation, accommodating to the patient's personal schedule. Select a time when the patient will be relaxed and be able to pay careful attention to detail. The patient's privacy is also important. Often you will have to teach the procedure to the patient. The more the irrigation in the hospital can be made to resemble the way it will be done at home, the easier the patient's transition will be.

The physician may decide which one of two general types of irrigation will be used, or your facility may have a policy regarding the type to be used.

The large-volume, enema-type irrigation stimulates the bowel to evacuate. Some patients using this method may have to irrigate only every 2 or 3 days. Its disadvantages include the retention of fluid and, later, dribbling; excessive distention of the colon; electrolyte depletion; and the prolonged amount of time required for the procedure. Also, some patients increase the volume of the irrigation beyond what is ordered or insert the tubing a long distance into the colon, both of which can damage the colon.

The small-volume, bulb-syringe method is used to stimulate the bowel to do its own emptying. Because the tip on the syringe is short, it is impossible for the patient to insert it too far *and cause bowel damage. A disadvantage of the method is that it may not empty the bowel adequately, so that stool might be excreted later.* Also, the *hard bulb may be too stiff for weak or arthritic elderly persons to squeeze.* In this case, the enema-type equipment is used for a smaller-volume irrigation. Usually the small-volume irrigation must be done daily.

Both methods are described below. Review the general procedure for enema administration outlined in Module 28, Administering Enemas, as a guide, with the following specific changes.

Assessment
1. Check the type of irrigation to be performed on the patient.
2. Find out if the patient is being taught to do his or her own irrigation.

Planning
3. Wash your hands *for infection control.*
4. Obtain the necessary equipment.
    a. For either large-volume method or bulb-syringe method:

(1) Bath blanket or large towel

(2) Water-soluble lubricant

(3) Clean gloves

(4) Container for soiled pouch or dressings

(5) Clean colostomy pouch or dressings

(6) Irrigation sleeve, or pouch

(7) Bedpan and two disposable protective pads (if the patient must remain in bed).

b. For large-volume method (Figure 38–5):

(1) Irrigation bag containing 1000 ml warm tap water or other solution as ordered. This bag is usually equipped with a flow regulator and a number 28 cone-tipped catheter. A cone may be substituted for the catheter. An advantage of the cone is that it cannot be inserted too far.

(2) IV pole or other hook

(3) Rubber nipple to prevent backflow. (This fits over the catheter. It is not necessary if a cone tip is on the tubing.)

c. For bulb-syringe method (Figure 38–6):

(1) 8-oz bulb syringe with a number 28 cone-tipped catheter attached. A large-sized ear syringe without a catheter may be substituted.

(2) Container filled with 750 ml warm tap water.

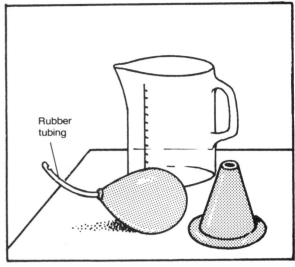

Figure 38–6. Cone catheter and bulb-syringe colostomy irrigating equipment.

5. Choose an appropriate location for the procedure. *The bathroom simulates the setting in which the patient will perform an irrigation at home. If the patient is weak or debilitated, the bedside is more appropriate.*

Implementation

6. Identify the patient *to be sure you are performing the procedure for the correct patient,* and explain what you are going to do.

7. Provide for the patient's privacy, either by closing the bed curtains or door (if done at bedside) or by taking the patient to the bathroom.

8. Put on clean gloves.

9. Remove the soiled pouch.

10. Wash around the stoma with soap and warm water. Dry well.

11. Place the irrigation bag or sleeve over the colostomy.

12. Position and drape the patient.

a. In the bathroom, the patient sits on the toilet or commode. Place the end of the irrigation bag between the legs, *so the bag can drain directly into the toilet.* You may drape a towel or bath blanket over the patient's lap *for warmth and modesty* (Figure 38–7).

b. In bed, position the patient on the side. Place the bedpan on a disposable protective pad on the bed. Then place the end of the irrigation sleeve in the bedpan (Figure 38–8). Use the other disposable pad to cover

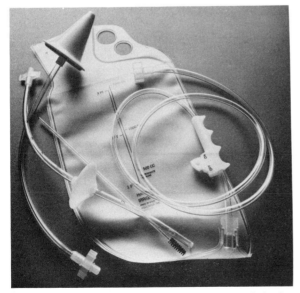

Figure 38–5. Equipment for large-volume colostomy irrigation. (*Courtesy Hollister Incorporated, Libertyville, Illinois*)

© **1992 by J.B. Lippincott Company**

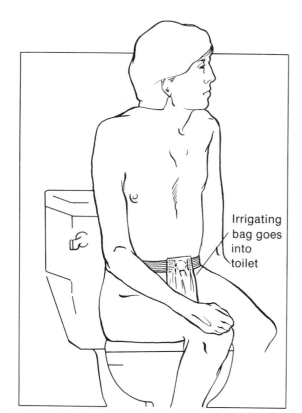

Figure 38-7. Patient sitting on a toilet for colostomy irrigation.

the bedpan as the colostomy empties, *to help contain odor.* Sometimes a patient who cannot sit on a commode but can sit in bed is placed in high Fowler's position. The bedpan is then placed beside the patient's hips.

13. Irrigate the colostomy.
 a. Large-volume method:
 (1) Hang the irrigation container on the IV pole, with the fluid level approximately 12–18 inches above the stoma. This positions the bottom of the container at the patient's shoulder *for appropriate pressure.*
 (2) Expel all air from the tubing.
 (3) Place the nipple over the end of the catheter, and push it down to 3–5 inches from the end, or attach the cone to the tubing.
 (4) Lubricate the tip of the catheter or the cone.
 (5) Lubricate your little finger.
 (6) Gently dilate the stoma by putting your lubricated finger through the open top of the irrigation sleeve (or the hole provided in the bag) into the opening. Check the direction of the lumen. If the colostomy is double-barreled (has two stomas), you will be irrigating the proximal loop.
 (7) Gently thread the catheter through the opening in the irrigation bag into the stoma. Insert the catheter only 3–5 inches. If you detect any obstruction, do not force the catheter. Rotate it gently, allowing a small amount of fluid to flow in. *This measure often opens the lumen.* If you still cannot insert the catheter, seek help. *It is possible to perforate a bowel or to traumatize the mucosa severely by forceful pushing.* The cone tip fits into the stoma only far enough to dam the flow of water.
 (8) Press the nipple or cone firmly against the stoma *to occlude the opening around the catheter.* If a nipple or cone is not available, press with the fingers *to close the stoma around the catheter.*

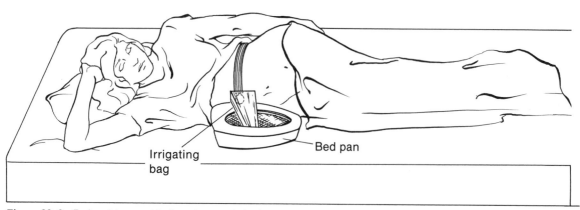

Figure 38-8. Patient lying on side for colostomy irrigation.

(9) Unclamp the tubing *to allow the fluid to flow into the bowel.* If cramping occurs, stop the flow and wait, as you would with a conventional enema.

(10) When all the fluid has been instilled, remove the catheter or cone *to allow the bowel to empty.*

b. Bulb-syringe (small-volume) method:

(1) Fill the syringe with water. Be sure to turn the opening up and expel all air.

(2) Dilate the stoma with your gloved and lubricated little finger.

(3) Gently insert the catheter of the syringe 3–5 inches into the stoma.

(4) Gently squeeze the bulb, instilling all the water, as you press around the stoma *to prevent backflow.* Do not allow the bulb to reinflate while in the stoma. There may be some return after the catheter is withdrawn.

(5) Remove and refill the syringe two more times, for a total of three syringes full (720 ml) of fluid. Do not instill more than this amount, even if some fluid is returned between instillations.

14. Have the patient sit for approximately 15 minutes *to allow the bowel to empty. You or the patient can encourage emptying* by gently massaging the abdomen.

15. Clean off the bottom of the irrigation sleeve, fold it up, and fasten it closed.

16. Wait an additional 30 minutes *to allow the colostomy to complete emptying.* During this time the patient can move around, shave, bathe, and so on.

17. Drain the irrigation sleeve again, then rinse and remove it.

18. Apply a clean pouch, using the procedure for changing a colostomy pouch above.

19. Clean all the equipment, dry it, and put it away for future use.

20. Remove gloves and wash your hands.

Evaluation

21. Evaluate using the following criteria:

a. The amount and consistency of stool returned.

b. If patient participated, understanding and ability to carry out the procedure.

Documentation

22. Record the irrigation, including the amount of fluid instilled and returned, a description of return, and the patient's reaction.

23. Document the patient's level of knowledge and ability to carry out the procedure by having the patient demonstrate the procedure.

Problems

1. *The fluid does not return* First, try to siphon fluid back. *Do not* instill additional fluid. Watch the patient carefully for later fluid return.

2. *No stool returns* If the bulb-syringe method is used, you may either repeat the procedure immediately, wait a few hours and repeat, or wait 24 hours and repeat, depending on the physician's decision and your facility's procedure. *Repeating the procedure immediately may excessively fatigue the patient.* A large-volume irrigation is not usually repeated without specific consultation with the physician *because of electrolyte depletion.*

3. *The fluid flows out as fast as you put it in* This action will not promote adequate emptying of the bowel. Stop the irrigation and devise a better way to occlude the stoma opening before you begin again.

4. *A patient with an old colostomy tells you he or she uses a lot more fluid than you are planning to use* Some patients increase the amount of fluid instilled on their own at home and have been known to instill 4000–5000 ml and to take 2 hours for an irrigation. Explain to the patient the rationale for the procedure as you are going to do it. Then consult with your team leader or head nurse. You may have to increase the amount of fluid *to obtain any results.* Also, inform the physician of the patient's current practice.

5. *The patient states that he or she always inserts the catheter 8 or 10 inches* Explain the rationale for the short distance and do not insert the catheter any further. One of the advantages of the bulb syringe (or cone) is that the patient cannot insert the device too far *because it is so short.*

PROCEDURE FOR CHANGING A URINARY DRAINAGE APPLIANCE

When working with a urinary diversion, you must pay particular attention to cleanliness *because of the potential for urinary tract infection.*

Assessment

1. Identify the type of urinary diversion the patient has and where the stoma is located.

2. Check skin integrity around the stoma and

whether a protective substance is being used on the skin.

3. Note the amount of urine in the pouch and any cloudiness or unusual odor.
4. Determine whether the patient is being taught self-care.

Planning

5. Wash your hands *for infection control.*
6. Obtain the following equipment:
   a. Adhesive solvent
   b. Cotton balls or small gauze squares
   c. Cleansing supplies
   d. Tissues
   e. Clean pouch of the type currently being used
   f. Adhesive
   g. Receptacle for the soiled pouch
   h. Protective spray for skin, if ordered
   i. Stoma guidestrip if available. *The guidestrip is a dissolvable paper material especially made for this purpose.*
   j. Container for emptying and measuring urine
   k. Clean gloves.
7. Plan how to involve the patient in the procedure.

Implementation

8. Identify the patient *to make sure you are performing the procedure on the correct patient,* and explain the procedure.
9. Empty the urine from the pouch, using the bottom closure, *to ensure that the urine will not be spilled while you are changing the pouch.* Measure the amount of urine *for the output record.*
10. Position the patient on his or her back and drape.
11. Remove the old appliance, following these steps:
    a. Remove the belt.
    b. Dip the cotton balls or small gauze squares in the adhesive solvent.
    c. Starting at one corner of the appliance, roll the applicator against the edge, loosening the adhesive.
    d. Push the skin away from the appliance as you gently pull it off. Do not try to pull off the appliance until the solvent has loosened the adhesive *or you may damage the skin.*
12. Clean the skin with clear warm water. Rinse thoroughly and pat dry. (*Soap can interfere with adhesive.*)

13. Place a folded tissue or 4 × 4 over the stoma to absorb any urine. Change as necessary *to keep the skin dry.*
14. Apply the protective spray to the skin if ordered.
15. Put adhesive on the appliance face only if needed.
16. When the adhesive on the appliance face has dried as much as the directions indicate, remove the covering from the stoma.
17. Place the guidestrip correctly over the stoma.
18. Center the appliance carefully over the stoma, using the guidestrip for placement. Make sure the skin is dry.
19. Press the appliance firmly into place. The guidestrip will drop into the appliance and dissolve.
20. Hook the belt into place.
21. Clean the used appliance according to your facility's procedure, and discard disposable equipment.
22. Remove gloves and wash your hands.

Evaluation

23. Evaluate using the following criteria:
    a. Security and placement of the appliance.
    b. Patient's level of knowledge and ability to carry out the procedure.
    c. Patient comfort.

Documentation

24. Record the appliance change, include your assessment of the urine, skin, and patient's reaction.
25. Document the patient's knowledge and ability.

PROCEDURE FOR CATHETERIZING AN ILEOLOOP

To obtain a sterile urine specimen or empty a continent ileoloop, it is necessary to catheterize the patient through the stoma. Before doing this procedure you should complete Module 35, Sterile Technique, and Module 39, Catheterization.

Assessment

1. Identify the type of urinary diversion the patient has.
2. Check the order for the catheterized specimen.

Planning

3. Wash your hands *for infection control.*
4. Obtain the equipment listed below. Some of these items may be included in a straight

catheterization set. *Sterile equipment is used to prevent introducing microbes into the urinary tract.*
   a. Sterile straight catheter
   b. Sterile gloves
   c. Sterile water-soluble lubricant
   d. Sterile container for the urine specimen
   e. Materials for applying a new appliance.

Implementation

5. Identify the patient *to make sure you are performing the procedure on the correct patient,* and explain what you are going to do.
6. Remove the existing drainage pouch from the stoma.
7. Open the sterile equipment packages.
8. Put on sterile gloves.
9. Prepare the sterile field and lubricate the catheter as described in Module 39, Catheterization.
10. Hold the sterile catheter approximately 3 inches from the tip *to provide good control while preserving sterility.*
11. Insert the catheter into the stoma until urine begins to flow out, but never insert it further than 2 inches. *This prevents trauma to the lining of the ileoloop.* If you meet resistance, do not force the catheter but gently rotate its tip to see if it will slide in with ease.

12. After the specimen has been obtained, remove the catheter.
13. Replace the appliance according to the above procedure.
14. Remove your gloves and clean all equipment.
15. Wash your hands.

Evaluation

16. Evaluate using the following criteria:
   a. Describe specimen for clarity and color.
   b. Patient's comfort during procedure.

Documentation

17. Record the catheterization of the ileoloop, the disposition of the specimen, and the drainage pouch change in the manner prescribed by your facility. This information may be placed on a flow sheet or added to the nurses' progress notes.
18. Document any significant response of the patient to the procedure.

References

Edwards, J. & Krouse, S. (1987). Helping the emergency colostomy patient through reality shock. *Nursing '87,* (7)17, 63–64.

Erickson, P. J. (1987). Ostomies: The art of pouching. *The Nursing Clinics of North America, 22*(2), 311–320.

Petillo, M. H. (1987). The patient with a urinary stoma. *The Nursing Clinics of North America, 22*(2), 263–279.

Performance Checklist

Changing a Colostomy or Ileostomy Pouch or Dressing	Unsat	Needs More Practice	Sat	Comments
Assessment				
1. Identify type and location of ostomy.				
2. Check skin integrity around the stoma.				
3. Note the amount of fecal drainage.				
4. Determine whether patient is being taught self-care.				
Planning				
5. Wash your hands.				
6. Gather the following equipment to change a pouch or dressing: a. Cleansing supplies				
b. Clean pouch of correct type				
c. Seal or adhesive				
d. Clean belt				
e. Dressing materials				
f. Receptacle for soiled pouch or dressing				
g. Protective spray				
h. Clean gloves.				
7. Determine whether patient is to participate and in what way.				
8. Choose appropriate location for procedure.				
Implementation				
9. Identify the patient and explain the procedure.				
10. Take the patient to the bathroom or provide privacy.				
11. Put on clean gloves and remove soiled dressing or appliance. (See specific instructions below.)				
12. Using warm water and soap, cleanse the skin around the stoma.				
13. Cover the stoma with a tissue.				

Changing a Colostomy or Ileostomy Pouch or Dressing *(Continued)*	Unsat	Needs More Practice	Sat	Comments
14. Dry the skin around the stoma.				
15. Apply skin protective.				
16. Allow skin to dry thoroughly.				
17. Remove the tissue and apply the clean pouch or dressing. (See specific instructions below.)				
18. Remove gloves and wash your hands.				
Evaluation				
19. Evaluate using the following criteria: a. Pouch or dressing secure.				
b. Area clean.				
c. Patient comfort.				
20. If the patient is being taught procedure, add: a. Able to change pouch, using correct technique.				
b. Verbalizes understanding.				
Documentation				
21. Record the following information: a. Amount, color and consistency of fecal material.				
b. Application of pouch and dressing change.				
c. Knowledge, understanding, and ability of patient's participation.				
Irrigating a Colostomy				
Assessment				
1. Check type of irrigation.				
2. Find out if patient is being taught self-care.				
Planning				
3. Wash your hands.				
4. Obtain the necessary equipment. a. For either large-volume method or bulb-syringe method: (1) Bath blanket or large towel				
(2) Lubricant				

Irrigating a Colostomy *(Continued)*	Unsat	Needs More Practice	Sat	Comments
(3) Clean gloves				
(4) Container for soiled pouch or dressing				
(5) Clean colostomy pouch or dressing material				
(6) Irrigation sleeve, or pouch				
(7) Bedpan and two disposable pads (for bed patient).				
b. For large-volume method: (1) Irrigation bag containing 1000 ml warm tap water				
(2) IV pole or hook				
(3) Rubber nipple if irrigation bag does not have a cone tip.				
c. For bulb-syringe method: (1) 8-oz bulb syringe with number 28 separate catheter				
(2) Container filled with 750 ml warm tap water.				
5. Choose an appropriate place for irrigation.				
Implementation				
6. Identify the patient and explain the procedure.				
7. Provide for patient's privacy.				
8. Put on clean gloves.				
9. Remove the old pouch.				
10. Wash around stoma with soap and warm water, then dry well.				
11. Place irrigation bag or sleeve over colostomy.				
12. Position and drape the patient, with end of bag in bedpan or toilet or commode.				
13. Irrigate the colostomy. a. Large-volume method: (1) Hang container on IV pole, with fluid 12–18 inches above the stoma.				
(2) Expel air from tubing.				

Irrigating a Colostomy *(Continued)*	Unsat	Needs More Practice	Sat	Comments
(3) Place nipple over end of catheter, approximately 3–5 inches from end, or attach cone.				
(4) Lubricate tip.				
(5) Lubricate little finger.				
(6) Gently dilate stoma and check direction of the lumen with lubricated finger.				
(7) Thread catheter into stoma 3–5 inches.				
(8) Press nipple or cone firmly against stoma.				
(9) Unclamp tubing and allow fluid to flow.				
(10) When all fluid has been instilled, remove catheter and allow bowel to empty.				
b. Bulb-syringe method: (1) Fill syringe with water after expelling all air.				
(2) Dilate the stoma with gloved and lubricated little finger.				
(3) Insert catheter 3–5 inches.				
(4) Gently squeeze bulb, instilling all the water. (During this step, press around the stoma to prevent backflow.)				
(5) Remove and refill the syringe two more times until 750 ml has been instilled.				
14. Have patient sit for 15 minutes to allow the bowel to empty.				
15. Clean off bottom of irrigation bag, fold it up, and fasten it closed.				
16. Wait an additional 30 minutes to allow complete emptying.				
17. Drain the irrigation sleeve again and remove it.				
18. Apply clean pouch.				
19. Clean all equipment, dry it, and put it away.				
20. Remove gloves and wash your hands.				

Irrigating a Colostomy *(Continued)*	Unsat	Needs More Practice	Sat	Comments
Evaluation				
21. Evaluate using the following criteria: a. Amount and consistency of stool returned				
b. Patient's understanding and ability to carry out procedure.				
Documentation				
22. Record the irrigation, including amount of fluid instilled and returned, description of return, and patient's reaction.				
23. Document patient's level of knowledge and ability to carry out procedure.				
Changing a Urinary Drainage Appliance				
Assessment				
1. Identify the type of urinary diversion and location of stoma.				
2. Check skin integrity and whether a protective substance is being used.				
3. Note amount of urine in the pouch.				
4. Determine whether patient is being taught self-care.				
Planning				
5. Wash your hands.				
6. Obtain necessary equipment. a. Adhesive solvent				
b. Cotton balls or small gauze squares				
c. Cleansing supplies				
d. Tissues				
e. Clean pouch				
f. Adhesive				
g. Receptacle for soiled pouch				
h. Protective spray for skin				
i. Stoma guidestrip				

Changing a Urinary Drainage Appliance (Continued)	Unsat	Needs More Practice	Sat	Comments
j. Container for emptying and measuring urine				
k. Clean gloves.				
7. Plan how to involve the patient.				
Implementation				
8. Identify the patient and explain the procedure.				
9. Put on clean gloves and empty urine, measuring for output record.				
10. Position patient on back and drape.				
11. Remove old appliance. a. Remove the belt.				
b. Dip applicators in adhesive solvent.				
c. Starting at one corner, roll applicator against edge to loosen adhesive.				
d. Pull off pouch as adhesive is loosened.				
12. Clean skin with clear water and pat dry.				
13. Place folded tissue or 4 × 4 over stoma and change as necessary.				
14. Apply protective spray to skin if ordered.				
15. Put adhesive on appliance face.				
16. When drying is at appropriate point, remove covering from stoma.				
17. Curl stoma guidestrip onto stoma opening.				
18. Center appliance over stoma, using the guidestrip.				
19. Press appliance firmly into place.				
20. Hook belt into place.				
21. Clean used appliance and discard disposable equipment.				
22. Remove gloves and wash your hands.				
Evaluation				
23. Evaluate using the following criteria: a. Security and placement of the applicance.				

Changing a Urinary Drainage Appliance (Continued)	Unsat	Needs More Practice	Sat	Comments
b. Patient's level of knowledge and ability to carry out the procedure.				
c. Patient comfort.				
Documentation				
24. Record appliance change, including assessment of urine, skin, and patient's reaction.				
25. Document patient's knowledge and ability.				
Catheterizing an Ileoloop				
Assessment				
1. Identify type of urinary diversion.				
2. Check order for catheterization specimen.				
Planning				
3. Wash your hands.				
4. Obtain the needed equipment. a. Sterile straight catheter				
b. Sterile gloves				
c. Sterile water-soluble lubricant				
d. Sterile container for urine				
e. Materials for applying new appliance.				
Implementation				
5. Identify the patient and explain the procedure.				
6. Remove existing appliance.				
7. Open sterile equipment packages.				
8. Put on sterile gloves.				
9. Prepare sterile field and lubricate catheter as described in Module 39, Catheterization.				
10. Hold sterile catheter 3 inches from tip.				
11. Insert catheter until urine begins to flow, but not further than 2 inches.				
12. After specimen has been obtained, remove catheter.				

Catheterizing an Ileoloop (Continued)	Unsat	Needs More Practice	Sat	Comments
13. Replace appliance according to above procedure.				
14. Remove and clean all equipment.				
15. Remove gloves and wash your hands.				
Evaluation				
16. Evaluate using the following criteria: a. Describe specimen for clarity and color.				
b. Patient's comfort during procedure.				
Documentation				
17. Record catheterization, disposition of specimen, and drainage pouch change.				
18. Document any significant response of patient.				

Quiz

Short-Answer Questions

1. What is an ileostomy? _____

2. What special problems does a patient with an ileostomy have?

   _____

3. Describe the appearance of a normal stoma. _____

   _____

4. How would you obtain a specimen from a urinary diversion? How would you obtain a specimen from a fecal diversion?

   _____

   _____

5. How is an ileoloop different from an ileostomy? _____

   _____

6. What is the best position for the patient having a colostomy irrigation?

   _____

7. How many milliliters of fluid are used for a large-volume colostomy irrigation? _____

8. How many milliliters of fluid are used for a bulb-syringe (small-volume) irrigation? _____

9. How far is the catheter inserted for a colostomy irrigation? _____

   _____

10. How long should the patient remain on the toilet after the irrigation fluid is instilled? _____

11. After the initial draining, how long should the irrigation pouch be left in place before the clean appliance is applied? _____

    _____

12. Why is special attention to cleanliness necessary when changing a urinary drainage appliance? _____

13. What are two important services provided by the home health nurse to the person with an ostomy who has been recently discharged from the hospital?

    _____

    _____

Module 39
Catheterization

Module Contents

Rationale for the Use of This Skill
Nursing Diagnoses
Preparing the Patient
Equipment
Procedure for Catheterization
 Assessment
 Planning
 Implementation
 Evaluation
 Documentation
Caring for a Patient With an Indwelling Catheter
Procedure for Removing a Foley Catheter
 Assessment
 Planning
 Implementation
 Evaluation
 Documentation

Teaching the Procedure for Intermittent Self-Catheterization
 Assessment
 Planning
 Implementation
 Evaluation
 Documentation
Procedure for Catheterization of a Urinary Diversion
 Assessment
 Planning
 Implementation
 Evaluation
 Documentation
Long-term Care
Home Care

Prerequisites

1. *Successful completion of the following modules:*

VOLUME 1

Module 1   An Approach to Nursing Skills
Module 2   Basic Infection Control
Module 3   Safety
Module 5   General Assessment Overview
Module 6   Documentation

VOLUME 2

Module 35 Sterile Technique

2. Review of the anatomy of the urinary system

101

Overall Objective

To insert a urinary catheter using correct sterile technique. To establish, maintain, and discontinue continuous urinary drainage when appropriate.

Specific Learning Objectives

	Know Facts and Principles	Apply Facts and Principles	Demonstrate Ability	Evaluate Performance
1. *Patient concerns*	State usual concerns of patient regarding catheterization.	Given a patient situation, identify what concerns have and have not been met.	In the clinical setting: a. Prepare patient by teaching. b. Provide privacy and drape. c. Allow time for patient's questions. d. Leave patient comfortable.	Evaluate own performance using Performance Checklist.
2. *Catheterization procedure*	List common ways contamination occurs in catheterization. Identify all items needed for catheterization of the bladder, urinary diversion, or self-catheterization and their purpose. State usual length of urethra in male and female. State rationale for sterile technique. Identify and explain principles of sterile technique used in catheterization.	Describe proper way to clean external meatus. Given a patient situation, state how to expose urinary meatus. Given a patient situation, state how far to insert catheter.	In the practice setting: a. Correctly set up equipment and arrange sterile field for catheterization. b. Carry out catheterization without contamination. c. Correctly identify meatus. d. Insert catheter correct distance.	Evaluate own performance using Performance Checklist and consulting with instructor.
3. *Maintaining continuous drainage*	List major concerns related to continuous drainage.	Given a patient situation, identify errors in continuous drainage setup.	In the clinical setting: a. Assess patient with continuous drainage to identify problems. b. Correct errors in continuous drainage setup.	Evaluate own performance using Performance Checklist.

(continued)

Specific Learning Objectives *(Continued)*

	Know Facts and Principles	Apply Facts and Principles	Demonstrate Ability	Evaluate Performance
4. *Removing a Foley catheter*	Describe procedure for removing Foley catheter.	Plan teaching regarding Foley catheter removal.	In the clinical setting: a. Teach patient regarding removal of Foley catheter. b. Remove Foley catheter correctly.	Evaluate own performance using Performance Checklist.
5. *Documentation*	List observations to be recorded.	Given a patient situation, identify information that should be recorded. Write nurses' progress note that would be appropriate for situation.	In the clinical setting: a. Record catheterization in appropriate places on patient chart.	Evaluate with instructor.

Learning Activities

1. Review the Specific Learning Objectives.
2. Read the section on the urinary system in the chapter on elimination in Ellis and Nowlis, *Nursing: A Human Needs Approach,* or comparable material in another textbook.
3. Look up the module vocabulary terms in the Glossary.
4. Review the anatomy of the urinary system.
5. Read through the module and mentally practice the specific procedure.
6. In the practice setting:
   a. Obtain a catheterization set.
   b. Open the set properly, noting the arrangement of all equipment. If more than one type or brand of equipment is available, compare the different sets.
   c. Repack the set as it was originally.
   d. Using the Performance Checklist as a guide, go through the entire procedure, improvising an area to represent a patient (pillows will work for this). Repeat the procedure until you feel comfortable with the equipment and you remember the steps.
   e. With a partner, arrange for a time to use a practice model.
   f. Take turns going through the procedure and evaluate each other's performance using the Performance Checklist.
   g. With a partner as the "patient," assume that an indwelling catheter is to be removed and do health teaching in the four appropriate areas.
   h. Have your instructor evaluate your performance.
7. In the clinical setting:
   a. Consult with your clinical instructor regarding an opportunity to perform a catheterization under supervision.
   b. Evaluate your own performance using the Performance Checklist.
   c. Consult your instructor regarding your performance.
8. If the opportunity arises, observe the teaching of a patient who is learning self-catheterization or learning to perform catheterization of a urinary diversion.

Vocabulary

catheter	perineum
catheterization	stoma
Foley catheter	straight catheter
foreskin	urethra
meatus	void
penis	

Catheterization

Rationale for the Use of This Skill

A catheter is used to drain urine from the bladder or to instill solution into the bladder. Patients' bladders are catheterized for various diagnostic and therapeutic reasons. It is the nurse's responsibility to carry out this task or delegate it to a skilled staff person. Because the inside of the bladder is sterile and provides direct access to the kidneys, the primary concern must be the prevention of contamination of the bladder. Urinary tract infections are common in those who have indwelling catheters in place. Even a single catheterization carries with it the danger of contaminating the urethra and/or bladder. Although bladder infections can be serious in themselves, they can also lead to infections of the kidneys, which may be life-threatening.

It is also the nurse's responsibility to know the anatomy of the urinary system to avoid damage to the urethra during catheterization. Once the catheter is in place, the nurse must establish correct drainage.

The patient with neuromuscular disease or obstruction that temporarily or permanently interferes with voluntary emptying of the bladder may be taught to perform self-catheterization. Patients who have had a surgical urinary diversion are taught to use the procedure of periodic stomal catheterization to empty the continent ileal pouch that has been surgically formed.

Not only is performing catheterization procedures effectively and safely important, but teaching and relieving anxiety is also a part of the nurse's responsibility.[1]

▶ *Nursing Diagnoses*

The following are common nursing diagnoses for the patient who is to be catheterized or the patient with an indwelling catheter:

Alteration in Urinary Elimination: Retention related to exposure to anesthesia

Dependence on Urinary Catheter: Related to incontinence

High Risk for Infection: Related to presence of indwelling catheter

[1] You will note that rationale for action is emphasized throughout the module by the use of italics.

PREPARING THE PATIENT

Many patients are anxious about catheterization, fearing pain and discomfort. They react emotionally to any procedure related to the genitourinary system—one that involves penetration of the body. Some facilities *protect privacy* by establishing a policy for male patients to be catheterized by male nurses and female patients to be catheterized by female nurses, unless the catheterization is an emergency. If an emergency occurs, and because there are relatively few male nurses, some facilities have specially trained male technicians or nursing assistants who can catheterize male patients. Always assess the patient's feelings about the procedure and review the policy of your facility *to cause the patient as little embarrassment as possible.* In preparing the patient, use a calm, straightforward, professional manner *to relieve the patient's anxiety.* Explain the procedure completely, and tell the patient what to expect. Give the patient an opportunity to ask questions and express concerns. Pay careful attention to privacy by closing doors, draping the patient, and exposing only the area involved in the procedure. *These actions show your concern for the patient's privacy and should alleviate some distress.*

EQUIPMENT

A catheterization set contains the basic equipment needed for the procedure (Figure 39–1). Some variation from one brand to another may occur, but usually the following items are included:

1. Sterile wrapper. When opened, the inside of the wrapper provides a sterile field. The outside is usually impervious to moisture.
2. Sterile gloves. These are usually on top, so all other items can be set up using sterile technique. As a beginner, you may want to have an extra pair of gloves in the room.
3. Sterile drapes. Two drapes are usually provided. One is a plain drape to slide under the female patient or to spread out under the penis. The other drape is often fenestrated (has a hole in it). The fenestrated drape is placed over the perineum, with the opening over the meatus for a female patient or around the penis of a male patient.
4. Sterile cleansing swabs. These may be cotton balls, or swabs with a short handle attached.
5. Thumb forceps, or pickups. You will need

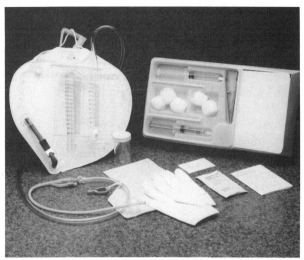

Figure 39–1. Foley catheterization set.
(*Courtesy American Hospital Supply Corp., McGaw Park, Illinois*)

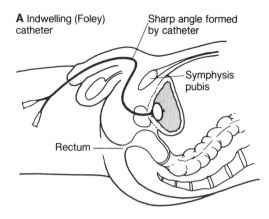

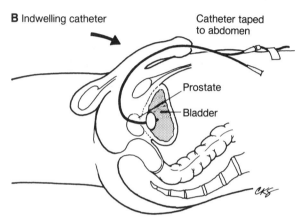

Figure 39–2. The inflated balloon holds the catheter in the bladder. **A:** Note the sharp angle formed at the penile-scrotal junction when the penis is directed toward the thigh. **B:** Note how correct taping of the catheter in the male patient eliminates the potential for abrasion and erosion at the penile-scrotal angle.

these to handle the cotton balls without contaminating your gloves.

6. Cleansing solution. A water-soluble povidone-iodine preparation is an excellent antibacterial agent for this purpose.

7. Syringe prefilled with sterile water. This is used to fill the retention balloon of a Foley catheter.

8. Water-soluble lubricant for lubricating the catheter.

9. Specimen container and label if necessary.

10. Safety pin and rubber band or plastic clamp. These are used to secure the catheter tubing to the bed if the catheter is to remain in place. If they are not in the set, you will have to obtain them separately. If it is policy to use tape, you will have to obtain this.

11. Catheter. Either a plain (straight) catheter or a Foley (indwelling) catheter can be used. *The indwelling catheter has a balloon at the end that can be inflated to hold the catheter in the bladder.*

Balloons are available in several sizes. Nurses most commonly insert catheters with balloons that hold 5 or 6 ml sterile water, depending on the manufacturer. Catheters with larger balloons are available and can be used for patients who have difficulty retaining the indwelling catheter. The larger sized balloon is needed to secure it in the bladder. During surgery, physicians sometimes insert catheters with balloons as large as 30 ml, which they secure with traction to provide hemostasis at a urologic surgical site (Figure 39–2). This type of catheter is used when continuous drainage is required. Catheters are available in sizes 8–20 French. (French is a method of sizing.) Size 8 French is used for infants and young children. Size 16 French is the size commonly used for adults. For patients who leak urine around an indwelling catheter, size 18 or 20 French is used.

It has been found that the selection of the smallest size of the catheter that will be effective *decreases the chance of infection. The reason is that larger catheters irritate the wall of the urethra causing it to be prone to invasion by microorganisms* (Ruge, 1987).

The type of catheter used also makes a difference in infection rates. Conti and Eutropius (1987) recommend the use of silicone catheters. *Silicone catheters are softer, cause less irritation than latex catheters, and therefore, can be left in place longer with less chance of infection.*

The balloon on a Foley catheter usually holds either 5 ml or 30 ml sterile water. An 8 French catheter, used for the pediatric patient, has a 3-ml balloon. The 5-ml balloon catheter is routinely used for urinary drainage of adult patients. The 30-ml balloon catheter is often ordered for a confused patient *who has pulled out a catheter with a smaller balloon.* Patients undergoing surgery of the prostate may have a 30-ml balloon catheter inserted before or during surgery and taped to the leg with traction *to provide hemostasis* (retard the tendency to bleed).

12. Drainage tubing and collection bag. These are often packaged with the Foley set. If not, obtain them separately.
13. Tape. Tape for securing the catheter to the patient is not included in the set. A disposable cloth peel-off patch with Velcro (Cath-Secure) or a leg strap can be used in place of tape.

PROCEDURE FOR CATHETERIZATION

Assessment

1. Check the order *to be sure that catheterization has been ordered for the patient.*
2. Determine whether the procedure is to be a straight or indwelling catheterization.
3. Find out whether a urine specimen is needed. When in doubt, always obtain a specimen. It can be discarded later if it is not needed.

Planning

4. Wash your hands *for infection control.*
5. Select the specific type and size of catheter to be used.
6. Collect the appropriate equipment, including the correct catheterization set, a good light if the room does not have adequate lighting (a portable gooseneck lamp or a flashlight may be used to improve existing lighting), a bath blanket or sheet *to drape the patient.* You may wish to have extra equipment available *in case something is contaminated.*

Implementation

7. Identify the patient *to be sure you are performing the procedure on the correct patient.* Explain the procedure to the patient and answer any questions.

8. Draw the bed curtains *for privacy,* and position and drape the patient.
   a. *For a pediatric patient or one who is disoriented and confused,* you will need another person (sometimes two others) *to hold the patient in the proper position.*
   b. Place a female patient in the dorsal recumbent position, with knees flexed and legs spread, *because it provides good visualization* (Figure 39–3) and is *usually most convenient.* Sometimes it is more comfortable for the patient to have her knees supported with pillows. Drape the bath blanket so that both legs are covered and only the perineum is exposed, *to protect modesty. If the patient cannot assume the dorsal recumbent position,* the Sims' position can be used.
   c. Place the male patient in the supine position (Figure 39–4). Expose only the penis and a small surrounding area (see Module 10, Assisting with Elimination and Perineal Care).
9. Set up the equipment.
   a. Arrange the lamp *so that you can see the perineum easily.* If the perineal area is soiled, perform perineal care, wearing clean gloves, with soap and water before you begin catheterization. You may also readily see the meatus during this procedure.
   b. Open the catheterization set and arrange the sterile field in a convenient location (on an overbed table at the foot of the bed, for the female patient, or beside the bed, for the male patient).
   c. Set up a receptacle for soiled cleansing swabs. The plastic bag that contained the set, a bedside bag, or several paper towels stacked together can be used for this purpose.
   d. If the drainage bag is in a separate package, open it and attach it to the bed.
   e. If a sterile drape is on top of the set, grasp it by one corner and open it with care, touching only the underside and edges to keep the top sterile. Ask the female patient to lift her hips and carefully slide the drape under the buttocks. The soft side should be up against the patient, and the shiny waterproof side should be down. Even though the drape is placed carefully, this area should be considered clean and not sterile throughout the procedure *since it is*

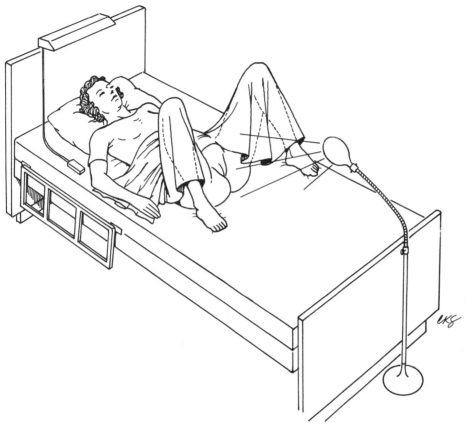

Figure 39–3. Female in dorsal recumbent position.

difficult to maintain sterility here. For the male patient, slide the drape under the penis, across the groin. This area can be considered sterile. Put on sterile gloves.

f. If sterile gloves are on top, put them on first, *so nothing is contaminated as you work.* Then, carefully take the first drape and

unfold it, keeping your gloved hands at the top of the drape. Grasp two adjacent corners of the drape and turn your hands, so that the drape covers as much of the gloves as possible *to protect them from contamination.* Next, place the drape as described above to provide a sterile field,

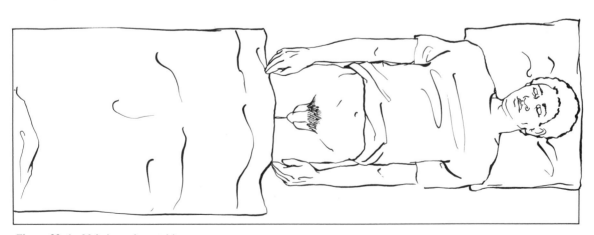

Figure 39–4. Male in supine position.

keeping the top sterile and not touching anything but the top side of the drape with your gloved hands.

g. Place the second drape *to secure and enlarge the sterile field*. If it is fenestrated, place the opening over the penis of the male patient. The drape can be placed over the meatus of the female patient, but many nurses find that it tends to fall forward, obscuring their vision and potentially contaminating the catheter. Thus, the drape is often folded in half and placed over the pubic area.

h. Open the cleansing solution and pour it over the swabs.

i. Open the lubricant and place it along the end of the catheter. *Lubricant minimizes trauma and discomfort to the urethra when the catheter is inserted.*

j. If a Foley catheter is being used, attach the prefilled syringe to the balloon port. Test the balloon by instilling all of the sterile water and then deflating it by withdrawing the water. Leave the syringe attached. (This is not essential but can simplify later work because you will want to hold the catheter in place with one hand, which leaves you only one hand to manipulate the syringe.) If the catheter is defective, ask someone else to get another catheter or take off your gloves and get both another catheter and another pair of gloves *in order to proceed.*

k. Set the specimen container and its cap upside down so that it is convenient and remains sterile.

l. If the drainage bag is in the set, connect the distal end of the catheter to the drainage tube. *This prevents urine spilling from a collecting container while you are performing the procedure.* If a specimen is needed, you can either not connect the catheter to the drainage tube at this time and use the specimen container or obtain a specimen from the drainage bag after you have finished.

10. Catheterize the patient.

a. Use your nondominant hand to expose the meatus. Remember that this hand is now contaminated and cannot be used to handle equipment again.

For a male, raise the penis at a 45° angle from the scrotum and retract the foreskin. For a female, separate both the labia majora and the labia minora. Retract the labia laterally and anteriorly. A common error is to place the fingers too high and too laterally to expose the meatus. If the meatus is not identifiable, move your hand for better exposure. Always identify the meatus before any other equipment is contaminated. Occasionally, when you are sure that the area of the meatus is well exposed—although you may not be positive of its exact location—cleaning will help you positively identify it. You may ask the patient to cough. *Coughing usually causes the meatus to open slightly and aids identification.*

b. After the meatus is exposed and identified, begin cleaning.

Use forceps to handle the cleansing swabs *to keep your dominant gloved hand completely sterile for handling the catheter.* Use each swab only once, and then discard in the prepared location, *where it will not contaminate your field.* Do not pass the used cotton balls over the sterile field *to prevent bacteria from falling onto the sterile field.*

For a male, clean in a circular motion, starting at the meatus, without retracing any area *to move bacteria away from the meatus* (Figure 39–5). For a female, use each swab from front to back, starting with the outside labia and moving toward the center (Figure 39–6). Clean one side first and then the other. The final stroke should be vertical to clean the meatus itself. The principle behind this pattern is to *move from the area of lesser accumulation of secretions and organisms (labia) to the area of greater concentration (meatus).* The last stroke, if done slowly, may pull the meatus slightly open, thereby assuring identification.

Some persons recommend that the first cleansing strokes be down the center, across the meatus, and that subsequent strokes move outward. The principle for this pattern is *to move from the area you want to be the cleanest area (meatus) to the area that is less critical (labia).*

Research has not identified which of these procedures is better. The most critical point seems to be that each swab be used only once and that the path of the swab be from anterior to posterior *to avoid moving microorganisms from the rectal area to the meatus.* For the pattern, follow the policy/procedure of your facility.

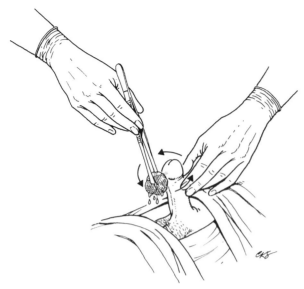

Figure 39-5. The nurse cleaning the male patient for catheterization. Clean the penis with circular strokes.

c. Use the sterile-gloved dominant hand to move the tray containing the catheter close to the patient (between the legs of the female patient and beside the male patient). Touch only the inside of the tray. Pick up the catheter several inches back from the tip *to keep the tip sterile.* If a collecting bag is not attached, be sure to keep the end of the catheter in the tray.

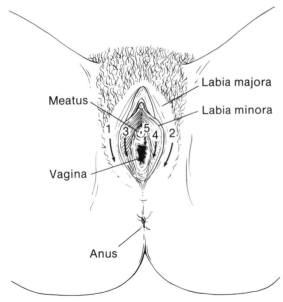

Figure 39-6. Cleaning the female for catheterization. Clean the genitalia from anterior to posterior.

d. Insert the lubricated catheter smoothly approximately 2–3 inches into the female and 6–9 inches into the male, beyond the urethra into the bladder. Do not use force. If you encounter resistance, ask the patient to breathe deeply (*to relax the muscles*) and gently rotate the catheter to see if it will penetrate. If it still will not enter, consult a physician before trying again. *It is possible to damage the urethra and the urinary sphincters by pushing against resistant tissue.*

The return of urine indicates that the catheter is in the bladder. To inflate a Foley balloon, insert the catheter 1 inch further after urine is returned, *to make sure that the balloon does not inflate in the urethra.*

11. If you are using a straight catheter, hold the catheter in place while you fill the specimen container.

12. If you are using a straight catheter, drain the bladder, pinch the catheter closed, *to prevent dribbling,* and remove the catheter quickly. Then proceed to step 15.

13. Recent research reveals that whichever type of catheter you use, it is not harmful to drain the bladder completely, regardless of the quantity. It was once thought that draining more than 1000 ml at one time could lead to a shocklike reaction. This does not appear to be true (Bristoll, 1989). Although there may be small changes in blood pressure and pulse, these are not usually clinically significant.

If you are using a Foley catheter, hold it in place while you fill the balloon. The catheter can continue to drain into the receptacle while this is done. Use the amount of fluid indicated on the catheter itself plus 4 or 5 ml. *Because the fluid must fill the tube leading to the balloon, as well as the balloon itself, you will need this extra amount, and manufacturers indicate that balloons will not overinflate or rupture from using this amount. If you use too little fluid, the catheter may slip out.*

Check for security by gently pulling the catheter until resistance is felt.

14. In most Foley catheter sets the bag is attached to the catheter. If it is not, connect the bag at this time. Be sure to maintain the sterility of the ends of the tubing at the connecting point. Place the tubing over the top of the thigh, *so the leg does not occlude the tubing.*

Hang the bag on the bed frame below the level of the bladder. Make sure the bag does not touch the floor.

15. Tape the catheter to the patient *to prevent pull on the neck of the bladder as the patient moves* (Figure 39–7). For a male, tape the catheter without tension to the side of the lower abdomen *to prevent the formation of a fistula at the penile-scrotal angle.* For a female, tape the catheter to the inner thigh. Some physicians prefer that the catheter not be taped.

Coil excess tubing flatly on the bed, *so that drainage is not impeded. Urine collecting in the tube provides a medium for bacteria to multiply and ascend.* Attach the tubing to the side of the bed with a plastic catheter clamp (which may be included in the set) or with a rubber band and safety pin. Wrap the rubber band around the tubing and pin it to the sheet (Figure 39–8).

16. Assist the patient to a comfortable position, straighten the bed, and open the curtains. The patient may have further questions or concerns. This is a good time to teach the patient about the Foley catheter. Tell the patient that the balloon will hold the catheter in place and that it is all right to move. Stress the need for fluids (if the patient's medical condition permits). *Because of the pressure of the balloon,* the patient with a Foley catheter usually feels as though he or she needs to void.

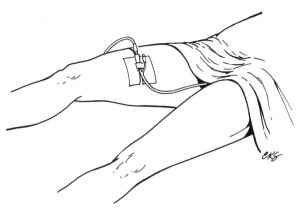

Figure 39–8. A cloth/Velcro peel-off patch or leg straps are also available commercially to secure the catheter and tubing.

Explain that this feeling will pass *as the tissue becomes less sensitive to the constant stimulation. Understanding this helps the patient to tolerate the discomfort.*

17. Gather and discard disposable equipment properly. If you have used nondisposable equipment, follow your hospital's procedure for cleaning.

18. Wash your hands *for infection control.*

Evaluation

19. Evaluate using the following criteria:
   a. Indwelling catheter draining properly.
   b. Patient comfortable.

Documentation

20. Document the following:
   a. The date and time of catheterization.
   b. The type and size of catheter inserted.
   c. Whether a specimen was obtained and sent to the lab.
   d. The amount of urine drained (add to the output record if appropriate).
   e. A description of the urine.
   f. The patient's response to the procedure.

CARING FOR A PATIENT WITH AN INDWELLING CATHETER

The urinary tract is normally sterile. *The introduction of organisms through the catheter is a common cause of urinary tract infection.* Various measures are used *to decrease the risk of infection.*

1. Place the patient on intake and output recording *to assess the functioning of the catheter.*

2. Encourage the patient to increase fluid intake. *Large intake causes a constant flow of urine out of*

A

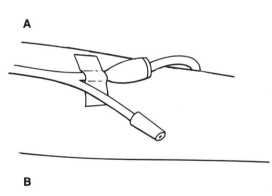

B

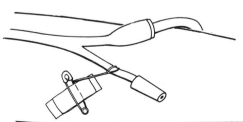

Figure 39–7. Taping a catheter. **A:** To decrease the chance of the tape pulling loose, the catheter is secured in a loop of tape before the ends are taped to the patient. **B:** Alternately, the catheter may be attached by using tape, a safety pin, and a rubber band.

DATE/TIME	
2/14/94 1600	#16 Fr indwelling catheter inserted per order, 600 ml clear, pale yellow urine obtained. Specimen to lab. Patient tolerated procedure well. ——————————— S. Frankle, RN

Example of Progress Notes Using Narrative Format

DATE/TIME	
4/19/94 0800	Perineal discomfort: ————————————
S "I feel like I have to go all of the time and I itch down there."
O Perineum reddened and catheter feels gritty when compressed between fingers. Urine dark amber in color, cloudy, and contains white sediment. ————
A Catheter collecting sediment and causing patient discomfort and potential for infection. ————
P Obtain order for replacement of indwelling catheter. Increase fluid intake to 2500 ml/24h. ——————— R. Sanders, RN

Example of Progress Notes Using SOAP Format

the kidneys and bladder, which tends to inhibit the upward movement of microbes. By increasing fluid intake, the system is being irrigated internally. Up to 3000 ml fluids per day (for the patient without circulatory problems and with no fluid restriction) is best. This quantity may be unrealistic for an elderly patient or child, but encourage any increase.

3. Maintain the closed system. *Every time the system is opened, microorganisms can enter.* Carry out all procedures so that the system is uninterrupted if possible. (See Module 18, Collecting Specimens, for a method of obtaining urine specimens without interrupting the system.)

4. Maintain external cleanliness around the catheter. *Secretions that build up are an optimum location for bacterial growth, which could ascend the outside of the catheter.* The basic necessity is thorough washing with soap and water. As an additional measure, some facilities follow the policy of cleaning the meatal area and the first several inches of exposed catheter with an antibacterial solution (povidone-iodine) and then applying an iodine ointment at the meatus around the catheter. Be sure to ask the patient if he or she is allergic to iodine before using the ointment. This policy is not recommended *because there is no evidence it decreases infection and there are allergic responses.*

5. Keep the catheter drainage bag below the level of the bladder at all times. *This prevents potentially contaminated urine from draining back into the bladder.* Some brands of collecting bags have one-way valves to prevent backflow.

6. Keep the tubing coiled by the patient's side. *Tubing that hangs off the bed in loops allows urine to sit in the tubing, creating a possible reservoir for microbes, which could then ascend.*

7. Keep the drainage bag off the floor. *If it touches the floor, the outside picks up microbes that can then move up the outside of the bag and the catheter.*

8. Tape or coil the catheter in a way that prevents pulling. *Pull irritates the patient's urethra and can actually dislodge the catheter and inflated balloon. In addition to causing the patient trauma and discomfort, irritation and inflammation predispose the tissue to infection.*

   Take extra care when moving or ambulating a patient. You must watch the position of the tubing and bag at all times *to prevent pulling.*

9. Observe for irritation at the meatal area. If any is found, report it to the physician.

10. Empty the bag at regular intervals (usually every 8 hours), *so that it does not overfill and cause urine backup in the tubing.* Empty more frequently *if large amounts of urine are being excreted.*

PROCEDURE FOR REMOVING A FOLEY CATHETER

Assessment

1. Verify the order to discontinue the indwelling catheter.
2. Determine whether a urine specimen is needed.

Planning

3. Wash your hands *for infection control.*
4. Obtain the necessary equipment.
   a. Several paper towels for wrapping the soiled catheter after removal
   b. A 10 ml syringe
   c. Padding and a small container to catch the fluid
   d. Clean gloves.

Implementation

5. Identify the patient *to be sure you are performing the procedure on the correct patient.*
6. Tell the patient that the catheter is to be removed and that the procedure is not painful. Health teaching should include four points.
   a. A mild burning sensation may accompany urination for a short period of time *because of the irritation caused by the catheter.* If this persists, it should be reported to the physician.
   b. Voiding may be more frequent and in smaller amounts than normal at first *because the bladder has been kept empty and may have to relearn how to respond to a sensation of fullness.* Again, if this persists, it should be reported to the physician because it may indicate infection.
   c. For the first 24 hours after the catheter is removed, the nurse should be called *to measure each voiding to facilitate assessment.* If the patient can go to the bathroom, explain how measurement is carried out.
   d. It is essential to continue increased fluid intake *to maintain proper kidney and bladder function.*
7. Draw the curtains and prepare the patient, draping the covers back to expose the catheter. Put on clean gloves.
8. Discontinue the catheter.
   a. Place paper towels under the catheter.
   b. Use the syringe *to remove fluid from the balloon.* In some facilities, nurses cut the balloon-filling tube of the catheter with

scissors *to remove the sterile water.* This is unwise, *because there is always some chance that the balloon will not deflate with this method.* If this occurs, the physician will have to introduce a special instrument *to deflate the balloon so that the catheter can be removed.*
   c. Pinch the catheter *to prevent leakage* and pull it out smoothly. This action should not cause discomfort but will be felt. Ask the patient to breathe in and out through the mouth to relax while you withdraw the catheter.
   d. With your free hand, wrap the end of the catheter in paper towel while you keep the catheter itself pinched closed.
   e. Hold the end of the catheter up *to allow urine to drain from the tubing into the bag.*
9. Assist the patient to a comfortable position, straighten the bed, and open the curtains.
10. Measure urine output.
11. Dispose of the equipment.
12. Remove gloves and wash your hands.

Evaluation

13. Evaluate using the following criteria:
    a. Catheter removed without difficulty.
    b. Patient is voiding in adequate amounts (approximately 250 ml each time) at regular intervals.
    c. Patient is continuing to increase fluid intake.

Documentation

14. On the patient's record, document the time the catheter was removed, the amount of urine output and the patient's response to the procedure.

TEACHING THE PROCEDURE FOR INTERMITTENT SELF-CATHETERIZATION

Intermittent self-catheterization is performed using clean rather than sterile technique. Conscientious handwashing is essential *to avoid infection.* Regular emptying of the bladder is another factor *for avoiding urinary tract infections.* The procedure is performed every 2–3 hours during the day and once during the sleeping hours, if necessary.

Assessment

1. Check the order to be sure that self-catheterization has been ordered for the patient.

2. Identify the medical diagnosis and whether the patient is learning the procedure for purposes of temporary or permanent urinary drainage.
3. Assess the patient's knowledge of own anatomy and any feelings of anxiety *that may interfere with learning.*

Planning
4. Wash your hands *for infection control.*
5. Collect the following equipment:
   a. A 14 or 16 French straight catheter (two or more)
   b. Lubricating jelly
   c. Small hand mirror (for the female patient)
   d. Small clean pan, container, or leakproof plastic bag
   e. Additional clean plastic bag for storing catheter.

Implementation
6. Identify the patient *to be sure you are teaching the procedure to the correct patient.*
7. Review the equipment you have selected with the patient, identifying each item, explaining its use, and answering any questions.
8. Review the steps of the procedure in detail.
9. Have the patient wash hands and clean the perineal area with soap and water.
10. Position the patient. If female, have the patient assume the dorsal recumbent position with the legs spread. Later, when the female patient has learned to perform catheterization without the use of a mirror, she can sit on a chair or on the toilet. If male, the patient can sit on a chair, toilet, or commode.
11. For the female, elevate the patient's head and position the mirror so that the patient can see the perineum. Spread the labia. You can point to the meatus with a sterile cotton-tipped applicator to help her identify the structure. The male patient is taught to retract the foreskin with one hand and elevate the penis with the other so that it is at a right angle to the body.
12. Lubricate the catheter with either lubricating jelly or clean water.
13. The lubricated catheter is introduced through the meatus, 2–3 inches for the female, 6–10 inches for the male or until urine begins to flow into the clean pan or a leak-proof plastic bag.
14. When the flow stops, the patient pinches the catheter *to prevent dribbling* and withdraws the catheter.

15. The patient can wipe away any urine that is on the perineum with a tissue, stand up, and reclothe.
16. The urine collected in the bag can be discarded in the toilet.
17. The patient washes the catheter in warm water with soap and rinses it thoroughly.
18. The catheter is then stored in a leak-proof plastic bag until its next use.

Evaluation
19. Evaluate according to the following criteria:
   a. Patient empties bladder completely.
   b. Patient maintains clean technique.
20. Have the patient give a repeat performance of the procedure later at least one more time.

Documentation
21. Document the following:
   a. That the patient performed self-catheterization.
   b. The degree of understanding and proficiency.
   c. Any problems with performing the procedure.

PROCEDURE FOR CATHETERIZATION OF A URINARY DIVERSION

The procedure for catheterizing the stoma of a urinary diversion is similar to that used for intermittent self-catheterization. Again, a clean technique is used. *The mucous membrane of the ileal pouch is fairly resistant to infection caused by microorganisms that may be introduced to the urinary tract. Also, the time interval between catheterization allows the patient's immune system to remain active in fighting off infection.* It must be remembered that resistance to pathogens is not as active in persons who are ill or debilitated.

Assessment
1. Follow steps 1–3 of the procedure for self-catheterization.

Planning
4. Follow steps 4 and 5 of the procedure for self-catheterization. You will not need a mirror for the female patient.

Implementation
6. Follow steps 6–8 of the procedure for self-catheterization.
9. Have the patient sitting in a comfortable position; this could be on a straight-backed chair or on the toilet or commode.

10. Instruct the patient to wash hands and the peristomal area.
11. Lubricate the catheter with either lubricating jelly or clean water.
12. Have the patient introduce the catheter through the urinary diversion stoma 2–3 inches or until the urine begins to flow into a small pan or a leak-proof plastic bag.
13. When the flow stops, the patient pinches the catheter to prevent dribbling and withdraws the catheter.
14. The patient can wipe away any urine that is on the skin with a tissue.
15. The urine collected in the bag can be discarded in the toilet.
16. The patient washes the catheter in warm water with soap and rinses it thoroughly.
17. The catheter is then stored in a leak-proof plastic bag until its next use.

Evaluation

18. Evaluate according to the following criteria:
    a. Patient empties the pouch completely.
    b. Patient maintains clean technique.

Documentation

19. Document the following:
    a. That the patient performed catheterization of a urinary diversion.
    b. The degree of understanding and proficiency.
    c. Any problems with performing the procedure.

LONG-TERM CARE

Some of the clients residing in long-term care facilities *have problems with incontinence* that necessitate their having a permanent indwelling catheter. Adaptations may have to be made when performing the catheterization procedure on women of advanced age *because they have difficulty maintaining the dorsal recumbent position for a period of time.*

Certainly, providing privacy is always essential for any patient being catheterized but for the elderly, this issue is particularly sensitive. Another problem may be the prevalence of urinary tract infections in the older person *due to a less active immune system than the person had when younger. Other reasons for urinary tract infections are poor hygiene and enlargement of the prostate, which partially obstructs drainage of the bladder.* One-half of institutionalized elderly people develop urinary tract infections at some time; this is particularly so in those with indwelling catheters (Pritchard, 1988).

To decrease the chance of urinary tract infection, the nurse in long-term care can see that perineal hygiene is properly done, that fluid intake is adequate, and that continual assessment for the presence of infection is provided.

🔲 Home Care

Because more chronically ill persons are being cared for in the home, the presence of persons with indwelling urinary catheters in the home is becoming more common. The patient may be discharged with a catheter in place or the home health nurse may insert one. In either case, meticulous care should be provided *to prevent complications.* It is recommended that patients be showered if possible. Showers do not carry any risk of infection and therefore, are preferable to tub baths. The policy in most long-term care settings and in the home is that the catheter should be changed every 30 days or *more often if there is evidence of sediment, crustations, or leakage.*

If the patient is able to be up in a chair or ambulating, the drainage system should be appropriate to the specific patient. Roe (1988) states that the drainage system for the patient who is not bedridden should be one that does not use rubber straps, is leak-proof, eliminates lengthy tubing, maintains correct positioning of the drainage bag, and is suited to the domestic environment.

For reasons of patient safety and comfort of the patient and family, ongoing assessment and advisement should be provided by the nurse in home health care.

References

Bristoll, S., Fadden, T., Fehring, R. J., Rohde, L., Smith, P. R., & Wohlitz, B. A. (1989). The mythical danger of rapid urinary drainage. *American Journal of Nursing, 89*(3); 344–345.

Conti, M. T. & Eutropius, L. (1987). Preventing UTIs: What works? *American Journal of Nursing, 87*(3), 307–309.

Pritchard, V. (1988). Geriatric infections: The urinary tract. *RN, 51*(5), 36–38.

Roe, B. H., Reid, F. J., & Brocklehurst, J. C. (1988). Comparison of four urine drainage systems. *Journal of Advanced Nursing, 13,* 374–382.

Ruge, C. A. (1987). Catheter-related U.T.I.s: What's the best way to prevent them? *Nursing '87, 17*(12), 50–51.

Performance Checklist

Performing Catheterization	Unsat	Needs More Practice	Sat	Comments
Assessment				
1. Check the order.				
2. Determine whether a urine specimen is needed.				
3. Find out whether catheter will be used only to empty bladder or continuous drainage will be established.				
Planning				
4. Wash your hands.				
5. Select specific type and size of catheter.				
6. Collect appropriate equipment, including catheterization set, light source, bath blanket or sheet for drape, and extra equipment as individually determined.				
Implementation				
7. Identify the patient and explain the procedure. Answer any questions.				
8. Draw bed curtains, and position and drape the patient. a. Pediatric patient or confused patient—seek an assistant.				
b. Female patient in dorsal recumbent position, with knees flexed, or in Sims' position				
c. Male patient in supine position				
9. Set up the equipment. a. Arrange the lamp.				
b. Open catheterization set and arrange sterile field.				
c. Set up receptacle for soiled cleansing swabs.				
d. If drainage bag is in separate package, open it and attach to bed.				
e. If sterile drape is on top of set, grasp drape by side that is to be nonsterile and place under patient. Then put on sterile gloves.				

Performing Catheterization *(Continued)*	Unsat	Needs More Practice	Sat	Comments
f. If sterile gloves are on top of set, put them on. Then grasp drape by side that is to be sterile and place under patient, protecting your gloves.				
g. Place second drape to enlarge sterile field.				
h. Open cleansing solution and pour over swabs.				
i. Open lubricant and place it on end of catheter.				
j. For a Foley, attach syringe and test balloon by instilling all of the sterile water and then deflating balloon by withdrawing water. Leave syringe attached.				
k. Set the specimen container and its cap upside down.				
l. If drainage bag is in set, connect distal end of catheter to drainage tubing.				
10. Catheterize the patient. a. Use nondominant hand to expose the meatus.				
b. After meatus is identified, cleanse the area surrounding the meatus, using swabs held in forceps. Use circular motion on males. Swab from anterior to posterior on females. Discard swabs away from sterile field.				
c. Use sterile hand to move tray containing catheter close to patient, and to pick up catheter.				
d. Insert catheter 2–3 inches into female or 6–9 inches into male, holding the penis at a 45° angle, until urine returns.				
11. Obtain a specimen.				
12. Drain the bladder.				
13. If using a Foley catheter, fill the balloon.				
14. Connect the bag to the catheter.				
15. Tape the catheter to the patient—for a male to the lower abdomen, for a female to the thigh or loosely over the leg without taping.				
16. Assist patient to comfortable position.				

Performing Catheterization (*Continued*)	Unsat	Needs More Practice	Sat	Comments
17. Gather and discard disposable equipment. Clean nondisposable equipment.				
18. Wash your hands.				
Evaluation				
19. Evaluate using the following criteria: a. Indwelling catheter draining properly.				
b. Patient comfortable.				
Documentation				
20. Document the following: a. Date and time.				
b. Type and size of catheter.				
c. Whether a specimen was obtained.				
d. Amount of urine.				
e. Description of urine.				
f. Patient's response to procedure.				

**Caring for a Patient
With an Indwelling Catheter**

	Unsat	Needs More Practice	Sat	Comments
1. Place patient on intake and output.				
2. Encourage increased fluid intake.				
3. Maintain closed system.				
4. Maintain external cleanliness around catheter.				
5. Keep catheter drainage bag below level of bladder.				
6. Keep tubing coiled by patient's side.				
7. Keep drainage bag off the floor.				
8. Tape catheter to prevent pulling.				
9. Observe for irritation at meatus.				
10. Empty bag at regular intervals.				

Removing a Foley Catheter	Unsat	Needs More Practice	Sat	Comments
Assessment				
1. Verify the order.				
2. Determine whether a urine specimen is needed.				
Planning				
3. Wash your hands.				
4. Obtain necessary equipment: a. Paper towels				
b. A syringe to remove the fluid from balloon				
c. A small container to catch urine				
d. Clean gloves.				
Implementation				
5. Identify the patient.				
6. Tell the patient that catheter is to be removed and what to expect.				
7. Prepare patient by proper draping. Put on clean gloves.				
8. Discontinue the catheter. a. Place paper towels under catheter.				
b. Use syringe to remove fluid from balloon.				
c. Pinch catheter and pull it out smoothly.				
d. Wrap catheter in paper towel.				
e. Hold end of catheter up to allow urine to drain from tubing.				
9. Assist patient to comfortable position.				
10. Measure urine output.				
11. Dispose of the equipment.				
12. Wash your hands.				
Evaluation				
13. Evaluate using the following criteria: a. Catheter removed without difficulty.				
b. Patient voiding adequate amounts (250 ml) at regular intervals.				

Removing a Foley Catheter *(Continued)*	Unsat	Needs More Practice	Sat	Comments
c. Patient is continuing to increase fluid intake.				

Documentation

14. Record time of catheter removal, urine output, and patient's response.				

Teaching the Procedure for Intermittent Self-Catheterization

Assessment

1. Check the order.				
2. Identify the medical diagnosis.				
3. Assess patient's knowledge.				

Planning

4. Wash your hands.				
5. Collect appropriate equipment, including a mirror for the female patient.				
6. Identify the patient.				
7. Review equipment, explaining use and answering questions.				
8. Review steps of procedure.				

Implementation

9. Position patient: female in dorsal recumbent, male sitting.				
10. Have patient wash hands.				
11. Position female so she can see perineal area in mirror. Have male retract foreskin and elevate penis so it is at right angle to the body.				
12. Lubricate the catheter with either lubricating jelly or clean water.				
13. Insert lubricated catheter 2–3 inches through the meatus until urine flows into a small pan or leak-proof plastic bag.				
14. When urine stops flowing, have patient pinch catheter and remove.				
15. Discard collected urine in toilet.				

Teaching the Procedure for Intermittent Self-Catheterization *(Continued)*	Unsat	Needs More Practice	Sat	Comments
16. The patient washes catheter in warm water with soap and rinses it thoroughly.				
17. Dry catheter and store in clean leak-proof plastic bag for future use.				
Evaluation				
18. Evaluate according to the following criteria: a. Patient empties bladder completely.				
b. Patient maintains clean technique.				
19. Have patient repeat procedure one time later.				
Documentation				
20. Document the following: a. That patient performed self-catheterization.				
b. Degree of understanding and proficiency.				
c. Any problems performing procedure.				

Performing Catheterization of a Urinary Diversion

	Unsat	Needs More Practice	Sat	Comments
Assessment				
1. Assess as in Checklist steps 1–3 of Procedure for Self-Catheterization (check order, identify diagnosis, assess patient's knowledge).				
Planning				
4. Plan as in Checklist steps 4 and 5 of Procedure for Self-Catheterization (wash hands, collect equipment).				
Implementation				
6. Implement as in Checklist steps 6–8 of Procedure for Self-Catheterization (identify patient, review equipment, review procedure steps).				
9. Have patient sitting in a comfortable position.				
10. Instruct patient to wash hands.				
11. Lubricate catheter.				
12. Have patient insert catheter 2–3 inches until urine flows.				

Performing Catheterization of a Urinary Diversion (Continued)	Unsat	Needs More Practice	Sat	Comments
13. When flow stops, patient pinches catheter and withdraws it.				
14. Wipe away any urine on the skin with a tissue.				
15. Discard the urine collected in the bag in the toilet.				
16. Catheter is washed in warm water with soap and rinsed thoroughly.				
17. Catheter is stored in clean, leak-proof, plastic bag until next use.				
Evaluation				
18. Evaluate using the following criteria: a. Patient empties the pouch completely.				
b. Patient maintains clean technique.				
Documentation				
19. Document the following: a. Patient performed catheterization of urinary diversion.				
b. Degree of understanding and proficiency.				
c. Any problems performing procedure.				

Quiz

Short-Answer Questions

1. Give three common concerns of patients being catheterized.

   a. _____

   b. _____

   c. _____

2. Mrs. Tigerson was to have a catheter inserted preoperatively. The nurse explained to Mrs. Tigerson what the procedure was, why it was being done, and what she should expect. The nurse then carried out the catheterization. What step in dealing with the patient's concerns did the nurse omit? _____

3. List the four important points to include when teaching the patient whose indwelling catheter is to be removed.

   a. _____

   b. _____

   c. _____

   d. _____

Multiple-Choice Questions

_____ 4. The length of the male urethra is approximately

   a. 4–5 inches.
   b. 6–9 inches.
   c. 7–8 inches.
   d. 8–10 inches.

_____ 5. The length of the female urethra is approximately

   a. ½–1 inch.
   b. 1½–2 inches.
   c. 2–3 inches.
   d. 3–4 inches.

_____ 6. When you are catheterizing a female patient, the catheter touches the meatus but then slides downward on the perineum and does not enter the urethra. Your next action should be to

   a. get better lighting.
   b. clean the area again.
   c. obtain a sterile catheter.
   d. clean the catheter with the remaining cleansing solution.

_____ 7. The most essential point of cleaning the female perineum for catheterization is to

   a. clean in a circular motion.
   b. clean from inner to outer areas.
   c. clean toward the anus.
   d. clean in any manner so long as you do it thoroughly.

_____ **8.** Which of the following items are usually part of a catheterization set? (1) drapes; (2) gloves; (3) catheter; (4) safety pin

  a. 1, 2, and 3
  b. 2, 3, and 4
  c. 1, 3, and 4
  d. All of the above.

_____ **9.** A drape with a hole in it is called

  a. fenestrated.
  b. sequestered.
  c. windowed.
  d. no special name.

_____ **10.** Which of the following must you chart after performing a catheterization?

  a. Only the name of the procedure and the time done
  b. Only those aspects that differed from a routine catheterization procedure
  c. Type and size of catheter, amount and description of urine, patient's response, and time of procedure

_____ **11.** The person with a urinary diversion should catheterize the stoma

  a. every hour.
  b. every 2–3 hours.
  c. once every 6 hours.
  d. only when necessary.

_____ **12.** The catheter used for self-catheterization should be stored between uses in

  a. a sterile pan in solution.
  b. the paper package it came in.
  c. a paper towel.
  d. a clean leak-proof plastic bag.

Unit 9
SUPPORTING OXYGENATION

MODULE 40
Administering Oxygen

MODULE 41
Respiratory Care Procedures

MODULE 42
Oral and Nasopharyngeal Suctioning

MODULE 43
Tracheostomy Care and Suctioning

MODULE 44
Caring for Patients With Chest Drainage

125

Module 40
Administering Oxygen

Module Contents

Rationale for the Use of This Skill
Nursing Diagnosis
Psychologic Problems for the Patient
Safety
Flowmeter
Regulator
Humidification
General Procedure for Administering Oxygen
  Assessment
  Planning

  Implementation
  Evaluation
  Documentation
Methods of Administration
  Nasal Cannula
  Nasal Catheter
  Oxygen Masks
  Oxygen Tents
  Self-Inflating Breathing Bag and Mask
Home Care
Long-term Care

Prerequisites

Successful completion of the following modules:

VOLUME 1
Module 1 An Approach to Nursing Skills
Module 2 Basic Infection Control
Module 3 Safety
Module 5 General Assessment Overview
Module 6 Documentation
Module 11 Hygiene
Module 13 Inspection, Palpation, Auscultation, and Percussion
Module 16 Temperature, Pulse, and Respiration

VOLUME 2
Module 41 Respiratory Care Procedures

127

Overall Objective

To administer oxygen to patients, using equipment appropriately in a safe and effective manner.

Specific Learning Objectives

	Know Facts and Principles	Apply Facts and Principles	Demonstrate Ability	Evaluate Performance
1. *Patients who need oxygen*	List general conditions that necessitate oxygen administration	Give rationale for oxygen administration when assigned a patient.	In the clinical setting, identify a patient's need for supplemental oxygen.	Evaluate patient's need for supplemental oxygen with instructor.
2. *Methods of administration*	Name five methods of oxygen administration.	Describe appropriate situation for use of each method. Determine methods used in a given facility.	In the clinical setting, identify appropriate method for a patient.	Evaluate choice of method with instructor.
3. *Psychologic support*	Know impact of fear and anxiety on breathing.	Assess level of anxiety in patient.	In the clinical setting, reassure and give adequate explanations to patient.	Evaluate patient's emotional status in terms of relaxation and decreased anxiety.
4. *Administering oxygen*	State hazards of oxygen.	Prepare room properly to prevent fire.	In the clinical setting, implement oxygen administration with emphasis on patient's comfort and safety.	Evaluate own performance using Performance Checklist.
5. *Documentation*	Know essential information to be documented.	Given a situation, indicate patient's potential physical and psychologic responses that should be documented.	In the clinical setting, document correctly.	Evaluate own performance with instructor.

Learning Activities

1. Review the Specific Learning Objectives.
2. Read the section on respiration in Ellis and Nowlis, *Nursing: A Human Needs Approach,* or comparable material in another textbook.
3. Look up the module vocabulary terms in the Glossary.
4. Read through the module and mentally practice the skills.
5. In the practice setting, if oxygen equipment is available:
   a. Inspect and handle the equipment.
   b. Practice applying a mask and a nasal cannula on a partner.
   c. Have your partner apply the mask and nasal cannula on you.
6. In the clinical setting:
   a. Become familiar with the oxygen equipment used in your clinical facility.
   b. By talking to a patient who is receiving oxygen, ascertain what he or she has been told regarding the procedure.
   c. Review the diagnoses of patients who are receiving oxygen.
   d. Observe the administration of oxygen on a specific patient. Were all safety precautions observed?
   e. Under supervision, plan and initiate oxygen therapy as ordered for a patient.
   f. Document the procedure properly, and share your notes with your instructor.

Vocabulary

ambient	combustion	humidifier	lumen
cannula	dyspnea	hypoxemia	prongs
catheter	explosive	hypoxia	tidal volume
claustrophobia	flowmeter	liter	uvula

Administering Oxygen

Rationale for the Use of This Skill

Oxygen is essential to life. An optimum level of oxygen must be maintained to sustain mental functioning. Approximately one fifth, or 20% of the air we normally breathe is oxygen.

In people who have respiratory tract disorders or systemic conditions that affect respiration, oxygen exchange in the lungs is often compromised, leading to a state of hypoxia. Trauma or injury (hemorrhage) can also interfere with oxygenation of the blood (hypoxemia). In such cases it is essential to administer additional oxygen to increase its concentration in the blood and thus the nurse must be familiar with the equipment and skilled in its use[1].

▶ *Nursing Diagnosis*

Oxygen therapy is used most often for the patient with the nursing diagnosis of "Impaired gas exchange" which may be related to a variety of factors such as excessive secretions in the lungs, hypoventilation, or a disease process that decreases the gas exchange surfaces in the lungs.

PSYCHOLOGIC PROBLEMS FOR THE PATIENT

The administration of oxygen, although a commonplace procedure, may make some patients anxious, which leads to difficulty in breathing. Some perceive the administration of oxygen as a lifesaving measure and are reassured by the therapy. Others perceive it as an indication that they are seriously ill and are made anxious by it. Still others find a mask or tent oppressive and experience claustrophobia during the process. By explaining the procedure (in simple terms) to the patient and the patient's family, as well as by maintaining a calm attitude, *you can help to allay many unnecessary fears. For this reason, even semicomatose patients should be given explanations.*

SAFETY

Certain dangers are inherent in the administration of oxygen. *Although oxygen itself is not explosive, it sup-*

[1] You will note that rationale for action is emphasized throughout the module by the use of italics.

ports combustion. This means that extremely rapid burning takes place in the presence of high oxygen concentration, almost as if the oxygen itself were explosive. Thus, it is essential that you prevent sparks or fire in an environment where oxygen is being used. Observe these precautions:

1. Prominently display a "no smoking" sign on the patient's door, *which cautions all persons in the room—including the patient—not to smoke.* Currently many institutions have a "no smoking" policy, which may make enforcement of this restriction easier. It is prudent to remove matches, lighters, and cigarettes from the bedside when oxygen is in use.
2. Inspect all electrical equipment in the immediate vicinity of the patient *for frayed cords and defective plugs that could cause sparks.* All electrical equipment should meet the safety standards of the health care facility.
3. Do not allow the patient to use any electrical equipment while oxygen is being administered.
4. Avoid using woolen blankets, *because they produce static electricity, another cause of sparks.*
5. Do not give electric or friction toys to children receiving oxygen in any form.
6. Take special precautions with patients in oxygen tents *because of the enclosed high concentration of oxygen.* Do not comb hair or allow electric call bells to be operated in a closed tent.

Oxygen can be stored in several ways. Most facilities have a piped-in system, with outlets on the wall by the bedside; gas flow is adjusted by means of a flowmeter that attaches to the wall outlet. This oxygen comes from a large holding tank that is usually located separate from the facility. When oxygen is not piped in, facilities use tanks that hold oxygen at more than 2000 lb of pressure per square inch. *Because of the extreme pressure,* these tanks should be handled with great care. Large tanks are chained to stands *to prevent falling and possible rupture of the valve.*

For outpatients who need intermittent therapy, smaller, portable tanks of liquid oxygen are available. These tanks can be wheeled by the patient or strapped to the body. Oxygen in this form is safe *because of its low pressure.*

Regardless of the method or appliance used, oxygen should always be turned on and checked before you administer it to a patient. *All oxygen is under pressure, and regulators and flowmeters do malfunction, so each time oxygen is to be started on a patient, check all equipment first.*

The physician usually writes an order for oxygen

that includes the date and time, the flow or concentration of oxygen to be delivered, and the type of equipment to be used. If at any time you assess that a patient is in a state of hypoxia (lacking oxygen), you can administer oxygen without a doctor's order, notifying the physician later. Such a decision requires skilled nursing judgment. Frequently a physician orders oxygen prn (as needed), so that the nurse can start or discontinue administration according to the patient's needs. This order may be written to give a variable amount of oxygen (i.e., up to 5 L) to maintain hemoglobin oxygen saturation at a specific level (i.e., 92%). In this instance, the nurse would measure hemoglobin saturation using pulse oximetry. Then the oxygen would be started, increasing the flow rate at intervals until the desired saturation is reached.

FLOWMETER

A flowmeter is a device that attaches to the oxygen outlet *to adjust the amount of oxygen being delivered* (Figure 40–1). Two types of flowmeters are available: mercury ball and gauge. Both types register the number of liters delivered per minute.

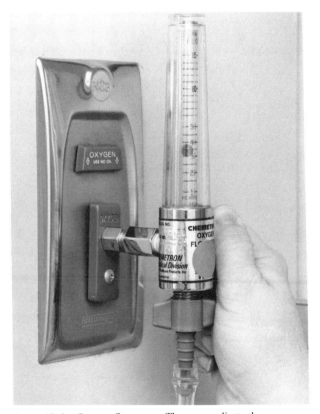

Figure 40–1. Oxygen flowmeter. The nurse adjusts the flowmeter, which registers the number of liters delivered per minute.

REGULATOR

An additional device, called a regulator, is attached to the valve of a tank of compressed gas (oxygen or air) *to reduce the pressure to a safe, functional working level.* The amount of gas registers on the gauge in pounds per square inch or PSI. When the tank is almost empty, the needle points to a red area, *warning that the tank must be replaced shortly.*

HUMIDIFICATION

The nasal mucosa is well designed to moisten air that moves through the nose to the lungs. The question of when additional moistening of inspired air or oxygen is necessary is an important one. *Anytime that oxygen is administered through a tracheostomy or through an endotracheal tube, so that the normal moistening mechanism is bypassed, humidification of the inspired air and oxygen is essential.*

Some experts believe that when oxygen is administered through the normal breathing route, humidification is unnecessary (Petty, 1982). Others believe that humidification is always important as a precautionary measure *to decrease the drying effect on the oronasal mucosa.*

Humidification is provided by containers of sterile water, which may be prefilled and disposable. They are attached to the oxygen delivery equipment. Oxygen flows through them and picks up moisture. The water must be sterile *to prevent infection from organisms that can grow in a moist environment.* Each facility has a policy on how frequently the container and the water are changed. Changing the container every 24 hours is common. Sterile water is added whenever the water level is low.

GENERAL PROCEDURE FOR ADMINISTERING OXYGEN

Assessment

1. Check the physician's order. If the patient's respiratory status is such that the patient is in danger, proceed with administering oxygen and obtain an order as soon as possible. Be cautious in administering oxygen to a patient with chronic obstructive pulmonary disease. A flow rate of greater than 2 L/min may cause the patient to stop breathing.
2. Assess the patient's immediate respiratory status. If the patient is anxious, have someone stay with the patient while you assess availability of equipment.

3. Identify the type of oxygen equipment and oxygen source in your facility.

Planning

4. Wash your hands *for infection control.*
5. Plan for any assistance needed. Often patients who are "oxygen hungry" become extremely restless and even disoriented. You may need a person to assist you *to ensure the patient's safety.*
6. Choose the appropriate equipment for the method of oxygen administration ordered. In an emergency, choose the method that best meets the patient's needs. For example, in some situations a breathing mask is necessary, whereas in others, when the patient is alert and in mild distress, a nasal cannula is sufficient and more comfortable. Obtain a flowmeter if one is not already attached to the wall outlet or tank.
7. Check the immediate environment carefully for any potential source of fire or sparks, such as smokers, electrical equipment, frayed cords. Eliminate any possible risk or, if necessary, move the patient to a safer area for oxygen administration.

Implementation

8. Identify the patient *to be sure you are performing the procedure for the correct patient.*
9. Carefully and calmly explain what you are going to do. Assure the patient that your actions will provide more comfort and that trying to relax and breathe more slowly and deeply helps.
10. Attach the oxygen supply tube to the mask, catheter, or cannula. Then turn on the oxygen and test the flow.
11. Follow the particular procedure for the equipment you are using, as outlined below in Methods of Administration.
12. Stay with the patient until you are sure the proper flow rate is maintained and the patient is calm enough to be left alone safely. Holding

the patient's hand is often very useful and comforting.

13. Assess the patient's breathing. Check the position of the mask, catheter, or cannula, and make any necessary adjustments.
14. Explain safety precautions to the patient and any family or visitors present. (Review Safety, above.)
15. Assess the patient's nose and mouth, and provide oronasal care. *Because oxygen dries the mucous membranes,* it is good nursing practice to administer frequent oronasal care to any patient receiving oxygen therapy. You can do this before you initiate oxygen therapy if the patient's respiratory status allows.
16. Post an "oxygen in use" sign on the patient's door.
17. Wash your hands.

Evaluation

18. Evaluate using the following criteria:
    a. Breathing pattern regular and at normal rate.
    b. Pink color in nail beds, lips, conjunctiva of eyes.
    c. No disorientation, confusion, difficulty with cognition.
    d. Patient resting comfortably.
    e. Laboratory measurement of arterial oxygen concentration (PaO_2) or hemoglobin oxygen saturation within normal limits.

Documentation

19. Record the following in a narrative progress note or on a flow sheet:
    a. Date and time oxygen started.
    b. Method of delivery.
    c. Specific oxygen concentration or flow rate in liters per minute.
    d. Subjective and objective observations of patient.
    e. Notification of the physician if appropriate.
20. Add oronasal care to the Nursing Care Plan.

DATE/TIME	
2/14/95 8:00 AM	Complained of mild dyspnea on ambulation. Respirations 34 and shallow after 30 min rest. O₂ at 3 L/min. started by cannula per standing order. Dr. Wilson notified. ———— S. Lester, SN

Example of Progress Notes Using Narrative Format

DATE/TIME	
3/7/95	*Impaired gas exchange; Dyspnea on exertion.*
1215	S *"Walking makes me short of breath."*
	O *Respirations 34 and shallow after 30 min rest period.*
	A *Dyspnea unrelieved by rest.*
	P *Administer O₂ 3 L/min by cannula per standing order.*
	Dr. Wilson notified.
	J. Hampton, SN

Example of Progress Notes Using SOAP Format

METHODS OF ADMINISTRATION

The administration of oxygen can be divided into two classifications. *Low flow oxygen systems* provide only part of the patient's total inspired air. Generally speaking they are more comfortable for the patient, but the delivery of oxygen varies with the breathing pattern of the patient. *High flow oxygen systems* provide the total inspired atmosphere to the patient. There is consistent oxygen delivery, which can be regulated precisely and does not vary with the patient's breathing pattern.

For each oxygen administration method discussed, except the self-inflating breathing bag and mask, steps 10 and 11 of the General Procedure are presented specific to that method. The detailed procedures, which include all the steps of the General Procedure as well as the individualized steps 10 and 11, are given in the Performance Checklist.

Nasal Cannula

The nasal cannula (also called nasal prongs) is the most common method of administering oxygen, *because it is effective, easy to apply, and comfortable for the patient. The patient receiving oxygen through a nasal cannula is able to communicate easily, to eat, and to engage in activities of daily living. These are all important factors in choosing this method of administration.* The nasal cannula is a low-flow system.

Although patients often mouth-breathe and appear as if they are not receiving the oxygen, they do receive a consistent supply. *The oxygen flows into the nose, and the entire upper airway (nose, oronasal pharynx, and mouth) becomes a reservoir for oxygen. In addition, some of the oxygen tends to flow down over the mouth, because it is heavier than air. Thus, when the patient breathes in, the inspired air provides a significant oxygen concentration.* The exact concentration inspired is determined by the interaction of the liter flow of oxygen,

the respiratory rate and pattern, and the volume of each inspired breath. Oxygen by nasal cannula may be given at 1–6 L/min and provides 22% to 50% oxygen in the inspired air. An excess of 6 L/min does not increase the oxygen delivery. It does increase the drying of mucous membranes and air swallowing, however. Oxygen by nasal cannula is most commonly used in low flow rates of 2 or 3 L/min.

Implementation
10. Attach the oxygen supply tube to the distal end of the nasal cannula.
    a. Allow 3–5 L oxygen to flow through the tubing *to make certain the equipment is working properly.* With flow rates over 4 L/min a humidifier must be used.
    b. Hold the cannula to the patient's face, and gently insert the prongs into the nostrils.
    c. Adjust straps either behind the head or around the ears and under the chin, and tighten to comfort (Figure 40–2).
    d. Adjust the flow rate to the ordered level.
    e. Pad the area where the straps rub the top of the ears, if necessary.

Nasal Catheter

The nasal catheter, a low flow oxygen system, is rarely used *because it can irritate a patient's nostrils, is unpleasant to have inserted, and must be changed every 8 hours.* If you need to insert a nasal catheter, measure from the tip of the patient's nose to the earlobe *to ascertain how far to insert the tube* and use water soluble lubricant *so that it is not hazardous if a small amount accidentally enters the lungs.*

Oxygen Masks

If is often necessary to use oxygen masks *to provide patients with adequate oxygen therapy* (Figure 40–3). There are, however, several disadvantages to their

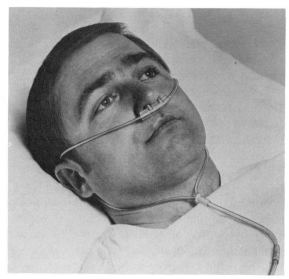

Figure 40–2. Nasal cannula. The patient can communicate easily, eat, and engage in activities of daily living while receiving oxygen.
(*Courtesy Ohio Medical Products, Madison, Wisconsin*)

use. The mask interferes with the patient's ability to communicate. It must be removed when eating, drinking, and taking medications and it makes some individuals claustrophobic. In addition, *because they are uncomfortable for many patients,* masks are not consistently left in place, thus making it impossible to guarantee the percentage of oxygen actually received by the patient.

The *simple mask* (or rebreathing mask) is a low-flow system. It has side vents and provides a reservoir over the face into which oxygen flows, so the patient breathes in air with a higher concentration of oxygen. It is usually used on a short-term basis when an ox-

ygen concentration of 30% to 60% is desired. (Oxygen dose is often abbreviated as FiO_2, which means fraction of inspired oxygen. Guidelines for estimating FiO_2 with simple masks are shown in Table 40–1.) This requires a flow rate of 6–8 L/min. The actual percentage of oxygen received by the patient depends on the patient's tidal volume, respiratory rate, the fit of the mask as well as the liter flow. *Because the patient breathes out into the same reservoir,* the carbon dioxide content of the inspired air tends to increase. This may actually stimulate respirations. However, *if the patient retains excess carbon dioxide,* this type of mask is contraindicated. The flow rate of 6–8 L/min assists in flushing CO_2 from the mask.

The *nonrebreathing mask,* a high flow system, has a bag attached to the bottom and can deliver 50% to 100% oxygen. The oxygen flows into the bag and accumulates there as a reservoir. When the patient breathes out, a special valve between the bag and the mask closes, and exhaled air exits through the vents in the side of the mask. When the person breathes in, the valve opens so that the inspired air comes from the bag and has a high concentration of oxygen. This overcomes the problem of excess carbon dioxide in the inspired air and prevents room air from diluting the oxygen. A flow rate of 12–15 L/min may be needed to keep the bag inflated.

The *Venturi mask,* another high flow system, is designed to deliver oxygen at a specific percentage between 24% and 40%. Pure oxygen delivered at a high rate flows past special vents, and the "Venturi effect" causes this oxygen to mix with the room air at a predictable level. The patient, therefore, receives a constant oxygen concentration, regardless of the rate or depth of respiration. A Venturi mask can be used with or without aerosol.

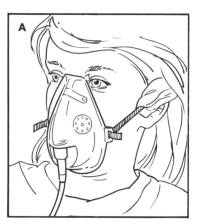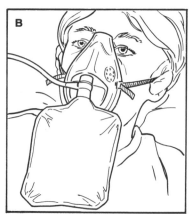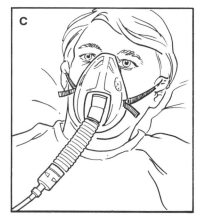

Figure 40–3. Oxygen masks. **A:** Simple mask. **B:** Nonrebreathing mask. **C:** Venturi mask.

Table 40–1 Guidelines for Estimating FiO₂ With Oxygen Masks

100% Oxygen Flow Rate in Liters	FiO₂
5–6	40%
6–7	50%
7–8	60%

Implementation

10. Attach the oxygen supply tube to the mask.
    a. Regulate the oxygen flow. With the nonrebreathing mask, be sure the bag is inflated before placing the mask over the patient's mouth and nose.
    b. Place the mask against the face, over the mouth and nose, and fit it securely, shaping the metal band on the mask to the bridge of the nose *to prevent leakage*.
    c. Adjust the elastic band around the patient's head and tighten. If the mask is not snug against the face, you may need to place gauze pads over the cheek area *to ensure a tight fit*.

Oxygen Tents

Tents are seldom used now, except for pediatric patients, because of several disadvantages. Some patients experience an unpleasant closed-in feeling when they are in an oxygen tent. They cannot move about freely in bed without disturbing the tucked edges. Tents require much more oxygen to maintain the desired concentration than other methods and are therefore more hazardous and costly to operate. Another disadvantage is the difficulty of maintaining a comfortable temperature for a patient in the tent. Tents are difficult to clean, although disposable canopies are now available.

For infants and young children, however, oxygen and humidity tents are commonly used. The mist tent or croup tent delivers cool saturated air *to keep the respiratory tract well hydrated* and is often used for patients with croup, pneumonia, or other upper respiratory diseases. There are several varieties of equipment. For larger children the "tent" consists of a transparent plastic canopy that is suspended from a frame. A high-output pneumatic nebulizer and reservoir and a high pressure hose with an oxygen or compressed air adapter are attached. A flowmeter and tubing may be needed for "bleeding in" oxygen and sterile distilled water will be necessary to mois-

turize the air or the oxygen. For small babies and infants a smaller piece of equipment constructed of hard plastic with transparent sides is used for the same purpose. One brand name is Croupette. Follow the manufacturer's instructions for the specific equipment used in your facility.

Implementation

10. Prepare the "tent" by attaching the metal frame to the bedsprings of the crib and

Home Care

Many patients require oxygen therapy at home. These patients or a family member must be taught the self-administration of oxygen as well as the care of the equipment. A "no smoking" sign should be posted on the outside door. It may, however, be more difficult to get people to cooperate with this restriction in the home than in a health care facility. Most people receiving oxygen at home use nasal prongs, but some will have had the option to choose transtracheal oxygen therapy. A small catheter is inserted into the trachea under local anesthesia. It is threaded underneath the patient's clothing to the waist where it is attached to the portable oxygen source. There are several advantages over the use of nasal prongs:

1. *Because the oxygen runs directly into the trachea,* a low flow rate is satisfactory. The therapy is, therefore, less costly.
2. Also *because the oxygen runs directly into the trachea,* there is no oxygen in the ambient air, making safety issues less of a problem.
3. *The catheter can be completely or partially covered by clothing.* The therapy is thus more socially acceptable and aesthetically pleasing.

The catheter does need to be irrigated on a daily basis with normal saline. This removes any secretions on the inside of the tubing. It is then flushed with air *to dry it*. The small insertion site is routinely cleaned in the bath or shower. Any secretions can be removed with a cotton-tipped applicator moistened with hydrogen peroxide.

suspending the canopy from the frame. Be certain that all access ports are closed.

- **a.** Tuck all sides of the canopy securely under the crib mattress.
- **b.** Be sure that the ice trough is filled with ice and the water jar with sterile water up to the indicator lines.
- **c.** Attach the tent to the oxygen or compressed air source.
- **d.** Turn on the oxygen and adjust the flow rate to 15 L/min for about 5 minutes.
- **e.** Open the valve that controls the mist output. Check the doctor's orders to see if it is to be left open continuously, left partially open, or opened intermittently.
- **f.** Adjust the oxygen flow rate to the ordered level of oxygen after 5 minutes.
- **g.** Place the child in the tent.

Damp bed linen and clothing should be changed as needed *to prevent the child from chilling.* Monitor the equipment and the child's response to treatment on a regular basis. Follow the policies and procedures in your facility.

Self-Inflating Breathing Bag and Mask

This device provides artificial ventilation to the person who is in respiratory arrest or is dependent on a ventilator for breathing. A face mask, which covers the mouth and nose and has a soft rim to make an airtight seal, is attached to a firm rubber or plastic bag. Manual compression of the bag forces air into the patient's nose and mouth. The breathing bag can be attached to oxygen in order to provide breaths with a higher oxygen concentration, or room air can fill the bag.

The self-inflating breathing bag and mask can be used to provide deep breaths of high oxygen concentration before suctioning, for rescue breathing, or as part of cardiopulmonary resuscitation. Humidification is not usually used with this method.

1. Apply the mask snugly over the patient's nose and mouth. Either hold the mask in place manually or fasten straps behind the patient's head.
2. Compress the bag as completely as possible to force air into the patient's nose and mouth.
3. Release the bag to allow expiration. Count 1, 2, 3, 4 to allow adequate time for expiration.
4. Repeat steps 2 and 3 in a rhythmic pattern to provide ventilation at a rate of 12 breaths/min or for the desired number of deep breaths. (See Module 32, Emergency Resuscitation Procedures, for complete directions for emergency resuscitation.)

LONG-TERM CARE

Residents in long-term care facilities may also require oxygen therapy—some continuously and some intermittently. Portable oxygen units can be attached to wheelchairs for residents who are not ambulatory and require constant oxygen. Care should be provided to the resident so that fatigue is prevented and mobility maintained. Techniques to decrease exertion might include the use of a bedside commode, small meals, or assistance with feeding and a calm, low-stress environment. The same safety considerations apply in long-term care as in acute care.

Reference

Petty, T. L. (1982). *Intensive and rehabilitation respiratory care* (3rd ed.). Philadelphia: Lea and Febiger.

Performance Checklist

Administering Oxygen	Unsat	Needs More Practice	Sat	Comments
Assessment				
1. Check physician's order or proceed in an emergency.				
2. Assess immediate respiratory status.				
3. Know oxygen equipment and source.				
Planning				
4. Wash your hands.				
5. Plan for any assistance needed.				
6. Choose appropriate equipment for patient's specific needs.				
7. Check environment for safety.				
Implementation				
8. Identify the patient.				
9. Explain what you are going to do.				
10. Attach oxygen supply tube to device you are using, turn on oxygen, and test flow.				
11. Follow procedure for equipment you are using.				
12. Stay with patient until safe to leave.				
13. Assess patient's breathing and adjust equipment if necessary.				
14. Explain safety precautions to patient and family or visitors present.				
15. Assess condition of nose and mouth and provide oronasal care if needed.				
16. Post an "oxygen in use" sign on the patient's door.				
17. Wash your hands.				
Evaluation				
18. Evaluate using the following criteria: a. Breathing pattern regular and at normal rate.				

Administering Oxygen *(Continued)*	Unsat	Needs More Practice	Sat	Comments
b. Pink color in nail beds, lips, conjunctiva of eyes.				
c. No disorientation, confusion, difficulty with cognition.				
d. Patient resting comfortably.				
e. Laboratory measurement of arterial oxygen (PaO_2), or hemoglobin oxygen saturation within normal limits.				
Documentation				
19. Record on the patient's chart: a. Date and time oxygen started.				
b. Method of delivery.				
c. Specific oxygen concentration or flow rate in liters per minute.				
d. Subjective and objective observations of patient.				
20. Add oronasal care to Nursing Care Plan.				
Nasal Cannula				
Assessment				
1. Follow Checklist steps 1–3 of the General Procedure for Administering Oxygen (check physician's order, assess respiratory status, and know oxygen equipment and source).				
Planning				
2. Follow Checklist steps 4–7 of the General Procedure (wash your hands, plan for any assistance needed, choose appropriate equipment, and check environment for safety).				
Implementation				
3. Follow Checklist steps 8 and 9 of the General Procedure (identify the patient and explain what you are going to do).				
4. Attach oxygen supply tube to distal end of nasal cannula. a. Allow 3–5 L oxygen to flow through tubing.				

Nasal Cannula *(Continued)*	Unsat	Needs More Practice	Sat	Comments
b. Hold cannula to patient's face and gently insert prongs into nostrils.				
c. Adjust straps and tighten to comfort.				
d. Adjust flow rate.				
e. Pad top of ears as needed.				
5. Follow Checklist steps 12–17 of the General Procedure (stay with patient until safe to leave, assess patient's breathing and adjust equipment if necessary, explain safety precautions, assess condition of nose and mouth and provide oronasal care, post an "oxygen in use" sign, and wash your hands).				

Evaluation

6. Evaluate using the criteria in Checklist step 18 of the General Procedure (breathing pattern, skin color, mental status, comfort, and oxygenation).				

Documentation

7. Document as in Checklist steps 19 and 20 of the General Procedure (date and time oxygen started, method of delivery, specific oxygen concentration or flow rate in liters per minute, subjective/objective observations of patient, notification of physician if appropriate, and add oronasal care to the Nursing Care Plan.				

Oxygen Masks

Assessment

1. Follow Checklist steps 1–3 of the General Procedure for Administering Oxygen (check physician's order, assess respiratory status, and know oxygen equipment and source).				

Planning

2. Follow Checklist steps 4–7 of the General Procedure (wash your hands, plan for any assistance needed, choose appropriate equipment, and check environment for safety).				

Oxygen Masks (Continued)	Unsat	Needs More Practice	Sat	Comments
Implementation				
3. Follow Checklist steps 8 and 9 of the General Procedure (identify the patient and explain what you are going to do).				
4. Attach oxygen supply tube to mask. a. Regulate oxygen flow.				
b. Fit mask over mouth and nose.				
c. Adjust elastic band around patient's head.				
5. Follow Checklist steps 12–17 of the General Procedure (stay with patient until safe to leave, assess patient's breathing and adjust equipment if necessary, explain safety precautions, assess condition of nose and mouth and provide oronasal care, post an "oxygen in use" sign, and wash your hands).				
Evaluation				
6. Evaluate using the criteria in Checklist step 18 of the General Procedure (breathing pattern, skin color, mental status, comfort, and oxygenation).				
Documentation				
7. Document as in Checklist steps 19 and 20 of the General Procedure (date and time oxygen started, method of delivery, specific oxygen concentration or flow rate in liters per minute, subjective/objective observations of patient, notification of physician if appropriate, and add oronasal care to the Nursing Care Plan.				
Oxygen/Humidity Tent				
Assessment				
1. Follow Checklist steps 1–3 of the General Procedure for Administering Oxygen (check physician's order, assess respiratory status, and know oxygen equipment and source).				
Planning				
2. Follow Checklist steps 4–7 of the General Procedure (wash your hands, plan for any assistance needed, choose appropriate equipment, and check environment for safety).				

Oxygen/Humidity Tent (Continued)	Unsat	Needs More Practice	Sat	Comments
Implementation				
3. Follow Checklist steps 8 and 9 of the General Procedure (identify the patient and explain what you are going to do).				
4. Prepare the tent (attach metal frame to crib, suspend canopy from frame, close access ports). a. Tuck all sides of canopy under mattress.				
b. Fill ice trough and water jar to indicator lines.				
c. Attach tent to oxygen or compressed air source.				
d. Turn on oxygen and adjust flow rate to 15 L/min for 5 minutes.				
e. Open valve that controls mist output and follow doctor's orders.				
f. Adjust oxygen flow rate to ordered level.				
g. Place child in tent.				
5. Follow Checklist steps 12–17 of the General Procedure (stay with patient until safe to leave, assess patient's breathing and adjust equipment if necessary, explain safety precautions, assess condition of nose and mouth and provide oronasal care, post an "oxygen in use" sign, and wash your hands).				
Evaluation				
6. Evaluate using the criteria in Checklist step 18 of the General Procedure (breathing pattern, skin color, mental status, comfort, and oxygenation).				
Documentation				
7. Document as in Checklist steps 19 and 20 of the General Procedure (date and time oxygen started, method of delivery, specific oxygen concentration or flow rate in liters per minute, subjective/objective observations of patient, notification of physician if appropriate, and add oronasal care to the Nursing Care Plan.				

Self-Inflating Breathing Bag and Mask	Unsat	Needs More Practice	Sat	Comments
1. Apply mask snugly over patient's nose and mouth.				
2. Compress bag.				
3. Release bag and count to four.				
4. Repeat sequence at rate of 12 breaths/min or for desired number of breaths.				

Quiz

Short-Answer Question

1. List four methods of delivering oxygen.

   a. _____

   b. _____

   c. _____

   d. _____

Multiple-Choice Questions

_____ 2. Oxygen is potentially dangerous because it

   a. burns rapidly.   c. supports combustion.
   b. is explosive.   d. combines with nitrogen

_____ 3. Regardless of the method used, it is important to test and regulate oxygen flow before applying to the patient because

   a. it is easier to observe the flow rates.
   b. it guards the patient from the danger of a malfunction.
   c. it guards the patient from an explosion.
   d. it limits the amount of oxygen intake.

_____ 4. Oxygen flow (liters per minute)

   a. should never exceed 3 L/min.
   b. should remain under 8 L/min.
   c. should be changed every 8 hours.
   d. is determined by the delivery method and the physician's order.

_____ 5. The self-inflating breathing bag is most likely to be used

   a. for routine oxygen administration.
   b. for rescue breathing.
   c. when an oxygen/humidity tent is not available.
   d. instead of a nonrebreathing mask.

_____ 6. The preferred method of oxygen/humidity treatment for infants and small children is the

   a. Venturi mask with aerosol.
   b. nasal cannula.
   c. croup tent.
   d. nasal catheter.

_____ 7. Frequent oronasal care should be given to the patient receiving oxygen primarily because

   a. of the patient's high anxiety level.
   b. oxygen dries mucous membranes.
   c. oxygen is irritating to the skin.
   d. secretions are increased.

_____ 8. Patients who receive oxygen therapy need explanations and reassurance because (1) the patient or family may think the patient is seriously ill when this is not so; (2) the patient may feel claustrophobic; (3) the patient has had no previous experience with it; (4) some oxygen appliances are uncomfortable to wear.

a. 1 only   c. 1, 2, and 4 only
b. 2 and 3 only   d. All of the above

_____ 9. A technique to decrease exertion in the long-term care resident on oxygen therapy is

a. serving the resident two meals per day.
b. having the resident use the bedpan instead of the bathroom.
c. providing a high-stress environment.
d. assisting the resident with eating.

_____ 10. A disadvantage of transtracheal oxygen therapy is

a. it is less safe.
b. it is more expensive.
c. it is less socially acceptable.
d. it requires a surgical incision.

Module 41

Respiratory Care Procedures

Module Contents

Rationale for the Use of This Skill
Nursing Diagnosis
General Procedure for Respiratory Care
  Assessment
  Planning
  Implementation
  Evaluation
  Documentation
Assisting the Patient With Deep Breathing
  Procedure for Deep Breathing
  Mechanisms for Encouraging Deep
    Breathing
    Incentive Spirometers
    Intermittent Positive Pressure Breathing
    (IPPB)

Teaching the Patient to Cough Productively
  Procedure for Coughing
Performing Postural Drainage
  Procedure for Postural Drainage
    Assessment
    Planning
    Implementation
    Evaluation
    Documentation
  Problems
Performing Percussion and Vibration
Long-term Care
Home Care

Prerequisites

1. *Successful completion of the following modules:*

VOLUME 1

Module 1 An Approach to Nursing Skills
Module 2 Basic Infection Control
Module 3 Safety
Module 4 Basic Body Mechanics
Module 5 General Assessment Overview
Module 6 Documentation
Module 8 Moving the Patient in Bed and Positioning
Module 13 Inspection, Palpation, Auscultation, and Percussion

2. *A review of the anatomy and physiology of the respiratory system, paying special attention to the physiology of the cough reflex.*

Overall Objective

To assist patients effectively with deep breathing, coughing, postural drainage, percussion, and vibration as necessary in their individual situations.

Specific Learning Objectives

	Know Facts and Principles	Apply Facts and Principles	Demonstrate Ability	Evaluate Performance
1. *Deep breathing*	State reasons for deep breathing. Identify patient situations in which deep breathing is needed. Describe procedure for deep breathing. State purposes for incentive spirometer and intermittent positive pressure breathing.	Given a patient situation, identify when deep breathing is needed.	In the clinical setting, assist patient to deep breathe effectively.	Evaluate effectiveness of deep breathing by checking depth of patient's respiration (identifying extent of rise and fall of abdomen and chest as breath is taken).
2. *Coughing*	Define *cough*. State reasons for encouraging patient to cough. Identify patient situations in which coughing is needed. Describe procedure for effective coughing.	Given a patient situation, identify when coughing is needed.	In the clinical setting, assist patient to cough effectively.	Evaluate effectiveness by checking for movement of secretions.
3. *Postural drainage*	Define *postural drainage*. Identify patient situations in which postural drainage is used. Describe positions used for postural drainage for all lung areas. Describe common problems of postural drainage.	Given a patient situation, identify which position for postural drainage would be most effective. Given a patient situation, identify problems occurring.	In the clinical setting: a. Assist patient in postural drainage. b. Recognize problems occurring during postural drainage and decide appropriate course of action related to problem.	Evaluate effectiveness of postural drainage by auscultation of lungs. Validate decision with instructor.

(continued)

Specific Learning Objectives *(Continued)*

	Know Facts and Principles	Apply Facts and Principles	Demonstrate Ability	Evaluate Performance
4. *Percussion and vibration*	State purpose of percussion and vibration. Describe procedure for percussion and vibration.	Identify situations where percussion and vibration might be helpful.	In the clinical setting, perform percussion and vibration correctly.	Evaluate own performance using Performance Checklist. Evaluate by checking amount of secretions raised.
5. *Documentation*	State information to be recorded regarding respiratory care procedures.		Record appropriate information when doing respiratory care procedures.	Evaluate with instructor.

Learning Activities

1. Review the Specific Learning Objectives.
2. Read the material on respiration and the chapter on health teaching in Ellis and Nowlis, *Nursing: A Human Needs Approach,* or comparable chapters in another text.
3. Look up the module vocabulary terms in the Glossary.
4. Read through the module and mentally practice the skills.
5. Using the module directions as a guide:
   a. Practice deep breathing until you can do deep abdominal breathing easily.
   b. Practice coughing until you can create an effective cough.
   c. Practice postural drainage at home on your own bed.
      (1) Use pillows to position yourself in a moderately slanted position.
      (2) Try the jackknife position.
      (3) Consider the fatigue and discomfort caused by these positions.
6. In the practice setting:
   Obtain a partner. Each of you, in turn, will be the patient while your partner is the nurse. Practice each skill as though you were instructing a patient with no previous knowledge or skill. The person representing the patient should do exactly as told, not what he or she knows to be correct.
   a. Teach one another deep breathing.
   b. Evaluate one another, using the Performance Checklist.
   c. Teach one another to cough effectively.
   d. Evaluate one another, using the Performance Checklist.
   e. Assist one another in postural drainage.
   f. While the "patient" is in each position, use percussion and vibration over the area being drained.
   g. When you can perform all skills correctly, ask your instructor to check your performance.
7. In the clinical setting:
   a. Ask your instructor for an opportunity to observe respiratory care being given.
   b. Ask your instructor for opportunities to use these skills.

Vocabulary

abdominal (diaphragmatic) breathing	diaphragm	lingula	postural hypotension
alveoli	expectorate	lobe	segment
atelectasis	expiration	lung	sputum
auscultation	gatched bed	mucous	Trendelenburg position
bronchiole	hyperventilation	mucus	vibration
cough	hypoventilation	nebulizer	
	inspiration	percussion	
	intermittent		

Respiratory Care Procedures

Rationale for the Use of This Skill
Respiratory care procedures prevent and treat respiratory complications that may occur as a result of bed rest, immobility, and a variety of illnesses. They are effective because they assist in inflating all alveoli and in removing secretions that are a place for microbial growth and that might interfere with gas exchange. Respiratory care departments may be responsible for some of this care but the nurse is always responsible for assessing, monitoring, and evaluating the patient's respiratory status and may be responsible for all respiratory care including teaching these measures.[1]

▶ *Nursing Diagnosis*

> These procedures are used for the patient who has the nursing diagnosis "High risk for altered respiratory function."

GENERAL PROCEDURE FOR RESPIRATORY CARE

Assessment
1. Count the individual's respiratory rate and assess for depth and chest expansion.
2. Auscultate the patient's lungs, especially noting areas where there are diminished breath sounds and areas where moisture is present.
3. Assess the individual's activity pattern.
4. Identify whether the patient is at risk for respiratory problems due to bed rest, inactivity, or surgical treatment.
5. Check the patient for pain or other factors *that may limit respiratory effort.*

Planning
6. Plan for pain relief, if necessary, before performing any respiratory care procedure.
7. Choose the appropriate respiratory care procedure. Some procedures require a physician's order. Deep breathing and coughing may be initiated by the nurse.
8. Plan an appropriate time for performing the

procedure as well as how often the procedure should be repeated.

Implementation
9. Wash your hands *for infection control.*
10. Identify the patient *to be sure you are performing the procedure on the correct patient.*
11. Explain to the patient why you are concerned about his or her respiratory status in a way that does not increase anxiety. Tell the patient which measures are necessary *to prevent or alleviate problems.*
12. Carry out the specific procedure as outlined below.

Evaluation
13. Evaluate, using the following criteria:
    a. Respiratory rate equal to or less than rate before procedure.
    b. Chest expansion equal to or greater than before procedure.
    c. Lungs clear to auscultation.
    d. Patient resting comfortably.

Documentation
14. On a flow sheet or in the nurses' progress notes, record the respiratory care procedure performed.
15. Note any changes in respiratory status or secretions produced.
16. Document the patient's response as evaluated.

Each of the following respiratory care procedures details step 12 of the general procedure specific to that technique. The detailed procedures, which include all of the steps of the general procedure as well as the individualized step 12, are found in the Performance Checklist.

ASSISTING THE PATIENT WITH DEEP BREATHING

All alveoli are not equally expanded during each breath taken. Normal respiration includes occasional deep breaths *which serve to fully expand all alveoli and encourage the movement of secretions.* Whenever a person is bedridden or otherwise immobile, continuous shallow respirations are common. This tends to encourage the retention of secretions and the collapse of alveoli (atelectasis).

Deep breathing is a planned part of the nursing care of every immobilized patient, especially those who have had increased secretions (persons who have inhaled respiratory anesthetics or who have respiratory disease).

---

[1] You will note that rationale for action is emphasized throughout the module by the use of italics.

For patients who have undergone abdominal or chest surgery, deep breathing may be difficult and even painful. You will have to provide a great deal of assistance and support when you help these patients to deep breathe.

PROCEDURE FOR DEEP BREATHING

12. Assist the patient with deep breathing as outlined below:

a. Instruct the patient. *Because the patient must carry out the procedure, he or she must understand what should be done and why. A person who understands and accepts the importance of deep breathing is more likely to cooperate and participate in the exercise.* As part of the instruction, you should demonstrate proper deep breathing for the patient. Remember to use the principles of health teaching as you plan for the patient's instruction.

b. Relieve the patient's pain. *A patient who has a surgical wound feels pain when moving the muscles that were cut during surgery. You can minimize this pain by holding the incisional area firmly, decreasing movement.* This is called *splinting.* You can spread your hands and hold them firmly over the incision, or the patient can hold the incision with his or her own hands, or a pillow can be held firmly over the incisional area to splint it. It may also be necessary to arrange for pain medication. Make sure that it is given in time to take effect before you begin the procedure.

c. Position the patient *for maximum expansion of the lungs.* To accomplish this, the chest should not be constricted. Having the patient sit on the edge of the bed or in a chair is ideal, but deep breathing can be done in any position necessitated by the patient's condition.

d. Have the patient inspire slowly. *This allows for more comfortable alveolar expansion. (Slow movement usually creates less discomfort than rapid movement does.)* It is helpful if you count slowly to two during inspiration.

e. *Because normal expiration is twice as long as inspiration,* have the patient expire slowly while you count to four. *This preserves the normal inspiratory-expiratory ratio and*

encourages maximum filling and emptying of the alveoli.

f. Watch the patient for chest and abdominal expansion. *Maximum expansion of the lungs occurs when both abdomen and chest expand during inspiration.* This is called *abdominal, or diaphragmatic, breathing. The expansion of the abdomen is caused by the diaphragm moving downward, displacing abdominal contents to allow complete lung expansion.* Observe the patient's breathing to see *whether complete lung expansion occurs.*

g. Correct the patient's breathing technique as necessary *to encourage complete lung expansion.*

h. Repeat the procedure, for a total of 10 deep breaths.

i. Record on the patient's chart. Usually there is a flow sheet on which deep breathing can simply be checked off. If not, make a brief progress note indicating the time respiratory care was given and the patient's performance (whether breaths were deep, how many were taken, and the patient's response).

Mechanisms for Encouraging Deep Breathing

Incentive Spirometers. Physicians often order an incentive sperometer (IS) *to encourage the patient to breathe deeply.* Several models of incentive spirometers are available, and *all have been developed to encourage the patient to deep breathe* (Figure 41–1). The volume-oriented or electronic device is set so that a signal is activated when the patient achieves a prescribed inspiratory volume. The patient is instructed in deep breathing, with particular emphasis on the long inspiratory effort. The patient expires normally, and then places the mouthpiece in the mouth and inspires only through the machine. If the inspiratory volume meets the preset amount, the signal is activated. Most incentive spirometers have counters to indicate the number of deep breaths taken.

The flow-oriented or mechanical incentive spirometer has plastic chambers with movable balls similar to Ping-Pong balls. The patient inhales through the nose, exhales through the mouth, and then inhales through the mouthpiece, attempting to keep the balls at the top of the chambers for 3 seconds. The patient is usually encouraged to do this exercise 10 times every 1 or 2 hours.

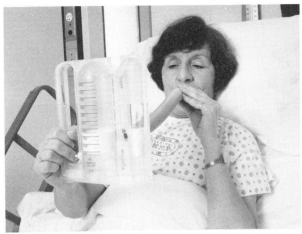

Figure 41–1. A mechanical incentive spirometer. The patient attempts to keep the balls at the top of the chambers for 3 seconds.

The incentive spirometer is based on the learning theory that immediate objective feedback about performance increases motivation to learn and results in quicker learning. When volume-oriented incentive spirometers are used, the achievement signal is set low at first, allowing the patient to master that level before moving higher. This also allows the patient to progress gradually. Spirometers are quite successful in that many patients do far more deep breathing using them.

Intermittent Positive Pressure Breathing (IPPB). The IPPB machine uses positive pressure to increase inspiration and to deliver nebulized moisture (with or without medication) deep into the lungs. Most often, IPPB is used for the patient with respiratory disease who needs to have a medication delivered to the lungs. A treatment usually lasts 5–10 minutes or as long as it takes to get all of the ordered medication delivered. In some cases, a short rest period may be needed during the treatment.

The actual procedure is specific to the brand of machine. The manufacturer provides a manual giving directions for use.

TEACHING THE PATIENT TO COUGH PRODUCTIVELY

Coughing is always combined with deep breathing, but deep breathing may be done without coughing. *Deep breathing fully expands the alveoli and enhances the normal respiratory function. Coughing raises respiratory* secretions so they do not plug the bronchioles (causing atelectasis) or provide a medium for bacterial growth. However, *coughing when the patient has no secretions to raise may collapse alveoli* and is therefore not recommended.

PROCEDURE FOR COUGHING

12. Teach the patient to cough productively as outlined below:
    a. Explain the reasons for coughing. *A patient who understands and accepts the reason for an activity is more cooperative in performing that activity.*
    b. Place the patient in a sitting position if possible. This is normally the most effective position for coughing. Other positions can be used, depending on the patient's needs.
    c. Splint, as described above in Deep Breathing, step b, if necessary.
    d. Have the patient deep breathe, following steps d and e in Deep Breathing.
    e. After the third deep breath, have the patient inspire and hold the breath 3 seconds.
    f. Have the patient expire forcefully against the closed glottis and then release the air abruptly while flexing forward. *Exhaling against the closed glottis builds up pressure, which tends to create a force that raises secretions. Flexion forward exerts abdominal pressure against the diaphragm, which increases the force of the expired air sufficiently to carry secretions.* (Use simpler language when explaining this to the patient. For example, instead of "Exhale against the closed glottis," say, "Hold your breath and then try to breathe out when your throat is closed.")
    g. Repeat for three deep coughs if possible, or repeat until mucus is expectorated. Do not prolong deep breathing and coughing, *because these actions can cause hyperventilation.* Watch for dizziness and tingling of the extremities, the most common symptoms of hyperventilation.
    h. Check the lungs by auscultation.
    i. Offer oral hygiene. *Sputum often leaves a disagreeable taste in the mouth.*
    j. Repeat deep breathing and coughing hourly as needed to clear the lungs of secretions, or as ordered.

PERFORMING POSTURAL DRAINAGE

When a large volume of secretions is present in the lungs, raising all of them by deep breathing and coughing may be impossible. *Postural drainage—positioning the patient so that the force of gravity helps drain the lung secretions*—may be required.

For most individuals, moderately slanted positions are successful in draining lungs. *Because of the branching structure of the lungs,* however, a variety of positions must be used *to drain all the lung segments adequately.*

When postural drainage is used for a patient with chronic respiratory problems but no current acute difficulty, each position needs to be held for only 15 seconds *to drain the lung segments adequately.* For a person with an acute problem, it is recommended that 5 minutes be spent initially in each position. When you have determined the position in which the majority of secretions are raised, you can shorten the time the patient spends in some positions and lengthen the time in other positions. Not all positions are necessary for every patient—*only those that drain specific affected areas.*

Postural drainage is best tolerated if done between meals, at least 2 hours after the patient has eaten, *to decrease the possibility of vomiting.* This will also allow the patient time to rest before the next meal. Even if you are not responsible for carrying out the postural drainage, you *are* responsible for coordinating all aspects of care in the patient's best interests.

The positions in the following procedure are moderate. Certain lung segments do not drain in these positions, but if the entire sequence is used, most do.

PROCEDURE FOR POSTURAL DRAINAGE

Assessment

1. Identify the specific segments of the lung to be drained. This step may be part of the physician's order, or the areas with excessive secretions may be identified by the physician in the progress notes. The areas with excessive secretions may be identified through auscultation or by checking the chest x-ray report.

   Most often, the lower lobes are drained. It is assumed that *most of the upper lobes drain in normal daily activity, but this would not be true for* a severely immobilized patient. The complex sequence is tiring and can be done with rest periods between positions. Pay particular attention to elderly patients with heart disease who may experience difficulty with the procedure.

Planning

2. Wash your hands *for infection control.*
3. Obtain pillows and a sputum cup and tissues for the patient to use for expectorated secretions. Wear clean gloves if the patient is unable to manage his or her own secretions.

Implementation

4. Identify the patient *to be sure you are performing the procedure for the correct patient.*
5. Explain to the patient the purpose and method of postural drainage, using the basic principles of health teaching.
6. Position the patient. Check the bed mechanism. Some beds can be "gatched" (raised in the middle) *to provide the correct position for postural drainage.* Some beds that cannot be gatched do have a foot section that can be lowered, in which case you can position the patient with his or her head at the foot of the bed and use the foot drop to achieve the desired position. Some beds can be placed in a headdown (Trendelenburg) position. You can use this position for postural drainage, but *raising the patient's feet may increase fatigue and is not essential to the procedure's effectiveness.* If the bed cannot be positioned properly, you will need one large or two small pillows to place under the patient's hips to provide the correct position. You will also need another pillow to support the patient in the side-lying position.
7. Drain the upper lobes.
   a. Have the patient sit up if possible. (Sitting in a fairly straight chair is ideal.) You can also raise the head of the bed to its maximum height.
   b. Have the patient lean to the right side for 5 minutes *to drain the left aspect of both upper lobes.* Support the patient with pillows if necessary.
   c. Then have the patient lean to the left side for 5 minutes *to drain the upper right lobes.* Again, support the patient with pillows if necessary.
   d. Have the patient lean forward at a 30°–45° angle and stay in this position for 5 minutes. *This position drains the posterior*

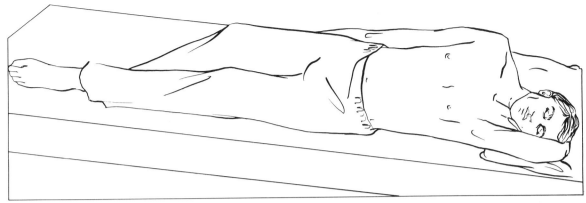

Figure 41–2. Draining the lateral basal segment of the right lower lobe. The patient lies on the left side with the head and thorax 30° to 45° down from the horizontal position.

segments of the upper lobes. Let the patient brace the elbows on the knees to maintain this position. Or you can pad an overbed table and place it in front of the patient to lean on.

e. Have the patient lean backward at a 30°– 45° angle for 5 minutes. *This position drains the anterior segments of the upper lobes.* Help the patient maintain the position by having him or her lean back in bed, with the headrest at the proper height.

f. Have the patient lie on the abdomen, back, and both sides while horizontal *to drain the remaining segments of the upper lobes.*

8. Drain the lower lobes. Use pillows or adjust the bed so that the patient's head and thorax are 30°–45° down from the horizontal position. *The 30° position is less tiring and creates fewer adverse circulatory effects than the 45° position does.*

Remember that there are six positions. Each can be achieved if the patient starts out lying on one side and gradually turns like a rotisserie. Use the same sequence of positions each time *to help you remember them easily. To identify which lung segments are drained with each position,* refer to the drawings in an anatomy text, which outline various lung segments. The patient should remain in each position for 5 minutes.

a. Have the patient lie on the left side, with the shoulders perpendicular to the bed. *This position drains the lateral basal segment of the right lower lobe* (Figure 41–2). Use pillows to support the patient, and place a small pillow under the head if essential to comfort.

b. Turn the patient halfway onto the back, so the shoulders are at a 45° angle to the bed (Figure 41–3). *This position drains the right middle lobe.* Again, use pillows to support this position.

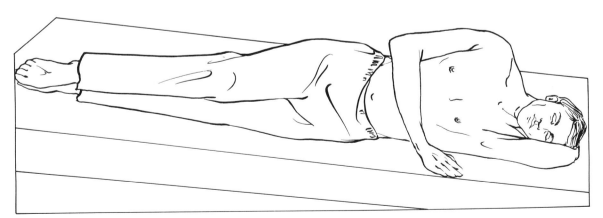

Figure 41–3. Draining the right middle lobe. The shoulders are at a 45° angle to the bed.

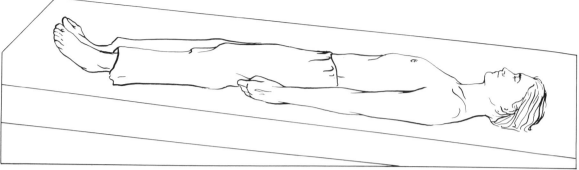

Figure 41–4. Draining the anterior basal segments of both lungs. The patient is flat on the back (supine) with thorax 30° to 45° down from the horizontal position.

c. Turn the patient flat on the back (Figure 41–4). *This position drains the anterior basal segments of the right and left lower lobes.*

d. Turn the patient halfway to the right side, so the shoulders are at a 45° angle to the bed (Figure 41–5). *This position drains the lingula of the left lower lobe.*

e. Turn the patient completely onto the right side, so the shoulders are again at a 90° angle to the bed (Figure 41–6). *This position drains the lateral basal segments of the left lower lobe.*

f. Have the patient turn onto the abdomen, with the head turned to the side (Figure 41–7). *This position drains the posterior basal segments of the lower lobes.* It is usually used last, *because secretions are often easier to cough out when the patient is on the abdomen.*

9. Have the patient cough forcefully (lying on the abdomen) *to expel secretions.*

10. Return the patient to a comfortable position and allow for a rest period. Provide mouth care when the patient so desires.

Evaluation

11. Evaluate, using the following criteria:
  a. Lungs clear to auscultation.
  b. Patient resting comfortably.

Documentation

12. On a flow sheet or in the nurses' progress notes, record the positions used for postural drainage.

13. Note any changes in respiratory status or secretions produced.

14. Document the patient's response as above.

Problems

Falling because of dizziness or fainting is a common concern when the patient is placed in postural drainage. Although this problem can occur when the patient is in the head-down position, it is more likely to occur when the patient is first returning to the normal position, *because of postural hypotension.* By changing the patient's position slowly, *you can help alleviate this problem. To protect the patient,* raise the side rails and

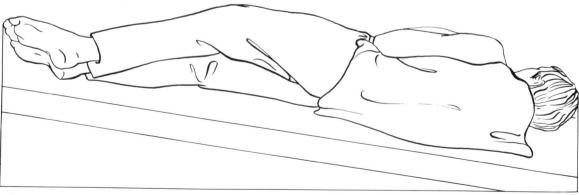

Figure 41–5. Draining the lingula of the left lower lobe. Pillows are used to support the shoulders at a 45° angle to the bed.

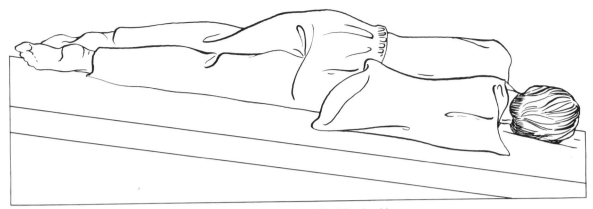

Figure 41–6. Draining the lateral basal segments of the left lower lobe. The shoulders are at a 90° angle to the bed.

make frequent observations during the procedure. Some patients cannot be left alone during the procedure, so use careful nursing judgment.

If a large volume of secretions is mobilized from the alveoli and small bronchioles at one time, a larger airway may be temporarily blocked, causing severe respiratory distress, anxiety, and fear. This experience may be so upsetting that the patient may resist future attempts at postural drainage. Explain what is happening and help the patient cough out the secretions. Support the patient with your continued presence and reassurance.

Sometimes it is necessary to use percussion (or clapping) and vibration (see below) to remove secretions. If the blockage is severe, suctioning may be required.

PERFORMING PERCUSSION AND VIBRATION

Percussion is the manual application of light blows to the chest wall. These blows are transmitted through the tissue and *help loosen secretions in the lung segment immediately below the area struck.* Percussion is done over areas that need to be drained. Percuss over a patient gown or other light clothing, not against the bare skin *to decrease friction.* While the patient is in the postural drainage position of choice, cup your hands and clap them over the chest wall (Figure 41–8). Correctly done, this action should produce a hollow sound and should not be painful for the patient. Instruct the patient to take slow deep breaths during percussion *to prevent tensing of the chest and to assist with the mobilization of secretions.*

Mechanical percussion devices that deliver percussion at a set force and rate are used by some respiratory therapists. These devices are not commonly available in nursing departments.

Vibration is performed for the same purpose as percussion and is as effective as percussion if done correctly. Ask the patient to exhale after a deep inspiration and vibrate as the patient exhales. Place your hands firmly against the chest wall, one over the other, and keeping your arms and shoulders straight, vibrate your hands back and forth rapidly (Figure

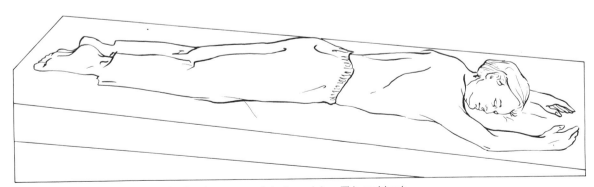

Figure 41–7. Draining the posterior basal segments of the lower lobes. This position is also used for coughing out secretions.

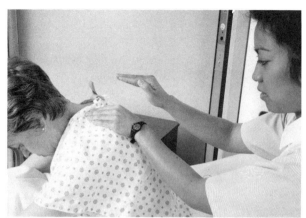

Figure 41–8. The hands are cupped and percussion is performed to help loosen mucus.

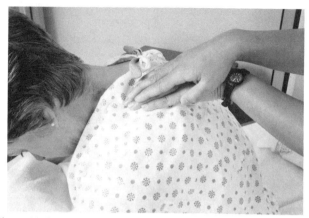

Figure 41–9. Vibration. The hands are placed firmly on the chest wall and vibration is performed while the patient exhales.

41–9). *The vibration is transferred through the tissues and loosens mucus.*

Mechanical vibrators also loosen secretions by transferring vibrations though the chest wall. Read the directions for the particular brand and model of vibrator available (generally you place the vibrating head firmly against the chest wall over the area where secretions are retained).

LONG-TERM CARE

Respiratory care procedures may be needed by those in long-term care facilities as well as by those in acute care. Treatments are the same, but may need to be modified for the older adult. For example, the resident may not be able to stay in a position for postural drainage as long and you may need to use a gentler touch with percussion and vibration techniques.

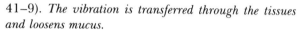 *Home Care*

> Patients may need to continue respiratory care procedures at home after discharge from the hospital or those with chronic respiratory problems may need to carry them out on a long-term basis. In any event, you will need to assess the home setting *to facilitate teaching of the patient* and family or care provider, supervise the treatments, and evaluate their effectiveness.

Performance Checklist

General Procedure for Giving Respiratory Care	Unsat	Needs More Practice	Sat	Comments
Assessment				
1. Count respiratory rate and assess depth and chest expansion.				
2. Auscultate the patient's lungs.				
3. Assess the individual's activity pattern.				
4. Identify whether the patient is at risk for respiratory problems.				
5. Check the patient for pain or other factors that may limit respiratory effort.				
Planning				
6. Plan for pain relief.				
7. Plan what respiratory care procedure is appropriate.				
8. Plan an appropriate time and frequency for the procedure.				
Implementation				
9. Wash your hands.				
10. Identify the patient.				
11. Explain to the patient why you are concerned and tell him or her which respiratory measures are to be used.				
12. Carry out the specific procedure.				
Evaluation				
13. Evaluate, using the following criteria: a. Respiratory rate equal to or less than rate before procedure.				
b. Chest expansion equal to or greater than before procedure.				
c. Lungs clear to auscultation.				
d. Patient resting comfortably.				

General Procedure for Giving Respiratory Care (Continued)	Unsat	Needs More Practice	Sat	Comments
Documentation				
14. Record the respiratory care procedure on the flow sheet or nurses' progress notes.				
15. Note any changes in respiratory status or secretions produced.				
16. Document patient's response as evaluated.				
Assisting the Patient With Deep Breathing				
Assessment				
1. Follow Checklist steps 1–5 of the General Procedure for Giving Respiratory Care. (Count respiratory rate and assess depth and chest expansion, auscultate lungs, assess activity pattern, identify whether the patient is at risk for respiratory problems, and check for pain or other factors that may limit respiratory effort.)				
Planning				
2. Follow Checklist steps 6–8 of the General Procedure. (Plan for pain relief, plan what respiratory care procedure is appropriate, and plan an appropriate time and frequency for the procedure.)				
Implementation				
3. Follow Checklist steps 9–11 of the General Procedure. (Wash your hands, identify the patient, and explain which respiratory measures are to be used and why.)				
4. Assist the patient with deep breathing as outlined below: a. Instruct patient, demonstrating if necessary.				
b. Relieve pain or splint if necessary.				
c. Position patient.				
d. Have patient inspire while counting slowly to two.				
e. Have patient expire while counting slowly to four.				
f. Observe patient for chest and abdominal expansion.				

Assisting the Patient With Deep Breathing
(Continued)

	Unsat	Needs More Practice	Sat	Comments
g. Correct patient's technique as necessary.				
h. Repeat for total of 10 deep breaths.				

Evaluation

5. Evaluate, using the following criteria: a. Respiratory rate equal to or less than rate before procedure.				
b. Chest expansion equal to or greater than before procedure.				
c. Lungs clear to auscultation.				
d. Patient resting comfortably.				

Documentation

6. Follow Checklist steps 14–16 of the General Procedure. (Record the procedure on the flow sheet or nurses' progress notes, note any changes in respiratory status or secretions produced, document patient's response as evaluated.)				

Teaching the Patient To Cough Productively

Assessment

1. Follow Checklist steps 1–5 of the General Procedure for Giving Respiratory Care. (Count respiratory rate and assess depth and chest expansion, auscultate lungs, assess activity pattern, identify whether the patient is at risk for respiratory problems, and check for pain or other factors that may limit respiratory effort.)				

Planning

2. Follow Checklist steps 6–8 of the General Procedure. (Plan for pain relief, plan what respiratory care procedure is appropriate, plan an appropriate time and frequency for the procedure.)				

Implementation

3. Follow Checklist steps 9–11 of the General Procedure. (Wash your hands, identify the patient, explain to the patient why you are concerned and which respiratory measures are to be used.)				

Teaching the Patient To Cough Productively *(Continued)*	Unsat	Needs More Practice	Sat	Comments
4. Teach the patient to cough productively as outlined below: a. Explain the reasons for coughing.				
b. Position patient (in sitting position, if possible).				
c. Splint if necessary.				
d. Have patient deep breathe.				
e. After third deep breath, have patient inspire and hold breath 3 seconds.				
f. Have patient expire forcefully against closed glottis and then release air abruptly while flexing forward.				
g. Repeat for three deep coughs or until mucus is expectorated.				
h. Auscultate lungs.				
i. Offer oral hygiene.				
j. Repeat hourly or as needed to clear lungs of secretions.				
Evaluation				
5. Evaluate, using the following criteria: a. Respiratory rate equal to or less than rate before procedure.				
b. Chest expansion equal to or greater than before procedure.				
c. Lungs clear to auscultation.				
d. Patient resting comfortably.				
Documentation				
6. Follow Checklist steps 14–16 of the General Procedure. (Record on the flow sheet or nurses' notes, note any changes in respiratory status or secretions produced, document patient's response as evaluated.)				

Performing Postural Drainage (Moderate Positions)	Unsat	Needs More Practice	Sat	Comments
Assessment				
1. Identify specific lung segments to be drained.				
Planning				
2. Wash your hands.				
3. Obtain pillows, sputum cup, tissues, and gloves, if necessary.				
Implementation				
4. Identify the patient.				
5. Instruct patient.				
6. Position patient.				
7. Drain upper lobes. a. Have patient sit up if possible.				
b. Have patient lean right (45° angle) for 5 minutes.				
c. Have patient lean left (45° angle) for 5 minutes.				
d. Have patient lean forward (30°–45° angle) for 5 minutes.				
e. Have patient lean backward (30°–45° angle) for 5 minutes.				
f. Have patient lie on abdomen, back, and both sides while horizontal.				
8. Drain lower lobes. a. Place patient in left side-lying position in bed. Use pillow or bed gatch to elevate hips higher than head. (Head should be approximately 30°–45° below horizontal level.)				
b. Have patient lie in each position for 5 minutes, breathing deeply.				
(1) On left side with shoulders perpendicular to bed				
(2) On left side with shoulders slanted backward at a 45° angle from bed				

Performing Postural Drainage (Moderate Positions) *(Continued)*	Unsat	Needs More Practice	Sat	Comments
(3) On back				
(4) On right side with shoulders slanted backward at a 45° angle from bed				
(5) On right side with shoulders perpendicular to bed				
(6) On abdomen with head turned to side				
9. While still on abdomen, have patient cough to raise secretions.				
10. Return patient to comfortable position and allow to rest.				
Evaluation				
11. Evaluate, using the following criteria: a. Lungs clear to auscultation.				
b. Patient resting comfortably.				
Documentation				
12. Record positions used for postural drainage.				
13. Note changes in respiratory status or secretions produced.				
14. Document the patient's response as above.				
Percussion				
1. Place patient in appropriate position for postural drainage.				
2. Use cupped hands.				
3. Clap rapidly over area being drained.				
Vibration				
1. Place patient in appropriate position for postural drainage.				
2. Use flat hands placed firmly against chest wall.				
3. Vibrate hands against chest while patient exhales.				

Quiz

Short-Answer Questions

1. Why is deep breathing necessary for the inactive or immobile patient?

2. What is the correct ratio of length of inspiration to length of expiration?

3. What is the purpose of postural drainage? _____

4. What five basic positions are used to drain the upper lobes?

   a. _____

   b. _____

   c. _____

   d. _____

   e. _____

5. What four positions are used to drain the left lower lobe?

   a. _____

   b. _____

   c. _____

   d. _____

6. What is the purpose of percussion and vibration? _____

7. What is the purpose of the incentive spirometer? _____

Module 42
Oral and Nasopharyngeal Suctioning

Module Contents

Rationale for the Use of This Skill
Nursing Diagnosis
Sterile Technique
Suction Catheters
Suction Source
Routes for Suctioning
Procedure for Oral and Nasopharyngeal Suctioning
    Assessment
    Planning
    Implementation

    Evaluation
    Documentation
Procedure for Bulb Suctioning an Infant
    Assessment
    Planning
    Implementation
    Evaluation
    Documentation
DeLee Infant Aspirator
Cleaning the Suction Apparatus

Prerequisites[1]

Successful completion of the following modules:

VOLUME 1

Module 1 An Approach to Nursing Skills
Module 2 Basic Infection Control
Module 3 Safety
Module 5 General Assessment Overview
Module 6 Documentation
Module 12 Basic Infant Care

VOLUME 2

Module 35 Sterile Technique
Module 40 Administering Oxygen
Module 41 Respiratory Care Procedures

---

[1] For tracheostomy suctioning, see Module 43, Tracheostomy Care and Suctioning.

164

Overall Objective

To suction patients safely and effectively using the oral or nasopharyngeal route.

Specific Learning Objectives

	Know Facts and Principles	Apply Facts and Principles	Demonstrate Ability	Evaluate Performance
1. *Patient explanation*	State information included in explaining suctioning to alert patient.	Given a patient situation, give adequate explanation.	In the clinical setting, explain procedure to alert patient.	Evaluate effectiveness with instructor.
2. *Equipment*	Know variety of equipment available for suctioning adults and infants.	Given a patient situation, select appropriate equipment.	In the clinical setting, select appropriate equipment for suctioning patient.	Evaluate selection with instructor.
3. *Routes for suctioning*	Name two routes for suctioning.	Given a patient situation, assess need for procedure and determine appropriate route.	In the clinical setting, determine appropriate route for suctioning.	Validate choice with instructor.

4. *Procedure*
  a. Sterile technique
  b. Patient position
  c. Inserting catheter
  d. Applying suction
  e. Safety
	Describe correct patient position and method to suction patient safely.	Given a patient situation, describe patient position and correct procedure for suctioning, using sterile technique and observing safety precautions.	In the clinical setting, carry out procedure safely on alert or comatose adult or an infant.	Evaluate performance with instructor using Performance Checklist.

5. *Assessment*	List assessments made before, during, and after suctioning.	Given a patient situation, identify specific assessment needed.	In the clinical setting, make significant observations.	Evaluate performance with clinical instructor.
6. *Documentation*	State information to be recorded.	Given a patient situation, document procedure and results correctly.	In the clinical setting, record data on patient's progress record.	Evaluate charting with clinical instructor.

Learning Activities

1. Review the Specific Learning Objectives.
2. Read the section on respiration in Ellis and Nowlis, *Nursing: A Human Needs Approach,* or comparable material in another textbook.
3. Look up the module vocabulary terms in the Glossary.
4. Read through the module and mentally practice the skills.
5. Review the Performance Checklist.
6. In the practice setting:
   a. Familiarize yourself with the suctioning equipment available.
   b. Using the available equipment and a mannequin, simulate oral and nasopharyngeal suctioning.
   c. Again, with available equipment and an infant mannequin, perform the bulb method and DeLee suction as used on an infant.
   d. Have your partner evaluate your performance, using the Performance Checklist.
   e. Compare your own evaluation with that of your partner.
   f. Reverse roles, and repeat steps b–e.
   g. Practice assessing and recording the suctioning procedure.
   h. When you feel you have practiced the procedure adequately, have your instructor evaluate your performance.
7. In the clinical setting:
   a. Consult with your clinical instructor regarding an opportunity to suction an alert adult, a comatose adult, and an infant.

Vocabulary

aeration	hypoxia	oropharynx
aspirate	inspiration	pharynx
bronchial	mucous	saliva
cough reflex	mucus	secretions
cyanotic	nasopharynx	trachea

Oral and Nasopharyngeal Suctioning

Rationale for the Use of This Skill

An abnormal increase in respiratory secretions can result from a variety of conditions. Among the more common causes are lung and bronchial infections, central nervous system depression, and exposure to anesthetic gases. In the newborn, saliva and amniotic fluid may be present in the mouth and throat in amounts the infant cannot expectorate. The premature newborn has an absent or decreased cough reflex and may be unable to raise secretions. In such situations the secretions must be removed mechanically to facilitate breathing.

In the conscious, alert adult, the cough reflex is activated when respirations are compromised, and secretions are then expectorated. Newborn, unconscious, or very ill patients are incapable of coughing and must rely on the nurse and the nurse's familiarity with the equipment and various techniques for suctioning to carry out this function for them.[2]

▶ *Nursing Diagnosis*

These procedures may be needed for the patient diagnosed as having Ineffective Airway Clearance.

STERILE TECHNIQUE

Because the respiratory tract is continuous and moist, pathogens can readily move downward from the area being suctioned. The bronchi and lungs of an ill person *are particularly susceptible to infection,* so sterile technique should be used for suctioning, whether performed orally or nasopharyngeally. If the suctioning route is changed for any reason (an obstruction), a new sterile catheter must be inserted.

Sterile gloves are used to perform suctioning. One gloved hand holds the portion of the catheter (*which is sterile*) in contact with the patient, while the other hand operates the machine or clean pieces of equipment. This hand becomes contaminated and is not used to touch sterile equipment.

[2] You will note that rationale for action is emphasized throughout the module by the use of italics.

Sterile water or saline is used *to flush the catheter and tubing. Tap water contains microorganisms that are not harmful to the well person but may cause infection of the respiratory tract in the ill person.*

In some settings clean technique is used for oral suctioning. Be aware that this is not the best procedure and make every effort to maintain an exceptional level of cleanliness.

SUCTION CATHETERS

Suction catheters are available with two types of tips (Figure 42–1). *Each has special advantages.* The *open-ended catheter* has a large opening at the end of the catheter and two opposite eyes. This type is effective *when large plugs of mucus are present,* but it does have a tendency to pull at tissue unless it is used carefully. The *whistle-tip catheter* has a large oblique opening in the end, *which has less of a tendency to grab or pull tissue than a side eye does.*

With any catheter, the system must be closed *to obtain suction, or pull.* Suctioning is easily controlled by using a Y-tube connector and placing the thumb over the open end of the Y *to close the system.* A button-type connector is also available. To use it, place the

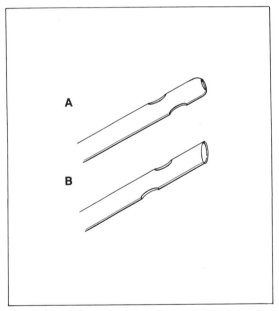

Figure 42–1. Suction catheters. **A.** Open-ended catheter. **B:** Whistle-tip catheter.

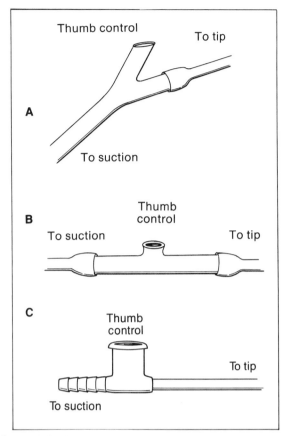

Figure 42–2. Suction controls **A:** Y-tube connector. **B:** Button-type connector attached to catheter. **C:** Button-type connector as integral part of suction catheter.

thumb over the opening in the protruding button (Figure 42–2).

SUCTION SOURCE

In many hospitals, each room has a suction outlet on the wall. In this case, only a length of clean tubing, a wall outlet control, and a reservoir are needed to connect to the outlet (Figure 42–3). If wall suction is not available, a portable suction machine (Figure 42–4) may be obtained from the central supply department.

The equipment should be tested before the procedure. *To be effective,* suction tubing must be tightly fastened to the outlet *to maintain a closed system.* The nurse should inspect all plugs and cords on portable units to make sure they are in good repair, *to prevent sparks. Remember that sparks can be hazardous when ox-*

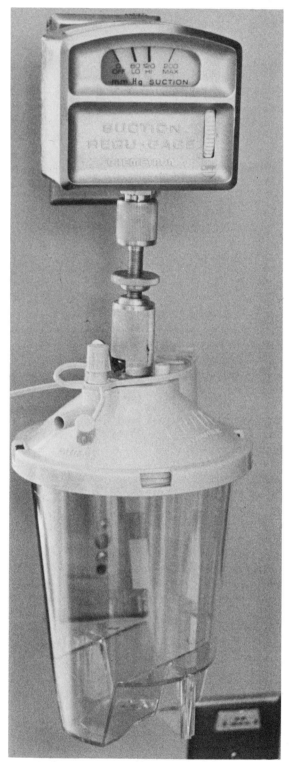

Figure 42–3. Wall outlet suction device. In many hospitals each patient unit has a suction outlet on the wall to which apparatus like this can be attached.
(*Courtesy Ivan Ellis*)

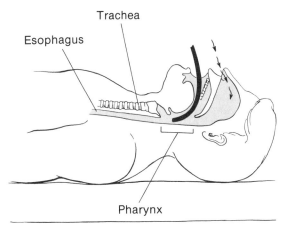

Figure 42–5. Oral suctioning. Placement of suction catheter in pharynx.

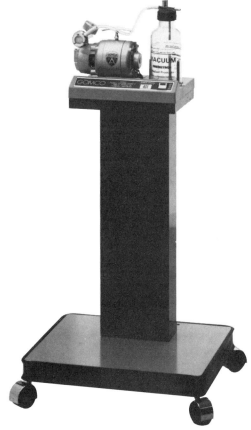

Figure 42–4. Portable suction machine. When wall suction is not available, a portable suction machine may be used. (*Courtesy Gomco Division, Allied Health Care Products, Inc., St. Louis, Missouri*)

ygen is in use, and often the patient who is ill enough to require suctioning is also receiving oxygen.

ROUTES FOR SUCTIONING

The suction catheter may be inserted orally (through the mouth to the back of the throat) or nasopharyngeally (through one of the nostrils). For an infant, suctioning is done orally, because the nostrils are too small for the introduction of a suction catheter. With oral suctioning, you can easily assess the length of catheter needed to aspirate the back of the throat (Figure 42–5). When using the nasopharyngeal route, the length for depth of insertion is generally the distance from the tip of the nose to the tip of the earlobe, or about 5 inches for an adult.

Tracheal or deep suctioning is done by a respi-

ratory therapist, a critical care nurse, or an experienced and skilled staff nurse who can perform this more complicated procedure safely. In tracheal suctioning the catheter is introduced past the glottis, deep into the trachea. *This route is used when a patient cannot raise deep secretions to the point where they can be suctioned out using another route.*

The cough reflex can be stimulated using either route. Although unpleasant for the conscious patient, *coughing raises deeper secretions, which can then be removed by suctioning.*

PROCEDURE FOR ORAL AND NASOPHARYNGEAL SUCTIONING

Assessment

1. In some facilities, a doctor's order is needed for suctioning. This order is usually written as a prn order. Increasingly, suctioning is a nursing decision. *If the patency of the patient's airway is threatened,* an emergency exists. Proceed with suctioning *to prevent respiratory obstruction.*

2. Carefully assess the patient before you proceed with suctioning unless the patency of the patient's airway is threatened. In such a situation, proceed without delay. Assess by listening to chest sounds and to sounds of the higher respiratory tract. You can sometimes hear gurgling sounds from the back of the throat. A patient with severely compromised respirations from the presence of copious secretions may appear cyanotic and have

labored breathing. It is important that you weigh the decision to suction a patient, *because the irritation of the catheter may intensify the buildup of secretions. Also, during suctioning the patient cannot breathe in oxygen. Suctioning performed too frequently can increase the accumulation of secretions and cause a degree of hypoxia.* Identify whether the patient needs a short period of hyperventilation with a high concentration of oxygen before suctioning. *This procedure is used for patients whose oxygenation level is critical.*

3. Be familiar with the suctioning equipment available and the details of the procedure prescribed by the facility.

Planning

4. Wash your hands *for infection control.*
5. Plan for any needed assistance from another staff person. Suctioning can cause the patient to become agitated *because of the feeling that breathing is being interfered with.*
6. Choose the appropriate equipment for the route of suctioning you plan. If you are not sure which route will be used, select two catheters for possible change of route (see Sterile Technique above). If a suction catheter kit (Figure 42–6) is not available, gather the following:
   a. Sterile catheter in the appropriate size
   b. Sterile gloves
   c. Sterile container or basin

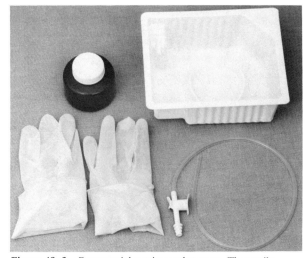

Figure 42–6. Commercial suction catheter set. The sterile water is in a container and ready to use, so no pouring is required.

d. Sterile water or sterile saline
e. Wall suction connector or portable suction machine (if wall suction is not available)
f. Tongue depressor (for oral suctioning)
g. Eye protection (goggles provide front and side protection, but most people who wear eyeglasses believe they provide adequate protection)
h. Mask, if desired
i. Suction trap, if a sputum specimen is needed (see Figure 43–8, page 192).

Implementation

7. Identify the patient *to be sure you are performing the procedure on the correct patient.*
8. Explain what you are going to do. Suctioning can be threatening to the alert patient. It is natural to resist foreign objects that enter the respiratory tract. *This is, in fact, the basis for our protective cough reflex.* You can alleviate the patient's fear and attain increased cooperation *by adequately explaining the procedure and the reasons for it.*

   Tell the patient that you will insert the catheter gently, and ask the patient to relax as much as possible. Inform the patient that coughing may be induced, but explain that this is all right *in that it may help to raise the secretions to a level where they can be suctioned.*
9. Secure adequate lighting *so you can see properly and suction safely.* If the room lighting is inadequate, have an assistant direct a gooseneck lamp or flashlight for you.
10. Place the patient in semi-Fowler's position with the head turned slightly toward you for oropharyngeal suctioning. For nasopharyngeal suctioning it is helpful to have the patient's neck hyperextended *to promote smooth insertion of the suction catheter.* Place the unconscious patient in the lateral position facing toward you *to promote drainage of secretions and prevent aspiration.*
11. Place the drape (from a suction catheter kit) or a clean towel across the patient's chest *to protect the gown.* If prior oxygenation is needed, do so at this time. Follow the procedure for using the self-inflating breathing bag and mask in Module 40, Administering Oxygen. It is good practice to routinely have the patient take two to three deep breaths before you start suctioning.
12. Open the suction kit, maintaining the sterile

technique. Use the wrapper as a sterile field. If you are not using a kit, use the inner surface of the sterile glove package *to provide a sterile field.*

13. If the sterile solution and container are not in the suction kit, set up the sterile container and open and pour the sterile solution into it at this time.

14. Turn on the wall suction mechanism or the suction machine.

15. Put on sterile gloves. Most kits now contain two sterile gloves *so that both hands are protected from contact with respiratory secretions and the patient is protected from microorganisms.* Reserve the glove on your dominant hand for contact with the suction catheter, and use the other hand for any other needs. *This action protects the patient from contact with outside microorganisms.* If the sterile solution and container are in the kit, open the container and fill it with solution.

16. Pick up the catheter with your dominant hand and attach the connector end to the suction tubing, which is held in your clean, gloved nondominant hand. Take care not to touch the tubing with the dominant hand *to avoid contamination.*

17. Test the wall unit or the machine by suctioning water once through the tubing and catheter. (*The water also serves to lubricate the catheter.*)

18. Insert the catheter either:
    a. Through the mouth, using a tongue blade if necessary *to hold the tongue aside for visibility.* Slide the catheter along the side of the mouth to the oropharynx.
    b. Through the nostrils. (If an obstruction is detected in one nostril, try the other side.) Slide the catheter gently along the floor of an unobstructed nostril to the nasopharynx. Never apply suction while you are inserting the catheter *because you could damage the mucous membranes and further deprive the patient of oxygen.* Use a catheter only for a single route. If you must change the route, obtain a new sterile catheter. For example, if you have attempted to suction a patient orally and have met with resistance, and then decide to proceed with the nasopharyngeal approach, discard the first catheter and obtain a second. If you are not using a kit, open separate sterile packs and proceed. Some facilities allow using the

same catheter for oral suctioning if the oral suctioning is done last.

19. Holding your thumb over the opening in the catheter, apply suction for no longer than 15 seconds. It is good practice as you begin to hold your breath during the suction period *to remember that the patient is not receiving oxygen or inspiring while you suction.*

    When suctioning orally, suction carefully in the cheeks, *where secretions tend to pool.*

20. Withdraw the catheter under suction with a rotating motion. *This action aspirates the secretions protruding from the catheter's tip.*

21. Flush the catheter with sterile water *to remove secretions.*

22. Using the nondominant hand, briefly turn off the suction *to listen to the patient's breath sounds and assess the need for repeated suctioning.* If the patient's breathing is not clear, repeat steps 17–21, allowing the patient to rest 20–30 seconds between suctioning periods if possible. It is also good practice to have the patient deep breathe and cough between suctioning periods *to get the secretions up where they can be reached by suctioning.* When the patient's breathing sounds clear, stop suctioning. You should never apply suction more than three times. Sometimes you will stop *because you have not been successful in reaching the secretions. At other times you may be forced to stop because the patient is actively fighting the procedure. Knowing when to stop suctioning requires good nursing judgment. Remember that this procedure can be tiring, as well as frightening, for the patient.*

23. With your nondominant hand, grasp the cuff of the sterile glove and pull it downward over the used catheter in your gloved hand. *This method neatly encloses the used catheter in the glove, making disposal more sanitary* (see Figure 42–7).

24. Detach the catheter from the tubing and dispose of it safely in a receptacle.

25. Reposition the patient *for comfort.*

26. Wash your hands.

27. Offer oral hygiene.

Evaluation

28. Evaluate, using the following criteria:
    a. Breath sounds clear.
    b. Patient comfortable and calm.

Documentation

29. Record the procedure on the patient's chart. Include date, time, and the amount and

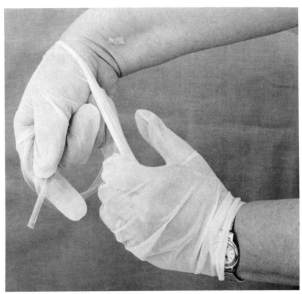

Figure 42–7. Disposing of the suction catheter. The nurse grasps the cuff of the glove and pulls it downward over the used catheter.

character of secretions removed. The patient's tolerance of the procedure should also be noted.

PROCEDURE FOR BULB SUCTIONING AN INFANT

Most infants have minimal secretions and are able to cough, *which effectively clears their air passages.* But

when amniotic fluid in the passages of the newborn or increased production of mucus in the infant causes breathing to become labored, suctioning must be done to maintain a patent airway.

Assessment

1. Usually you do not need a doctor's order for bulb suctioning an infant.
2. Assess the rate and depth of the infant's respirations, as well as breath sounds and chest movements. Note also the pulse rate and skin color. Check the mouth and nose for the presence of secretions.

Planning

3. Wash your hands *for infection control.* Good medical asepsis is all that is necessary in this procedure, *because you are only suctioning in the mouth and nostrils.* Deeper suctioning is usually performed in the nursery by specially prepared nurses.
4. Gather the necessary equipment.
   a. Sterile bulb syringe. (You should begin with a sterile syringe. If frequent suctioning is needed, rinse the bulb well and place it in a clean towel at the side or foot of the crib for further use. *This is often done to decrease response time when suctioning is needed.*)
   b. Clean diaper or towel to place under the infant's chin *to protect chest area.*
   c. Kidney basin *as a waste receptacle for secretions.*
   d. Clean gloves.

DATE/TIME	
8/20/94 4:20 AM	Unresponsive to painful stimuli. Gurgling sounds with respirations. Nasopharyngeal suctioning done with moderate amount thick green mucus obtained. ———— K. Jones, RN

Example of Progress Notes Using Narrative Format

DATE/TIME	
8/20/94 0420	Ineffective airway clearance ————
	S
	O Unresponsive to painful stimuli. Gurgling sounds with respirations. Moderate amount thick green mucus obtained by nasopharyngeal suctioning. ————
	A Unable to cough up secretions independently. ————
	P Recheck respirations hourly and suction prn. ———— K. Jones, RN

Example of Progress Notes Using SOAP Format

DATE/TIME	
4/1/94 1115	Ineffective airway clearance S
	O Frequent coughing and restlessness. Mildly dusky. Turning head with cough and "spitting" moderate amounts of mucus.
	A Increased secretions, partially interfering with aeration. Possible upper respiratory infection.
	P Observe q 15min and bulb suction prn. — M. Schultz, RN

Example of Progress Notes Using SOAP Format

Implementation

5. Put on clean gloves to protect against contact with respiratory secretions.
6. Wrap the infant in a warm blanket *to prevent chilling.*
7. Position the infant. You can swaddle, or wrap, the infant with a small sheet if necessary (see Module 12, Basic Infant Care). The infant's head should be flat on the surface of the crib. A newborn can be held "football" fashion, with the head slightly downward. *Gravity will help move secretions from the back of the throat to the mouth, where they can be suctioned more readily.* If the infant is held during the suctioning, swaddling *for restraint* is usually not necessary.
8. Compress the bulb before inserting the syringe tip into the infant's mouth. *Any compression with the syringe tip in the mouth may force secretions deeper into the respiratory tract.*
9. Insert the syringe tip into the mouth and release the bulb to aspirate (Figure 42–8).
10. Remove the syringe and compress the bulb, expressing the contents into the basin.
11. Repeat steps 8–10 until the infant's cheeks and mouth are clear.
12. Carefully suction the nostrils, placing the syringe tip just at each opening. You can use the same syringe, *since it is not entering the nasal passages.*
13. Place the infant on the side after suctioning *so any remaining secretions can drain freely.*

Evaluation

14. Evaluate, using the following criteria:
    a. Breath sounds clear.
    b. Mouth and nose free of secretions.

Documentation

15. Bulb suctioning the infant—particularly the newborn—is often a routine procedure and is not recorded each time it is performed. In some facilities, suctioning is included in a checklist for the infant. If your facility uses such a checklist, enter "bulb" in the method column. Any significant observations (unusual color or amount of secretions) should be entered in the nurses' notes.

DeLEE INFANT ASPIRATOR

A device called a DeLee infant aspirator has traditionally been used to suction newborn infants. This device uses mouth suction applied to a tubing to achieve the suction pressure (Figure 42–9). Secretions fall into a small receptacle attached to the tub-

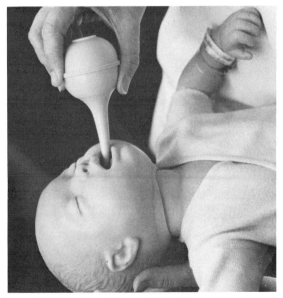

Figure 42–8. Bulb suctioning an infant. Compress the bulb before inserting the syringe tip into the infant's mouth. (*Courtesy Ivan Ellis*)

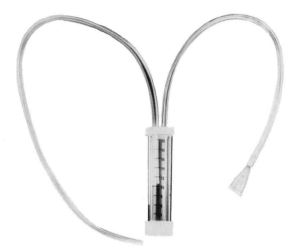

Figure 42-9. Delee infant aspirator. This device uses mouth suction to achieve the suction pressure. (*Courtesy Sherwood Medical, St. Louis, Missouri*)

ing. The same general procedure used for bulb suctioning can be used for the DeLee infant aspirator.

Although the DeLee method is very effective, there is some question as to whether it is appropriate if one considers the potential it creates for spreading microorganisms. Although the secretions do not reach the mouth of the nurse who is aspirating, *air passes through the secretions and could potentially transmit microorganisms.* It is prudent practice not to use this device on any infant suspected of having an infection.

CLEANING THE SUCTION APPARATUS

The receptacle for suction secretions should be emptied frequently, *because it has the potential for growing many pathogenic microorganisms. In addition, it is esthetically unpleasant for patients and visitors.* Certainly it should be emptied once each shift, but emptying after each use is preferable. When emptying the suction secretion container, empty it into the toilet in the room or take it to a utility sink. Do not empty it into a sink in the patient's room. *The secretions tend to stay in the sink and are difficult to rinse away.* Always rinse the container with cold water. *Hot water tends to coagulate protein and make the secretions more difficult to rinse off.* It is prudent practice to wear clean gloves while emptying the container *to protect yourself from contact with the secretions.* The container itself should be replaced frequently. Check your facility's policy to determine frequency.

Performance Checklist

Oral and Nasopharyngeal Suctioning	Unsat	Needs More Practice	Sat	Comments
Assessment				
1. Check for doctor's order if this is facility's policy.				
2. Carefully assess patient's need for suctioning before proceeding.				
3. Be familiar with equipment available and details of procedure as performed in the facility.				
Planning				
4. Wash your hands.				
5. Plan for any needed assistance.				
6. Choose appropriate equipment for route of suctioning planned.				
Implementation				
7. Identify the patient.				
8. Explain what you are going to do.				
9. If room lighting is inadequate, secure gooseneck lamp or flashlight with assistance.				
10. Position patient. a. Oropharyngeal suctioning: Semi-Fowler's with head toward you.				
b. Nasopharyngeal suctioning: Semi-Fowler's with neck hyperextended.				
c. Unconscious: Lateral position facing you.				
11. Place drape or clean towel across patient's chest and hyperoxygenate the patient if needed.				
12. Provide a sterile field.				
13. Set up sterile container and pour solution (if not in kit).				
14. Turn on suction.				
15. Put on sterile gloves. Set up and pour solution (if in kit).				
16. Attach suction catheter to tubing from suction source.				

Oral and Nasopharyngeal Suctioning
(Continued)

	Unsat	Needs More Practice	Sat	Comments
17. Test equipment by suctioning water through tubing and catheter.				
18. Insert catheter, using either the oral or the nasopharyngeal route and described procedure.				
19. Apply suction by closing the system.				
20. Withdraw catheter.				
21. Flush catheter with sterile water to remove secretions.				
22. Turn off suction and listen to patient's breath sounds. Repeat suctioning if needed.				
23. Pull glove downward over used catheter, enclosing it for disposal.				
24. Detach catheter from tubing and discard it.				
25. Reposition patient for comfort.				
26. Wash your hands.				
27. Offer oral hygiene.				
Evaluation				
28. Evaluate, using the following criteria: a. Breath sounds clear.				
b. Patient comfortable and calm.				
Documentation				
29. Record procedure and pertinent observations.				

Bulb Suctioning an Infant

Assessment

	Unsat	Needs More Practice	Sat	Comments
1. Doctor's order usually not needed.				
2. Assess rate and depth of infant's respirations, breath sounds, and chest movements. Check pulse rate, skin color, and mouth and nose for secretions.				
Planning				
3. Wash your hands.				
4. Gather necessary equipment.				

Bulb Suctioning an Infant *(Continued)*	Unsat	Needs More Practice	Sat	Comments
Implementation				
5. Put on clean gloves.				
6. Wrap infant in warm blanket.				
7. Either swaddle infant or hold "football" fashion for stability.				
8. Compress bulb before inserting syringe tip in infant's mouth.				
9. Insert syringe tip into mouth and release bulb to aspirate.				
10. Remove syringe and compress bulb, expressing contents into basin.				
11. Repeat steps 8–10 until tract is clear.				
12. Carefully suction nostrils, placing tip just at each opening.				
13. Place infant on his or her side.				
Evaluation				
14. Evaluate, using the following criteria: a. Breath sounds clear.				
b. Mouth and nose free of secretions.				
Documentation				
15. Record any pertinent observations or according to the facility's policy.				

Quiz

Short-Answer Questions

1. List two reasons why the patient must be given an adequate explanation of the suctioning procedure.

   a. _____

   b. _____

2. When using a suction catheter, why must you maintain sterility?

   _____

3. Why does a newborn or infant usually need to be suctioned?

   _____

4. When you are operating the suctioning equipment, why must the system be closed? _____

5. In what position should you place the unconscious patient for suctioning? _____

6. What are two reasons for placing the unconscious patient in this position?

   a. _____

   b. _____

7. What is the maximum length of time you should suction on each insertion of the catheter? _____

8. Ideally, what is the maximum number of times you should suction a patient? _____

9. When might oxygenating a patient with a self-inflating rebreathing bag and mask before suctioning be indicated?

   _____

10. In what situation would it be prudent practice *not* to use the DeLee infant aspirator? _____

Module 43
Tracheostomy Care and Suctioning

Module Contents

Rationale for the Use of This Skill
Nursing Diagnoses
Tracheostomy
  Tracheostomy Tubes
  Safety Measures
Procedure for Suctioning the Tracheostomy
  Assessment
  Planning
  Implementation
  Evaluation
  Documentation
Procedure for Administering Tracheostomy Care
  Assessment
  Planning

Implementation
Evaluation
Documentation
Procedure for Changing the Tracheostomy Dressing
  Assessment
  Planning
  Implementation
  Evaluation
  Documentation
Obtaining a Sputum Specimen Through a Tracheostomy
Long-term Care
Home Care

Prerequisites

Successful completion of the following modules:

VOLUME 1

Module 1 An Approach to Nursing Skills
Module 2 Basic Infection Control
Module 3 Safety
Module 5 General Assessment Overview
Module 6 Documentation
Module 11 Hygiene

VOLUME 2

Module 35 Sterile Technique
Module 37 Wound Care
Module 40 Administering Oxygen
Module 42 Oral and Nasopharyngeal Suctioning

179

Overall Objective

To care for patients with tracheostomies correctly and to perform suctioning through the tracheostomy safely and effectively.

Specific Learning Objectives

	Know Facts and Principles	Apply Facts and Principles	Demonstrate Ability	Evaluate Performance
1. General considerations				
a. Definition	Define *tracheostomy*.			
b. Indications for tracheostomy	State two reasons for tracheostomy.	Given a patient situation, state rationale for tracheostomy.	In the clinical setting, state why a patient has a tracheostomy.	Evaluate with instructor.
c. Types of tracheostomy tubes	Name two types of tracheostomy tubes and advantages and disadvantages of each.	In the practice setting, identify various types of tubes.	In the clinical setting, identify type of tube in use for a particular patient.	Evaluate own performance with instructor.
d. Safety factors	State three important safety measures and rationale for each.	Given a patient situation, state safety measures appropriate to that situation.	In the clinical setting, carry out measures safely with patient.	Evaluate performance with instructor.
2. Tracheostomy suctioning				
a. Equipment	Describe equipment used in tracheal suctioning.	In the practice setting, select and adapt equipment correctly.	In the clinical setting, use appropriate equipment in manner described.	Evaluate with instructor.
b. Procedure	State information to be given to patient.	In the practice setting, role play appropriate patient teaching and nurse–patient interaction.	In the clinical setting, carry out appropriate nurse–patient interaction and patient teaching.	Evaluate interaction with instructor.
	Know correct positioning. Explain use of sterile technique. State distance catheter is inserted for shallow or deep suctioning. Describe method and how long to apply pressure.	In the practice setting, correctly plan and carry out tracheostomy suctioning on a mannequin.	In the clinical setting, correctly suction the patient with a tracheostomy.	Evaluate own performance with instructor using Performance Checklist.

(continued)

Specific Learning Objectives *(Continued)*

	Know Facts and Principles	Apply Facts and Principles	Demonstrate Ability	Evaluate Performance
c. Documentation	State what needs to be recorded.	Given a patient situation, identify pertinent information to be charted.	In the clinical setting, record accurately on patient's chart.	Evaluate charting format and content with instructor.
3. Cleaning and dressing				
a. Equipment	Name equipment needed for cleaning and dressing tracheostomy.	Given a specific situation, select and assemble equipment correctly.	In the clinical setting, correctly use equipment and materials.	Evaluate with instructor.
b. Procedure	State explanation to be given to patient. Know correct positioning. Explain use of sterile equipment. List steps in cleaning and dressing procedure.	In the practice setting, correctly clean and dress a tracheostomy.	In the clinical setting, carry out cleaning and dressing procedure.	Evaluate own performance with instructor using Performance Checklist.
c. Documentation	State items to be recorded.	Given a patient situation, identify pertinent information to be charted.	In the clinical setting, record accurately on patient's chart.	Evaluate charting format and content with instructor.

Learning Activities

1. Review the Specific Learning Objectives.
2. Read the section on the respiratory system in the chapter on basic vital functions in Ellis and Nowlis, *Nursing: A Human Needs Approach,* or comparable material in another textbook.
3. Look up the module vocabulary terms in the Glossary.
4. Read through the module and mentally practice the skills.
5. Review the Performance Checklist.
6. In the practice setting:
   a. Examine the various tracheostomy tubes available.
   b. Select and gather the equipment for suctioning a tracheostomy.
   c. If a tube can be attached to a mannequin, use the Performance Checklist as a guide and practice suctioning the tracheostomy.
   d. Gather the equipment for cleaning a tube and changing a dressing.
   e. Following the Performance Checklist, practice cleaning the tube and changing the dressing.
   f. When you think you have mastered these skills, ask your instructor to evaluate your performance.
7. In the clinical setting:
   Consult with your instructor for an opportunity to give care to and suction a patient with a tracheostomy.

Vocabulary

apnea	clockwise	hypoxia	prophylactic
asphyxiation	counterclockwise	inflatable cuff	respirator
aspirate	dead-air space	lumen	suction
bronchi	fenestrated	mucus	trachea
button	tracheostomy	necrosis	tracheal ring
cannula	tube	obturator	tracheostomy
catheter	hydrogen peroxide		

Tracheostomy Care and Suctioning

Rationale for the Use of This Skill

Because patients with tracheostomies are often cared for on the general hospital unit, the nurse must be familiar with the special care required and the variations needed for suctioning such patients. Normally, the upper respiratory passages protect the trachea, filtering out foreign material and providing some protection from microorganisms. However, the trachea is highly susceptible to infection. Because the tracheostomy opens directly into the trachea, a thorough knowledge of sterile technique is required. In addition, safety involves the constant maintenance of a patent airway.[1]

▶ Nursing Diagnoses

High Risk for Respiratory Infection is always present in the patient with a tracheostomy *because the protection of the upper airway has been eliminated.* Much of the care described in this module is directed at preventing infection through correct technique in care of the tracheostomy.

Suctioning is a skill needed for the individual with a nursing diagnosis of Ineffective Airway Clearance. The tracheostomy tube irritates the respiratory tract and causes an increase in secretions. If the patient is not able to effectively cough these secretions out, this nursing diagnosis is present and you will need to suction the patient to remove secretions.

The patient with a tracheostomy tube in place is unable to speak except for when a fenestrated tube is in use or when the regular tracheostomy tube is "buttoned" or occluded. For this reason, the nursing diagnosis of Impaired Verbal Communication is often appropriate.

TRACHEOSTOMY

A tracheostomy is a surgical incision into the trachea *for the purpose of inserting a tube through which the patient* can breathe more easily and secretions can be removed. At one time, the procedure was performed only as an emergency measure *to allow a critically ill patient to breathe when life was imminently threatened by respiratory obstruction.*

In current practice, a tracheostomy is performed more commonly *as a prophylactic procedure, so that secretions in the respiratory tract can be removed more effectively before a patient's breathing is severely compromised.* A tracheostomy may also be performed *to decrease the amount of dead-air space in the airway and thus to reduce the effort of breathing.* In some instances the procedure is done *so that a respirator can be used to breathe for the patient.*

The procedure is performed by a physician, usually in the critical care unit or the operating room. A small, horizontal incision is made just below the first tracheal ring, and a tracheostomy tube is inserted. In most cases this is a temporary measure. Once the patient can tolerate temporary closure, or buttoning, from brief to more prolonged periods, the tracheostomy tube is removed and the incision heals over.

Tracheostomy Tubes

Tracheostomy tubes are composed of three parts. An outer cannula fits through the tracheostomy opening. This cannula is curved and has a flange near the upper opening, which rests against the surface of the neck. Ties attached to this flange are used to fasten the outer cannula securely. Inside the outer cannula is an inner cannula, which has a slightly smaller diameter. A latch usually holds this cannula securely, and allows it to be removed for cleaning. An obturator with a smooth, oval end fits inside the inner cannula and protrudes from the end. *This makes it easier to insert the tracheostomy tube through the opening into the trachea* (Figure 43–1) and is removed once the tube is in place.

The size of the tube used is usually the choice of the physician who performs the procedure and inserts the tube. Most tubes are available in standard sizes: 0–12 or French 24–44, from smaller to larger.

Tracheostomy tubes are most commonly made of plastic, but metal tubes are also available. The plastic tube has a larger lumen and is softer than the metal tube. It molds more easily to the trachea; therefore it causes less irritation and is more comfortable for the patient. Plastic tracheostomy tubes are disposable; metal tubes may be cleaned, sterilized, and reused.

Cuffed tracheostomy tubes are plastic tubes with

---

[1] You will note that rationale for action is emphasized throughout the module by the use of italics.

© 1992 by J.B. Lippincott Company

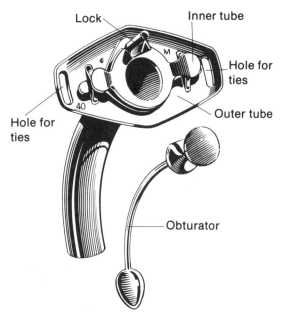

Figure 43-1. The parts of a tracheostomy tube. (*Courtesy Pilling Company, Fort Washington, Pennsylvania*)

an inflatable cuff that enables medical personnel to seal the tube into the trachea. *This is necessary to provide a closed system in which a ventilator can operate through the tracheostomy tube. It also helps to guard against aspiration of secretions or vomitus from the upper airway into the lungs* (Figure 43-2).

A fenestrated tracheostomy tube is designed with openings that allow air to pass through the larynx and into the upper airway from the lungs. A fenes-

trated tube allows an individual to talk while the tracheostomy is in place. It can also be used as a step toward removal of the tracheostomy (Figure 43-3).

One approach to determining whether an individual can function without a tracheostomy tube in place is to close the tube with a cork or "button," which requires air to move around the sides of the tracheostomy tube (or through the fenestration) as it passes from the upper airway to the lungs and back out (Figure 43-4).

Safety Measures

Crucial to the care of a tracheostomy is the prevention of infection, not only to the wound, but to the bronchi and lungs as well. If a patient has a new or recent tracheostomy, sterile technique is used when cleaning or dressing. In home settings and some long-term care facilities, good handwashing and clean technique are used when cleaning or dressing a tracheostomy of long standing. Regardless of how long a patient has had the tracheostomy, sterile technique is always used when suctioning.

Emergency equipment should be kept at the bedside *in case the tracheostomy tube becomes dislodged or is coughed out, allowing the opening to close.* It is procedure in some facilities to keep at the bedside an extra tracheostomy set, which contains a clamp *that the nurse can quickly insert into the opening to maintain patency.* A new sterile tube is then inserted. If a complete set is not available, a sterile clamp and a

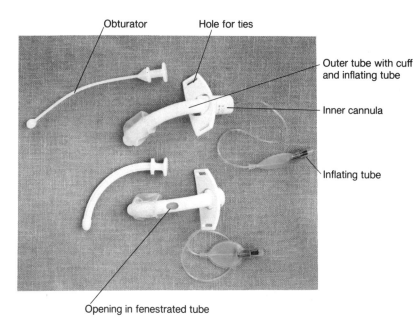

Figure 43-2. Two types of plastic cuffed tracheostomy tubes.

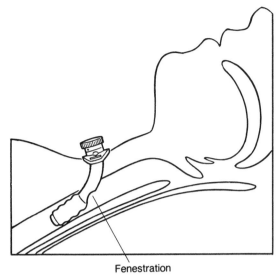

Fenestration

Figure 43-3. A fenestrated tracheostomy tube (often called a "talking trach").

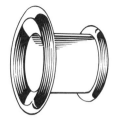

Figure 43-4. Tracheostomy button. When a "button" is in place, air moves around the sides of the tracheostomy tube as it passes from the upper airway to the lungs and back out. (*Courtesy Pilling Company, Fort Washington, Pennsylvania*)

tube of the correct size and type should always be kept at the bedside.

If cloth material or gauze is used in tracheostomy care, it must be lint-free *to avoid the possibility of aspirating particles into the respiratory tract.* For this reason, the nurse should not use cut cloth or cut gauze in tracheostomy care.

If a patient has a tube with a firm inflatable cuff, the cuff can be deflated *to prevent pressure necrosis or erosion of the tracheal lining.* The cuff is usually deflated for 10 minutes of each hour or as the physician orders. Any accumulated oral secretions should be suctioned before the cuff is deflated *to prevent them from going deeper into the trachea when the cuff is deflated.* During the time the cuff is deflated, take special precautions to ensure that the tapes are secure and that the tracheostomy tube is in the proper position, *so it is not coughed out.* This is not a problem if the tube has a double cuff, *because one cuff remains inflated while the other is deflated, providing alternating pressure areas and preventing necrosis.* Many tubes have soft, pliable cuffs that can remain inflated. Other cuffs are inflated with atmospheric pressure. The nurse should check the tube for the type of cuff and follow the procedure recommended by the manufacturer or the facility. To check a cuff for correct pressure, attach a gauge to the cuff port.

A patient with a tracheostomy requires constant, careful watching. It is also a matter of safety to place a call bell within easy reach of the alert patient at all times, *so help can be summoned if respiratory difficulty occurs.*

PROCEDURE FOR SUCTIONING THE TRACHEOSTOMY

The procedure for tracheal suctioning is similar to that described for nasopharyngeal suctioning, in Module 42, Oral and Nasopharyngeal Suctioning. If the patient with a tracheostomy is on a respirator, the procedure is more complex and requires advanced skills not included in this module.

Suctioning the trachea and bronchi decreases the oxygen available to the lungs and also causes collapse of alveoli. The result is hypoxemia (a lowered blood oxygen level). *To prevent hypoxemia,* you must hyperventilate the patient with 100% oxygen immediately before and after suctioning. Many ventilators can be set to provide hyperventilation when it is needed, or you can use a breathing bag attached to oxygen. Some equipment is structured so that the breathing bag can be attached directly to the tracheostomy or endotracheal tube. In other cases the breathing bag is attached to a T-shaped piece on the tracheostomy tube.

To use the breathing bag effectively and still maintain sterility of the suction catheter, two people should work together on tracheostomy suctioning, although an experienced individual who is very dexterous may be able to do this procedure effectively alone. The procedure presented here is for two persons working together. The individual handling the suction equipment is designated person #1, and the individual handling the breathing bag is designated person #2. All steps are done by person #1 except those that specify person #2.

In instances when the patient is very stable, hyperventilation may be omitted. If you are not using hyperventilation, simply omit the steps that refer to person #2.

Assessment

1. Assessing the needs of a patient with a tracheostomy for suctioning and cleaning is an

important function for the nurse. *This assessment is especially critical because many of these patients are comatose, and most conscious patients cannot talk because of the tracheal opening.*

If suctioning, cleaning, and dressing are all needed, suction first, *so the cleaned tube and dressing will stay cleaner longer.* While giving care, always observe the incision for redness and swelling, which *can be symptoms of infection or irritation. Remember that suctioning removes oxygen, causes tissue irritation, and increases secretions,* so use discretion when performing this procedure. Also, for tracheostomies, do not suction longer than 10 seconds at any one time.

To assess the patient, listen to the breath sounds. They should be quiet, not labored. If the respirations are labored and you hear the movement of secretions (a gurgling sound), the patient needs suctioning. You can also observe the condition of the tubes.

Planning

2. Wash your hands *for infection control.*
3. Obtain the necessary equipment. Commercial suctioning kits are available that contain the essential items you will need. If the kits are not used in your facility, gather the following:
   a. Sterile gloves
   b. Sterile suction catheter
   c. Sterile basin
   d. Sterile water or sterile normal saline
   e. Sterile syringe and normal saline if saline is to be instilled
   f. Sterile gauze squares
   g. Portable suction machine if wall suction is not available
   h. Self-inflating breathing bag and mask
   i. Eye protection (goggles or eyeglasses)
   j. Mask if desired
   k. Suction trap, if a sputum specimen is needed.

Implementation

4. Identify the patient *to be sure you are performing the procedure on the correct patient.*
5. Pull the curtain around the patient's bed *to provide privacy.*
6. Explain the procedure. If the patient is responsive, it is imperative to explain the procedure carefully. *Without proper psychologic preparation, the patient may fear choking or bleeding to death.* A brief explanation should also be given to the unresponsive patient,

because the patient may understand even though unable to respond. The responsive patient should be asked to cough *to raise secretions so they are more easily suctioned.*

7. *Because the patient with a tracheostomy usually cannot speak,* it is important to establish a way of communicating. *Being able to communicate greatly relieves the patient's feeling of helplessness.* Provide a slate or pencil and paper for the alert patient so he or she can respond to you during the procedure. If the patient cannot write, establish a yes-or-no signal system.

   Tell the patient *that the tracheal opening prevents air from reaching the vocal cords, so speech is not possible.* Later, the patient will be able to speak by placing a button or finger over the opening, thus forcing air around the tube. Of course, the patient with a fenestrated tracheostomy tube is always able to speak, *because air is able to reach the vocal cords.*

8. Test the suction apparatus.
   a. Turn on either the wall suction or the portable suction machine.
   b. Place your thumb over the end of the unsterile tubing that is attached to the suction equipment and test for "pull."
   c. Keep the suction regulated to a range of efficiency, usually low to medium.

9. Place the patient supine or in mid Fowler's position. Turn the patient's head slightly toward you *so the chin is out of the way and you can see better.* Place the unconscious patient in the lateral position facing you.

10. Put on eye protection.

11. Prepare 5 ml sterile saline in a syringe, if it is ordered. *The properties of normal saline may help liquefy thickened respiratory secretions,* although this is not supported by research. Remove the needle *for safety.*

12. Open the sterile suction set and prepare the equipment. Place the drape from the kit or a clean towel over the patient's chest to *protect the gown or clothing.* Most kits contain a packet of saline solution, sterile gloves, the sterile suction catheter, and sterile gauze squares. If your kit contains all this equipment, put on the gloves and pour the saline into the basin. Hold the catheter in your dominant hand and use the nondominant hand to hold the suction tubing, to control the suction, and to handle any other nonsterile object. *The nondominant hand is now contaminated* and cannot touch the catheter. *The glove will protect you from contact*

e solution is not in the kit,
t up the basin carefully,
outside, and move the glove
le. Pour the saline from the
into the basin and then put
s on and proceed. Rinse the
ormal saline solution.

hes the breathing bag to the
and prepares to ventilate the

ches the breathing bag to the
tube and provides three deep
inated with the patient's
tern.
dominant, nonsterile gloved hand
normal saline into the
iy if this is ordered.
nondominant, nonsterile-gloved
e suction tubing and control button.
dominant, sterile-gloved hand on the
proceed to suction.
the catheter 4–5 inches into the
eostomy without occluding the port on
ction catheter, so that suction is not
applied. *Suctioning at this time would
er deprive the patient of oxygen.*

b. Apply suction by closing the system. This is usually done by placing your thumb over the port or side opening at the base of the catheter. The patient may cough *in response to the irritation caused by the catheter, which helps to raise secretions.* Persistent coughing *can indicate tracheal spasm,* in which case you should stop the procedure.

c. Apply suction for only 10 seconds (per entry). *Remember that the patient cannot breathe during the procedure.* (You can hold your own breath while suctioning *to help you time the procedure.*) If oxygen is ordered, administer after each period of suctioning.

d. Withdraw the catheter, rotating it gently while you continue suctioning, *so higher*

secretions are removed and are not tracked through the lumen of the tracheostomy.

e. Rinse the catheter with sterile water or normal saline.

f. Person #2 provides ventilation immediately after the suction catheter is removed *to supply needed oxygen.*

17. Observe the patient for dyspnea and skin color changes.

18. If these symptoms of hypoxia occur, person #2 immediately provides deep breaths of oxygen *to reverse hypoxia.*

19. Turn off the suction and listen for clear breath sounds.

20. If breathing is not clear, repeat steps 16 a–e.

21. If the breathing sounds clear, person #2 immediately uses the breathing bag to provide three or four deep breaths of oxygen *to oxygenate the patient fully.*

22. Detach the catheter.

23. Grasp the cuff of the sterile glove and pull the glove down over the used catheter. *This method makes disposal of the equipment more sanitary.* Remove eye protection.

24. Discard all disposable equipment and take nondisposable equipment to the appropriate place for cleaning.

25. Wash your hands.

26. Offer oral hygiene.

Evaluation

27. Evaluate, using the following criteria:
   a. Tracheostomy tube securely in place.
   b. Respiratory rate and depth normal.
   c. Breath sounds clear.
   d. Patient resting comfortably.

Documentation

28. Record the procedure and your observations on the patient's chart. The entry should include the amount and description of secretions, as well as the patient's tolerance of the procedure.

DATE/TIME	
10/2/94 9:15 AM	*Respirations noisy and labored. Not coughing. Tracheostomy suctioned. 5 ml normal saline instilled. Mod am't thick, white mucus obtained. Respirations quiet after suctioning. Vital signs remained stable. Skin reddened around tube. — B. Cook, RN*

Example of Progress Notes Using Narrative Format

DATE/TIME	
10/2/94	Ineffective airway clearance
9:15 AM	S
	O Respirations noisy and labored. Not coughing up secretions. Tracheostomy suctioning with 5 ml normal saline instilled to liquefy secretions produced mod am't thick, white sputum. Respirations quieted. Vital signs remained stable. Skin reddened around tube.
	A Continues unable to clear airway. Secretions decreasing in amount. Irritation around stoma increasing.
	P Increase frequency of changing tracheostomy dressing to q 4h. Notify Dr. Ryan of increasing irritation. Continue plan for tracheostomy suctioning.
	— B. Cook, RN

Example of Progress Notes Using SOAP Format

PROCEDURE FOR ADMINISTERING TRACHEOSTOMY CARE

Assessment

1. Check the tracheostomy frequently, *because the opening can become obstructed by the buildup of crusts and secretions.* Never allow the patient to reach the point of laborious breathing. Clean by necessity, not by a definite schedule. *Some patients have more secretions than others.* Cleaning and dressing the tracheostomy once per shift may be adequate for some patients, whereas other patients may need care two or three times per shift.

Planning

2. Wash your hands *for infection control.*
3. Gather the equipment you will need. Commercial tracheostomy care kits that contain the necessary items are available (Figure 43–5). If your facility does not use such kits, obtain the following equipment:
   a. Sterile gloves, if the tracheostomy has recently been performed, *to prevent the wound from becoming infected*
   b. 4 × 4 gauze squares
   c. Cleansing solution (often a hydrogen peroxide mixture or saline)
   d. Basin
   e. Tracheostomy brush, pipe cleaners, or swabs *to clean the cannula surfaces*
   f. Sterile water.
   If you plan to change the tracheostomy dressing at this time, you will want to gather

the equipment for that procedure, too, *to avoid making another trip out of the room for needed supplies.* Add the equipment listed in step 3 of the Procedure for Changing the Tracheostomy Dressing, page 190.

Implementation

4. Identify the patient *to be sure you are performing the procedure on the correct patient.*
5. Pull the curtain around the patient's bed *to provide privacy.*
6. Explain what you are going to do. *Many patients are afraid the tube may become dislodged during care. By demonstrating competence you can reassure the patient.*
7. Provide a slate or pencil and paper to the alert patient *for communication,* as for suctioning.
8. Place the patient supine or in mid Fowler's position *to promote comfort and visibility.*
9. Set up the supplies.
10. Put on sterile or clean gloves as necessary.
11. To clean a cannula-type tracheostomy tube:
    a. Hold the outer tube carefully in place with one hand as you turn the lock clockwise with your other hand *to unfasten the inner cannula.*
    b. Slide the inner cannula out by curving it toward you.
    c. Place the inner cannula in the basin.
    d. Immerse the cannula in the cleansing solution for a few minutes *to soften crusts.*
    e. Apply friction to the cannula with brush, pipe cleaners, or swabs *to remove mucus and crusts.*

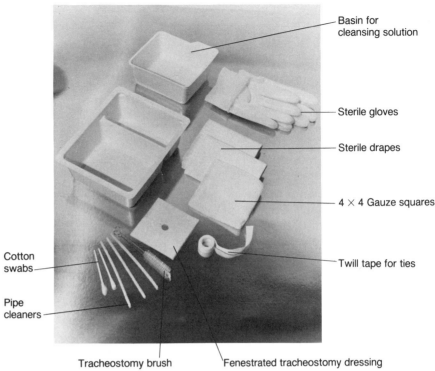

Figure 43-5. A commercially prepared tracheostomy care kit. (*Courtesy Sherwood Medical, St. Louis, Missouri*)

f. Rinse the cannula well in cold sterile water.

g. Dry the cannula thoroughly with sterile, lint-free gauze or towel.

h. If the patient's secretions are copious, or if the patient coughs while you are cleaning the inner cannula (so that the secretions come in contact with the inside surface of the outer cannula), remove the secretions and thoroughly dry the inner surfaces as described in step 11 *to prevent the surfaces of the two cannulas from adhering.*

i. Hold the outer cannula and replace the clean inner cannula.

j. Turn the lock counterclockwise *to secure.*

k. *Test to make sure the inner cannula is secure.*

12. If a plastic tube with no inner cannula is being used, carefully clean the inner surfaces with pipe cleaners or swabs dampened, but not saturated, with normal saline *to prevent aspiration.*

13. If you are planning to change the tracheostomy dressing, move on to step 6 of the Procedure for Changing the Tracheostomy Dressing. If not, complete this procedure.

14. Dispose of the equipment.

15. Wash your hands.

Evaluation

16. Evaluate, using the following criteria:
   a. Tracheostomy tube securely in place.
   b. No secretions present.
   c. Breath sounds clear.

Documentation

17. The procedure is usually recorded in conjunction with the dressing change that follows. (See next procedure.)

PROCEDURE FOR CHANGING THE TRACHEOSTOMY DRESSING

Ideally, this is a two-person procedure, although a single person can, by working carefully, carry it out alone. It is most commonly done at the time of cleaning but in some situations may be needed more frequently.

Assessment

1. *Because a tracheostomy is prone to infection,* dressings should be changed frequently. The dressing should be changed routinely after giving tracheostomy care and at other times when you assess the patient and find any appreciable amount of drainage or soiling of the dressing.

Planning

2. Wash your hands *for infection control.*
3. Obtain a tracheostomy care kit, or gather following items:
   a. 4×4 gauze squares or special tracheostomy dressings
   b. Twill tape ties
   c. Scissors
   d. Swabs
   e. Cleansing solution
   f. Oral care equipment
   g. One pair clean gloves/one pair sterile gloves
   h. Bag for soiled dressings.

Implementation

4. Identify the patient *to be sure you are performing the procedure on the correct patient.*
5. Pull the curtain around the bed *to provide privacy.*
6. Explain what you are going to do.
7. Put on clean gloves and remove the old dressing and discard it.
   a. *Two persons* Have an assistant hold the tube while you remove the old dressing.
   b. *One person* Place one hand gently around the tube *to keep it secure* as you carefully remove the soiled gauze.
8. Remove gloves and wash hands.
9. Put on sterile gloves.
10. With sterile swabs moistened in saline or hydrogen peroxide solution, clean around the edges of the tracheostomy opening.
11. Notice any redness or swelling of the wound margins.
12. Prepare the dressing. Use a precut tracheostomy dressing or a 4×4 gauze square.
    a. Open the first fold of a 4×4 gauze square if you are using plain gauze squares.
    b. Fold it in half lengthwise.
    c. Fold each end toward the center (Figure 43–6).
    d. Place it around the tube with the ends up. This type of dressing eliminates the need to cut the material, *which might expose the patient to free lint that could be inhaled.*
13. Remove the soiled holding tape and replace.
    a. *Two persons* Have an assistant apply light pressure to the tube *to prevent dislodging it* while you cut the tape, remove it, and discard.

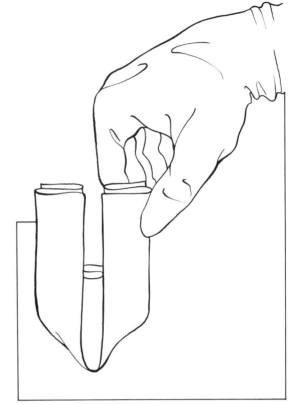

Figure 43–6. Tracheostomy dressing. Open a 4×4 gauze square, fold it in half lengthwise, and place it around the tube with the ends up.

Carefully slip the prepared dressing, ends extending up, around the tube. With the tube held in place, apply tapes (Figure 43–7).
(1) Make a slit near the end of the twill tape.
(2) Thread the tape through the flange on one side of the tube.
(3) Pass the end through the tape slit and pull until it is snug.
(4) Bring the tape around the back of the patient's neck.
(5) Thread the loose end through the remaining flange. Tie the tapes at the side of the neck *tightly enough so the tube is held securely, but loosely enough so there is not undue pressure on tissues.* It is helpful if the assisting nurse holds a finger under the tape as it is tied *to allow for slack.*

b. *One person* *To stabilize the tube,* leave the twill tapes in place while you remove the soiled dressing and place the new one. Cut and prepare both ties. Thread the new ties

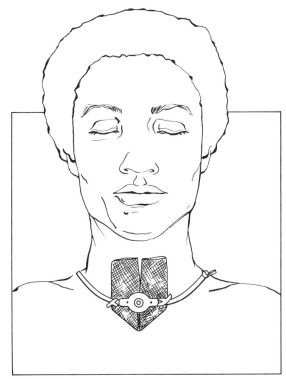

Figure 43–7. Tapes holding the tracheostomy tube in place. The knot is to the side to prevent rubbing and pressure when the patient is lying back.

through the slits above the old ties, and tie the new ties. Then cut and remove the old ties. Or you can ask an alert, oriented patient to hold the tube in place while you change the tapes.

It is possible to develop the dexterity to hold the tracheostomy tube with the nondominant hand and use the dominant hand to remove the old tape and fasten the new. After you have attached both new tapes, hold the ties firmly while you tie them around the neck. The knot should be to the side *to prevent rubbing when the patient is lying back.*

14. Check the placement of the tube.

15. Perform oral care, following the guidelines in Module 11, Hygiene. *Because a patient with a tracheostomy has a changed breathing pattern (without air moving freely through the mouth), the oral cavity becomes dry and there is a buildup of sordes and crusts. This condition can cause odor, which is distressing to both the patient and those providing care. Because the patient needs meticulous oral care frequently, make this procedure part of the general tracheostomy care, so it is neither forgotten nor neglected.*

16. Dispose of the equipment.

17. Wash your hands.

Evaluation

18. Evaluate, using the following criteria:
   a. Tracheostomy tube securely in place.
   b. No redness or swelling present.
   c. No secretions present.
   d. Dressing and tapes clean and dry.
   e. Absence of stale or foul-smelling breath.

Documentation

19. Record the procedure and any observations.

Example of Progress Notes Using Narrative Format

DATE/TIME	
9/17/95 2:15 PM	Tracheostomy stoma cleaned with H_2O_2. Clean drsg applied. Small amount of serosanguineous exudate noted on old drsg. Skin around stoma intact with no redness or edema. S. Burns, NS

Example of Progress Notes Using SOAP Format

DATE/TIME	
9/17/95 1415	Impaired skin integrity: new trach stoma
	S
	O Small amount serosanguineous exudate on old drsg. Stoma cleaned with H_2O_2 and clean drsg applied. Skin around stoma intact with no redness or edema.
	A Stoma healing.
	P Continue with cleansing and drsg changes q4h. S. Burns, NS

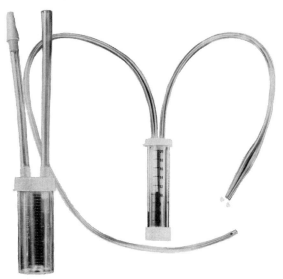

Figure 43–8. A suction trap for obtaining a sputum specimen. (*Courtesy Sherwood Medical, St. Louis, Missouri*)

OBTAINING A SPUTUM SPECIMEN THROUGH A TRACHEOSTOMY

A sputum specimen may be obtained when you are suctioning a tracheostomy. Use a special sputum trap (Figure 43–8) with two outlets. One outlet is attached to the suction catheter, and the other is attached to the tubing from the suction source. As the sputum is suctioned out, it drops into the trap and remains there. The entire container is then sent to the labo-

ratory. This protects the specimen from the possibility of outside contamination, and it protects health care workers from contact with the sputum.

LONG-TERM CARE

The same general procedures for suctioning, caring for, and dressing a tracheostomy are used in long-term care settings and acute care settings. Clean technique may be used when cleaning or dressing a tracheostomy that has been in place for a long time. Sterile technique should always be used for suctioning.

Home Care

Caring for the patient who returns home with a tracheostomy requires that the patient and family be taught not only how to perform the various aspects of care, but also the signs and symptoms that should be reported and how to respond in an emergency. Initially, they may feel inadequate to the task, but complete written instructions as well as opportunities to observe and then practice the skills can result in skilled and knowledgeable care.

Performance Checklist

Suctioning the Tracheostomy	Unsat	Needs More Practice	Sat	Comments
Assessment				
1. Assess needs of patient for suctioning by listening to breath sounds and involving patient.				
Planning				
2. Wash your hands.				
3. Obtain a tracheostomy suctioning kit or gather the following: a. Sterile gloves				
b. Sterile suction catheter				
c. Sterile basin				
d. Sterile water or sterile normal saline				
e. Sterile syringe and normal saline if saline is to be instilled				
f. Sterile gauze squares				
g. Portable suction machine if wall suction is not available				
h. Self-inflating breathing bag and mask				
i. Eye protection				
j. Mask				
k. Sputum trap, if needed.				
Implementation				
4. Identify the patient.				
5. Pull the curtain around the patient's bed.				
6. Explain procedure carefully to the patient.				
7. Establish a way patient can communicate with you.				
8. Test suction apparatus.				
9. Position the patient: Supine or mid Fowler's with head slightly toward you if conscious, lateral position facing you if unconscious.				
10. Put on goggles.				

Suctioning the Tracheostomy *(Continued)*	Unsat	Needs More Practice	Sat	Comments
11. Prepare 5 ml sterile saline in a syringe; remove needle.				
12. Prepare equipment: a. Open kit and place drape or towel over patient's chest.				
b. Put on gloves.				
c. Open and pour saline.				
d. Attach catheter to suction tubing and moisten catheter in normal saline solution.				
13. Person #2 attaches breathing bag to oxygen source.				
14. Person #2 attaches breathing bag to tracheostomy tube and provides three breaths.				
15. Instill saline into tracheostomy.				
16. Suction: a. Insert catheter 4–5 inches without applying suction.				
b. Close system to apply suction.				
c. Apply suction for 10 seconds.				
d. Rotate catheter while withdrawing it.				
e. Rinse catheter in sterile water or normal saline.				
f. Provide ventilation immediately after suction catheter removed.				
17. Observe for dyspnea and skin color changes.				
18. If necessary, person #2 provides deep breaths.				
19. Turn off suction and listen to respirations.				
20. If breathing is not clear, repeat steps 16 a–e.				
21. When breathing is clear, person #2 provides three or four deep breaths.				
22. Disconnect the catheter from the suction tubing.				
23. Pull sterile glove over catheter to cover it and remove eye protection.				
24. Discard disposable equipment and take nondisposable equipment to appropriate place for cleaning.				

Suctioning the Tracheostomy (Continued)	Unsat	Needs More Practice	Sat	Comments
25. Wash your hands.				
26. Offer oral hygiene.				
Evaluation				
27. Evaluate, using the following criteria: a. Tracheostomy tube securely in place.				
b. Respiratory rate and depth normal.				
c. Breath sounds clear.				
d. Patient resting comfortably.				
Documentation				
28. Record procedure and observations.				

Administering Tracheostomy Care

Assessment				
1. Check condition of tracheostomy and need for cleaning.				
Planning				
2. Wash your hands.				
3. Obtain tracheostomy care kit or gather: a. Sterile gloves (or clean gloves for long-standing tracheostomy in long-term care facility)				
b. 4 × 4 gauze squares				
c. Cleansing solution, according to policy of facility				
d. Basin				
e. Tracheostomy brush, pipe cleaners, or swabs				
f. Sterile water.				
Implementation				
4. Identify the patient.				
5. Pull curtain around patient's bed.				
6. Explain what you are going to do.				
7. Provide method of communication for patient.				

Administering Tracheostomy Care *(Continued)*	Unsat	Needs More Practice	Sat	Comments
8. Place patient in mid Fowler's position.				
9. Arrange supplies.				
10. Put on sterile gloves.				
11. To clean cannula-type tube: a. Hold outer tube with one hand and turn lock clockwise with other hand.				
b. Slide inner cannula out by sliding toward you.				
c. Place cannula in basin.				
d. Immerse in cleansing solution for several minutes.				
e. Apply friction with brush, pipe cleaners, or swabs				
f. Rinse well in sterile water.				
g. Dry thoroughly.				
h. If necessary, carefully clean and dry inner aspect of outer cannula.				
i. Hold outer cannula and replace inner cannula.				
j. Turn lock counterclockwise to engage.				
k. Test to make sure cannula is secure.				
12. If plastic tube does not have an inner cannula, clean inner surfaces of tube.				
13. If you plan to change dressing, move to step 6 of procedure for changing tracheostomy dressing. If not, complete this procedure.				
14. Dispose of equipment.				
15. Wash your hands.				

Evaluation

	Unsat	Needs More Practice	Sat	Comments
16. Evaluate, using the following criteria: a. Tracheostomy tube securely in place.				
b. No secretions present.				
c. Breath sounds clear.				

Administering Tracheostomy Care *(Continued)*	Unsat	Needs More Practice	Sat	Comments
Documentation				
17. Record procedure in conjunction with dressing change.				
Changing the Tracheostomy Dressing				
Assessment				
1. Although done routinely after tracheostomy care, assess the patient's dressing for drainage or soiling.				
Planning				
2. Wash your hands.				
3. Gather the following items:				
a. 4 × 4 gauze squares				
b. Twill tape ties				
c. Scissors				
d. Swabs				
e. Cleansing solution				
f. Oral care equipment				
g. Two pair clean gloves				
h. Bag for soiled dressings.				
Implementation				
4. Identify the patient.				
5. Pull curtain around patient's bed.				
6. Explain what you are going to do.				
7. Put on gloves and remove old dressing and discard. a. With two persons, have assistant hold tube while you remove dressing.				
b. With one person, place your fingers on tube while you remove dressing.				
8. Remove gloves and wash hands.				
9. Put on fresh gloves.				
10. With sterile, moistened swabs, clean around edges of tracheostomy opening.				

Changing the Tracheostomy Dressing
(Continued)

	Unsat	Needs More Practice	Sat	Comments
11. Note any redness or swelling.				
12. Prepare the dressing. Precut or as follows: a. Open first fold of 4 × 4 gauze square.				
b. Fold in half lengthwise.				
c. Fold each end toward the center.				
d. Place around tube with ends up.				
13. Remove the soiled holding tape and replace. a. With two persons, have assistant secure tube while you cut tape, remove it, and discard. Carefully slip prepared dressing, ends extending up, around tube. With tube held in place, apply tape.				
(1) Make slit near end of twill tape.				
(2) Thread tape through flange on one side of tube.				
(3) Pass the end through tape slit and pull until snug.				
(4) Bring tape around back of patient's neck.				
(5) Thread loose end through remaining flange and tie tapes.				
b. With one person, prepare new ties and thread with old ties in place and tie tapes. Then cut old ties.				
14. Check placement of tube.				
15. Perform oral care, following Module 11, Hygiene.				
16. Dispose of equipment.				
17. Wash your hands.				
Evaluation				
18. Evaluate, using the following criteria: a. Tracheostomy tube securely in place.				
b. No redness or swelling present.				
c. No secretions present.				
d. Dressing and tapes clean and dry.				

Changing the Tracheostomy Dressing *(Continued)*	Unsat	Needs More Practice	Sat	Comments
e. Absence of stale or foul-smelling breath.				
Documentation				
19. Record procedure and any observations.				

Quiz

Multiple-Choice Questions

_____ 1. Which of the following are purposes of a tracheostomy?

(1) It allows a critically ill patient to breathe when threatened by respiratory obstruction.

(2) It provides an avenue for nutrition when the patient cannot take food and fluids orally.

(3) It may be done to remove secretions before a patient's breathing is severely compromised.

(4) It may be done so that a respirator can be used.

a. 1 and 2
b. 1, 2, and 3
c. 1, 3, and 4
d. All of the above

_____ 2. The patient with a tracheostomy cannot talk because

a. he or she is too ill.
b. air does not reach the vocal cords.
c. there is swelling of the trachea.
d. of the presence of secretions.

_____ 3. Emergency equipment that should always be kept at the bedside of a tracheostomy patient includes (1) tape, (2) clamp, (3) tracheostomy tube, (4) oxygen.

a. 2 and 3
b. 1, 2, and 3
c. 2, 3, and 4
d. All of the above

_____ 4. The primary reason for periodically deflating a cuffed tracheostomy tube is to

a. promote the patient's comfort.
b. adjust the position of the tube.
c. remove and clean the tube.
d. prevent tissue necrosis.

_____ 5. Disadvantages of suctioning the trachea and bronchi include:

(1) It may cause the patient to cough.
(2) The oxygen available to the lungs is decreased.
(3) It causes the collapse of alveoli.
(4) It increases secretions.

a. 1 and 4
b. 1, 2, and 3
c. 2, 3, and 4
d. All of the above.

_____ **6.** When performing shallow tracheal suctioning, how far should the catheter be inserted?

    a. 1 inch
    b. 3 inches
    c. 5 inches
    d. 8 inches

_____ **7.** The primary reason for tying the tapes holding the tracheostomy in place loosely is to prevent

    a. undue pressure that could cause respiratory obstruction.
    b. skin irritation.
    c. circulatory impairment.
    d. discomfort.

_____ **8.** The greatest threat to the patient with a tracheostomy is the danger of

    a. hemorrhaging.
    b. pneumonia.
    c. infection.
    d. asphyxiation.

Module 44

Caring for Patients With Chest Drainage

Module Contents

Rationale for the Use of This Skill
Anatomy and Physiology
Hemothorax, Pneumothorax, and
     Hemopneumothorax
Purpose of Chest Tubes
Procedure for Assisting with the Insertion
     of Chest Tubes
    Assessment
    Planning
    Implementation
    Evaluation
    Documentation
Stripping or Milking the Tubing

Waterseal Drainage
    One-Bottle System
    Two-Bottle System
    Three-Bottle System
    Commercial Chest Drainage Units
Alternative to Chest Tubes
Caring for Patients with Chest Tubes
Problems Related to Chest Drainage
Procedure for Assisting with the Removal of
     Chest Tubes
    Assessment
    Planning
    Implementation
    Evaluation
    Documentation

Prerequisites

1. *Successful completion of the following modules:*

VOLUME 1

Module 1 An Approach to Nursing Skills
Module 2 Basic Infection Control
Module 3 Safety
Module 5 General Assessment Overview
Module 6 Documentation
Module 13 Inspection, Palpation, Auscultation, and Percussion
Module 16 Temperature, Pulse, and Respiration
Module 17 Blood Pressure
Module 19 Assisting with Examinations and Procedures

VOLUME 2

Module 35 Sterile Technique
Module 37 Wound Care

2. *Review of the anatomy and physiology of the respiratory system, especially the dynamics of breathing.*

© 1992 by J.B. Lippincott Company

Overall Objective

To care for patients with chest drainage safely and appropriately, ensuring proper functioning of the chest drainage system.

Specific Learning Objectives

	Know Facts and Principles	Apply Facts and Principles	Demonstrate Ability	Evaluate Performance
1. *Rationale for chest tube insertion*	State three reasons for insertion of chest tube(s).	Given a patient situation, state the reason for the placement of the chest tube(s).	In the clinical setting, identify the reason(s) for the placement of chest tube(s) in a designated patient.	Evaluate with instructor.
2. *Anatomy and physiology*	Describe the anatomy of the pleural space. Describe what happens when the negative pressure in the pleural space is disturbed.			
3. *Hemothorax, pneumothorax, and hemopneumothorax*	Define hemothorax, pneumothorax, and hemopneumothorax. Differentiate between open pneumothorax and closed, or tension, pneumothorax.	Given a patient situation, state which of these is the problem.		Evaluate with instructor.
	Explain the reason for location of a chest tube to remove air and one to remove fluid. State two reasons why it is preferable to connect chest tubes to individual drainage systems when two are placed in a single patient.	Given the location of a chest tube in a hypothetical situation, state the probable reason for its insertion.	In the clinical setting, identify the reason for a chest tube, according to its location. In the clinical setting, connect chest tubes appropriately.	Using facility procedure, evaluate with instructor.
4. *Insertion of chest tubes*	List equipment that might be needed for chest tube insertion on the clinical unit.	Adapt equipment list to your assigned clinical facility.	Select appropriate equipment for chest tube insertion in your clinical facility.	Evaluate using Performance Checklist and facility procedure.

(continued)

Specific Learning Objectives *(Continued)*

	Know Facts and Principles	Apply Facts and Principles	Demonstrate Ability	Evaluate Performance
5. *Stripping or milking the tubing*	Describe how to strip chest tubing. State rationale for stripping tubing. State rationale for stripping tubing gently and only when necessary.	In the practice setting, practice the technique for stripping chest tubing.	In the clinical setting, strip chest tubing gently and only as ordered.	Evaluate with instructor.
6. *Waterseal drainage*	Describe how waterseal drainage works. State two reasons for locating waterseal drainage system *below* the level of the patient's chest.		Keep waterseal drainage system below the level of the patient's chest at all times.	Evaluate with instructor.
a. *One-bottle system*	Describe the one-bottle system of waterseal drainage. State the function of the two pieces of glass tubing.	Explain why the vent must be kept open at all times.	In the practice or clinical setting, set up one-bottle waterseal correctly.	Evaluate with instructor using diagrams.
b. *Two-bottle system*	Describe the two-bottle system of waterseal drainage. Identify one advantage of the two-bottle system when fluid is being drained from the pleural space.		In the practice or clinical setting, set up two-bottle chest drainage correctly.	Evaluate with instructor using diagrams.
c. *Three-bottle system*	Describe the function of the third bottle in the three-bottle system of waterseal drainage.		In the practice or clinical setting, set up three-bottle chest suction correctly. In the clinical setting, check any chest drainage systems to be sure they are set up correctly.	Evaluate with instructor using diagrams.
d. *Commercial waterseal chest drainage systems*	Compare the chambers of the commercial waterseal system to the three-bottle system.		In the clinical setting, set up a commercial waterseal system correctly.	Evaluate with instructor.

(continued)

Specific Learning Objectives *(Continued)*

	Know Facts and Principles	Apply Facts and Principles	Demonstrate Ability	Evaluate Performance
7. *Care of patients with chest tubes*	Know facts and principles related to the care of patients with chest tubes connected to one-, two-, or three-bottle systems.	Given a patient situation, identify appropriate action(s) for that situation.	Under supervision, care for patients with chest tubes.	Evaluate performance with instructor.
8. *Assisting with the removal of chest tubes*	List equipment that might be needed for chest tube removal on the clinical unit. Discuss items that would be included in your explanation to a patient about to undergo chest tube removal. Name two specific things for which you would observe after the removal of chest tubes.	Adapt equipment list to your assigned facility.	Select appropriate equipment for chest tube removal in your clinical facility. Given an opportunity in the clinical setting, prepare a patient for the removal of chest tubes. Make appropriate observations after chest tube removal.	Evaluate with instructor.
9. *Documentation*	State information and observations that need to be documented with the insertion, maintenance, and removal of a chest tube.	Given a patient situation, record data as though on a chart.	Document procedure and observations accurately.	Evaluate with instructor.

Learning Activities

1. Review the Specific Learning Objectives.
2. Read the material on thoracentesis in Appendix J in Ellis and Nowlis, *Nursing: A Human Needs Approach,* or comparable material in another textbook.
3. Look up the module vocabulary terms in the Glossary.
4. Read through the module and mentally practice the specific procedure.
5. In the practice setting:
   a. Examine any chest tube insertion materials available, for example, trocars of various sizes, rubber and plastic chest tubes.
   b. Using your partner as a patient, simulate the explanation and positioning appropriate for chest tube insertion. Have your partner evaluate your performance.
   c. Examine any chest tube drainage bottles or systems available.
   d. Explain to a partner how each of the above systems works.
6. In the clinical setting:
   a. Consult with your instructor for an opportunity to assist with the insertion or removal of a chest tube and to care for a patient with a chest tube(s) in place.

Vocabulary

atelectasis	mediastinum	stab wound	thoracentesis
fibrin	parietal pleura	subcutaneous	tidaling
hemopneumo-thorax	pleural space	emphysema	visceral pleura
	pneumothorax	tension	waterseal drainage
hemothorax	rubber-shod	pneumothorax	

Caring for Patients With Chest Drainage

Rationale for the Use of This Skill
Trauma, surgery, or disease may allow air or fluid to enter the pleural space, leading to impaired breathing and eventually to collapse of the affected lung. Chest tubes are used to drain air or fluid from the pleural cavity and to restore the normal negative intrapleural pressure. The nurse should be able to anticipate the needs of the patient and physician during the insertion and removal of chest tubes, as well as to care safely for the patient with a chest drainage system.[1]

ANATOMY AND PHYSIOLOGY

The pleural space is a *potential* space formed by the visceral and parietal pleura. It contains only enough lubricating fluid to allow the two surfaces to slide smoothly over each other during inhalation and exhalation. On inspiration, the negative pressure is approximately -8 cm water and remains negative on expiration but somewhat less so, at about -4 cm water (Erickson, 1989). The pleural space does not normally contain air or fluid except for the small amount of lubricating fluid.

HEMOTHORAX, PNEUMOTHORAX, AND HEMOPNEUMOTHORAX

A collection of blood in the pleural space is a *hemothorax.* An accumulation of air in the pleural space is a *pneumothorax.* The presence of blood and air is a *hemopneumothorax.*

If any air enters the space or any fluid accumulates, breathing is compromised *because the space normally occupied by the expanded lung is filled with the air or fluid.* This increased pressure in the pleural space may also interfere with the filling of the ventricles of the heart, *leading to circulatory problems.* If too much space is occupied by fluid or air and the pressure exerted is great enough, *the lung may collapse completely.*

In an open pneumothorax, breathing is compromised *by the presence of air in the pleural space.* In a *closed* or *tension pneumothorax,* air gets trapped in the pleural space (usually because of an abnormal opening

[1] You will note that rationale for action is emphasized throughout the module by the use of italics.

such as a gunshot wound or puncture wound that allows passage of air through the chest wall) and cannot escape, leading to a buildup of pressure, which in turn collapses the lung and pushes the structures in the mediastinum toward the opposite side of the chest (mediastinal shift). This condition can result in the collapse of the other lung and can rapidly compromise circulatory and respiratory function.

PURPOSE OF CHEST TUBES

In hemothorax, pneumothorax, or hemopneumothorax, a chest tube is inserted through a surgical cut in the chest after the skin has been anesthetized. This is sometimes referred to as a "stab wound." The insertion of the tube or tubes is done *to remove the air or bloody fluid and allow for reexpansion of the lung and restoration of the normal negative pressure in the pleural space. Because air rises,* a chest tube inserted to remove air is usually placed anteriorly through the second intercostal space. A chest tube inserted to remove fluid is placed posteriorly in the eighth or ninth intercostal space, *because fluid tends to flow to the bottom of the pleural space.* If both air and fluid are in the pleural space, two chest tubes may be inserted. Sometimes tubes are inserted through a stab wound low on the chest, and the end of one tube is threaded high in the pleural cavity *to remove air.*

A chest tube inserted at surgery may be brought out of the chest through the incision or through a stab wound. A chest tube placed for reasons other than surgical trauma is inserted through a stab wound. If two chest tubes are inserted, they can be connected to each other with a Y connector and connected to the same waterseal drainage. It is preferable to leave the chest tubes separate for two reasons: (1) *fluid or air and drainage may be observed and measured individually,* and (2) *one tube can be removed without disturbing the other tube or the rest of the waterseal setup.*

PROCEDURE FOR ASSISTING WITH THE INSERTION OF CHEST TUBES

To assist the physician with the insertion of a chest tube, you should review Module 19, Assisting with Examinations and Procedures, especially noting the procedure for thoracentesis, under Diagnostic and Therapeutic Procedures.

Assessment
1. Check to see if a consent form has been signed by the patient. If not, notify the physician who is to perform the procedure.

2. Measure vital signs (temperature, pulse, respirations, and blood pressure) *to use as a baseline.*

Planning

3. Wash your hands *for infection control.*
4. Obtain a chest tube tray. After you have ascertained which items are included on the tray in your clinical setting, you can add other needed items, such as the chest tube, local anesthetic, antiseptic, suture materials, and sterile gloves. Knowing the specific preferences of the physician inserting the tube is useful and *will help the procedure to go more smoothly.*

Implementation

5. Identify the patient *to be sure you are performing the procedure on the correct patient.*
6. Explain the procedure to the patient in general terms.
7. If ordered, administer mild sedation.
8. Assist the patient to the upright position, *so the pull of gravity consolidates the chest fluid in the lower portion of the affected lung.* This positioning may be accomplished in any of the following ways:
   a. Pad the back of a straight chair *for comfort,* and have the patient straddle the chair, leaning the arms on the padded back.
   b. Have the patient sit upright in bed and lean forward, resting on the overbed table.
   c. Have the patient sit at the edge of the bed, leaning on the overbed table.
9. Open the chest tube tray and assist the physician as indicated. Most necessary items are included on the tray. You may be asked to assist in any of the following ways:
   a. Pour antiseptic over the cotton balls.
   b. Hold the vial of local anesthetic as the physician withdraws the proper dosage.
   c. Apply an occlusive dressing to the tube insertion site(s) or dry sterile gauze and tape.

   d. Have the requested drainage system available.
   e. Make sure a chest film is ordered following the procedure *to check proper placement of the chest tube.*
10. Reassure and observe the patient throughout the procedure.
11. If a specimen of fluid is obtained, label it and send it to the laboratory.
12. Return the patient to a comfortable position.
13. Recheck pulse, respirations, and blood pressure and notify the physician of any significant changes.
14. Allow the patient to rest.
15. Care for the equipment appropriately.
16. Wash your hands.

Evaluation

17. Evaluate, using the following criteria:
    a. Patient vital signs stable.
    b. Patient comfortable.
    c. Chest tube system functioning properly.

Documentation

18. Record appropriate data, including the physician's name, before-and-after vital signs, type of drainage system in use, and the response of the patient.

STRIPPING OR MILKING THE TUBING

Milking and stripping chest tubes means that the tubes are manually compressed and released *to maintain the patency of the tubes.* Both procedures have been studied and found to be potentially hazardous. Milking should only be done if there is evidence of clots in the tube. However, it is the policy in some facilities to milk the tubing every hour or as needed.

Milking may be done in various ways, but basically it means compressing the tubing gently by running the fingers along it, moving away from the patient

DATE/TIME	
5/21/94 1400	Chest tube inserted in left lower chest by Dr. Martin and attached to low suction under waterseal. Breath sounds decreased in left lower lobe. Respirations 28, shallow but regular. See parameter sheet for record of vital signs. Patient resting comfortably and states only slight discomfort at insertion site. ——— S. O'Riley, RN

Example of Progress Notes Using Narrative Format

toward the collection bottle. The tubing is stabilized with one hand while the other hand does the milking. Sometimes an alcohol swab or lotion is *used to enhance the sliding action, but the nurse needs to be alert to any deterioration of the tubing resulting from the use of these agents.*

Recent research indicates that negative pressures created by chest tube stripping are considerably higher than the suction pressures of -15 to -20 cm water usually applied to chest drainage systems.

Stripping *has been reported to produce negative pressures as high as -350 cm water* (Carroll, 1986). Therefore, it is now recommended that stripping not be done as a general practice *to prevent potential tissue injury.* It should also be noted that when air alone is being evacuated from the chest, there is no logical reason to strip the tubing *since there is no potential for obstruction.*

WATERSEAL DRAINAGE

The chest tube (or tubes) is connected to plastic or rubber tubing, which is attached to waterseal drainage—a tube submerged in a container of water *that allows air to escape through a vent (Figure 44–1) but prevents air from traveling back up the tube and into the pleural space.* The waterseal drainage system is placed below the level of the patient's chest, *which takes advantage of the force of gravity to promote drainage and prevents backflow of bottle contents into the pleural space.*

One-Bottle System

The one-bottle system provides waterseal drainage using gravity only, with a single bottle serving as both waterseal and collection container (see Figure 44–1). A long glass or plastic tube is inserted through a rubber stopper and is submerged about 2 cm in the sterile water or saline. Air from the chest passes through the chest tube and bubbles out through the water into the bottle. Also inserted through the rubber stopper is a short tube, which acts as an escape valve or vent and allows air to escape from the bottle, *thus preventing pressure buildup in the bottle. Increased pressure could lead to backup of the water or saline in the bottle toward the chest.*

Because the single bottle is serving a dual purpose, it must be marked at the original (2 cm) fluid level and again at the end of each shift, *to keep track of the amount of drainage.* A long strip of tape can be attached vertically to the bottle for this purpose (Figure 44–2). *When the amount of fluid in the bottle is increased by*

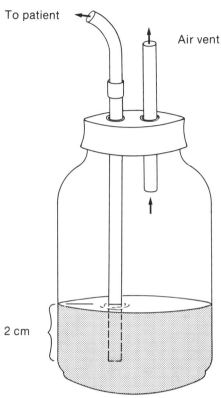

Figure 44–1. One-bottle system (note vent).

drainage, more of the tube is submerged, creating more resistance to drainage. For this reason, some physicians use the one-bottle system for pneumothorax only.

Two-Bottle System

The two-bottle system consists of a fluid collection bottle plus a waterseal bottle as described above (Figure 44–3). *Because the level in the waterseal bottle remains constant,* the amount and type of drainage may be observed and described more accurately than with the one-bottle system. Gravity drainage or suction may be used. If suction is used, the air vent tube on the waterseal bottle is attached to a suction source. The suction level is regulated by a wall gauge or a gauge attached to the suction source.

An alternative two-bottle system consists of one bottle that is both a fluid collection bottle and a waterseal and a second bottle that controls suction (see Three-Bottle System below and Figure 44–4).

Three-Bottle System

Even though the suction is set to a certain level, *it is possible for a higher level of suction to be reached at the end of the attached tubing if the tubing is blocked by tissue.*

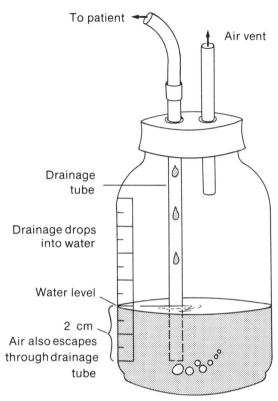

To patient

Air vent

Drainage tube

Drainage drops into water

Water level

2 cm
Air also escapes through drainage tube

Figure 44–2. One-bottle system with vertical tape to measure drainage. Tape can be marked hourly or by the shift to check the amount of drainage.

To prevent this possibility, a three-bottle system is used. The three-bottle system consists of the two-bottle system plus a third bottle, *which controls the amount of suction applied to the chest tube by the suction source.* The amount of suction applied is determined by the depth to which the long tube in the third bottle is submerged in the sterile water or saline (Figure 44–5). Mechanical suction applied is responsible for the negative pressure but will not rise above the amount of suction (usually 10–20 cm) set by the third bottle.

Commercial Chest Drainage Units

Two of several plastic, disposable chest drainage units available commercially are the Pleur-evac® (Figure 44–6) and the Argyle double-seal unit. The Pleur-evac® is essentially a three-bottle system, with a positive pressure release valve to prevent the buildup of excessive pressure in the system. The Argyle double-seal unit is similar to the Pleur-evac® but has a fourth chamber that prevents possible pressure buildup (Figure 44–7). In these units, separate plastic chambers serve the purpose of each bottle in the traditional bottle systems. The units are lightweight, unbreaka-

ble, and can hang from the bedframe so they are not in the way. Settings for suction level and for measuring drainage are clearly marked.

ALTERNATIVE TO CHEST TUBES

An alternative to chest tubes for the treatment of pneumothorax is to insert a chest catheter, which can provide immediate relief of symptoms and correction of the underlying problem. The distal 3 inches of the catheter has multiple perforations *to allow air to flow into the tubing.* A Luer-Lok connector at the proximal end allows staff to connect a three-way stopcock after the chest catheter is inserted and to remove the air from the pleural space with a 50-ml syringe. The proximal end of the catheter is then connected to a Heimlich drainage valve, which permits a one-way flow of air away from the pleural cavity (Figure 44–8). This system can be connected to waterseal drainage and/or suction if necessary. The pneumothorax catheter is not recommended for patients who have large amounts of fluid or hemorrhage, *because of its small internal diameter.*

CARING FOR PATIENTS WITH CHEST TUBES

To provide safe care for the patient with a chest tube or tubes in place, you should follow these guidelines.

1. The chest tube insertion site should be protected with a sterile dressing. The dressing is removed and the site inspected for signs of infection before it is replaced (Figure 44–9).
2. The tubing between the patient and the waterseal bottle should be long enough *to allow the patient to move and turn* (usually about 6 feet). It should be coiled and fastened to the bed (or chair if the patient is up) *so as not to form dependent loops or kinks that would inhibit free drainage.*
3. The patient should be positioned in good alignment and should be encouraged to change positions frequently *to prevent complications of immobility.* When the patient is lying on the affected side, *the tubing can be occluded by the patient's weight.* You can prevent this occlusion by placing rolled towels beside the tubing.
4. The patient should be encouraged to cough and deep breathe at least once hourly *to prevent*

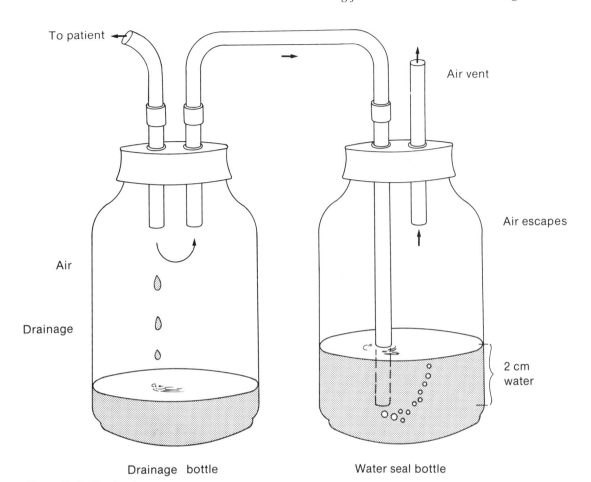

Figure 44–3. Two-bottle system.

atelectasis and to assist in removing air or fluid from the pleural space.

5. The end of the long tube in the waterseal bottle must be submerged approximately 2 cm into the water *to prevent air from going back into the pleural space.* Putting the waterseal bottle in a special holder will prevent it from being tipped. Visitors should be cautioned to avoid the bottle(s). If the bottle is accidentally tipped over, return it to the upright position as rapidly as possible, and ask the patient to take several deep breaths *to help force out air that might have entered the pleural cavity when the waterseal was not intact.* If drainage bottles are on the floor, be careful not to lower a high-low bed or side rails onto the bottles, which should be kept 2–3 feet below the patient's chest.

6. A vent must be present *to allow air to escape.* Except for this vent, the system should be airtight *to prevent air from entering the pleural space.* In many facilities it is the policy to tape all connections and to check the system on a

routine basis *to be sure that the waterseal is in operation, that the air vent is open, and that all connections are intact.*

7. The bottles are kept below the level of the patient's chest at all times *to prevent any backflow of fluid from the bottle into the pleural space.* If the bottles are accidentally raised above the level of the patient's chest, they should be lowered immediately, the physician notified, and the patient observed for signs of further lung collapse and mediastinal shift.

8. Fluctuation (tidaling) of the water level should occur in the long tube in the waterseal bottle. The water level rises when the patient inhales and falls when the patient exhales. Shallow breathing results in slight fluctuation. When it is difficult for the patient to breathe—for example, when secretions are retained—fluctuation is greater. *Continuous bubbling in the waterseal bottle can mean either persistent leakage of air from the lung or a leak in the system* and should be reported immediately.

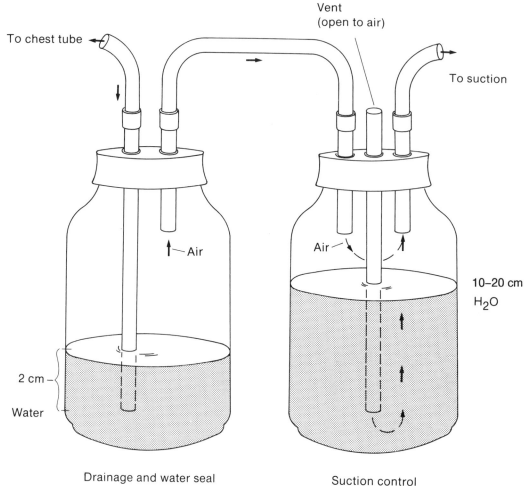

Figure 44–4. Alternative two-bottle system. This system is connected to a suction source.

9. A number of observations should be made and recorded for the patient who has chest drainage. Lung assessment and the level of suction applied are essential parts of this data. Amount, character, and rate of accumulation of drainage must be observed *to identify excessive bleeding, beginning infection, or tube blockage.* This observation is usually made hourly immediately after chest tube insertion and less often thereafter—at least every 8 hours.

   For an example of a chest tube parameter flow sheet, see Figure 44–10.

10. If suction is ordered, the level must be kept at the amount ordered at all times. *Excessive levels of suction may damage tissue, whereas an inadequate level may delay lung reexpansion.* A piece of tape placed at the level of solution in the suction control bottle or at the ordered levels on a gauge can be a helpful reminder.

11. If a suction control bottle is used, check for gentle, continuous bubbling. *Gentle bubbling indicates that suction is constantly reaching the desired level but cannot go higher.* The fluid level in the bottle should be checked periodically *to be sure it is the proper depth to provide the amount of suction ordered.* If it is not the proper depth, sterile water or saline must be added. Likewise, sterile water or saline is added if the physician orders the amount of suction increased. *The higher the fluid level, the more suction develops before the seal is broken and the bottle bubbles.*

12. Two large, rubber-shod hemostats or Kelly clamps for each chest tube should be kept at the bedside *to clamp the chest tube(s) if necessary.* A chest tube is clamped *to determine the cause of*

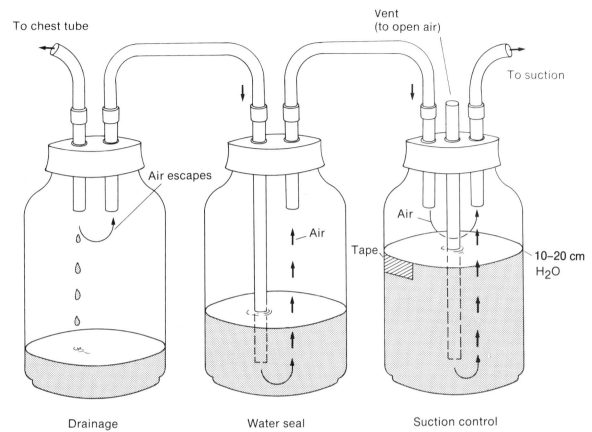

Figure 44–5. Three-bottle system. Top of tape marks suction line.

an air leak when there is bubbling in the waterseal bottle and the patient is on chest suction. It is also necessary to clamp a chest tube *to empty the collection bottle or replace a broken or cracked bottle in the system.* If the lung is leaking air into the pleural space, do not leave the tubes clamped for more than a few minutes. *Air would accumulate in the pleural space, collapsing the lung and causing pressure on the mediastinum.*

13. You do not need to clamp chest tubes to transport a patient to another department or for the patient to ambulate. When transporting or ambulating a patient, you must take care:
   a. to keep the waterseal bottle upright (*the waterseal is intact as long as the long tube is kept below the fluid in the bottle*).
   b. to keep the bottle(s) below the level of the patient's chest *to prevent backflow into the chest.*
   c. to maintain an airtight system (taping all connections and preventing tension or pulling on the tubing helps in this effort) *to prevent air from entering the system.*

When clamps are used, be careful not to cover them with the sheet or blanket *to avoid the possibility of the chest tube(s) being clamped and forgotten.* If clamps are forgotten and left in place for too long a period of time, pressure can build up in the pleural space, *causing a tension pneumothorax.*

   d. A Vaseline gauze should be readily available to provide an airtight dressing should the chest tube inadvertently be pulled out of the chest cavity.

PROBLEMS RELATED TO CHEST DRAINAGE

1. *The drainage is copious and bright red.* Take vital signs and immediately call the physician.
2. *Fluctuations and drainage suddenly stop.* This may indicate a blood or fibrin clot within the tube. Other causes could be kinking of the tube or the patient lying on the tube. A more gradual

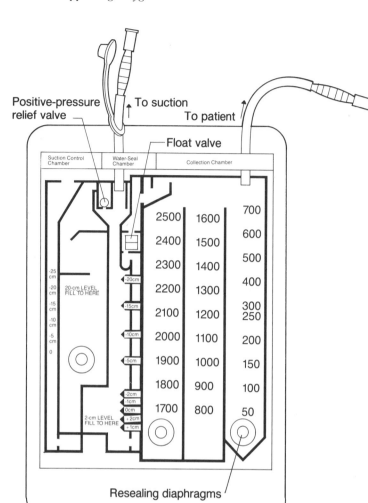

Figure 44–6. Pleur-Evac.® A commercial chest drainage system.

cessation of fluctuation or drainage could indicate that the lung has reexpanded.

3. *The drainage quickly fills the collection chamber.* Briefly clamp the tube and connect to a new, sterile system. If water is used, it must be sterile water. Remove clamp and reinstate the suction.

4. *The drainage bottle or plastic system has broken.* Clamp briefly and replace as described above.

5. *The chest tube has pulled out.* Immediately place an occlusive dressing such as a sterile vaseline gauze (which should be available in the room) over the site to prevent room air from entering the pleural space and call the physician.

6. *Increase in bubbling with inspiration and expiration.* Inspect system, including taped connections, for a leak.

7. *The patient's anxiety increases.* First, assess the drainage system for problems and the patient's respiratory status. If the system is working

properly and respiratory status is stable, spend time with the patient. Explain how the drainage system works and why the sounds of the suction are important and beneficial.

8. *Patient experiences moderate pain when moving.* Medicate the patient liberally per physician's order.

PROCEDURE FOR ASSISTING WITH THE REMOVAL OF CHEST TUBES

To assist the physician with the removal of a chest tube, you should again refer to Module 19, Assisting with Examinations and Procedures. The physician may order an analgesic premedication, or you can give the patient the ordered pain relief medication about 30 minutes before the chest tube is removed.

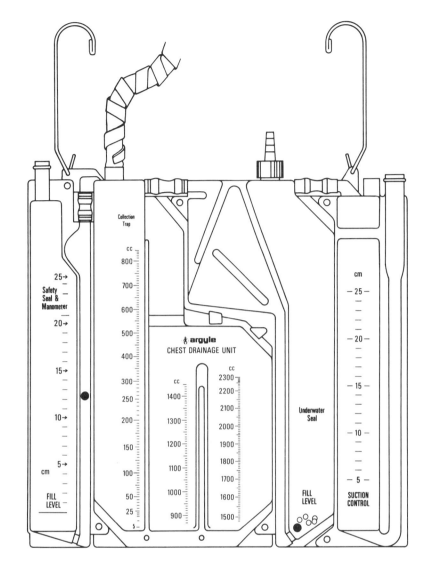

Figure 44-7. Argyle "double-seal" commercial chest drainage unit. (*Courtesy Argyle Division of Sherwood Medical, St. Louis, Missouri*)

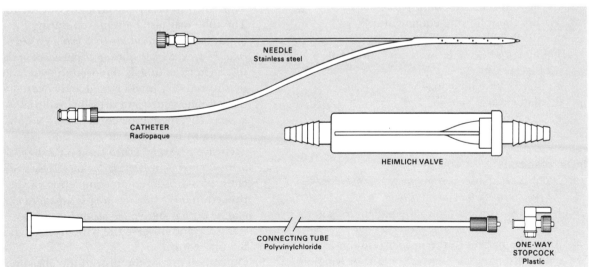

Figure 44-8. Pneumothorax catheter set. (*Courtesy Cook Critical Care, Bloomington, Indiana*)

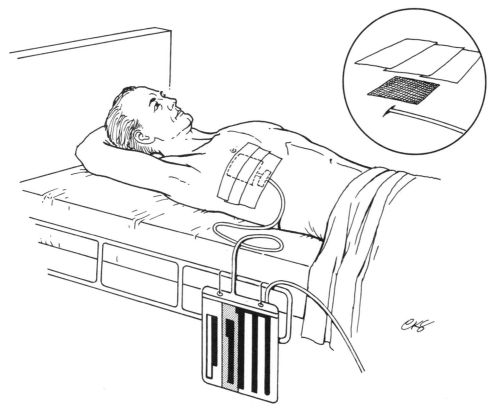

Figure 44–9. The chest tube insertion site is protected by a gauze and tape dressing.

Assessment

1. Measure vital signs (pulse, respirations, and blood pressure) to use as a baseline.

Planning

2. Wash your hands *for infection control.*
3. Gather the following equipment:
   a. Sterile gloves
   b. Suture set (or sterile scissors and sterile forceps)
   c. Sterile Vaseline gauze
   d. Skin closure material
   e. Dressing material
   f. Wide tape.

Implementation

4. Identify the patient *to be sure you are performing the procedure on the correct patient.*
5. Explain the procedure to the patient in general terms.
6. Assist the patient to the proper position— either sitting at the edge of the bed or lying on the unaffected side.

7. Open the sterile packages and assist the physician as indicated. First the physician removes any dressing materials and then cuts the sutures. The patient is asked to take a deep breath and bear down (Valsalva maneuver) while the physician quickly pulls out the tube. The tube may also be removed during expiration, *to prevent air from being pulled back into the pleural space during the removal of the tube.* After the tube is removed the wound may be sutured or clipped closed and covered with the vaseline gauze and dressing material, which is securely taped in place, or it may simply be covered with petrolatum gauze and an occlusive dressing, *which forms an airtight seal to prevent air from reentering the chest.* Usually a chest film is ordered on completion of the procedure *to be sure the lung is expanded and that no air has entered the pleural space.*
8. Reassure and observe the patient throughout the procedure.
9. On completion of the procedure, auscultate breath sounds and watch for indications of

Suction Device ___Waterseal___

Location of chest tube A. (L) lower lobe

B. ___—___

Key

1. Character of resp: normal, symmetry, shallow, deep labored
2. Sputum: character, amount, color
3. Drainage: character, amount, color
4. Pain scale: 0=non; 1=mild; 2, 3=moderate; 4,5=severe
5. Anxiety: none, minimal, moderate, severe
6. Air leak: none, small, medium, large bubbling
7. Dressing: dry, intact, loose, reinforced
8. Equipment function: yes/no, check q8°

*Document in nursing progress notes any notable changes & q8° evaluative statement.

Date	Time	lung assessment	character of respirations	character of sputum	drainage	dressing	level of suction	equipment function	air leak	pain	anxiety		init.
6/10/92	0700	↓ LLL	reg.	sm. white	mod.	change	20 cm	✓	Ø	1+	min		J.B.
6/10	1500	↓ LLL	reg.	mod. white	mod	—	20 cm	✓	Ø	2	min	medi-cated	SW
6/10	2300	—	—	—	—	change	—	✓	Ø	1	Ø		SW
6/11	0200	↓ LLL	—	sm. white	mod.	—	20 cm	✓	Ø	1	Ø	sleeping	DD

Identify Initials with Signature:	4.	8.
1. Jean Bennett, RN	5.	9.
2. Sue Williams, RN	6.	10.
3. Donna Davis, RN	7.	11.

ADDRESSOGRAPH:

WARNER, Steven   M

754 56 2354   27

SWEDISH HOSPITAL MEDICAL CENTER
Seattle, Washington

Figure 44–10. Chest drainage observations can be made by the nurse on a special parameter sheet.

DATE/TIME	
2/25/95	Interim Note
1400	S "I'm glad to have that out."
	O Chest tube removed by Dr. Martinez. Stab wound sutured and covered with petrolatum gauze and occlusive dressing. Portable chest film ordered. VS stable. Breath sound clear bilaterally. No respiratory difficulty.
	A Chest tube removed without difficulty.
	P Continue to assess respiratory status.
	J. Ross, RN

Example of Progress Notes Using SOAP Format

pneumothorax (dyspnea, tachypnea, chest pain) and subcutaneous emphysema (air trapped in the subcutaneous tissue that crackles when palpated) *to identify complications that might occur.*

10. Recheck vital signs and notify the physician of any significant changes.
11. Allow the patient to rest.
12. Care for the equipment appropriately.
13. Wash your hands.

Evaluation
14. Evaluate, using these criteria:
    a. Patient vital signs stable.
    b. No indication of pneumothorax or subcutaneous emphysema.
    c. Patient comfortable.

Documentation
15. On the patient's chart, record appropriate data, including physician's name, before-and-after vital signs, the response of the patient, and any other significant observations.

References

Carroll, P. F. (1986). The ins and outs of chest drainage systems. *Nursing '86, 16*(12), 26–33.

Duncan, C., & Erickson, R. (1982). Pressure associated with chest tube stripping. *Heart and Lung, 11*(2), 166–171.

Erickson, R. (1989). Mastering the ins and outs of chest drainage, Part I. *Nursing '89, 19*(5), 36–43; Part II. *Nursing '89, 19*(6), 45–50.

Palau, D. (1987). Test your skill at troubleshooting chest tubes. *RN, 50*(6), 20–25.

Performance Checklist

Assisting With the Insertion of Chest Tubes	Unsat	Needs More Practice	Sat	Comments
Assessment				
1. Check to see if consent form has been signed.				
2. Measure vital signs.				
Planning				
3. Wash your hands.				
4. Obtain chest tube tray and add other needed items.				
Implementation				
5. Identify the patient.				
6. Explain the procedure.				
7. Administer mild sedation, if ordered.				
8. Assist patient to one of the following positions: a. Patient straddles chair, leaning on the padded back.				
b. Patient sits upright in bed, resting on overbed table.				
c. Patient sits at edge of bed, leaning on overbed table.				
9. Open tray and assist physician as indicated. a. Pour antiseptic over cotton balls.				
b. Hold vial of local anesthetic as physician withdraws proper dosage.				
c. Apply an occlusive dressing to tube insertion site(s).				
d. Have requested drainage system available.				
e. Make sure chest film is ordered to check tube placement.				
10. Reassure and observe patient throughout.				
11. Label any specimen and send to lab.				
12. Return patient to a comfortable position.				
13. Recheck vital signs and report any significant changes.				

Assisting With the Insertion of Chest Tubes
(Continued)

	Unsat	Needs More Practice	Sat	Comments
14. Allow patient to rest.				
15. Care for the equipment.				
16. Wash your hands.				
Evaluation				
17. Evaluate, using the following criteria: a. Patient vital signs stable.				
b. Patient comfortable.				
c. Chest tube system functioning properly.				
Documentation				
18. Record appropriate data, including physician's name, vital signs, response of patient.				

Caring for the Patient With a Chest Tube

	Unsat	Needs More Practice	Sat	Comments
1. Protect insertion site with sterile dressing. Inspect regularly for signs of infection.				
2. Coil and fasten tubing so as not to form dependent loops or kinks.				
3. Position patient in good alignment and encourage frequent position change.				
4. Encourage patient to cough and deep breathe every hour.				
5. Make sure end of long tube in waterseal bottle is submerged in approximately 2 cm water.				
6. Check that vent is present and all connections are intact.				
7. Keep bottles below chest level of patient at all times.				
8. Note fluctuations in the long tube in waterseal bottle.				
9. Observe amount, character, and rate of accumulation of drainage as ordered or at least every 8 hours.				
10. Keep suction at level ordered at all times.				
11. Check suction control bottle for continuous bubbling.				

Caring for the Patient With a Chest Tube
(Continued)

	Unsat	Needs More Practice	Sat	Comments
12. Keep two large, rubber-shod hemostats or Kelly clamps for each chest tube at bedside. Clamp chest tubing a. to determine the cause of an air leak when there is bubbling in the waterseal bottle and the patient is on chest suction.				
b. to empty the collection bottle or replace a broken or cracked bottle in the system.				
13. When transporting or ambulating patient, take care a. to keep the waterseal bottle upright and waterseal intact.				
b. to keep the bottle(s) below the level of the patient's chest.				
c. to maintain an airtight system.				

Assisting With the Removal of Chest Tubes

Assessment

1. Measure vital signs.				

Planning

2. Wash your hands.				
3. Gather equipment. a. Sterile gloves				
b. Suture set (or sterile scissors and sterile forceps)				
c. Sterile Vaseline gauze				
d. Skin closure material				
e. Dressing material				
f. Wide tape.				

Implementation

4. Identify the patient.				
5. Explain the procedure.				
6. Assist patient to proper position—either sitting at edge of bed or lying on unaffected side.				

Assisting With the Removal of Chest Tubes (Continued)	Unsat	Needs More Practice	Sat	Comments
7. Open sterile packages and assist physician by having suture materials ready, applying vaseline gauze and occlusive dressing, and checking to see if chest film is ordered.				
8. Reassure and observe patient throughout procedure.				
9. Observe patient for indications of pneumothorax and subcutaneous emphysema.				
10. Recheck vital signs and report any significant changes.				
11. Allow patient to rest.				
12. Care for equipment.				
13. Wash your hands.				
Evaluation				
14. Evaluate, using the following criteria: a. Patient vital signs stable.				
b. No indication of pneumothorax or subcutaneous emphysema.				
c. Patient comfortable.				
Documentation				
15. Record appropriate data, including physician's name, before-and-after vital signs, response of patient, and any other significant observations.				

Quiz

Short-Answer Questions

1. List three reasons for insertion of chest tubes.

   a. _____

   b. _____

   c. _____

2. Define pneumothorax. _____

3. A chest tube placed to remove air is usually located _____

4. The reason for the location of a chest tube placed to remove air is that

   _____

5. List two reasons for locating the waterseal drainage system below the level of the patient's chest.

   a. _____

   b. _____

6. Describe the function of the third water bottle in the three-bottle system of waterseal drainage. _____

7. List three things to check when observing a chest drainage system.

   a. _____

   b. _____

   c. _____

8. Clamps should be used on chest tubes briefly and only when necessary to prevent a _____

9. Patients who have chest tubes may experience _____ and _____ .

10. A chest film is often ordered after a chest tube is removed to be sure that and _____ .

Unit 10

SPECIAL THERAPEUTIC AND SUPPORTIVE PROCEDURES

MODULE 45
Nasogastric Intubation

MODULE 46
Preoperative Care

MODULE 47
Postoperative Care

MODULE 48
Irrigations: Bladder, Catheter, Ear, Eye, Nasogastric Tube, Vaginal, Wound

225

Module 45
Nasogastric Intubation

Module Contents

Rationale for the Use of This Skill
Types of Nasogastric Tubes
  Standard Nasogastric Tubes
  Salem Sump Tube
  Small-Bore, Silicone Rubber Tubes
    Keofeed Tube
    Duo-Tube
    Dobbhoff Tube
  Special Purpose Tubes
    Ewald Tube
    Cantor Tube
    Miller-Abbott Tube

Procedure for Inserting a Nasogastric Tube
  Assessment
  Planning
  Implementation
  Evaluation
  Documentation
Intubating the Unconscious Patient
Procedure for Removing a Nasogastric Tube
  Assessment
  Planning
  Implementation
  Evaluation
  Documentation

Prerequisites[1]

Successful completion of the following modules:

VOLUME 1
Module 1   An Approach to Nursing Skills
Module 2   Basic Infection Control
Module 3   Safety
Module 5   General Assessment Overview
Module 6   Documentation
Module 11 Hygiene
Module 15 Intake and Output
Module 29 Tube Feeding

[1] For nasogastric irrigation, see Module 48, Irrigations: Bladder, Catheter, Ear, Eye, Nasogastric Tube, Vaginal, Wound. For feeding through a nasogastric tube, see Module 29, Tube Feeding.

227

Overall Objective

To insert nasogastric tubes for the purpose of feeding, instilling medications, irrigating the stomach, or initiating gastric suction.

Specific Learning Objectives

	Know Facts and Principles	Apply Facts and Principles	Demonstrate Ability	Evaluate Performance
1. *Types and uses of tubes*	Identify characteristics of nasogastric tubes.	Know when to ice tubes and how to lubricate.	Ice tube if needed. Lubricate tube correctly.	Evaluate own performance with instructor.
2. *Equipment*	Recognize types of equipment needed and whether it should be clean or sterile.		Select appropriate equipment and assemble tray.	Evaluate own performance with instructor.
3. *Psychologic support*	Know importance of preparing patient for procedure.	Given a patient situation, identify psychologic problems present.	In the clinical setting, explain procedure and elicit cooperation from patient.	Review interaction with instructor.
4. *Inserting tube*	Describe placement of tube in pharynx and esophagus. Explain how to ascertain correct distance to insert tube.	Given a patient situation, identify appropriate nursing action in response to patient problems during nasogastric tube insertion.	Under supervision, insert nasogastric tube.	Evaluate using Performance Checklist.
5. *Placing tube properly*	List three methods for determining proper placement.	Identify which method is most reliable.	Use a reliable method to determine correct placement. Do not proceed until sure.	Evaluate placement of tube with instructor.
6. *Attaching suction equipment*	Know types of suction equipment used in facility.	Take safety factors into account in planning.	Attach suction equipment only after testing.	Have procedure checked by staff nurse or instructor.
7. *Carrying out irrigation*	State purposes of gastric irrigation.	Select proper solution and equipment.	Instill solution slowly and aspirate with care.	Evaluate own performance with instructor.
8. *Documentation*	State observations to be made and data to be included when documenting the procedure.	List data for documenting specific patient situation.	Make routine data entries as well as specific observations for given patient.	Have instructor review entries.

Learning Activities

1. Review the Specific Learning Objectives.
2. Read the section on the effects of immobility in the chapter on activity and rest and the section on the essentials of nutrition in the chapter on nutrition in Ellis and Nowlis, *Nursing: A Human Needs Approach,* or comparable material in another textbook.
3. Look up the module vocabulary terms in the Glossary.
4. Review the anatomy of the upper gastrointestinal tract.
5. Read through the module and mentally practice the skill.
6. In the practice setting:
   a. Inspect the various nasogastric tubes available. Note the differences in size and lumen.
   b. After carefully reading over the procedure and the Performance Checklist, report to the practice setting at your appointed time and insert a nasogastric tube into a mannequin.

c. Give instructions and explanations to the mannequin as if it were an actual patient.
7. In the clinical setting:
   a. Observe the insertion of a nasogastric tube by either your instructor or a staff nurse. Were the steps followed precisely? What was the patient's response?
   b. Familiarize yourself with the kind of nasogastric suction used in your facility. If the patient in step a, above, is to have suction applied, observe how this is done.
   c. When you are ready and with your instructor's supervision, perform the following activities in the clinical area:
      (1) Insert a nasogastric tube.
      (2) If ordered, attach it to suction.
   d. After performing each procedure, again review the Performance Checklist and evaluate your skills.
   e. Consult your instructor regarding any problems you encounter.

Vocabulary

alimental	gag reflex	mercury	silicone
asepto syringe	gavage	nasogastric tube	sternum
aspirate	intubation	peristalsis	stylet
dyspnea	lavage	pharynx	trachea
enteral	Levin tube	pylorus	xiphoid process
enteric	lumen		

Gastric Intubation

Rationale for the Use of This Skill

Nasogastric tubes are inserted for a number of reasons: for instilling liquid feedings and medications for the patient who cannot swallow without aspirating or eat by mouth; for decompressing the abdomen before or after surgery; or for washing out, or lavaging, the stomach.

Because many patients cannot take food orally after surgery, long-term tube feeding in convalescence is sometimes necessary. Feeding the patient in this manner is called gastric gavage. Also, physical and muscular debilitation caused by stroke or cerebrovascular accident (CVA) or by other conditions may necessitate tube feeding for some length of time.

Nausea and general discomfort can occur after surgery. Distention is not only uncomfortable, but it can place tension on an abdominal suture line. To prevent these conditions, physicians may order a nasogastric tube inserted through a nostril and into the stomach. A nasogastric tube can also prevent nausea and vomiting when gastric or bowel surgery is performed and peristalsis is absent. When suction is applied to the tube, gastric secretions and any accumulated gas are removed, leaving the postop patient more comfortable.

In some medical conditions, such as bowel obstruction, pancreatitis, and cholecystitis, normal peristalsis is lost and intestinal secretions accumulate, causing distention and discomfort. A nasogastric tube is inserted and attached to suction that removes these accumulated secretions and gas. This stops nausea and vomiting and makes the patient more comfortable.

A nasogastric tube is also used if a patient has ingested toxic substances and the stomach must be emptied and washed. The term for this procedure is lavage.

Most facilities consider the use of the nasogastric tube a routine procedure. But it can be frightening and unfamiliar to patients. It is the nurse's responsibility to help patients overcome their anxieties about the tube's insertion and to make it as comfortable as possible.[2]

TYPES OF NASOGASTRIC TUBES

Several types of nasogastric tubes are available. They may be made of rubber, plastic, or silicone. Diameters also vary. Some tubes have very small lumens, whereas others have quite large lumens.

Several models are designed with a stylet or fine

[2] You will note that rationale for action is emphasized throughout the module by the use of italics.

metal wire that threads through the center of the tube. *This makes the tube more rigid and easier to pass. Stylets are also radiopaque and can be viewed by x-ray if placement is a concern.* The distal ends of some nasogastric tubes are weighted *so that they settle in the lower portion of the stomach, where secretions or gas collects.* If necessary, weighted tubes can pass further down the alimentary tract into the small intestine. In this module we will discuss several of the common tubes.

Standard Nasogastric Tubes

The standard nasogastric tube may be used for either suctioning gastric contents or administering tube feedings. Often called a Levin tube, it comes in a variety of sizes from 5 French (very small) to 18 French (very large). All are approximately 50 inches long. Sizes 5–12 are customarily used for children and sizes 12–18 are used for adults. Most facilities carry only one or two sizes. The portion inserted into the stomach has a large opening at the tip and several side openings located near the end. The external end is slightly funnel shaped to allow easy connection to a suction tubing or to a feeding set. All are disposed of after use.

All standard nasogastric tubes cause some irritation to the nares and to the throat through which they pass. They also keep the cardiac sphincter of the stomach from closing tightly and may predispose to regurgitation of stomach contents into the esophagus or on up to be aspirated into the lungs.

The most common type is made of rigid, clear plastic with a series of black marks to denote tube length for insertion. Red rubber tubes of the same design are also available. Some physicians prefer them *because they cause less irritation in the back of the throat and the nose.* Red rubber tubes are more expensive and in the past were cleaned and resterilized. Many nurses find the red rubber tubes easier to insert if they are chilled in a pan of ice for 15–20 minutes before insertion. *This makes them more rigid and less likely to coil in the back of the throat on insertion.*

Pediatric-sized nasogastric tubes may be used for some adults, *because they are less irritating than larger tubes.* Pediatric tubes are the type most commonly used for unconscious adults *but these tubes tend to coil rather than move down smoothly,* and insertion is often difficult. To facilitate passage of a pediatric tube into an adult patient, first obtain both a pediatric and an adult tube and half of an empty gelatin capsule. Fill the empty capsule half full with water-soluble lubricant (*in case the patient aspirates*) and insert the ends of both tubes into the capsule. Pass both tubes together into the patient. *The large tube facilitates passage of the small tube.* After the tubes are in the stomach, the gelatin capsule will dissolve. Then the large tube can be withdrawn, leaving the small tube in place.

Salem Sump Tube

The Salem sump tube is a variation of the standard nasogastric tube that is especially designed for gastric suctioning. The Salem sump tube has a double lumen, with two distinct tubes at the distal portion. Its advantage over the Levin tube is that its smaller, open end (color-coded blue) is open to room air, *allowing equalization of pressure and therefore continuous, steady suction without pull on the tissues* (Figure 45–1). *Suction pull above the level of capillary fragility, which can cause damage to tissues, is prevented.*

One nursing precaution you should take is to position the open end of the air-vent tube above the patient's midline *to prevent leakage of stomach contents* when low suction is on and the pull pressure is not sufficient to maintain flow through the drainage tube. An antireflux valve device *that allows the Salem sump to be equalized by air but prevents leakage of gastric secretions* is available (Figure 45–2).

The nurse should irrigate the tube using the

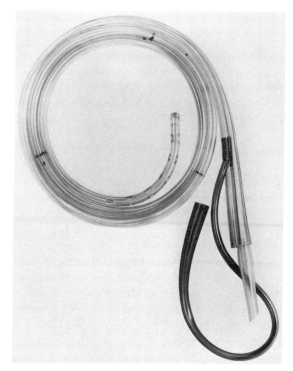

Figure 45–1. Salem sump tube with second lumen to act as an air vent.

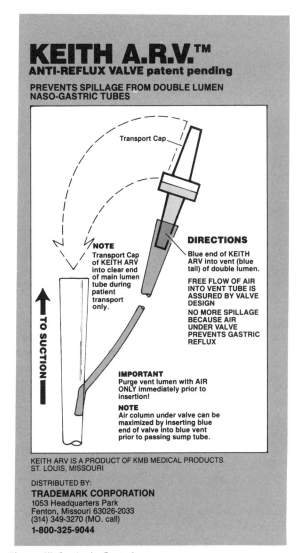

Figure 45–2. Antireflux valve.
(*Courtesy Trademark Corp., Fenton, Missouri*)

larger or primary tube, because the vented air tube *may become occluded with the irrigation solution or secretions.* If it is necessary to irrigate the vent lumen to clear secretions, always follow the solution by instilling air to restore the open vent.

Small-Bore Silicone Rubber Feeding Tube

A variety of small-bore silicone rubber feeding tubes are available. Their soft material and small size decrease the irritation of nose and throat. In addition, the cardiac sphincter closes more tightly around them, lessening the possibility of regurgitation and aspiration. The softness and small size that make them desirable for the patient also make them somewhat more difficult to insert. Most of the special features designed into these tubes are to facilitate their insertion.

Keofeed Tube

The Keofeed tube is small in diameter and made of soft Silastic (silicone), with a weighted end. Because its flexibility makes insertion difficult, the tube comes from the manufacturer with a firm stylet threaded through its lumen *to facilitate insertion.* Final positioning is usually verified by x-ray with the stylet in place. Then the stylet is removed. The stylet should be saved because the tube might be removed or pulled out and have to be reinserted. Lubricating the stylet well with water-soluble lubricant *facilitates its reinsertion so the tube can be reinserted into the patient.*

Because the end of the tube is weighted, it will move with peristalsis into the small intestine if the tube is not taped with tension to the nose. This feature makes it especially suitable for delivering alimentary feedings. Alimentation is the instillation through a tube of a liquid diet composed of substances that can be directly absorbed without digestion.

Duo-Tube

Another variation of a weighted tube is the Duo-Tube. This clear vinyl tube surrounds a silicone radiopaque catheter. The silicone catheter comes with either a silicone weight *for gastric feeding* or a mercury weight *if passage into the pylorus is desired for diagnostic or feeding purposes.* After lubrication with a water-soluble lubricant, the Duo-Tube is inserted into the stomach in the same manner as other nasogastric tubes. The inner tube is advanced approximately 2 inches by attaching a water-filled bulb (which comes with the set) to the distal end of the tube and squeezing. This maneuver can be repeated until the tube is inserted the desired length. Then the clear tube is carefully withdrawn. It remains attached to the inner tube and forms a continuous long tube. It can be either attached to a feeding set or shortened. The inner tube, then, directly attaches to the feeding set (Figure 45–3).

Dobbhoff Tube

Another type of weighted tube is the Dobbhoff tube, which is made of soft plastic material and coated on both its inner and outer surfaces with a water-soluble lubricant. The stylet is hollow *so that air can be injected*

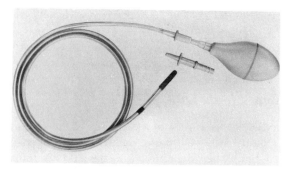

Figure 45–3. Duofeed tube with bulb to advance inner tube. (*Courtesy Argyle Division of Sherwood Medical, St. Louis, Missouri*)

through it to check tube placement before the stylet is removed. The distal end of the tube is weighted with tungsten rather than mercury. If a rupture occurs (which is rare), *tungsten is considered less hazardous to the patient than mercury.* The Dobbhoff tube is designed to be passed from the stomach into the small intestine, which minimizes the chance of regurgitation, which can lead to aspiration (Wilson, 1986).

Special Purpose Tubes

Some tubes are used for special functions not routine suctioning or feeding. These include the Ewald, the Cantor, and the Miller-Abbott tubes.

Ewald Tube

Like the Levin tube, the Ewald tube has a large lumen, but it is uncommon on the general nursing unit. It ranges in size from 26 to 30 French and is *used for lavage, usually for a patient who has ingested poisonous agents. The Ewald tube is also used for diagnostic tests.*

Cantor Tube

The Cantor tube is a long, single-lumen rubber tube with a rubber bag attached to its distal tip (Figure 45–4). Just before insertion, medical personnel inject approximately 30 ml mercury into the bag, using a needle and syringe. Insertion of this tube is uncomfortable, *because the bag is large.* This tube is usually inserted by a physician, who uses a topical anesthetic in the nose and posterior pharynx *to make insertion more tolerable for the patient.* The weight of the mercury *facilitates passage of the tube into the small bowel and may also help overcome an obstruction.* When the Cantor tube is removed, a flashlight is used *to observe the back of the throat.* When the bag reaches that level, a pair of forceps is used to grasp the bag and pull it out

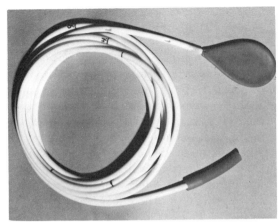

Figure 45–4. Cantor tube with balloon to hold mercury. (*Courtesy American Hospital Supply Corp., McGaw Park, Illinois*)

through the mouth. The bag is then cut off and the tube pulled out through the nose. *This prevents the possibility of this large, heavy bag damaging the inside of the nose.*

When the Cantor tube is used, a safety consideration should be *to protect the patient and the nurse from the mercury, which can cause poisoning through skin absorption and inhalation of mercury vapor as well as through ingestion.* The container should be kept covered and care taken not to spill the mercury. Do not touch the mercury with bare hands. Before the mercury is inserted, inspect the bag for holes. When the tube is removed, do not throw the mercury away but return it in a sealed container through appropriate hospital channels for correct disposal. *Mercury is very expensive,* so care should be taken not to waste it.

Miller-Abbott Tube

The Miller-Abbott tube is a long, double-lumen rubber tube. One lumen leads to a rubber bag at the tube's end. This lumen can be filled with air or fluid *to provide a larger object at the end so that peristalsis can advance the tube into the small intestine.* The other lumen is used for suction and irrigation. The Miller-Abbott tube is inserted in the same manner as a conventional nasogastric tube. Once the tube is positioned in the stomach, the bag is inflated with air or fluid through its lumen. If the tube is not secured with tape to the patient's nose, it will gradually advance into the small bowel. This is desirable when small bowel obstruction is suspected. It is important to keep the openings to each lumen clearly marked *so suction is attached correctly.*

PROCEDURE FOR INSERTING A NASOGASTRIC TUBE

Assessment

1. Check the physician's orders *to determine the type of tube to be inserted and the reason (feeding, suction).*
2. Assess the patient's capabilities for assisting or cooperating with the procedure.
3. Determine where the needed equipment is located. Some may be kept on the unit. Other items may need to be ordered from central services.

Planning

4. Wash your hands *for infection control. Because the gastrointestinal tract is not sterile, it is appropriate to use clean but not sterile technique.*
5. Gather the equipment. If the tube is to be used for feeding or suction, also obtain the appropriate feeding set or suction apparatus.

   In addition to the tube, you will need clean gloves and a water-soluble lubricant, which, if aspirated, *will not cause aspiration pneumonia.* An emesis basin, tape, tissues, a towel, a glass, a straw, a stethoscope, and a large syringe with an adapter or an asepto syringe should also be at hand. A rubber band and safety pin are often used to attach the tube to the patient's gown.
6. Plan for any assistance that might be necessary.
7. If a special or weighted tube is being used, review the manufacturer's directions for insertion. If a Levin or unweighted tube is to be inserted, continue with the next steps.

Implementation

8. *Identify the patient to be sure you are performing the procedure for the correct patient.*
9. Explain the procedure to the patient and why it is needed. *Because the patient is apt to be anxious,* do not explain the procedure too far in advance. Tell the patient that the procedure will not be painful but may be a little uncomfortable. Explain how the patient can help. For example, *relaxation is important,* so ask the patient to breathe deeply, and explain as you proceed. *Your confidence will also help the patient to relax.*
10. Place the patient in high Fowler's position if possible, *so gravity aids insertion of the tube.* Put a clean towel over the patient's chest *to protect the linen.* If the patient's skin is oily, you may

use an alcohol swab to cleanse the nose for later tape application. A skin prep may also be used on the nose to increase tape adherence.

11. Some manufacturers mark the length for insertion, for both pediatric and adult use, on the tube. If the tube you are using is not marked, stand to the patient's right, if you are right-handed, and measure the portion of tube to be inserted by extending it from the tip of the patient's nose to the earlobe and from the nose to the xiphoid process. Experience has shown that in tall people, it may be necessary to add 2 inches to the length of the tube *to ensure entrance into the stomach.* If you are measuring the nasogastric tube for an infant, extend it from the tip of the nose to the earlobe and then from the nose to a point halfway between the xiphoid process and the umbilicus, *because the body proportions are different in infants and adults.* Mark the tube with a piece of tape.

12. Put on gloves and squeeze a water-soluble lubricant from the package onto the tube. Lubricate the portion of the tube from tip to

marking *so as not to damage the nasopharyngeal mucosa when you insert the tube.*

13. Flex the patient's head slightly forward. *In this position the tube is less likely to pass into the trachea because the glottis closes the trachea in this position.* Grasp the tube with your right hand, about 3 inches from the end, and gently insert it into the nostril, guiding it straight back along the floor of the nose.

14. Have a basin in the patient's lap and tissues handy. If orders allow, have the patient sip water and swallow while you gently but steadily advance the tube. There may be some temporary gagging, *caused by the gag reflex,* but this should subside as the tube is progressed. If any coughing persists or dyspnea occurs, remove the tube immediately *because you may have entered the trachea.*

15. Using tape, secure the tube to the patient's nose. Place a vertical strip down the bridge of the nose. Cut the lower end of the tape into two "tails" and wrap them around the tube (Figure 45–5). *This method is comfortable for the patient and prevents irritation of the side of the*

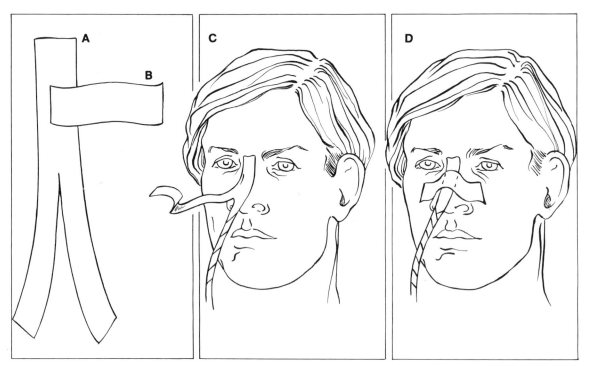

Figure 45–5. Securing the nasogastric tube. **A:** Tape torn lengthwise for several inches, to be placed lengthwise on nose, with tails hanging beyond end of nose. **B:** Second tape, to be placed crosswise over bridge of nose to secure tape A. **C:** Tape A in place, one tail wrapped around tube in a spiral. **D:** Second tail of tape A wrapped around tube, spiraling in opposite direction; tape B has been placed across bridge of nose, securing tape A.

nostril. Fasten the length of tube to the patient's gown with a rubber band and safety pin, *so the patient can move freely in bed without pulling or dislodging the tube.*

Flexible tape bandages may also be used to attach the tube to the nose. Figure 45–6 gives an example of one type.

16. Check to see if the end of the tube is in the stomach. *If it is curled in the back of the throat, it is uncomfortable and ineffective.* You can easily check this by asking the patient to open the mouth or by holding down the tongue with a tongue depressor. Using a flashlight, you can see if the tube is curled in the back of the throat. *The possibility that it is partially in the trachea, so that fluids would enter the lungs and cause serious complications, is more dangerous.* You can check the tube's position in several ways. Some are more reliable than others.

In a conscious patient who is able to swallow a nasogastric tube, identifying incorrect tube placement is usually quite straightforward. If the patient swallows the tube voluntarily, the epiglottis closes over the tracheal opening preventing the tube from entering the trachea. Although the patient may gag or vomit *from the stimulation of the pharynx by the tube,* this is usually easy to differentiate from the coughing and choking that occur if the tube does enter the trachea. The patient

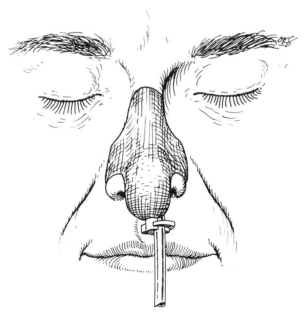

Figure 45–6. Commercial nasogastric suction tube attachment devices are also available.

will be unable to talk *because the tube will interfere with vocal cord movement.* The general skin color may change, becoming dusky *as the person does not receive enough oxygen.* These indications of misplacement are usually enough to cause you to immediately withdraw the tube.

These indications of tube misplacement may be completely absent in the unconscious patient or in the patient with neurologic deficits. Verifying accurate tube placement (i.e., clearly with the end in the stomach or small intestine as desired) is much more difficult and many different bedside methods have been used by nurses throughout the years. Most of these methods have not been confirmed by research data. If the tube will be used only for suction, these bedside methods may be considered adequate and the tube simply repositioned if it is not functioning adequately.

The only positive method of guaranteeing correct placement is through x-ray. Bedside methods are used as a tentative indication of correct placement and then the x-ray is done for verification when feedings are going to be inserted into the tube because *instilling feedings where they might be aspirated is a serious danger.*

The following bedside methods are used to check for tube placement:

a. **Aspiration of visually recognizable gastrointestinal secretions.** This is usually considered an excellent method *because in most instances gastric secretions are clearly identifiable by their greenish brown, mucoid appearance. This method is less reliable if the patient has had bleeding in the respiratory tract, making respiratory secretions dark, or if the patient has been receiving dilute tube feedings that might give a frothy white appearance to gastric contents that is mistaken for respiratory secretions. This method may not work with small-bore silicone rubber feeding tubes because they often collapse when suction pressure is applied. Sometimes the stomach is empty and it is not possible to aspirate any fluid.*

b. **Auscultation of air insufflated through the nasogastric tube.** The nurse auscultates over the epigastrium as he or she pushes 10–15 ml air into the tube with a syringe. *The air makes a gurgling, bubbling noise that can be heard clearly. This is more discernable through a large-bore tube. Through a small tube* *the sound may be muffled and it may be difficult to distinguish between air in the stomach or air in the esophagus.*

   c. **pH testing of aspirates.** This method may be valuable. *The pH of the stomach is low (very acid) and the pH of the small intestine is higher (more alkaline).* This method might help to identify when the tube entered the stomach and then when it was passed on into the duodenum. However, no data are available clearly documenting the pH that is reliable. *Such factors as the administration of drugs whose purpose is to lessen gastric acidity, the recent administration of other drugs that affect pH, and the effect of tube feedings may all need to be considered. This method does rely on the ability to obtain secretions when aspirating.*

   d. **Observing for coughing and choking.** As previously discussed, this method will be useful for identifying misplacement when working with an alert patient who has all neurologic responses intact. It is not reliable for the unconscious or neurologically impaired patient. This method does not verify whether the end of the tube is placed in the esophagus, stomach, or duodenum.

   e. **Testing for ability to speak.** This method has worked with large-bore tubes placed in alert, neurologically intact patients. However, there are reports of patients with small silicone rubber tubes in the trachea who could still talk. It is not useful for the unconscious or nonalert patient. Again it may identify misplacement but will not verify correct placement.

   f. **Observing for bubbling when the tip of the tube is held under water.** This method is considered unreliable *because air bubbles may come out of the stomach as well as out of the respiratory tract. Also, the patient who is breathing very shallowly with little force may not force air out of the tube through the water and therefore would not create bubbles even if the tube were in the lungs.*

     Metheny (1988) reviewed the research data available regarding bedside methods of verifying nasogastric and nasointestinal tube placement. She concluded that research in this area is clearly needed and that until such research is done, x-ray verification be considered the only accurate method.

17. *To prevent air from entering the stomach, which could cause distention,* keep the free end of the tube plugged at all times, except when checking position, feeding, or irrigating.
18. To irrigate the tube:
      a. Slowly instill 10–20 ml solution, usually water or normal saline, with a syringe. The physician may order a larger volume to be used for irrigation.
      b. Gently aspirate. If any bleeding is apparent, stop the aspiration and report your observations to the physician. Carefully measure all gastric secretions, which must be considered output (see Module 48, Irrigations: Bladder, Catheter, Ear, Eye, Nasogastric Tube, Vaginal, Wound).
19. To suction:
      a. Turn on the equipment *before* attaching it to the nasogastric tube. This way, *if the suction is too strong or the device malfunctions, the patient is not harmed.* Test the suction by placing your finger over the suction tube opening and feeling the amount of pull. Unless otherwise ordered, always begin with the low setting when applying suction, *so tissues are not damaged.*
      b. Attach the suction to the patient's nasogastric tube, using an adapter.
      c. Check the equipment regularly *to make sure suction is occurring and the proper suction level is being maintained.*
20. Help the patient to a position of comfort.
21. A patient with a nasogastric tube in place needs frequent oronasal care. *This is because the tube irritates the nostrils and the back of the throat, producing a drying condition. Also, the mouth becomes particularly dry because the patient is mouth-breathing and is neither eating nor taking fluids.*
22. Dispose of gloves and wash your hands.

Evaluation
23. Evaluate using the following criteria:
      a. Patient is comfortable.
      b. No irritation at nostrils.
      c. Normal breathing pattern, rate, and rhythm.
      d. No indications of nausea or regurgitation.
      e. Tube properly placed.

Documentation
24. Record the following on the patient record:
      a. Type and size of tube inserted.

DATE/TIME	
2/14/94 1430	*Salem sump tube inserted. Attached to low intermittent suction. Resting quietly with no discomfort. — T. Kent, SN*

Example of Progress Notes Using Narrative Format

b. Amount and characteristics of any drainage returned.

c. Suction pressure applied.

d. Patient response to procedure.

25. Add information to the Nursing Care Plan relative to care needed.

INTUBATING THE UNCONSCIOUS PATIENT

An unconscious patient may require insertion of a nasogastric tube *to relieve gastric distention or to receive liquid feedings.*

Observe all the principles described in the procedure above, with the following important adaptations: Place the patient in low to mid Fowler's position, again with the head flexed forward slightly *to facilitate passage past the trachea. The main danger is the possible insertion of the tube through the bronchus into the lung. The unconscious patient may have lost both gag and cough reflexes,* so you may not accurately know the position of the tube *because the patient will not cough if the tube is positioned incorrectly.* An easy but effective way to avoid this problem is to insert an oropharyngeal airway into the patient's mouth. *The distal end of the airway acts as a guide,* moving the tube smoothly down into the esophagus (Figure 45–7). Even if you have used an airway, carefully check tube placement. Once you are sure the location is correct, remove the airway.

PROCEDURE FOR REMOVING A NASOGASTRIC TUBE

Assessment

1. Verify that the tube is no longer needed and that the physician has ordered its removal.

Planning

2. Wash your hands *for infection control.*

3. Obtain clean gloves and a towel *for handling and covering the soiled tube.*

Implementation

4. Identify the patient *to be sure you are performing the procedure for the correct patient.*

5. Explain to the patient that although removing the tube will be uncomfortable, it will be over quickly, *so the patient will not be frightened.*

6. If suction is operating, turn it off and disconnect the tube. *If suction is on while you are removing the tube, patient discomfort may be increased.*

7. Put on gloves and pinch the tube closed or plug it *to prevent secretions from dribbling into the esophagus and pharynx. The secretions in the tube are stomach acids and therefore irritating.*

8. Withdraw the tube rapidly in a continuous, smooth motion. *Any nausea and gagging that occurs is increased by pulling the tube slowly, which stimulates the posterior pharynx.*

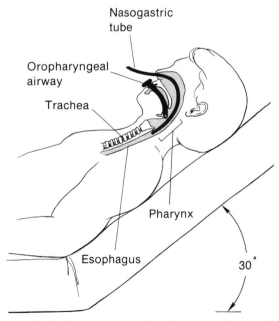

Figure 45–7. Nasogastric intubation of an unconscious patient. The oropharyngeal airway prevents the nasgastric tube from coiling forward, so the tube passes easily into the esophagus.

DATE/TIME	
2/17/95 *2200*	*Nasogastric tube removed per order. 1100 ml cloudy, light green drainage in suction bottle. Abdomen soft, bowel tones present.*
	T. Kent, SN

Example of Progress Notes Using Narrative Format

9. Place the soiled tubing in the towel and cover it, for *it is aesthetically unpleasant.*
10. Make the patient comfortable and give mouth care.
11. Measure any output remaining.
12. Dispose of the equipment and gloves properly.
13. Wash your hands.

Evaluation

14. Evaluate using the following criteria:
    a. Patient is comfortable.
    b. No abdominal distention present.

Documentation

15. In the manner prescribed by your facility, record the time the tube is removed, the amount of fluid measured, and the patient's tolerance of the procedure.

References

Metheny, N. (1988). Measures to test placement of nasogastric and nasointestinal feeding tubes: A review. *Nursing Research, 37*(6), 324–328.

Wilson, V. How to Make a Feeding Tube Go Down Easily, *RN (November 1986)*: 40–43.

Performance Checklist

Inserting a Nasogastric Tube	Unsat	Needs More Practice	Sat	Comments
Assessment				
1. Check physician's order.				
2. Assess patient's capabilities for cooperating.				
3. Determine availability of equipment.				
Planning				
4. Wash your hands.				
5. Gather equipment.				
6. Plan for any assistance necessary.				
7. If weighted or special tube is to be used, review manufacturer's directions for insertion.				
Implementation				
8. Identify the patient.				
9. Explain procedure to patient.				
10. Place patient in high Fowler's position with head flexed forward. (Prepare nose skin for tape.)				
11. Determine length of tube to be inserted and mark.				
12. Put on gloves and lubricate tube.				
13. Gently insert into nostril.				
14. Using prescribed procedure, advance tube.				
15. Secure tube to bridge of nose.				
16. Check to see if tube is in stomach.				
17. Plug end of tube.				
18. If irrigating, follow directions.				
19. If applying suction, follow directions.				
20. Make patient comfortable.				
21. Give oronasal care.				
22. Dispose of gloves and wash your hands.				

Inserting a Nasogastric Tube (Continued)	Unsat	Needs More Practice	Sat	Comments
Evaluation				
23. Evaluate using the following criteria: 　a. Patient is comfortable.				
b. No irritation at nostrils.				
c. Normal breathing.				
d. No indications of nausea or regurgitation.				
e. Tube properly placed.				
Documentation				
24. Record the following on the patient record: 　a. Type and size of tube inserted.				
b. Amount and characteristics of any drainage returned.				
c. Suction pressure applied.				
d. Patient response to procedure.				
25. Add information to the Nursing Care Plan relative to care needed.				
Removing a Nasogastric Tube				
Assessment				
1. Verify that tube is to be removed.				
Planning				
2. Wash your hands.				
3. Obtain towel for handling and covering tube.				
Implementation				
4. Identify the patient.				
5. Explain procedure to patient.				
6. If suction is on, turn it off.				
7. Put on gloves and pinch tube closed.				
8. Withdraw tube rapidly and smoothly.				
9. Place soiled tube in towel and cover.				
10. Make patient comfortable.				

Removing a Nasogastric Tube *(Continued)*	Unsat	Needs More Practice	Sat	Comments
11. Measure any output.				
12. Dispose of equipment and gloves.				
13. Wash your hands.				
Evaluation				
14. Evaluate using the following criteria: a. Patient is comfortable.				
b. No abdominal distention present.				
Documentation				
15. Record time of procedure, amount of any drainage, and patient's tolerance.				

Quiz

Short-Answer Questions

1. List three reasons why a nasogastric tube would be inserted.

   a. _____

   b. _____

   c. _____

2. Why is the nasogastric tube lubricated? _____

3. Removing a nasogastric tube smoothly but swiftly prevents _____

   and/or _____ .

Multiple-Choice Questions

_____ 4. To determine the proper distance to insert the nasogastric tube for the adult patient, measure

   a. from the tip of the earlobe to the cricoid.
   b. from the nose to the umbilicus.
   c. from the tip of the nose to the earlobe, and then to the lower sternum.
   d. from the tip of the earlobe to the nose, and then to the umbilicus.

_____ 5. When passing the tube, have the patient's head

   a. in extension.
   b. in flexion.
   c. turned to one side.

_____ 6. The nasogastric tube is passed more easily if the patient is

   a. in low Fowler's position.
   b. flat in bed.
   c. in high Fowler's position.
   d. positioned on the left side.

_____ 7. In checking the position of the tube, which of the following methods is most reliable?

   a. Introduce a small amount of air into the tube and listen with a stethoscope over the gastric region for the entrance of air into the stomach.
   b. Aspirate the gastric contents gently with a syringe.
   c. Place the end of the tube in a glass of water.
   d. Obtain an x-ray.

_____ 8. A primary safety factor to remember when applying suction to a patient's nasogastric tube is to

   a. turn the equipment on to the *low* position always.
   b. test the functioning of the equipment *before* attaching it to the patient's tube.
   c. *be sure* the seals on the collection bottle are tight.
   d. *never* use extension cords.

Module 46
Preoperative Care

Module Contents

Rationale for the Use of This Skill
Scheduling Preoperative Care
  Role of the Anesthesiologist
  Role of the Surgeon
  Preoperative Interview
Procedure for Preoperative Interview
  Assessment
  Planning
  Implementation
  Evaluation
  Documentation
Rationale for Preoperative Teaching
Procedure for Preoperative Teaching
  Assessment
  Planning
  Implementation
  Evaluation
  Documentation
Procedure for Preoperative Interventions
  Assessment
  Planning
  Implementation
  Evaluation
  Documentation

Preoperative Skin Preparation
  Bath
  Scrub of the Surgical Site
  Shave
    When to Shave
    Wet versus Dry Shaving
    Depilatories
Procedure for Wet Shaving
  Assessment
  Planning
  Implementation
  Evaluation
  Documentation
The Night Before Surgery
Procedure for Immediate Preoperative Care
  Assessment
  Planning
  Implementation
  Evaluation
  Documentation
Ambulatory Surgery

Prerequisites

1. *Successful completion of the following modules:*

VOLUME 1
Module 1   An Approach to Nursing Skills
Module 2   Basic Infection Control
Module 3   Safety
Module 4   Basic Body Mechanics
Module 5   General Assessment Overview
Module 6   Documentation
Module 14   Admission, Transfer, and Discharge
Module 16   Temperature, Pulse, and Respiration
Module 17   Blood Pressure
Module 18   Collecting Specimens

243

© 1992 by J.B. Lippincott Company

VOLUME 2

Module 41 Respiratory Care Procedures

2. *The following modules are not essential, but their successful completion will allow you to carry out more complete care for selected patients.*

VOLUME 1

Module 28 Administering Enemas

VOLUME 2

Module 39 Catheterization

Module 45 Nasogastric Intubation

Module 48 Irrigations: Bladder, Catheter, Ear, Eye, Nasogastric Tube, Vaginal, Wound

Module 49 Administering Oral Medications

Module 51 Giving Injections

Overall Objective

To prepare patients physically and psychologically for anesthesia and surgery.

Specific Learning Objectives

	Know Facts and Principles	Apply Facts and Principles	Demonstrate Ability	Evaluate Performance
1. *Initial preoperative planning and care* *a. Interview*	List information to be obtained through preoperative interview.	Given a patient situation, identify information indicating potential problem.	Carry out preoperative interview correctly.	Evaluate own performance using Performance Checklist.
b. Teaching	State information to be included in preoperative teaching.	Adapt teaching plan to meet individual patient's concerns.	Carry out preoperative teaching correctly.	Evaluate own performance using Performance Checklist.
2. *Preoperative skin preparation*	State three objectives of preoperative skin preparation.			
a. Bath	State rationale for bathing/showering before surgery and for using an antimicrobial agent.	Explain to patient rationale for preoperative bath or shower.	Assist patient with preoperative bath or shower.	Evaluate with instructor.
b. Scrub of surgical site	State rationale for scrub of the surgical site before selected surgeries.	Explain to patient rationale for scrub of surgical site.	Carry out preoperative scrub of surgical site when ordered.	Evaluate with instructor.
c. Shave *(1) Timing shave*	State rationale for timing preoperative shave.	Given a time schedule for surgery, identify appropriate time for shave preparation.		
(2) Wet versus dry shave	List advantages and disadvantages of wet and dry shaving.			
(3) Depilatories	List advantages and disadvantages of using chemical depilatories.			

(continued)

Specific Learning Objectives *(Continued)*

	Know Facts and Principles	Apply Facts and Principles	Demonstrate Ability	Evaluate Performance
d. *Shaving procedure*	List equipment needed for preoperative shave.	Given a patient situation, describe correct area to be shaved by naming perimeters.	Correctly and safely complete preoperative shave.	Evaluate shave by checking skin with strong light for hair removal and irritation. Evaluate own performance using Performance Checklist.
3. *Immediate preoperative care*	List aspects of physical care given during immediate preoperative period.	In the practice setting, simulate immediate care of patient.	Carry out immediate care of preoperative patient.	Evaluate own performance using Performance Checklist.
4. *Checklist*	State information included on preoperative checklist.	In the practice setting, complete preoperative checklist.	In the clinical setting, complete patient's preoperative checklist.	Evaluate with instructor.

Learning Activities

1. Review the Specific Learning Objectives.
2. Read the chapters on health teaching and hygiene and the section on anxiety in the chapter on mental health in Ellis and Nowlis, *Nursing: A Human Needs Approach,* or comparable material in another textbook.
3. Review the material in your medical-surgical nursing textbook that relates to preoperative care.
4. Look up the module vocabulary terms in the Glossary.
5. Read through the module and mentally practice the skills.
6. In the practice setting:
   a. Using a partner as a patient, practice performing the assessment interview. Include preoperative teaching and record your data.
   b. Have your partner evaluate your performance using the Performance Checklist.
   c. Reverse roles, and have your partner interview you and perform preoperative teaching.
   d. Evaluate your partner's performance.
   e. Observe the equipment used for the preoperative shave.
   f. Again, with your partner, role-play the immediate preoperative period using the Performance Checklist as a guide.
   g. Have your partner evaluate your performance.
   h. Reverse roles, and repeat step f.
   i. Evaluate your partner's performance.
   j. Demonstrate making a postop bed.
7. In the clinical setting:
   a. Perform initial preoperative planning and care.
      (1) Review your facility's procedure manual for initial preoperative planning and care.
      (2) Consult with your instructor when you are ready to perform initial preoperative planning and care.
   b. Perform preoperative skin preparation.
      (1) Review your facility's procedure for preoperative skin preparation, paying special attention to the areas to be shaved for designated surgeries.
      (2) Ask for an opportunity to observe a preoperative shave.
      (3) Consult with your instructor regarding an opportunity to do a preoperative shave. (Shaving for abdominal surgery is a wise choice for a beginning experience.)
   c. Perform immediate preoperative care.
      (1) Review your facility's procedure for giving immediate preoperative care.
      (2) Examine the checklist used.
      (3) Request an opportunity to give immediate preoperative care, including the completion of the checklist.

Vocabulary

ambulatory surgery
anesthesia
anesthesiologist
anesthetic
anesthetist

antiembolic stockings
antimicrobial
aspirate
complete blood count

depilatory
diuretic
endotracheal tube
epithelial
inpatient
laparotomy

lather
NPO
outpatient
perineal
TEDs
thoracotomy

Preoperative Care

Rationale for the Use of This Skill
An important factor that contributes to safe and successful surgery and an uneventful convalescence is the conscientious preparation of patients by the registered nurse. Remember that the patient is traumatized not only by the surgical procedure, but by exposure to anesthetic agents as well. In addition, surgery is emotionally stressful, causing degrees of fear and anxiety. Preoperative care, therefore, must include adequate health teaching, physical preparation, and psychologic support. Although portions of preoperative care may be undertaken by other members of the health care team, it remains the nurse's primary responsibility.[1]

SCHEDULING PREOPERATIVE CARE

Traditionally patients entered the hospital at least one day before a scheduled surgery to ensure that there was adequate time for preoperative care. (Surgeries scheduled ahead of time are called *elective* surgeries.) In some instances, such as those in which bowel preparation must begin in the evening before surgery, this is still true. However, to limit hospital costs through decreasing the days of stay, many patients now enter the hospital the morning of surgery. This practice termed "AM admission" has often resulted in limited time for preoperative care. Nurses working in units with morning surgical admissions have to develop excellent organizational skills and plan carefully to complete all the preoperative care described in this module. Often more than one task is accomplished at the same time.

Preadmission patient visits are used in some hospitals to ensure adequate time for preoperative care. This is especially true for patients scheduled for major surgery involving lengthy recovery periods and for children undergoing surgery. During these visits the initial patient interview, laboratory work, and consent forms are completed. In addition, the nurse begins preoperative teaching. This may be done on a one-to-one basis or special programs may be structured for groups of patients undergoing similar procedures.

These programs are directed and instructed by nurses with special surgical and teaching skills. Patients receive health teaching regarding what to expect after surgery and how to participate in regaining

---

[1] You will note that rationale for action is emphasized throughout the module by the use of italics.

independence. With the help of booklets and visual aids they are taught deep-breathing exercises, leg and foot exercises, and how to move in bed and are shown types of equipment that may be used. Some programs include a tour of the surgical unit and introductions to the staff. *It is recognized that such programs are helpful in reducing anxiety and decreasing complications after surgery.* Many hospitals also have visual materials available to the nurse and the patient for preoperative teaching. Often the patient entering the unit has already been to the laboratory, where blood and urine samples have been collected for laboratory studies such as a complete blood count (CBC) and urinalysis (UA). The consent-for-surgery form may have been signed and witnessed in the admitting office. If it has not, the physician or nurse will ask the patient to sign the form on the unit (see Module 14, Admission, Transfer, and Discharge, for general admitting procedure).

When a patient needs emergency surgery (a surgery not scheduled ahead of time), the nurse will need to determine what parts of preoperative care are essential for this particular situation and what parts can be omitted or abbreviated. Sometimes there are several hours from the time an emergency surgery is scheduled until it is performed. On other occasions the patient moves from the emergency room directly to the operating room.

Preoperative care varies from facility to facility. At points throughout the module you may have to check the policies of the facility in which you practice and adapt your care to those policies.

Role of the Anesthesiologist

The *anesthesiologist* is a medical doctor whose specialty is administering local, regional, and general anesthetic agents. An *anesthetist* is a nurse with specialized training to administer anesthetics under the supervision of an anesthesiologist. One of these persons will visit the patient before surgery—usually the evening before or morning of surgery. The purpose of the visit is to (1) assess the patient for the dosage and appropriate anesthetic to be used, (2) give the patient information about the anesthetic that is to be given, and (3) write the orders for the preoperative medication.

Role of the Surgeon

When surgery is planned, the surgeon is responsible for obtaining informed consent for the procedure. This may be done before the patient enters the hospital or in the hospital the patient will sign a consent for surgery and a nurse may witness that signature. The nurse in this situation is not responsible for informing the patient about the surgery; that remains the responsibility of the surgeon. The nurse should notify the surgeon if assessment reveals that the patient is not adequately informed.

Because surgery is a highly technical and complex field that changes rapidly, the surgeon has the ultimate responsibility for determining what preoperative care is needed specific to the surgery itself. Although every facility will have certain routine procedures, the individual surgeon may alter these. Therefore, the nurse working on a surgical unit must have a close collaborative relationship with the surgeons to ensure that the patient receives the best possible care.

Preoperative Interview

The initial step in preoperative care is the preoperative interview. If the patient has not been admitted to the hospital prior to the time you begin your preoperative interview, you will also need to perform an admission physical assessment (see Modules 5, Assessment, and 14, Admission, Transfer, and Discharge).

PROCEDURE FOR PREOPERATIVE INTERVIEW

Assessment

1. Verify the type of surgery, the date and time surgery is scheduled, and the name of the surgeon. You can do this by checking the operative schedule form that comes to the unit from the operating room or one that is entered into the computer. A specific time will usually be listed, or the abbreviation TF may be used. This means your patient's surgery is "to follow" a previous procedure and the exact time is undetermined.

2. Check the preoperative orders *to determine your responsibilities toward preparing the patient for surgery.* Some surgeons use a stamp for their routine orders on a specific procedure and add any special orders for the individual patient.

Planning

3. Consult the procedure book of your facility regarding the type of surgery, the preparation needed, and the surgeon's preferences. Some

facilities maintain a Kardex or file that lists surgeons' preferences.

4. Check the patient's chart for the history and physical (H&P) and the signed consent form. A CBC and/or UA may also be needed, depending on physician's orders. The H&P and the completed consent form must be on the record before surgery, *to protect the patient, the physician, and staff.* Depending on the health of the patient and type of surgery, other tests may also be performed. In some facilities it is permissible to go ahead with the surgery if the H&P is not on the record but has been performed and dictated. You may have to check on this. Surgery cannot proceed (except in a life-threatening emergency) without a properly completed consent form. Know your facility's policy regarding consent.

5. Arrange to complete the forms and procedures listed in step 4 if they are not on the record. Inform the laboratory or physician about any missing data.

6. Plan sufficient uninterrupted time to carry out the preoperative interview.

Implementation

7. Using the appropriate form, perform the interview.

   a. *Verification of patient's identity To practice safely,* always validate the patient's identity by comparing the wristband to the name and hospital number on the chart. At a preoperative visit the patient will not have a wristband. Ask the patient to spell his or her name to ensure correct identification.

   b. *General appearance and physical condition* A description of the patient's general appearance and physical condition is objective data. Record the patient's height and weight, *which is sometimes used to compute the amount of anesthetic agent to be administered.*

   c. *Anxiety level* Communication with the patient during the interview *will usually tell you something about the patient's level of anxiety.* Look for restlessness, fidgeting, rapid respirations and pulse, and statements indicating anxiety.

   d. *Knowledge level regarding current surgery* Ask the patient what he or she knows about the surgery. The physician may have adequately explained the procedure. If not, you should give a general explanation. As with all health teaching, gear any necessary explanation to the level of the individual patient. *Remember that explicit details can raise the patient's anxiety level.* Any questions regarding specific points of the surgical procedure or expected results of surgery should be answered by the physician.

e. *Previous surgeries* List all previous surgeries. *They may have both physical and psychologic consequences for the current surgery.* Never assume that the patient who has had multiple surgeries needs less preparation. There may still be anxiety and inadequate knowledge.

f. *Smoking habits* Note whether the patient is a smoker or nonsmoker. *The lung tissue of a patient who smokes is more sensitive to anesthetic gases because of mild irritation.* Discourage smoking just before surgery. Many hospitals are nonsmoking environments. Not being able to smoke may increase anxiety in some smokers.

g. *Drug and alcohol intake* List all medications the patient is taking, including vitamin preparations, birth control pills, and nonprescription drugs. Some patients do not think to mention long-term medications, such as diuretics or daily birth control pills. Emphasize the importance of a complete list *because anesthetic agents and other medications ordered may interact with the medications the patient is already taking.* Certain medications (for example, anticonvulsant drugs) will be continued throughout the operative period, *because interruption would cause adverse effects for the patient.*

A reliable alcohol history is also essential. *Heavy use of alcohol has multiple effects on the body that can change the patient's response to anesthesia, surgery, and recovery.*

h. *Support system data* *Because the family and significant others are concerned about the patient, may be involved in the health teaching, and often care for the patient after discharge,* it is important to list on the form the names and relationships of close family members and friends along with telephone numbers.

8. Encourage the patient to ask questions about the procedure, the policies of the hospital, or aspects of care. If you do not know the answers to specific questions, consult the appropriate resource person.

9. Provide emotional support. *To add to the patient's confidence,* demonstrate your competence to care for the patient and help him or her learn what to expect. Refer to your basic text for techniques for handling anxiety.

Evaluation

10. Evaluate the completeness of your interview by reviewing the data for completeness. If you need more information in any area, return to the patient and clarify.

Documentation

11. Attach the interview form to the patient's chart where you and others can refer to it as you begin the written plan of care.

Rationale for Preoperative Teaching
Well-planned, individualized preoperative teaching prepares the patient for intelligent participation in the activities surrounding the surgery and results in fewer postoperative complications and a smoother postoperative course. You must incorporate your knowledge of the principles of teaching and learning into the routines of the facility and with the physician's orders to plan a teaching strategy that will best meet the needs of the individual patient and ensure the best outcome for the patient.

PROCEDURE FOR PREOPERATIVE TEACHING

Assessment

1. Carefully review once again the preoperative orders, *so you can give appropriate information.*

2. If you interviewed the patient, you have some knowledge of his or her language level, educational background, and level of anxiety. If you are not familiar with the patient, spend some time assessing these areas.

Planning

3. Plan to allow considerable uninterrupted time, *so you will not be hurried in your instruction and the patient will feel more relaxed.*

4. If family members or significant others are present, include them if the patient and they so wish and you think it is appropriate and helpful to the patient. *During the postoperative period these persons can often reinforce what has been taught.*

Implementation

5. Provide a quiet, nonstressful environment in which to teach. This includes providing comfortable chairs for those present, turning off the television set, and using an empty day room or conference room if the teaching could disturb a roommate.

6. You may design your own teaching plan or use one provided in your clinical setting (Figure 46–1), but be sure to include these points as appropriate to the specific surgery planned:

a. *Preoperative routines* Outline the routines for the patient in clear, understandable terms. You may do this by systems, describing preoperative care of the gastrointestinal tract, skin, and so on, or by going through the preparation sequentially.

b. *Postoperative routines* Explain what will be done, with what frequency, and why.

TEACHING MAY INCLUDE: Pathophysiology, Treatments, Nutrition, Medications, Side Effects, Procedures, Symptoms to report, Home Management, Preventative Health, etc.

TEACHING CONTENT PRE-OPERATIVE TEACHING	PATIENT RESPONSE			
	Indicates Understanding	Needs Reinforcement	Return Demonstration	Able to Perform Independently
1. Understands surgical procedure and expected outcome.	3/14 PB			
2. Immediate Post-op				
a. Recovery room	3/14 PB			
b. Frequent monitoring of vital signs	3/14 PB			
c. Return to floor/ICU	3/14 PB			
3. Diet				
a. Pre-op (i.e., clear liquids)	3/14 PB			
b. NPO after midnight	3/14 PB			
c. Progression after surgery	3/16 JE	3/14 PB		
4. Medications				
a. Sedation at H.S.	3/14 PB			
b. Pre-op medication day of surgery	3/14 PB			
c. Post-op medications (analgesics, antibiotics, other)	3/14 PB			
5. Pre-op Preparation				
a. Skin prep	3/14 PB			
b. Bowel prep				
c. Other				
6. Equipment				
a. Intravenous	3/14 PB			
b. Foley catheter	3/14 PB			
c. Naso-gastric tube				
d. Drains				
e. Dressings	3/14 PB			
f. Cast/splints				
g. Other				
7. Activity Post-Op				
a. Positioning				
b. Exercise	3/16 JE	3/14 PB	3/14 PB 3/16 JE	3/16 JE
c. Restrictions				
8. Pulmonary Care				
a. Turn, cough, deep breathe	3/14 PB		3/14 PB	3/14 PB

Identify Initials with Signature:	2. J. Ellison, R.N.	4.		6.	
1. P. Boyd, R.N.	3.	5.		7.	

ADDRESSOGRAPH:

THE SWEDISH HOSPITAL MEDICAL CENTER
SEATTLE, WASHINGTON

Figure 46–1. Patient education flow sheet.

(1) *Vital signs* Blood pressure, pulse, and respiration are checked every 15 minutes *for early identification of any problems.*

(2) *Dressing checks* These are made to observe *the kind and amount of drainage.*

(3) *Progressive surgical diet* List the usual progression—from ice chips, to clear liquids, to full liquids, to a soft diet, and finally to a regular diet. *The surgical patient can regain normal eating patterns sooner if this progression is followed.* For some surgeries, such as an extremity, the full progression will not be used.

(4) *Special procedures* Specific procedures (irrigation, respiratory therapy, casting, brace fitting) may be necessary for particular surgeries. Explain any special or unusual procedures that will be ordered *so the patient will know what to expect.*

c. *Pain management* All surgical patients want to be as free from pain as possible after surgery. By encouraging the patient before the surgery to participate in planning for pain management, *you relieve the patient's fear that pain will not be controlled.* Tell the patient about available pain medications. Instruct the patient to alert a nurse before the pain becomes moderate or acute. *It is recognized that avoiding pain medication "peaks" and "troughs" consistently results in more effective pain management. It is difficult to control pain that has become severe.* Allay possible fears of medication overuse by explaining that after the first few postsurgical days the pain will subside and large doses of injectable medications will no longer be necessary. The physician will then order oral pain medications *so the patient can maintain a comfort level that will help increase mobility.* A patient-controlled analgesia (PCA) pump may be ordered for postoperative pain control. In this case, the patient should be told how the unit functions and what he or she needs to do to self-medicate. See Module 54, Administering Intravenous Medications, for a more detailed explanation of PCA.

d. *Postoperative appliances, tubes, and equipment* Inform the patient of any equipment or appliances that will be in place after surgery. These might include a catheter, an IV infusion, or a suction apparatus.

e. *Deep breathing and coughing* If the patient is going to have a general anesthetic, *the medication and the immobility of surgery will cause secretions to build up in the lungs.* Therefore, teach the patient how to breathe deeply and cough. (For instructions, consult Module 41, Respiratory Care Procedures.) In some hospitals, this teaching, as well as that regarding the use of the incentive spirometer and/or other special equipment, is done by a respiratory therapist.

f. *Methods for moving* These methods include moving in bed and getting in and out of bed, as appropriate for the patient's postoperative condition and expected physician's orders. *The purpose of teaching the patient to move with as little discomfort as possible is to encourage the action.* Turning in bed and getting in and out of bed *prevent circulatory problems, stimulate the respiratory system, and decrease discomfort from gas.* Review your medical-surgical text for the use of pillows for splinting, side rails for support, and body mechanics adaptations.

g. *Leg exercises* *These exercises facilitate venous return in the lower extremities and prevent stasis and clot formation.* They are often augmented by the use of antiembolic hose, *which provide continuous support to the veins, decreasing venous stasis and promoting venous return.* Three exercises are most commonly taught:

(1) *Calf pumping* Instruct the patient to alternately dorsiflex and plantar flex the foot. *This causes the calf muscles to contract and relax.*

(2) *Quadriceps setting* Instruct the patient to alternately contract the anterior thigh muscles and allow them to relax.

(3) *Gluteal setting* Instruct the patient to alternately contract the posterior thigh and gluteal muscles and allow them to relax.

These exercises should be done 10 times each hour as soon as possible after surgery. If appropriate to the patient's surgery, active range-of-motion exercises can be substituted for these isometric exercises.

When teaching steps e–g, first *explain* what you want the patient to do and why it is important; then *demonstrate* for the patient; and last, ask the patient to *return the demonstration.* Give positive feedback to the

Example of Progress Notes Using Narrative Format

DATE/TIME	
4/16/94 10:30 AM	*Preoperative teaching done, including coughing and deep breathing, moving in bed, leg exercises, and pain management. Return demonstrations and clarification of questions show good patient understanding. Family present. —— M. Davies, RN*

patient when the return demonstration is correct and encourage the patient if extra practice is needed.

Evaluation

7. Evaluate the effectiveness of your health teaching by asking the patient to summarize with you the points you have covered. You may also involve the family and significant others. Clarify any false information or reemphasize points missed or misunderstood.

Documentation

8. Some facilities have a preoperative form that provides space for noting preoperative teaching (see Figure 46–1). If your facility does not have such a form, make an entry in the nurses' progress notes.

PROCEDURE FOR PREOPERATIVE INTERVENTIONS

Assessment

1. Check to see if any new preoperative orders have been written, and if so, incorporate them into your care plan.
2. Assess the patient's readiness for procedures. Delay the procedure if the patient has visitors or is eating the light diet usually ordered the evening before surgery. However, you may need to ask visitors to step out to enable you to complete tasks in a timely manner.

Planning

3. Plan time for carrying out the tasks ordered.
4. Wash your hands for *infection control.*
5. Review a manual or any modules necessary to carry out any ordered procedures, such as Module 28, Administering Enemas, and Module 48, Irrigations.

Implementation

6. Identify the patient *to be sure you are performing the procedure for the correct patient.*
7. Administer an enema, douche, or irrigation as ordered.

Evaluation

8. Evaluate using the following criteria:
   a. Patient comfortable.
   b. Patient states questions were answered.
   c. Procedure completed successfully.

Documentation

9. Consult the appropriate modules and record as indicated.

PREOPERATIVE SKIN PREPARATION

The effective preparation of the skin before an operation *is an important aspect of preventing infection in the postoperative patient. Because the skin—the first line of defense against invasion by microorganisms—will be opened, additional measures to prevent the invasion of microbes are necessary.*

The main objective of preparing the skin is *to remove dirt, oils, and microorganisms. A second objective is to prevent the growth of microorganisms that remain. A third objective is to leave the skin undamaged, with no irritation from the cleansing and shaving procedure.*

Bath

In most facilities the preoperative patient is asked to shower or bathe, using an antimicrobial cleansing agent, on the evening before or the morning of surgery. If possible, the patient should shampoo at the time of the bath. *Bathing removes gross contamination and soil and reduces colonization of typical wound pathogens. The antimicrobial agent leaves a residue on the skin that serves to decrease the overall bacterial count.*

Scrub of the Surgical Site

Sometimes a surgeon orders that a surgical site be scrubbed for a predetermined length of time (for example, 5 minutes) daily for several days before the surgery. This is most commonly done for elective orthopedic (bone) surgery *because of the high risk of in-*

fection. The process results in a significantly lower bacterial count on the surgical site at the time of surgery. Because the procedure is so time-consuming and because infection is not as frequent and serious in other kinds of surgeries, it is not performed routinely for most surgeries. A scrub procedure may also be ordered to be done after the preoperative shave.

Shave

Because microorganisms are found in large concentrations on hairs, the removal of skin hair at and near the operative site cuts down the number of these organisms. The smooth skin can then be cleaned more completely. To have the skin as clean as possible, a shave preparation is routine before surgery. However, *since shaving with a razor can potentially injure skin and thereby increase the risk of infection,* clipping hair, using a depilatory, or no shaving at all has been suggested. Consult the policy or procedure book in your facility.

When to Shave. Although the timing can be ordered by the surgeon, it may be determined by hospital routine. If you have an opportunity to participate in the planning, you should understand the differences in infection rate that result from changes in timing of the preoperative shave in relationship to the time of surgery. *Any time interval between the shaving and the actual surgery allows hair to begin to regrow and microorganisms to multiply.* Although the practice for many years was to perform the preoperative shave the evening before surgery, *recent studies have demonstrated that the overall infection rate is reduced by moving the time of the shave closer to the time of surgery.* In some hospitals, the shave is done early in the morning on the day scheduled for surgery. Increasingly, hospitals are going a step further: in many the preoperative shave is being done immediately before the surgery, in a special preparation area or in the induction room in the operating room suite. Not all hospitals have the facilities to make this type of change in procedure, but where it is possible, it is wise practice.

Wet Versus Dry Shaving. Wet shaves are done using warm water and lather; dry shaves are done on dry skin. Most patients feel that the wet shave is more comfortable. *The water and lather serve as lubricants to the razor, decrease the pull, and lessen the chance of nicks or cuts. In addition, the use of antibacterial soap is one more technique to decrease the skin count of microorganisms.*

Recent evidence indicates that fewer epithelial cells

are removed by using a dry shave. Also, the skin is clearly visible, making a very close shave possible. When you perform a dry shave, it is imperative to use a sharp razor *to avoid nicks and cuts.* In fact, you may have to change the blade during the procedure *if you are cutting thick hair.* You can use powder as a lubricant. Some facilities specify that clippers be used for a dry shave. Usually, hospital policy determines whether a wet or dry shave is used, but the surgeon may also decide.

Depilatories. Depilatories are chemicals that destroy the hair below the skin level, *causing the hair to break off, leaving the skin freer of hair than is possible with a razor and free from cuts.* If a patient is not sensitive to depilatories, using them is a safer method of hair removal than shaving. To use a chemical depilatory, read the instructions carefully and follow them exactly.

PROCEDURE FOR WET SHAVING

Assessment

1. Verify the surgeon's order. Do not perform a shave preparation unless it has been ordered by a surgeon. The order may indicate the specific area to be "prepped," although in many facilities a standard routine is followed unless the surgeon specifically describes another preparation area. If the order simply reads, "Prep for gastric surgery," you will have to refer to your facility's procedure book to identify the exact area to be prepped.
2. Assess the patient's readiness for the procedure.

Planning

3. Wash your hands *for infection control.*
4. Obtain the necessary equipment. In most settings the preoperative shave is done using disposable equipment that is originally sterile. Although the procedure itself is a clean procedure, *starting with sterile equipment ensures that new microorganisms from the hospital environment are not introduced to the patient's skin at this critical time.* If disposable equipment is not available, carefully clean the reusable items and send them to the central supply department for resterilization.
   a. Bath blanket to drape the patient. Top linen is sometimes substituted for the bath blanket, but it can cause subsequent

discomfort if small hairs drop in the bed or if the linen becomes wet or soiled.

  b. Shaving equipment. A prepackaged shave preparation kit usually contains most of the necessary items, but be sure to check the label. If you are not using a prepackaged kit, obtain the following:

    (1) Small basin of warm water

    (2) Antibacterial soap for lather

    (3) Razor with a new blade

    (4) Sterile gauze squares

    (5) Antibacterial cleansing agent

    (6) Cotton swabs.

  c. If the instructions for the shave preparation in your facility include covering the area with a sterile towel after shaving, include one in the equipment.

5. Plan the area to be shaved. Obviously, you will include the area of the incision itself, but you will also include a large area beyond the incisional site. *This is done to decrease the possibility that microorganisms will move from unprepared areas to the surgical site. In addition, this provides a safeguard if the physician must enlarge the surgical area during the surgery beyond what was originally planned.*

Implementation

6. Identify the patient *to be sure you are performing the procedure for the correct patient.*

7. Explain the procedure to the patient. *Because a patient might be upset at the idea of the shave preparation,* carefully explain the exact nature and extent of the preparation.

8. Provide for the patient's privacy. To do a thorough job, you will have to expose the patient, but do make sure that the drapes and bed curtains are closed.

9. Arrange for adequate lighting.

10. Drape the patient with a bath blanket *to provide as much warmth and privacy as possible.* Base the draping technique on the area to be exposed.

The areas to be shaved presented here are the long-standing, wide preparation approach that has been used for many years. Some surgeons prefer a smaller area of preparation because it is more comfortable for the patient and there is little evidence to document a difference in infection rates between widely prepared areas and more limited prepared areas. Use the areas presented here as a general guideline but follow the policy in your facility or the specific orders of the surgeon.

  a. *Head and neck surgeries* If the scalp must be shaved, it is best to wait until the person has been anesthetized. *Shaving the head can be psychologically traumatic.* If it must be done earlier, provide a head covering *to lessen the patient's embarrassment. Since the patient may wish to keep the hair removed,* especially if it is long, be sure to get this information in advance.

Do not shave the eyebrows unless expressly ordered by the surgeon. *Eyebrows may not grow back in or may grow in irregularly. This can significantly alter a patient's appearance* and should be avoided unless it is essential.

The prepared area extends from above the eyebrows over the top of the head, and includes the ears and both anterior and posterior areas of the neck (Figure 46–2). The face is not shaved.

  b. *Lateral neck surgery* The prepared area extends from the midline of the back, from the scapula to a line level with the top of the ear, around the operative side, across the front of the neck, and to the top of the opposite shoulder. Anteriorly, the preparation area slants down from the top of the ear on the operative side across the chin line, and extends down below the clavicle across the thorax (Figure 46–3).

  c. *Chest surgery* For a lateral thoracotomy, prep the chest from the center of the sternum, extending from the neck to the

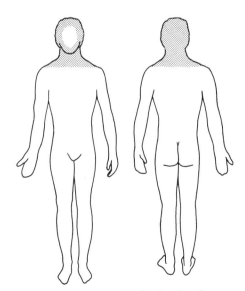

Figure 46–2. Preparation area for head and neck surgery.

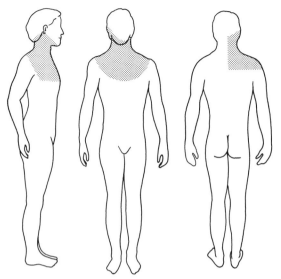

Figure 46–3. Preparation area for lateral neck surgery.

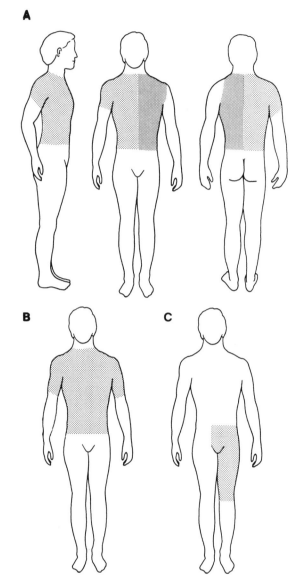

Figure 46–4. Preparation area for chest surgery. **A:** Lateral thoracotomy. **B:** Sternal incision. **C:** Femoral artery access needed.

bottom of the rib cage. Continue to prep on the posterior side to the center of the back at the same level. The arm on the operative side is also prepped to the middle of the forearm. In some instances the prep is extended across the entire back and chest (see Figure 46–4**A**).

For a midline or sternal incision, the preparation extends from the neck to the pubic bone and to the midaxillary line on each side (Figure 46–4**B**).

For access to the femoral artery, extend the preparation to include the area prepped for femoral artery surgery on the designated side (Figure 46–4**C**).

d. *Abdominal surgery* The abdomen is prepared from a line level with the axillae to the pubic bone. The area extends on each side to the mid-axillary line (Figure 46–5).

e. *Perineal surgery* The perineal preparation includes shaving all the pubic area. The area begins above the pubic bone in the front and extends beyond the anus posteriorly. Shave the inner thighs approximately one third of the way to the knees (Figure 46–6).

f. *Cervical spine surgery* Prep the back from the line level with the bottom of the ears down to the waist. Include the shoulders. The back area is prepped to the midaxillary line on each side (Figure 46–7).

g. *Lumbar spine surgery* Prep the back from a line level with the axillae, down onto the buttocks, to the midgluteal level. The area extends to the midaxillary line on each side (Figure 46–8).

h. *Rectal surgery* Shave the buttocks from the iliac crest down the posterior thigh, to a line one third of the way to the knee. Include the anal area. The area extends to the midline on each side (Figure 46–9).

i. *Flank incision* Prep from just beyond the midline anteriorly, around the designated side, to beyond the midline posteriorly. Include the axilla, from the upper level at

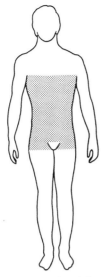

Figure 46–5. Preparation area for abdominal surgery.

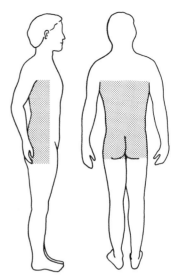

Figure 46–7. Preparation area for cervical spine surgery.

the nipple line in the front to the scapula in the back. Shave the back down to the middle of the buttocks. In the front, the pubic area and the upper thigh are shaved (Figure 46–10).

j. *Hand and forearm surgery* Prep the entire circumference of the arm, to the axilla (Figure 46–11).

k. *Entire lower extremity surgery* Prep the entire leg, including the toes and the foot. Extend posteriorly up over the buttocks, and anteriorly over the pubis up to the umbilicus (Figure 46–12).

l. *Lower leg surgery* Prep the leg and foot, extending the area to midthigh (Figure 46–13).

11. Shave the area as follows:
   a. Make sure the water is warm. *Warm water makes the patient more comfortable, produces better lather, and helps soften the hair.* Lather the area well. *The suds soften the hair and also provide lubrication so the razor moves easily.*
   b. Shave carefully. Hold the skin taut *to prevent nicks* and shave by stroking in the direction of hair growth. Use short strokes, *which are more easily controlled.*
   c. Rinse the razor frequently *to remove hairs that have accumulated on the blade. These hairs could interfere with the cutting action of the razor.*

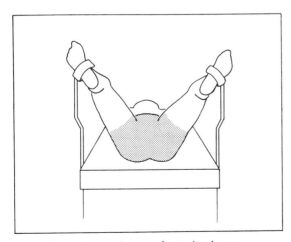

Figure 46–6. Preparation area for perineal surgery.

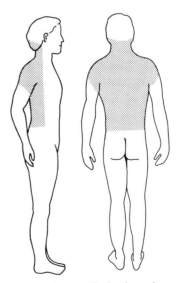

Figure 46–8. Preparation area for lumbar spine surgery.

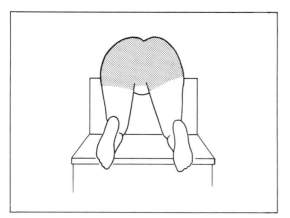

Figure 46–9. Preparation area for rectal surgery.

d. Wipe off excess hair from the skin as it is removed *to allow you to see the skin clearly and the razor to operate more freely.*

e. After all the hair has been removed, scrub the area with an antibacterial cleaner, keeping the cleansing agent in contact with the skin for 5 minutes *"in order to kill or inhibit more adherent, deep, resident flora"* (Garner, 1985). Check your facility's procedures, *because some omit this step.*

f. Clean any body orifice or crevice in the prep area (the umbilicus, the ear canals, under the fingernails), using cotton swabs.

g. Rinse the area with clean water.

h. Blot the skin dry—do not rub vigorously. *Vigorous rubbing can traumatize the skin.*

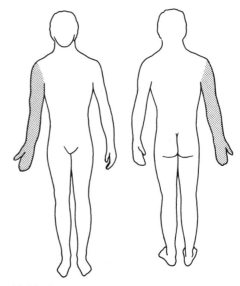

Figure 46–11. Preparation area for hand and forearm surgery.

i. Observe the general condition of the skin. Any abnormal skin irritation, infection, or break in the skin's integrity on or near the operative site should be reported to the surgeon, *as it might be a contraindication to surgery.*

j. Cover the area with a sterile towel if necessary.

k. Remove the bath blanket carefully *to prevent small hairs from dropping into the bed and causing discomfort.* Replace top linen.

12. Make the patient comfortable.

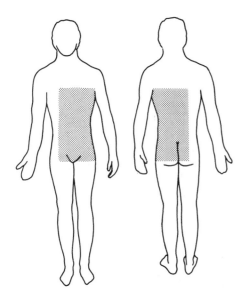

Figure 46–10. Preparation area for flank incision.

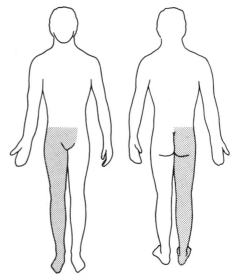

Figure 46–12. Preparation area for entire lower extremity surgery.

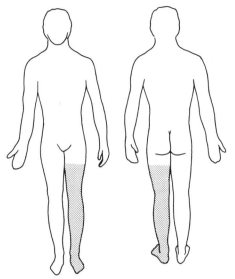

Figure 46–13. Preparation area for lower leg surgery.

13. Dispose of the equipment.
14. Wash your hands.

Evaluation

15. Evaluate using the following criteria:
    a. Skin free of hair.
    b. Skin free of nicks.
    c. Skin shows no evidence of irritation.

Documentation

16. Record the procedure either on a flow sheet or the progress notes, according to the policy of your facility.

THE NIGHT BEFORE SURGERY

Understandably, many patients are anxious the night before surgery. Plan to spend time with the patient, and allow the patient to share any feelings or fears about the procedure. A quiet time with the patient, after visitors have left, *can be reassuring and supportive.*

Administer any sleeping medication ordered. *It is important for the patient to understand that unfamiliar surroundings may prevent a good night's rest before surgery.* Explain that patient will not be given anything by mouth after midnight. *This is to ensure that the stomach is free of contents that could be vomited and aspirated.* At midnight, remove the water pitcher and glass from the patient's bedside and post an NPO sign.

PROCEDURE FOR IMMEDIATE PREOPERATIVE CARE

Assessment

1. Determine the precise time scheduled for the surgery.
2. Check the chart for any changes or additions in orders.
3. Check to be certain that the operative permit has been signed. If it has not, take action to see that consent is obtained as soon as possible, *since it must be done before the patient receives any preoperative sedation.* "If the patient's sensorium is clouded by medications, such as narcotics, or if he does not know the essential information pertaining to the surgery, he cannot give valid consent for it." (Creighton, 1981). Remember also that the patient has the right to withdraw consent after it is given. Contact the surgeon if this occurs.

Planning

4. Plan ample time to complete the tasks necessary before the patient leaves the unit for surgery.

Implementation (Consult Individual Modules for Specific Procedures)

5. Record the patient's vital signs. Blood pressure, pulse, and respirations may be increased *because of anxiety,* but if the patient's temperature is at all elevated, report this to the surgeon at once. *An elevated temperature can mean an infection, and the surgeon will have to decide whether to proceed with the surgery.* By recording the vital signs, *you also establish a baseline for future measurements.*
6. Administer or assist the patient with oral care. *Oral care is necessary because the mouth tends to dry during the unconscious period with the administration of anesthetic gases.* Caution the patient not to swallow water, but only to rinse the mouth. You may have to perform oral care for some patients.
7. Insert a nasogastric tube if ordered (see Module 45, Intubation).
8. Have the patient remove all items of clothing, including underwear, and put on a clean gown, untied. If the gown is untied, *it can be changed or removed easily when the patient is unconscious.*
9. Have the patient void, or insert a Foley catheter if ordered. *The bladder is emptied to*

avoid incontinence or injury during surgery. If the surgery is of short duration, voiding is usually sufficient. If a Foley catheter is ordered, consult Module 39, Catheterization. Some physicians prefer to have gastric intubation and catheterization done in surgery after the patient has been anesthetized.

10. Remove colored nail polish, *so the anesthesiologist can observe the nail beds during surgery for circulatory assessment.*

11. Remove any makeup, *so skin color can be assessed during surgery.*

12. Remove hairpins and hairpieces. *These can cause pressure on the patient's scalp during the unconscious period.*

13. Remove all prostheses, such as eyeglasses, contact lenses, hearing aids, and partial or complete dentures, and store them appropriately. Usually patients go to surgery without their dentures in place. Some anesthesiologists, however, prefer that dentures be kept in place *to provide a better seal around the endotracheal tube that delivers the anesthetic agent.* If the patient has natural teeth or is a child, check for loose teeth *that might be dislodged and aspirated during surgery.* Note the presence of crowned or capped teeth or a permanent bridge.

14. Remove and store the patient's jewelry. Jewelry can be given to the family during surgery. Religious medals are often sent with the patient *for comfort.* If a patient does not want to have a wedding band removed, tape it in place *to guard against loss.* If the ring contains a stone, use a Band-Aid, *so that the stone is in contact with the gauze instead of with the sticky tape.*

15. Put antiembolism stockings (TEDs) on the patient if ordered. *These stockings compress the peripheral leg tissue, increasing venous return during the immobile period.*

16. Ascertain the location of the patient's family or friends during surgical procedures, *so they can be reached in an emergency or can be informed when the patient moves to the recovery room.*

17. Check the chart for the preoperative medication order. Review the preop checklist for completion prior to giving the preop medication.

18. Prepare medications as ordered, administer, and document. More than one medication is usually given, and you must be certain all drugs are compatible and measured accurately (see Module 51, Giving Injections).

19. Caution the patient to remain quietly in bed once medication has been given.

20. Put the side rails up *for safety.* In some facilities you might place the bed in the high position, *so the stretcher can be brought up to the side of the bed to transfer the patient.* In most facilities, the bed is left down until the stretcher arrives.

21. Place the call bell within the patient's reach.

22. Wash your hands. Complete the preoperative checklist (Figure 46–14). Check the form used in your facility. You should also record the location of glasses or contact lenses, dentures, and jewelry.

23. Follow the proper procedure for patient identification as the patient leaves the unit. In most facilities the operating room transport person reads the patient's identifying data off of the patient's wristband while another hospital employee checks the chart. *This is a legal precaution to verify identification.*

24. Send the patient's chart and x-rays with the patient. *The surgeon may need to refer to them during surgery.*

Evaluation

25. Evaluate using the following criteria:
    a. All actions/procedures ordered were completed on time.
    b. Patient ready for surgery on time.

Documentation

26. Record all pertinent data.
    a. Preop checklist completed and signed.
    b. All nursing actions taken to prepare the patient for surgery and the patient's response.
    c. Any articles sent with the patient to surgery.
    d. Time and mode of transportation to operating room.

AMBULATORY SURGERY

Patients having ambulatory surgery—also called short-stay, day, or outpatient surgery—need the same preparation as inpatients do. These patients have their history and physical exam, laboratory tests, and other necessary preop examinations (such as electrocardiograms) on an outpatient basis, usually within

	YES	NO	N/A
1. Consent signed and witnessed	JE		
2. Time of last oral intake liquids _2400_ solids ____			
3. Preop lab work CBC ____	JE		
Blood Ordered ____	—	JE	
Here ____			
Other ____			
Urinalysis	JE		
4. Preoperative bath or shower	JE		
5. Makeup and nail polish removed	JE		
6. Bobby pins, combs, hair pieces & wig removed	JE		
7. Rings, earrings, jewelry, watch (Disposition) c̄ *husband*	JE		

8. Prosthesis
    artificial eye—in - out
    contact lens—in - out
    pacemaker
    other
			JE

9. Teeth
    natural ____
    artificial   upper ____
           lower ____
           bridges ____
           partial plate ____
    loose teeth ____
	JE		

10. Describe size and location of any skin lesion, burns, abrasions, etc. *None JE*			
11. Surgical Prep		JE	

12. Apparent preop mental condition of patient
    within normal limits ____   excited ____
    depressed ____   apprehensive _JE_
    irritable ____ other ____			

13. Location of family
   Rotunda ____
   Home _X – Will return at 1000_
   Office ____

14. Allergies   _None_

15. Pre-op vital signs
   TPR ___ 98⁴ – 88 – 24
   B/P ___ 136/88
   Wt. ___ 149 #

16. Voided
   Yes _0715_   No ____   NA ____

17. Retention Catheter
   Yes ____   No _JE_   NA ____

18. Pre-op Medication
   Ordered _None_
   Given ____

Form completed by:

X   _Jean Estes R.N._
Signature

Date _4/22/94_

Patient identification on unit
A.   Person from surgery calling for patient
   1.   Ask for patient by name & check identification band.
   2.   Check patient's chart with nursing personnel on unit according to procedure.

Signature:

X   _Holly Martin LPN_
Nursing Unit

X   _John Peters_
Surgery Personnel

NURSING UNIT PREOPERATIVE CHECK LIST

Figure 46–14. Preoperative checklist.

72–96 hours ahead of their planned surgery. They are responsible for their own night-before-surgery preparation, which might be as little as remaining NPO after midnight, or might include as much as the administration of special medications, enemas, and the like. Careful preoperative teaching and instructions are the best insurance for a successful outcome of the surgery.

References

Atkinson, L. J., & Kohn, M. L. (1978). *Berry & Kohn's introduction to operating room technique* (5th ed.) (p. 223). New York: McGraw-Hill.

Creighton, H. (1981). *Law every nurse should know* (4th ed.) (p. 199). Philadelphia: W. B. Saunders.

Garner, J. S. (1985). *Guideline for prevention of surgical wound infections* (p. 5). Atlanta: Centers for Disease Control.

Performance Checklist

Procedure for Preoperative Interview	Unsat	Needs More Practice	Sat	Comments
Assessment				
1. Verify type and exact time of surgery.				
2. Check preoperative orders.				
Planning				
3. Consult facility procedure book regarding specific type of surgery and preparation.				
4. Check patient's chart for history and physical, signed consent form, and results of required lab tests.				
5. Complete or secure any information listed above in planning.				
6. Plan sufficient time to carry out preoperative interview.				
Implementation				
7. Using appropriate form, perform interview, including the following areas: a. Verification of patient's identity				
b. General appearance and physical condition				
c. Anxiety level				
d. Knowledge level regarding proposed surgery				
e. Previous surgeries				
f. Smoking habits				
g. Drug and alcohol intake				
h. Family data.				
8. Encourage patient to ask questions and answer any inquiries.				
9. Provide emotional support.				
Evaluation				
10. Check data for completeness.				
Documentation				
11. Attach interview form to patient's chart.				

Procedure for Preoperative Teaching	Unsat	Needs More Practice	Sat	Comments
Assessment				
1. Review preoperative orders.				
2. Assess patient's language level, educational background, and anxiety level.				
Planning				
3. Plan considerable uninterrupted time for teaching.				
4. Include family members present if they so wish.				
Implementation				
5. Provide a quiet, nonstressful environment.				
6. Design your own plan but include as appropriate: a. Preoperative routine, including procedures and skin prep				
b. Postoperative routine and what is included in postoperative care				
c. Principles of pain management				
d. Explanation of postoperative equipment and appliances that may be used				
e. Deep-breathing exercises and coughing				
f. Methods for moving				
g. Leg exercises. (Remember to demonstrate and request a return demonstration of such things as breathing and leg exercises and methods for moving postoperatively.)				
Evaluation				
7. Evaluate teaching by: patient able to summarize points you have covered.				
Documentation				
8. Record on health teaching form or patient's chart, according to policy of your facility.				

Procedure for Preoperative Interventions	Unsat	Needs More Practice	Sat	Comments
Assessment				
1. Check for new orders before proceeding.				
2. Assess patient's readiness for procedures.				
Planning				
3. Plan time for carrying out procedures unhurriedly.				
4. Wash your hands.				
5. Review manual or modules for any skill you are undertaking.				
Implementation				
6. Identify the patient.				
7. Carry out procedures, such as enema, douche, or irrigations.				
Evaluation				
8. Evaluate using the following criteria: a. Patient comfortable.				
b. Patient states questions were answered.				
c. Procedure completed successfully.				
Documentation				
9. Record as directed by facility policy.				

Procedure for Wet Shaving				
Assessment				
1. Verify surgeon's order to determine area to be prepared.				
2. Assess patient's readiness for shaving.				
Planning				
3. Wash your hands.				
4. Obtain necessary equipment: a. Bath blanket for draping				

Procedure for Wet Shaving (Continued)	Unsat	Needs More Practice	Sat	Comments
b. Shaving equipment: basin of warm water, soap for lather, razor, sterile gauze squares, cleansing agent, cotton swabs				
c. Sterile towel to cover area after shaving.				
5. Plan area to be shaved.				
Implementation				
6. Identify the patient.				
7. Explain procedure to patient.				
8. Provide privacy.				
9. Arrange for adequate lighting.				
10. Drape patient with bath blanket.				
11. Shave area.				
12. Make patient comfortable.				
13. Dispose of equipment.				
14. Wash your hands.				
Evaluation				
15. Evaluate using the following criteria: a. Skin free of hair.				
b. Skin free of nicks.				
c. Skin shows no evidence of irritation.				
Documentation				
16. Record according to facility policy.				
Procedure for Immediate Preoperative Care				
Assessment				
1. Determine precise time scheduled for surgery.				
2. Check chart for any changes or additions in orders.				
3. Check to see that the operative permit has been signed.				

Procedure for Immediate Preoperative Care (Continued)	Unsat	Needs More Practice	Sat	Comments
Planning				
4. Plan ample time to complete tasks before time of surgery.				
Implementation				
5. Record vital signs and report any unusual findings.				
6. Administer or assist with oral care.				
7. Insert nasogastric tube if ordered.				
8. Have patient remove all clothing and put on clean gown, untied.				
9. Have patient void or, if ordered, insert Foley catheter.				
10. Remove colored nail polish.				
11. Remove any makeup.				
12. Remove hairpins or hairpieces.				
13. Remove all prostheses, including eyeglasses, contact lenses, hearing aids, and partial or complete dentures, and store them appropriately. Leave dentures in if indicated by anesthesiologist.				
14. Remove jewelry and store or give to family.				
15. If ordered, assist patient to put on TEDs.				
16. Ascertain location of family during surgery.				
17. Check orders for preoperative medication.				
18. Prepare, administer, and document medications as ordered.				
19. Caution patient to remain quietly in bed after medication is given.				
20. Put side rails in up position after injection of medications.				
21. Place call bell or light within patient's reach.				
22. Wash your hands.				
23. Follow facility policy for final identification of patient before leaving unit for surgical suite.				
24. Send patient's chart and x-rays with patient.				

Procedure for Immediate Preoperative Care (Continued)	Unsat	Needs More Practice	Sat	Comments
Evaluation				
25. Evaluate using the following criteria: a. All actions/procedures ordered were completed on time.				
b. Patient ready for surgery on time.				
Documentation				
26. Record all pertinent data. a. Preop checklist completed and signed.				
b. Nursing actions taken and patient's response.				
c. Any articles sent with patient to surgery.				
d. Time and mode of transportation to surgery.				

Quiz

Short-Answer Questions

1. What is the difference between elective and emergency surgery?

   _____

2. How does this difference affect your care? _____

3. List three activities you would teach a patient preoperatively.

   a. _____

   b. _____

   c. _____

4. Why is the patient usually placed on NPO at midnight the night before surgery? _____

5. List three objectives of preoperative skin preparation.

   a. _____

   b. _____

   c. _____

6. Why is the shave often done immediately before surgery?

   _____

7. What are two advantages of a wet shave?

   a. _____

   b. _____

8. List two reasons why vital signs are taken during the immediate preoperative period.

   a. _____

   b. _____

9. Name three aspects of immediate preoperative care that aid the anesthesiologist.

   a. _____

   b. _____

   c. _____

10. List two reasons why you should know the family's location during surgery.

    a. _____

    b. _____

Multiple Choice Questions

_____ 11. During the preoperative interview you assess that the patient does not understand the expected outcomes of the scheduled surgery. The appropriate nursing action would be:

   a. Explain the expected outcome of the surgery.
   b. Notify the surgeon of the patient's lack of understanding.
   c. Notify the anesthesiologist of the patient's lack of understanding.
   d. Cancel the surgery.

_____ 12. You note that the preoperative orders include meperidine. During the preoperative interview the patient tells you that she is allergic to meperidine. The correct nursing action would be:

   a. Give it anyway because the doctor knows about the patient.
   b. Hold the medication and put a note on the chart to that effect.
   c. Notify the surgeon of the problem.
   d. Notify the anesthesiologist of the problem.

_____ 13. The patient expresses worry over the outcome of the upcoming surgery and states "I guess I'm just scared that it will turn out to be cancer." The best nursing action in this situation is:

   a. Sit down with the patient and encourage him or her to express his or her feelings.
   b. Request a psychiatric consultation for the patient based on severe anxiety.
   c. Ask the surgeon to visit the patient for reassurance.
   d. Reassure the patient that it is unlikely to be cancer.

_____ 14. The patient asks you why he or she cannot have anything to drink before surgery. Your best answer is:

   a. Because the surgeon ordered that.
   b. Because it will make you nauseated.
   c. To prevent the possibility of vomiting and aspiration during anesthesia.
   d. To more closely monitor fluid balance through the use of intravenous fluids only.

Module 47
Postoperative Care

Module Contents

Rationale for the Use of This Skill
Postoperative Care
Ambulatory Surgery
Preparing the Postoperative Nursing Unit

Procedure for the Immediate Care of a
   Postoperative Patient
Assessment
Planning
Implementation
Evaluation
Documentation
Ongoing Care of the Postoperative Patient

Prerequisites

1. *Successful completion of the following modules:*

VOLUME 1

Module 1   An Approach to Nursing Skills
Module 2   Basic Infection Control
Module 3   Safety
Module 4   Basic Body Mechanics
Module 5   General Assessment Overview
Module 6   Documentation
Module 7   Bedmaking
Module 8   Moving the Patient in Bed and Positioning
Module 10 Assisting with Elimination and Perineal Care
Module 11 Hygiene
Module 13 Inspection, Palpation, Auscultation, and Percussion
Module 15 Intake and Output
Module 16 Temperature, Pulse, and Respiration
Module 17 Blood Pressure
Module 23 Ambulation
Module 24 Range-of-Motion Exercises

VOLUME 2

Module 41 Respiratory Care Procedures

2. *The following modules are not essential, but their successful completion will allow you to carry out more complete care for selected patients in the postoperative state:*

VOLUME 1

Module 28 Administering Enemas
Module 30 Caring for Patients with Casts and Braces
Module 31 Applying and Maintaining Traction

VOLUME 2

Overall Objective

To give comprehensive postoperative care designed to prevent complications when possible, identify complications that occur, institute treatment rapidly, and thereby facilitate the surgical patient's return to health.

Specific Learning Objectives

	Know Facts and Principles	Apply Facts and Principles	Demonstrate Ability	Evaluate Performance
1. *Postoperative nursing unit*	Discuss items to be included in postoperative nursing unit.	Given a patient situation, state which items should be included in postoperative nursing unit.	In the clinical setting, prepare unit to receive postoperative patient.	Evaluate with instructor using Performance Checklist.
2. *Initial observations*	List observations to be made immediately when postoperative patient arrives from recovery room.	Given a patient situation, state appropriate initial observations.	In the clinical setting, make complete initial observations on postoperative patient. Record initial observations correctly.	Evaluate with instructor using Performance Checklist.
3. *Information from chart*	State information to be obtained from chart after initial observations are made.	Given a sample patient's chart, obtain appropriate information about patient, following recovery room period.	In the clinical setting, check chart of postoperative patient for specific items of information after initial observations are made.	Evaluate for completeness of information with instructor.
4. *Potential problems*	Discuss observations, preventive actions, and treatment for potential postoperative problems.	Given a patient situation, state appropriate observations and preventive actions.	In the clinical setting, make appropriate observations and take appropriate actions to prevent postoperative problems.	Evaluate own performance with instructor.

Learning Activities

1. Review the Specific Learning Objectives.
2. Read the section on hypothermia in the section on neurologic function and the section on surgery and sexuality in the chapter on sexuality in Ellis and Nowlis, *Nursing: A Human Needs Approach,* or comparable material in another textbook.
3. Read the material in your medical-surgical nursing textbook that relates to postoperative care.
4. Look up the module vocabulary terms in the Glossary.
5. Read through the module and mentally practice the skills.
6. In the practice setting:
   a. Set up a postop unit using the Performance Checklist.
   b. Using another student as the patient, practice receiving your "patient" from the postanesthesia recovery room (PARR) and make all the appropriate initial observations. Use the Performance Checklist as a guide.
   c. Practice recording the information gathered in your initial observations, using the format used in your clinical facility.
7. In the clinical setting:
   a. Ask your instructor for an opportunity to assist a staff member in receiving a patient from the PARR. Notice how the patient is moved. Compare your initial observations with those of the staff person.
   b. Ask your instructor to arrange for you to receive a patient from the recovery room under supervision. Compare your initial observations with those of your instructor.

Vocabulary

atelectasis
collaborative
  problem
dehiscence
evisceration
hemorrhage
Homan's sign

hypoventilation
intensive care unit
  (ICU)
paralytic ileus
pneumonitis
postanesthesia
  care unit
  (PACU)

postanesthesia
  recovery room
  (PARR)
pulmonary
  embolus
purulent
recovery room
  (RR)

second-intention
  healing
shock
singultus
thrombophlebitis

Postoperative Care

Rationale for the Use of This Skill
Patients who have just returned from the recovery room are, in most instances, dependent. They may depend on the nurse for all aspects of care after major surgery, or for only selected aspects of care after minor surgery. In either event the nurse must make frequent and astute observations of these patients to provide for their comfort and safety, to prevent the many potential problems, and to act appropriately when problems are identified.[1]

POSTOPERATIVE CARE

Immediately after surgery, the patient is usually taken to the recovery room (RR), or postanesthesia recovery room (PARR), where skilled care is provided by experienced nurses until the patient has recovered from the anesthetic or can respond to stimuli. Usually, a minimum of one hour is spent in the recovery room, but this time can be considerably longer. Patients who have had complex surgery or who develop complications may be taken to the intensive care unit (ICU) for a stay of several days.

In this module we deal with the care of patients on their return to the regular nursing unit. For a complete understanding of the problems mentioned, consult your medical-surgical nursing text.

AMBULATORY SURGERY

The person having ambulatory surgery returns home within 24 hours of admission to the hospital. This is sometimes referred to as *day surgery*. Many hospitals now have a special unit for these patients. Here the patient is admitted, sent to surgery, received back from the PARR, monitored until stable, and discharged home with planned transportation. If complications occur or the patient remains unstable, he or she is then admitted to the hospital for ongoing care.

The same directions for care apply as in inpatient surgery; however, the potential for problems is usually less. In particular, the patient is usually not immobile so the problems of immobility that follow major surgeries are less of a concern.

The nurse spends a greater percentage of nursing

[1] You will note that rationale for action is emphasized throughout the module by the use of italics.

time teaching the patient and family or other caregivers how to manage at home than would be used for teaching inpatient surgical patients. Written instructions are particularly important *because this is a stressful time for those involved and complex instructions are easily forgotten or confused.* Many hospitals have standardized forms of home care instructions for common surgical procedures. These may be modified for the individual. When standard instructions are not available, the nurse is responsible for identifying the important teaching material. These instructions might include activity, wound care, diet, hygiene, and pain management, as well as signs and symptoms of complications and how to seek help if any problems arise.

A nurse from the facility may make a follow-up telephone call to the patient the day after the surgery to see if any difficulties are being encountered and to answer questions.

PREPARING THE POSTOPERATIVE NURSING UNIT

Before a patient is received from the recovery room, the room is prepared *to facilitate efficient care.* The postoperative bed is made up to receive the patient (see Module 7, Bedmaking). The postoperative bed should have extra protection at the head (a pad or bath towel) and in the middle (plastic draw-sheet, pad, or Chux) *to make changing easier in case of vomiting or soiling.* A turning sheet is also helpful if the patient is going to need assistance with positioning.

Tissues, an emesis basin, equipment for taking vital signs, and an IV stand are usually standard equipment in the postoperative unit. A pencil and paper for making notes are also helpful. Special equipment appropriate to the type of surgery the patient has undergone should be placed in the room *to prevent disorganization at the time of the patient's arrival.* This might include traction equipment for a patient who has undergone an orthopedic procedure or a tracheostomy tray for a patient who has had thyroid surgery.

PROCEDURE FOR THE IMMEDIATE CARE OF A POSTOPERATIVE PATIENT

You can use this general approach to care for any postoperative patient. It can be modified as appropriate for the needs of a specific patient.

1. Move the patient carefully from the stretcher

to the postoperative bed. *Rough or precipitous handling can contribute to sudden changes in pulse and blood pressure.* Use of a device such as a roller board can make the move safer and more comfortable for both nurse and patient. You may also wish to review Module 22, Transfer. Leave in place the blanket that covered the patient en route to the unit, *to help prevent chilling.*

Assessment

2. Receive the report from the PARR nurse. *This report will give you information about the patient's stay there and serve as a baseline for your own assessment.* In some facilities, PARR personnel telephone a status report to the nursing unit before the patient leaves the PARR to assist the nurse in preparing for the arrival of the patient.
3. Make the following initial observations:
   a. Time of arrival on unit
   b. Responsiveness (to what does the patient respond and how does the patient respond, for example, to name call)
   c. Vital signs:
      (1) Temperature
      (2) Pulse
      (3) Respirations
      (4) Blood pressure
   d. Skin:
      (1) Color
      (2) Condition (dryness or moisture)
   e. Dressing:
      (1) Clean
      (2) Dry
      (3) Intact
      Look and feel under patient to detect pooling of blood.
   f. Presence of an IV infusion:
      (1) Type of solution
      (2) Amount left in bottle
      (3) Drip rate
   g. Presence of bladder catheter:
      (1) Unclamped
      (2) Connected to drainage bag or bottle
      (3) Freely draining
      (4) Characteristics and amount of urine
   h. Presence of other drainage tubes:
      (1) Unclamped
      (2) Attached appropriately to bottle or suction
      (3) Tubes not kinked or under patient
      (4) Characteristics and amount of drainage

   i. Safety and comfort:
      (1) Presence of pain, nausea, or vomiting
      (2) Position appropriate for surgical procedure
      (3) Side rails up and bed in low position and call light within reach
4. Check the chart for the following information (some of which may have been included in the report from the PARR nurse):
   a. Operation performed
   b. Postoperative diagnosis
   c. Anesthetic agents used
   d. Estimated blood loss (EBL)
   e. Blood or fluid replacement given during surgery and PARR stay
   f. Type and location of drains
   g. Vital signs when patient left PARR (for use as a baseline)
   h. Medications administered in the PARR:
      (1) Time
      (2) Type
      (3) Amount
      (4) Response of the patient
   i. Output:
      (1) Urine
      (2) Other drainage
      (3) Vomitus
   j. Physician's orders:[2]
      (1) Frequency of vital signs
      (2) Diet
      (3) Activity
      (4) IV orders
      (5) Medications (amount and frequency of pain and other medications)
      (6) Laboratory or respiratory therapy orders
      (7) Orders specific to type of surgery or other problems of patient
   Some institutions use a recovery room nursing record, which can be very helpful to the nurse who is taking over the care of the patient on the nursing unit (Figure 47–1).
5. Identify any problems present.

Planning

6. Plan actions to resolve and/or monitor problems identified.
7. Wash your hands *for infection control.*
8. Determine the equipment necessary.

---

[2] In most facilities, postoperative orders automatically cancel all previous written orders. These must be reordered by the physician after surgery if still wanted.

Group Health Cooperative
POSTANESTHESIA RECORD

Schwartz, Mabel
000-92-7654
Dr. Jenkins

ADMISSION	1410	DISCHARGE	1520	ANESTHESIA	general

SURGERY cholecystectomy

NURSE I. Hubbard RN

OR TOTAL INTAKE	OR TOTAL OUTPUT	PERTINENT MEDICAL DATA		O₂ L/M 2 LPM	
Fluid— 275 ml	EBL— 350 ml	No significant medical history		⊠ AIRWAY dcd @ 1430	⊠ INTUBATED dcd @ 1420
Blood— 0	Urine— 100 ml			VENTILATOR 0	

☐ ECG   ☐ 12-LEAD ECG   ☐ ART. LINE   ☐ CVP   ☐ SWAN GANZ   ☐ X-RAY

NO	SOLUTION	VOL.	ADDITIVE	TIME	TOTAL ABSORBED	TUBES	LOCATION DESCRIPTION	INTAKE	OUTPUT
1	D5LR	1000	—	1200	400 ml	FOLEY/CYSTO CATH.	—	—	75 ml
						CBI/IBI			
						HEMOVAC/JP			
						PLEUREVAC/EMERSON			
						NASO GASTRIC 0			
						EMESIS 0			
						DRESSINGS 0			

ALDRETE SCORING

COLOR	AWAKE	VENTILATION	BP	MOVEMENT
2 PINK	2 AWAKE-AWARE	2 DEEP BREATHS & COUGHS	2 BP 20% ANESTH	2 MOVES 3 LIMBS
1 PALE-DUSKY-BLOTCHY	1 ROUSABLE-ORIENTED	1 SHALLOW BREATH AIRWAY	1 BP 20 - 50%	1 MOVES 2 LIMBS
0 CYANOTIC	0 NOT RESPONDING	0 APNEA/OBSTRUCTED	0 BP 50%	0 MOVES 0 LIMBS

ALLERGIES

COLOR:	2	2	2	2	2
AWAKE	0	0	1	1	2
VENTILATION	1	1	2	2	2
BP	1	2	2	2	2
MOVEMENT	0	1	1	2	2

VITAL SIGNS

• PULSE
ᐱ CUFF BP
ˣ MONITOR BP

MEDICATIONS

	AMT.	TIME
Demerol	50 mg	1425

RESP.	14	16	16	18	18
TEMP.	97.6				
SAB					
CVP					
URINE					
PAIN	0	0	5	5	2

ABGS	PH	PCO²	PO²	% SAT	HCO³	B.E.	TESTS

Figure 47–1 Postanesthesia record.

9. Gather the appropriate equipment not already in the room.

Implementation

10. Identify the patient *to be sure you are performing the procedure for the correct patient.*
11. Explain to the patient what you plan to do.
12. Carry out procedure(s) deemed necessary according to assessment.

Evaluation

13. Evaluate, using appropriate criteria.

Documentation

14. Record appropriately, on flow sheet(s) or on the narrative record.

ONGOING CARE OF THE POSTOPERATIVE PATIENT

The ongoing care of the postoperative patient is largely preventive in nature. We present it here in chart form, using a human needs approach (pages 278–282).

In the first column, the general category of nursing diagnoses and the pertinent assessment observations are listed. The second column lists nursing diagnoses and collaborative problems. Nursing diagnoses are patient problems that the nurse is able to identify and to treat independently. Nursing diagnoses are in NANDA terminology. Collaborative problems are those patient problems that the nurse must assess for and report to the physician who must order the treatment. Collaborative problems are stated as "Potential complications." The third column lists the defining characteristics for the problem. Defining characteristics indicate that the problem is currently present. The fourth and fifth columns provide information on selected nursing actions. This is not meant to be an exhaustive list of all possible nursing actions, but outlines the most important ones. The actions listed in the fourth column are those that will help prevent the patient problem. Actions listed in the fifth column will either correct the problem or refer it for corrective measures.

Ongoing Care of the Postoperative Patient

Human Needs Area	Nursing Diagnoses/ Collaborative Problems	Defining Characteristics	Selected Nursing Actions	
			Prevention	Treatment
1. Circulation Potential Alterations in Circulation Assess: Blood pressure, pulses, color of mucous membranes, peripheral circulation, temperature and color of lower legs, pain, visible bleeding	a. Potential complication: Hypovolemic shock related to blood loss	External or internal hemorrhaging; drop in blood pressure; rapid, weak pulse; cold, clammy skin	Avoid sudden movements; get patient up slowly; maintain IVs per physician's orders; keep warm.	Place flat with legs elevated; report changes in patient status to physician immediately; be prepared to administer medications, start oxygen, administer blood and/or IV fluids per physician's orders.
	b. Potential complication: Thrombophlebitis related to venous stagnation	Localized pain, heat, and swelling, usually in lower extremities; positive Homan's sign	Encourage early ambulation or bed exercises, active or passive; encourage fluids; provide elastic hose per physician's orders.	Provide bed rest; notify physician and prepare to apply hot moist packs; administer drug therapy per physician's orders.
	c. Alteration in tissue perfusion: Peripheral venous stasis related to immobility	Legs immobile; dilated superficial veins; edema	Teach patient the importance of active exercise of legs while in bed and early ambulation; teach value of fluids in maintaining blood viscosity.	Encourage early ambulation or bed exercises, active or passive; encourage fluids; provide elastic hose per physician's orders.
	d. Fluid volume deficit related to inadequate fluid intake	Decreased urine output, dry mucous membranes, hypotension, fever, increased urine specific gravity, thirst	Maintain IV fluids at ordered rate; encourage adequate fluid intake as soon as oral intake permissible.	Readjust IV fluids based on policy and physician's orders; offer oral fluids of the patient's choice every hour.
	e. Fluid volume excess related to rapid infusion of IV fluids	Rapid, bounding, full pulse; moist sounds on auscultating lungs; puffy areas around eyes, sacrum, ankles	Maintain IV fluids at ordered rate.	Slow IV fluids according to policy or physician's orders; notify physician and be prepared to administer medications as ordered.
2. Oxygenation/Aeration Potential Alterations in Respirations Assess: Respiratory rate, depth, chest excursion, respiratory effort, breath sounds, color of	a. Potential complication: Pulmonary embolus	Rapid respirations; sudden chest pain; shortness of breath; anxiety; shock	Prevent thrombophlebitis (see above); *do not* massage lower extremities.	Notify physician. Administer drug therapy and oxygen per physician's orders; place patient in Fowler's position.

278

© 1992 by J.B. Lippincott Company

mucous membranes, nail beds, and conjunctiva

	Assessment		Interventions
b. Ineffective breathing pattern: Hypoventilation related to pain and immobility	Rapid shallow breathing; diminished breath sounds	Preoperative teaching regarding the importance of deep breathing; pain management	Encourage turning, deep breathing and coughing at least every 2 h. Encourage fluids and early ambulation.
c. Ineffective airway clearance: Retained secretions related to painful coughing or decreased cough reflex secondary to narcotics	Presence of adventitious lung sounds; use of accessory muscles for respiration	Preoperative teaching regarding the importance of coughing up secretions; pain management	Increase frequency of turning, deep breathing and coughing; use suction if patient cannot cough out secretions. Notify physician for possible respiratory therapy.
d. Potential complication: Atelectasis related to ineffective breathing pattern	Areas of absence of breath sounds, low grade fever in first 24 h postoperatively; ineffective breathing pattern; ineffective airway clearance	All of the above treatments for ineffective airway clearance and ineffective breathing pattern	Notify physician for possible respiratory therapy; continue with treatment for ineffective airway clearance as above, increasing frequency.
e. Potential complication: Hypostatic pneumonia	Rapid, noisy respirations; elevated temperature; increased pulse rate; restlessness; pain; cough	All the above treatments for ineffective airway clearance and ineffective breathing pattern	Administer respiratory therapy and antibiotics per physician's orders.
3. *Comfort* Potential Alterations in Comfort Assess: Patient subjective statements regarding comfort, willingness to engage in ADLs, facial expressions, vital signs			
a. Alteration in comfort: Pain related to incision/surgical procedure	Complaint of pain, grimacing; immobility (guarding wound); restlessness; blood pressure drop not accompanied by signs of blood loss	Administer pain medication *before* pain becomes severe; enhance pain medication with nursing measures (change of position, back rub, reassurance, information as to how long it will take pain medication to work); inspect for edema, tight dressings, or tight casts.	Administer medication per physician's orders; splint when moving; move slowly.
b. Alteration in comfort: Nausea and vomiting related to anesthetic agents, pain, medications	Complaint of nausea; emesis	Urge patient to breathe in and out through mouth; keep area well ventilated and free of odors.	Position patient on side to prevent aspiration; provide frequent oral care; give antiemetic medication before meals per physician's orders; NPO and nasogastric tube per physician's orders (for persistent vomiting).

(continued)

279

Ongoing Care of the Postoperative Patient (Continued)

Human Needs Area	Nursing Diagnoses/ Collaborative Problems	Defining Characteristics	Selected Nursing Actions	
			Prevention	Treatment
	c. Alteration in comfort: Abdominal discomfort related to retained gas	Complaint of discomfort; drumlike distention of abdomen (palpate and percuss)	Encourage early ambulation.	Continue to encourage active movement and ambulation; encourage hot fluids (ice can increase problem); administer rectal tube, return-flow enema (Harris flush), or medication per physician's orders.
	d. Alteration in comfort: Hiccoughs (singultus) related to phrenic nerve stimulation secondary to dilation of the stomach or irritation of the diaphragm	Complaint of hiccoughs		Have patient rebreathe own carbon dioxide (inhaling and exhaling into paper bag held tightly over nose and mouth); administer medication per physician's orders.
4. *Skin integrity/Hygiene* Potential Alterations in Skin Integrity Assess: Wound appearance, temperature of skin around wound, wound drainage	a. Potential complication: Wound infection related to wound contamination or decreased resistance	Local signs of infection (redness, heat, swelling, pain, purulent drainage); generalized signs of infection (fever, increased pulse and respiratory rate)	Keep dressing clean and dry; pay conscientious attention to caring for patient's hygiene needs; change linen at least daily; follow strict aseptic technique when changing dressing; administer antibiotics per physician's orders.	Administer antibiotics per physician's orders.
	b. Potential complication: Dehiscence related to delayed healing	Separation of skin edges	Apply abdominal binder (scultetus binder) per physician's orders.	Keep sterile dressings over wound; notify physician (surgical reclosure may be needed or the wound may be left open to heal by second intention).
	c. Potential complication: Evisceration related to delayed healing	Complaint of "giving" sensation in area of incision; sudden leakage of fluid from wound; wound open with abdominal contents protruding	Apply abdominal binder per physician's orders.	Cover open wound with sterile, warm saline packs; keep patient quiet; observe for signs of shock; notify physician; notify surgery (emergency surgical treatment

280

d. Impairment of skin integrity related to surgical wound	Surgical wound not yet intact		usually required); stay with patient for psychological support. Use sterile technique in care of wound, encourage optimum nutrition as permitted.
5. *Elimination* Potential Alterations in Elimination Assess: Bowel tones, abdominal palpation, passing flatus?, stool appearance, urinary output, color and clarity of urine a. Alteration in bowel elimination: Constipation related to inadequate fluids and bulk, decreased activity, and effects of anesthesia and analgesics	Complaint of no bowel movement or small amounts of hard, dry stool; abdominal discomfort; abdominal distention	Encourage early ambulation; encourage fluids; administer stool softeners per physician's orders.	Administer enema per physician's orders (if no bowel movement in first 4 or 5 days); administer stool softeners per physician's orders.
Potential complication: Paralytic ileus	Abdominal distention and discomfort, no flatus, absence of bowel tones	Encourage early activity and ambulation, use narcotics with care.	Notify physician; NPO and nasogastric tube per physician's orders (if paralytic ileus exists); administer medication to stimulate peristalsis per physician's orders.
b. Alteration in urinary elimination: Retention related to recumbent position, effects of anesthetic and narcotics	Urine output (measure); bladder distention (palpate); complaint of discomfort	Encourage early activity and ambulation, use narcotics with care.	Attempt measures to encourage voiding; pass urinary catheter per physician's orders (if no voiding for 8–12 h after surgery).
Potential complication: Urinary tract infection related to catheterization or urinary stasis	Elevated temperature; cloudy and/or dark urine; burning on urination	Maintain adequate fluid intake; if catheter in place, give thorough catheter care.	Encourage fluid intake; administer medications per physician's orders.
6. *Activity and rest* Potential Alterations in Activity Assess: Ability to move and participate in ADLs a. Impaired physical mobility related to general muscle weakness secondary to decreased mobility; and pain and soreness secondary to surgical procedure	Weakness; dizziness; fatigue	Encourage early ambulation, or active or passive range of motion if ambulation not possible; encourage adequate nutrition.	Same as preventive actions.

(continued)

281

Ongoing Care of the Postoperative Patient (Continued)

Human Needs Area	Nursing Diagnoses/ Collaborative Problems	Defining Characteristics	Selected Nursing Actions	
			Prevention	Treatment
7. *Psychosocial* Potential Alterations in Coping Assess: Ability to make decisions, willingness to assume responsibility for self care, ability to identify resources for support	a. Ineffective individual coping: related to diagnosis, physical status, hospitalization	Asocial behavior; malaise; listlessness; sleep disturbance	Encourage early ambulation; assist patient with personal needs; encourage patient's participation as appropriate; keep patient and patient's unit neat and free of odor; be available as listener; perform patient teaching.	Same as preventive actions; also arrange consultation per physician's orders.
Potential Alterations in Emotional Integrity Assess: Expression of feelings, facial expressions, and body posture	b. Anxiety related to pain and discomfort or possible outcome of surgery	Rapid pulse and respiration, elevated blood pressure, fidgety movement, states feels anxious or "nervous"	Preoperative teaching; stay with patient; encourage presence of significant others who are supportive; meet needs promptly.	Provide explanation and let patient know anxiety is normal response; encourage expression of feelings; help patient to name feelings, consider previous coping strategies, challenge unrealistic expectations of self, instruct in relaxation methods.
	c. Depressed mood related to illness, surgery, change in body image, or effect of medications	Crying, withdrawal, sad appearance, indecision, apathy	Encourage participation in care, encourage use of support persons, point out indications of progress, listen to concerns, teaching expected course of recovery.	Encourage activity as possible; point out progress in recovery; spend time with patient; encourage visits from significant others; inform that these feelings are common in postoperative period and resolve as recovery progresses.

282

© **1992 by J.B. Lippincott Company**

Performance Checklist

Preparing the Preoperative Nursing Unit	Unsat	Needs More Practice	Sat	Comments
1. Make postoperative bed. a. Extra protection at head				
b. Extra protection and turn sheet in middle				
2. Obtain necessary equipment. a. Tissues				
b. Emesis basin				
c. For vital signs:				
(1) Thermometer				
(2) Stethoscope				
(3) Blood pressure cuff				
(4) Sphygmomanometer				
d. IV stand				
e. Pencil and paper				
f. Special equipment				

Procedure for the Immediate Care of a Postoperative Patient

	Unsat	Needs More Practice	Sat	Comments
1. Move patient carefully from stretcher to postoperative bed.				

Assessment

	Unsat	Needs More Practice	Sat	Comments
2. Receive report from the recovery room nurse.				
3. Make following initial observations: a. Time of arrival on unit				
b. Responsiveness				
c. Vital signs:				
(1) Temperature				
(2) Pulse				
(3) Respirations				
(4) Blood pressure				

Procedure for the Immediate Care of a Postoperative Patient *(Continued)*	Unsat	Needs More Practice	Sat	Comments
d. Skin:				
(1) Color				
(2) Condition				
e. Dressing:				
(1) Clean				
(2) Dry				
(3) Intact				
f. IV infusion:				
(1) Type of solution				
(2) Amount left in bottle				
(3) Drip rate				
g. Bladder catheter:				
(1) Unclamped				
(2) Connected to drainage bag or bottle				
(3) Freely draining				
(4) Characteristics and amount of urine				
h. Other drainage tubes:				
(1) Unclamped				
(2) Attached appropriately to bottle or suction				
(3) Not kinked or under patient				
(4) Characteristics and amount of drainage				
i. Safety and comfort				
(1) Side rails up, bed in low position, call bell within reach				
(2) Appropriate position				
(3) Pain, nausea, and vomiting				
4. Check the chart for the following information: a. Operation performed				
b. Postoperative diagnosis				
c. Anesthetic agents used				

Procedure for the Immediate Care of a Postoperative Patient *(Continued)*	Unsat	Needs More Practice	Sat	Comments
d. Estimated blood loss (EBL)				
e. Blood and/or fluid replacement				
f. Type and location of drains				
g. Vital signs when patient left RR				
h. Medications administered in the RR				
(1) Time				
(2) Type				
(3) Amount				
(4) Response of patient				
i. Output				
(1) Urine				
(2) Other drainage				
(3) Vomitus				
j. Physician's orders				
(1) Frequency of vital signs				
(2) Diet				
(3) Activity				
(4) IV orders				
(5) Medications				
(6) Laboratory and/or respiratory therapy orders				
(7) Orders specific to type of surgery or other problems				
5. Identify any problems present.				
Planning				
6. Plan actions to resolve and/or monitor problems identified.				
7. Wash your hands.				
8. Determine equipment necessary.				
9. Gather appropriate equipment not already in room.				

Procedure for the Immediate Care of a Postoperative Patient *(Continued)*	Unsat	Needs More Practice	Sat	Comments
Implementation				
10. Identify the patient.				
11. Explain to patient what you plan to do.				
12. Carry out procedure(s).				
Evaluation				
13. Evaluate, using appropriate criteria.				
Documentation				
14. Record appropriately.				

Quiz
Short-Answer Questions

1. List four types of equipment that are usually included in the items gathered for a postoperative nursing unit.

   a. _____

   b. _____

   c. _____

   d. _____

2. List six general areas of concern that are included in the initial observation of the patient after his or her return from the postanesthesia recovery room.

   a. _____

   b. _____

   c. _____

   d. _____

   e. _____

   f. _____

3. If a bladder catheter is present when a patient returns from surgery, what four observations should you make?

   a. _____

   b. _____

   c. _____

   d. _____

4. Write a sample nursing note in the space below, using the format of your clinical facility. Include five items of information appropriate to any postoperative patient.

   _____

   _____

   _____

   _____

5. List seven of the items of information that are obtained from the patient's chart after the initial observations are made.

   a. _____

   b. _____

   c. _____

   d. _____

   e. _____

    f. _____

    g. _____

6. List three observations the nurse can make to identify thrombophlebitis.

    a. _____

    b. _____

    c. _____

7. List three actions that can help to prevent postoperative constipation.

    a. _____

    b. _____

    c. _____

8. List three of the nursing actions that might help to prevent depressed mood in the postoperative patient.

    a. _____

    b. _____

    c. _____

9. List three nursing actions that should be taken if postoperative hemorrhage is identified.

    a. _____

    b. _____

    c. _____

10. Name two potential nursing diagnoses in the area of elimination that are pertinent to the postoperative patient.

    a. _____

    b. _____

11. What are two major reasons for preoperative teaching?

    a. _____

    b. _____

12. What defining characteristics would indicate that the patient is anxious?

_____

_____

_____

Module 48

Irrigations: Bladder, Catheter, Ear, Eye, Nasogastric Tube, Vaginal, Wound

Module Contents

Rationale for the Use of This Skill
Nursing Diagnoses
Asepsis
Safety
Patient Teaching
Observation
Documentation
General Procedure for Irrigation
    Assessment
    Planning
    Implementation
    Evaluation
    Documentation

Bladder and Catheter Irrigation
    Closed Technique
        Y Connector and Fluid Reservoir
        Syringe-and-Needle Method
    Open Technique
    Three-Way Irrigation
Irrigating the Ear
Irrigating the Eye
    Small-Volume Irrigation
    Large-Volume Irrigation
Nasogastric Tube Irrigation
Vaginal Irrigation (Douche)
Irrigating Wounds
Long-Term Care
Home Care

Prerequisites

1. *Successful completion of the following modules:*

VOLUME 1

Module 1   An Approach to Nursing Skills
Module 2   Basic Infection Control
Module 3   Safety
Module 5   General Assessment Overview
Module 6   Documentation
Module 15 Intake and Output

2. *The following may be needed for some irrigations:*

VOLUME 2

Module 35 Sterile Technique
Module 37 Wound Care
Module 49 Administering Oral Medications
Module 50 Administering Medications by
    Alternative Routes

289

Overall Objective

To know the purpose of an irrigation, to plan the correct technique needed to accomplish that purpose, and to carry out the irrigation safely and correctly.

Specific Learning Objectives

	Know Facts and Principles	Apply Facts and Principles	Demonstrate Ability	Evaluate Performance
1. Purposes	List two general purposes for irrigation.	In a specific situation, identify purpose of irrigation.	Identify purpose of irrigation before proceeding.	
2. General concerns *a. Clean versus sterile technique* *b. Safety*	Identify irrigations that require sterile technique. List factors in irrigation that may irritate or damage tissue.	Given an example of an irrigation, determine whether clean or sterile technique is needed.	In the clinical setting, use correct technique for situation. Use correct pressure, solution, and temperature for irrigation.	Evaluate own performance with instructor using Performance Checklist.
3. Performing irrigations	State procedure for each irrigation discussed in module.	Modify procedure for individual situation. Explain procedure to patient.	Carry out specific irrigation correctly.	Evaluate own performance with instructor using Performance Checklist.
4. Observations	State important observations to be made during irrigation.	Identify observations that are most critical for particular situation.	Make appropriate observations while performing irrigations.	Evaluate appropriateness of observations with instructor.
5. Documentation	State what needs to be recorded.	Given an example of an irrigation, identify what should be recorded.	Record appropriate information on narrative record or flow sheet.	Evaluate using Performance Checklist.

Learning Activities

1. Review the Specific Learning Objectives.
2. Read the chapter on dependent nursing functions in Ellis and Nowlis, *Nursing: A Human Needs Approach,* or a comparable chapter in another textbook.
3. Look up the module vocabulary terms in the Glossary.
4. Read through the module and mentally practice the specific procedure.
5. Arrange for time to practice irrigations.
6. In the practice setting:
   a. Review the equipment available for irrigations.
   b. Identify the various types of syringes and any prepackaged sets for specific types of irrigations.
   c. Try using each piece of equipment to make sure you understand its function and can handle it.
   d. Review the recording of irrigations in sample situations given in the module.
7. In the clinical setting:
   a. Seek opportunities to observe irrigations done by others.
   b. Perform irrigations with supervision.

Vocabulary

asepto syringe
canthus
catheter tip
   syringe
cerumen
concentration of
   solution
douche
exudate
instill
irrigate
mucous
mucus
pinna
Toomey syringe

Irrigations: Bladder, Catheter, Ear, Eye, Nasogastric Tube, Vaginal, Wound

Rationale for the Use of This Skill

Generally, irrigations are done for two purposes. The first is to clean the passage or body area. Small or large amounts of solution can be used to remove secretions, small clots, foreign material, and microorganisms. The solution used may be one that simply flushes particles away or may contain special cleansing agents.

The second purpose is to instill medication. The medication may be an antibacterial agent, a soothing agent, or an agent that exerts another specific therapeutic effect, such as changing acidity. Sometimes an irrigation serves both purposes at the same time (see Module 50, Administering Medications by Alternative Routes, regarding instilling medications).

The nurse must also understand that frequent or excessive irrigation of some body cavities with hypotonic solutions can lead to electrolyte imbalance. Irrigations may be ordered by the physician specific to the needs of the patient or in some institutions, there is a standing order for irrigations at the nurse's discretion. There are many similarities in the way these irrigations are done, but the differences are critical. The nurse must be able to plan an appropriate procedure and to carry it out correctly.[1]

▶ *Nursing Diagnoses*

A number of nursing diagnoses would require irrigation intervention. Examples are:

Alteration in Elimination: Urinary retention related to occlusion of the indwelling urinary catheter due to sediment

Sensory Alteration, Auditory: Decreased hearing bilaterally related to increased collection of wax within ears

High Risk for Injury: Left eye related to presence of small foreign body

Alteration in Comfort: Abdominal distress related to nonfunctioning of nasogastric tube

[1] You will note that rationale for action is emphasized throughout the module by the use of italics.

ASEPSIS

Sterile technique must be used on all areas of the body that are normally sterile. These include the bladder, the kidney pelvis, and open wounds. Sterile technique is also used for irrigations involving the eye *because of the potential for serious injury from even a minor eye infection.*

Clean technique is used for all other irrigations, including irrigations of the throat, ear, vagina, bowel, and stomach. In an instance of surgery on any of these organs, sterile technique is necessary, *because the surgical incision has broken the intact tissue that provides a barrier to microbes.*

SAFETY

The nurse wears clean gloves when performing most irrigations *to provide protection from the patient's body secretions.* Sterile gloves are worn when it is necessary to touch an open wound or sterile equipment. *Most body tissue is sensitive to excessive pressure. Because fluid under pressure can cause spasms of an organ, such as the bladder, and actual tissue damage to a structure as sensitive as the eye,* use gentle pressure only. If the patient feels discomfort, reduce the pressure. *Remember that by decreasing the height of the container you decrease the pressure.*

Medications or chemicals may also irritate or cause tissue reaction. This is especially true if the wrong concentration is used for a particular tissue. For example, a benzalkonium chloride solution, suitable for use on instruments, is far too strong for mucous membranes. Therefore, carefully check both the type and the concentration of solution used to make sure they are correct.

Most irrigations are done with solutions at room temperature. *To increase the patient's comfort,* you can warm solutions to body temperature. Do not use extreme temperatures, however. *Very high temperatures can burn tissues. Low temperatures can produce a shocklike reaction as the body attempts to maintain homeostasis.*

PATIENT TEACHING

Teaching the patient about the procedure and what to expect is essential. *This allows the patient to participate in care as much as possible.*

To begin, find out what the patient knows. Then explain what the patient does not understand. If an irrigation has been done previously, it is important to find out what the previous procedure was and the patient's response. It may upset the patient to have each nurse proceed in a different manner. The irrigation technique should be noted in the Nursing Care Plan *to facilitate continuity of care.*

Allow time for the patient to ask questions and to express personal feelings about the procedure. Some persons fear that the irrigation will cause pain. Additionally, many irrigation procedures produce anxiety. You will, therefore, have to take action *to decrease the patient's anxiety by listening and expressing concern.*

OBSERVATION

During an irrigation, it is important that you observe the area being irrigated as much as possible. Of course, certain internal areas cannot be observed directly, but the opening into the area can be observed. Notice any drainage or exudate, and describe the amount, color, consistency, and odor of it. Also, observe the irrigation fluid for secretions that may be washed out with the fluid.

DOCUMENTATION

When recording, note the area irrigated, the type and amount of solution used, and the time of irrigation, as well as the patient's response to the procedure.

All fluid used for irrigating should be returned. If the fluid fails to return, note that fact in the chart and record the amount retained on the intake worksheet.

GENERAL PROCEDURE FOR IRRIGATION

Assessment
1. Verify the following:
   a. Type of irrigation ordered
   b. Amount, temperature, type, and concentration of solution ordered.

Planning
2. Decide whether the irrigation is to be clean or sterile.
3. Wash your hands *for infection control.*
4. Identify and gather the equipment needed for the specific irrigation, including:

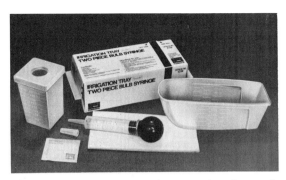

Figure 48-1 A commercial irrigation set consists of a container that holds the solution and bulb syringe, an alcohol wipe, protective pad, and a receptacle for collecting the irrigation fluid.
(*Courtesy American Hospital Supply Corp., McGaw Park, Illinois*)

a. Solution
b. Irrigating device (Figures 48–1 and 48–2)
c. Receptacle for used irrigating fluid
d. Protective padding (towels or disposable waterproof pads *to keep the patient and the environment dry*)
e. Clean gloves *to protect yourself if body secretions are contacted.* It is also important to protect the patient from microorganisms that you may harbor in small cracks in your skin or on a minor abrasion. All nurses should become accustomed to wearing clean gloves while performing irrigations for patients *because there is current evidence that organisms can be transferred during any procedure.*

Implementation
5. Identify the patient *to be sure you are performing the procedure for the correct patient.*
6. Explain the procedure to the patient.
7. Provide privacy by closing curtains and adequately draping the patient as appropriate for the specific irrigation *to safeguard the patient's modesty.*
8. Position the patient as needed for the irrigation.
9. Place protective padding where needed.
10. Put on gloves and carry out the irrigation according to the specific procedure outlined below.
11. Make sure the patient is dry and comfortable.
12. Dispose of the used equipment following the policy of your facility. If the equipment is reusable, you may have to wash it thoroughly or return it to central supply for processing. If

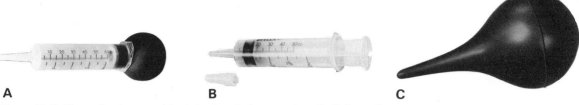

A   **B**   **C**

Figure 48–2 Types of syringes used for irrigations **A:** Asepto syringe. **B:** Catheter-tip syringe. **C:** Ear syringe (bulb syringe).
(*Courtesy American Hospital Supply Corp., McGaw Park, Illinois*)

it is disposable, you may have to discard it in a specific place.

13. Wash your hands.

Evaluation

14. Evaluate using the following criteria:
  a. Area of irrigation was thoroughly cleaned.
  b. Medication contacted desired area.
  c. Patient resting comfortably.

Documentation

15. Document the following in the record:
  a. Type of irrigation.
  b. Type, concentration, and amount of fluid used.
  c. Appearance and odor of any secretions washed away.
  d. Results of the procedure.
  e. Patient's response to the procedure.

DATE/TIME	
2/10/94 1600	3 cm open sacral decubitus ulcer irrigated with 100 ml half-strength hydrogen peroxide. Solution returned with large amount yellow-green exudate. Wound surface still not clear of exudate. States there is no discomfort with irrigation. — K. Thorsen, RN

Example of Progress Notes Using Narrative Format

DATE/TIME	
2/10/94 1600	Alteration in Skin Integrity: Sacral decubitus ulcer
	S States no discomfort associated with ulcer or irrigation
	O Wound irrigation with 100 ml half-strength hydrogen peroxide returned large amount of yellow-green exudate. Wound surface still not clear of exudate.
	A Infection of decubitus ulcer persists.
	P Continue with irrigations each shift. Keep wound covered with dressing between irrigations. Continue to isolate wound drainage and follow specific isolation procedures. Consult physician regarding treatment of infection. — K. Thorsen, NS

Example of Progress Notes Using SOAP Format

DATE	Time	Procedure	Result
2/10/94	1600	Irrigation of decubitus ulcer 100 ml 1/2 st H_2O_2.	Large amount of yellow-green drainage.

Example of Flow Sheet

Any necessary modifications are presented for each of the following specific irrigation procedures. The complete procedure, which includes all steps of the general procedure as well as necessary modifications, is found in the Performance Checklist.

BLADDER AND CATHETER IRRIGATION

The terms *bladder irrigation* and *catheter irrigation* are often used interchangeably. They are not the same, so when either is ordered you should check carefully as to the purpose of the irrigation. A *catheter irrigation* is performed to keep the catheter patent. A *bladder irrigation* is performed to clean or medicate the bladder itself. Much of the technique is identical for both procedures and both procedures require sterile technique, *because the inside of the bladder is sterile.*

An open or closed technique can be used for intermittent irrigations. It is highly recommended that if at all possible, the closed technique be used *so that the system is not interrupted, which could allow microorganisms to enter the sterile environment of the urinary tract.* Today, the closed technique is being used increasingly *to maintain the urinary drainage as a closed system, preventing the introduction of microorganisms that might cause infection.* (For a further discussion of catheter care, see Module 39, Catheterization.)

Closed Technique

This method can be carried out in three ways. Two are described below. A third closed technique—three-way irrigation—will be described later.

Y Connector and Fluid Reservoir. One method of closed technique is using the Y connector on the catheter and a fluid reservoir. A sterile Y connector is placed between the catheter and the drainage tubing. A large bottle or bag of sterile irrigating solution is hung on an IV standard with a sterile tubing attached. This is the same setup used for the solution for a three-way irrigation (Figure 48–3). The fluid tubing is attached to one arm of the Y connector.

1. Gather the necessary equipment.
   a. Container of sterile irrigating solution, as prescribed by the physician
   b. Sterile Y connector
   c. Sterile tubing to connect the solution bottle to the Y connector
   d. Clean gloves

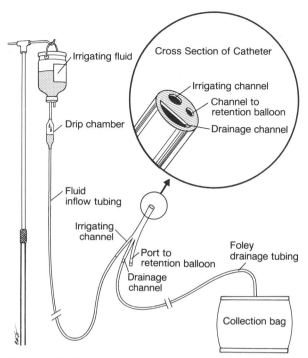

Figure 48–3 Three-way irrigation set-up.

2. Set up the irrigating system.
   a. Open sterile packages *so that the contents are available.*
   b. Connect the fluid tubing to the fluid container, maintaining sterility of the ends of the tubing.
   c. Expel air from the tubing and clamp it closed *to avoid instilling air into the bladder.*
   d. Put on clean gloves *to protect yourself from contact with urine* and wipe connection site with alcohol *to promote infection control.*
   e. Disconnect the catheter from the drainage tubing, being careful to maintain sterility of the end of the tubing and the end of the catheter.
   f. Insert the Y connector into the catheter and attach it to the drainage tubing.
   g. Attach the fluid tubing to the third arm of the Y connector.
3. Irrigate the catheter as follows.
   a. Clamp the drainage tubing.
   b. Unclamp the fluid tubing and allow the prescribed quantity of fluid to flow into the catheter. *Remember that you will be filling the bladder, so you have to watch carefully to avoid causing the patient discomfort or injury.* If the amount is not specified, use 50–100 ml fluid.

c. Clamp off the fluid tubing.

d. Unclamp the drainage tube and allow the fluid to flow out into the drainage bag.

e. Observe the returning fluid.

f. The fluid used for irrigation is not part of the patient's urinary output so you must remember to subtract the amount of solution used to do the irrigation from the total amount in the collection bag when you measure it.

Syringe-and-Needle Method. Another way to irrigate the catheter through a closed system is to use the syringe-and-needle method.

1. Gather the necessary equipment.
   a. 20- to 30-ml syringe with needle (19 gauge)
   b. Alcohol wipe
   c. Solution ordered
2. Draw up the solution into the syringe, using sterile technique (see Module 51, Giving Injections, for techniques for filling the syringe).
3. Use the alcohol wipe *to clean the entry port on the drainage tubing.* This is a soft, resealable rubber area. Most commercial catheters now have an entry port. If the drainage tubing does not have an entry port, use the portion of the Foley catheter distal to the entry to the balloon as an entry area, *so you do not inadvertently enter the balloon channel.*
4. Insert the needle into the entry port.
5. Clamp the tubing distal to the needle entry area, *so the fluid can flow only to the bladder.*
6. Inject the fluid into the catheter.
7. Remove the syringe and needle.
8. Release the catheter and allow the fluid to drain into the drainage bag.
9. Observe the fluid returning.
10. Repeat as necessary *to use the amount of fluid ordered or to clear the catheter.*
11. Note the amount of fluid used for the irrigation on the intake and output worksheet, according to the policy of your facility.

Open Technique

1. Gather the necessary equipment.
   a. Sterile irrigation set (asepto syringe, container for irrigating fluid, drainage receptacle, alcohol wipe)
   b. Solution (normal saline is commonly used, but acidifying or antibacterial solutions can also be ordered)
   c. Clean gloves
2. Open the set, maintaining sterile technique. You can touch the exterior of the fluid container, the exterior of the receptacle, and the bulb of the syringe, to set them up conveniently, *because these areas will not touch the sterile inside surface of the catheter or the sterile fluid.*
3. Pour the solution from the bulk container into the irrigating bottle *to maintain sterility of the original container as you work and to facilitate drawing up the fluid.*
4. *To reduce the possibility of contamination,* clean the junction of the catheter and drainage tubing with an alcohol swab before disconnecting them. Some sets contain a sterile cleansing wipe in a foil package for this purpose. If the set does not contain one, obtain separately.
5. Put on clean gloves and disconnect the catheter from the drainage tubing, and hold the catheter end over the drainage fluid receptacle, *so the fluid will drain into the receptacle.* Some receptacles have a notched end to hold the catheter firmly, *so it doesn't touch anything and become contaminated.*
6. Protect the end of the drainage tubing from contamination, *so it will be sterile when reconnected.* You can do this in many ways. For example, you can fold a sterile gauze square over the end of the drainage tubing and secure it with a rubber band. You can slip the end of the drainage tubing inside the foil package that contained the cleansing wipe (it is sterile inside) and secure it with a rubber band. Also, a sterile drainage tubing cap may be included in the set or may be available separately.
7. Instill the fluid.
   a. For a catheter irrigation:
      (1) Fill the asepto syringe with 30–60 ml solution.
      (2) Insert the tip of the asepto into the catheter and instill the fluid with gentle pressure.
      (3) Pinch the catheter closed and hold it closed while you withdraw the syringe, *so you do not put suction on the bladder and cause trauma.*
      (4) Allow the fluid to drain into the drainage receptacle.
      (5) Observe the drainage for color and sediment.

      (6) Repeat this procedure until the catheter is clear of sediment. Usually three times is sufficient.

      Do not aspirate the fluid into the asepto syringe, *because it can traumatize the bladder lining or even collapse the bladder.*

  b. For bladder irrigation:

      (1) Instill the ordered fluid into the bladder.

      (2) Clamp the tubing, *so the solution remains in the bladder for several minutes.*

      (3) Allow the fluid to drain out.

8. Reconnect the catheter to the drainage tubing.

Three-Way Irrigation

Insert a special three-way catheter when this type of irrigation is needed (see Figure 48–3). The catheter has a channel for fluid to be instilled, as well as the usual channels for drainage and for inflating the balloon in the bladder. This type of irrigation is most frequently done after surgical procedures on the bladder.

The patient having prostatic surgery often returns to the surgical unit with a three-way catheter in place. Rather than insert the catheter, it is your responsibility to perform irrigations as ordered by the physician or following the policy of the facility. Other names sometimes used for a three-way catheter are "through and through" and "CBI," continuous bladder irrigation.

1. You will need the following equipment:
  a. IV standard
  b. Solution
  c. Tubing

2. Hang a reservoir of the ordered sterile fluid, which looks much like an IV solution, from an IV pole.

3. Expel all air from the tubing before you attach it, *so air is not instilled into the bladder.*

4. Attach the tubing to the inflow channel of the catheter.

5. Attach the other channel of the catheter to the drainage tubing.

6. Regulate the irrigation as a continuous drip with a clamp on the tubing.

The physician may order a specific rate of flow in milliliters per hour or may simply order that a slow continuous drip be used. The nurse is responsible for monitoring and maintaining this flow. Larger quantities of fluid can be run through as needed *to keep the catheter open and the bladder free of debris.*

The most critical concern is that large quantities of fluid not be put into the bladder if the drainage tubing is clogged or inadvertently clamped. *This causes severe pain and could rupture the patient's bladder.* Closely watch the output of the catheter *to see that it corresponds to the amount of fluid being instilled plus any other intake.*

Again, remember to record the amounts of all irrigation solution used to subtract it from the total amount in the collection bag. A separate record of the amount of fluid instilled can be kept to make this easier for you.

IRRIGATING THE EAR

Before irrigating the ear, you must examine it with an otoscope *to check the tympanic membrane.* This may have been done by the physician, but if not, you should do it. If the tympanic membrane (eardrum) is not intact, do not irrigate the ear. *The fluid could enter the middle ear and cause an infection.*

An ear syringe is usually used to instill the fluid, although some facilities use a water pressure device, commercially known as a Water Pik (a machine that delivers a pulsating water stream), on low pressure. This is a clean procedure.

1. Gather the necessary equipment.
  a. Ear syringe or water pressure device
  b. Emesis basin
  c. Clean towels
  d. Clean gloves
  e. Solution, warmed to body temperature

2. Position the patient sitting or lying with the head tilted away from the side to be irrigated *so the ear is accessible.*

3. Place the basin under the patient's ear *to catch the solution.*

4. Place a towel across the patient's shoulder *to keep the patient dry.*

5. Put on clean gloves.

6. Fill the syringe with fluid.

7. Straighten the ear canal in the adult by gently pulling the pinna upward and back. The ear canal in the child *is much straighter than in the adult* and should be gently pulled downward and back.

8. Direct the tip of the syringe toward the top of the patient's ear canal (Figure 48–4), so that a circular current is set up with fluid flowing in along the top and out along the bottom. With

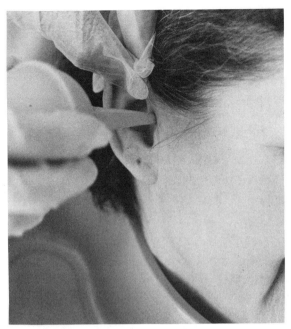

Figure 48–4 To irrigate the ear, the nurse straightens the ear canal by gently pulling the pinna upward and back, directing the flow from the bulb toward the upper part of the canal. (*Courtesy Ivan Ellis*)

this action, *cerumen or foreign material will be irrigated out.*

Be careful! Severe discomfort and dizziness can result from fluid directed onto the eardrum. *Cold fluid increases the chance of adverse effects.*

9. Irrigate until either the ear canal is clean or the ordered volume is used.
10. Dry the ear with a clean sponge or towel.
11. Remove your gloves and assist the patient to a comfortable position on the affected side *to drain out excess fluid.*

IRRIGATING THE EYE

This is a sterile procedure, *because eyes are easily damaged by infection.* Use a sterile syringe and sterile fluid. If both eyes are to be irrigated, use separate sets for each eye *to prevent cross-contamination.*

Small-Volume Irrigation

1. Gather the necessary equipment.
   a. Sterile syringe
   b. Sterile solution (normal saline is most common)
   c. Emesis basin
   d. Sterile cotton balls
   e. Sterile gloves
2. Place the patient in the supine position. Turn the patient's head to the side of the eye that is to be irrigated. (The patient can be seated with the head tilted back and supported.)
3. Place an emesis basin beside and below the eye.
4. Put on sterile gloves and hold the eye open with the thumb and forefinger of your nondominant hand. (Resting your hand on the patient's forehead may make this easier.)
5. Fill the syringe with 30–60 ml fluid.
6. Gently release the fluid onto the lower conjunctival sac at the inner canthus, allowing it to flow across the eye and then into the basin. *Do not touch the irrigator to the eye, because this may injure the eye.* Keep the tip close to the eye *so fluid pressure is not increased by the height of the fluid container.*
7. Continue the procedure until the eye is clean or until the fluid ordered has been used.
8. Dry the eyelid, wiping it from the inner canthus to the outer canthus, using a sterile cotton ball. Use each cotton ball only once, and discard. *This protects the opposite eye and moves any infected material away from either eye.*

Large-Volume Irrigation

For large-volume irrigation (1000 ml), use a sterile IV container of normal saline with IV tubing.

1. Adjust the IV standard to its lowest height *to keep pressure low.*
2. Hang the solution on the IV standard.
3. Fill the tubing with fluid *so it will flow evenly.* Eliminate the air from the tubing.
4. Position the patient with a drainage basin by the eye. If the fluid is to be given continuously, it is wise to have a large bath basin available in which *to empty the drainage basin partway through the irrigation. This prevents it from overflowing onto the patient.*
5. Open the control valve or clamp on the IV tubing and allow the fluid to flow slowly across the eye, directing fluid into the lower conjunctival sac at the inner canthus. A continuous flow is important *for thorough cleansing, but the pressure should never cause discomfort.* It may be necessary to hold the eye open *to allow the fluid to flow directly onto the eye itself rather than onto the eyelid.*

NASOGASTRIC TUBE IRRIGATION

Clean technique is used *because the acid environment of the stomach is resistant to bacteria* except when there has been surgery on the stomach, in which case sterile technique may be required.

1. Obtain the necessary equipment.
   a. Prepackaged irrigation set or conventional syringe with an adapter, an asepto syringe, or a catheter-tip syringe
   b. Solution (*normal saline is preferred because it reduces electrolyte depletion*)
   c. Emesis basin
   d. Clean gloves
2. Turn off suction and disconnect the nasogastric tube from the connecting tubing.
3. Fill the syringe with the fluid.
4. Gently instill approximately 30 ml fluid into the tubing. If the fluid will not enter the tubing, the outlet eyes may be against the mucosa. Untape the tube from the nose and move it in and out gently (not over 1 inch either way) unless the patient has had gastric surgery and moving the tube may disrupt the operative site. *This can release the end of the tube and allow you to proceed with the irrigation.* Be sure to retape the tube before you continue with the procedure, *so the tube does not come out.*
5. Aspirate the fluid back and discard it in the basin. If the fluid does not return after several attempts at aspiration, instill another 30 ml fluid. Do not continue to instill fluid after this if none is returning. *You may cause excessive distention.* Report the situation to the nurse in charge.

   In some facilities the fluid is not aspirated. After instillation the tubing is reconnected and the suction machine aspirates the fluid. The fluid must then be added to the intake record or to a separate record of the irrigating fluid. That amount is subtracted from the suction amount when output is figured. Follow the policy of your facility.
6. Repeat the procedure, instilling and aspirating fluid, *until the tubing is cleared of clotted material or thick mucus.*
7. Reconnect the tubing to the suction machine. If the suction does not appear to be functioning and you have cleared the nasogastric tube, the tubing to the machine itself may be clogged. Squeeze this tubing between your fingers *to*

loosen the material and allow the machine to clear the tubing (see Module 45, Nasogastric Intubation, for the care of a patient with a nasogastric tube in place).

VAGINAL IRRIGATION (DOUCHE)

This procedure is also called a *vaginal douche.* Clean technique is used, *because the vagina is not sterile.*

1. Gather the necessary equipment.
   a. Douche set with a special douche tip
   b. Solution (approximately 1000 ml) at body temperature
   c. IV standard (*although it is possible to hold the fluid container during the procedure, you will find it is inconvenient to do so*)
   d. Waterproof pad
   e. Bedpan
   f. Tissues
   g. Clean gloves
2. Have the patient void before beginning, *because the fluid on the vulva may cause a desire to void.*
3. Position the patient flat on her back in bed. *If the patient sits up, fluid will drain out too quickly and not contact all the tissue.*
4. Place a waterproof pad under the patient's hips *to protect the bed.*
5. Place a bedpan under the patient.
6. Drape the patient in the lithotomy position, with the perineal area exposed.
7. Put on gloves and wash the patient's perineal area if necessary.
8. Fill the fluid container.
9. Hang the container on the IV standard 18–24 inches above the vagina *to provide appropriate pressure.*
10. Run the fluid through the tubing *to clear the air from the tubing.*
11. Moisten the douche tip *to lubricate it.*
12. Run a small amount of fluid over the patient's labia *to check that the temperature of the solution is comfortable.*
13. With the tubing clamped, insert the tip 3–4 inches into the vagina, at an angle toward the base of the spine, *the plane at which the vagina lies.*
14. Unclamp the tubing and allow the fluid to flow.
15. Rotate the tip, *so the fluid contacts all vaginal tissue.*
16. Remove the tip.

17. Help the patient to sit on the bedpan *to allow any remaining fluid to drain out.*
18. Provide tissue *for drying the perineum.*

IRRIGATING WOUNDS

Always use sterile technique for wound irrigations, *because the body's defense created by intact skin is not present.*

1. Gather the necessary equipment. This will vary according to the wound, but commonly, you will need the following:
   a. Irrigating set (asepto syringe, solution container, receptacle for used solution). A special water pressure device may be used to irrigate seriously contaminated traumatic wounds, but this is usually done in the emergency room or in the operating room. A catheter may be attached to a syringe to facilitate irrigating a very deep wound.
   b. Sterile gloves (*if the wound is to be touched*)
   c. Materials for applying a new sterile dressing (including gauze squares)
   d. Solution (as ordered by the physician)
   e. Waterproof linen protector
2. Open the sterile set and pour the sterile fluid into the container.
3. Remove the soiled dressing, using gloves *to protect yourself.*
4. Position the patient *so the solution will flow from the upper end of the wound to the lower, and then into the receptacle.*
5. Position the receptacle.
6. Position the padding.
7. Fill the syringe with fluid.
8. Put on a sterile glove if it is necessary to touch the wound. The gloved hand is then used to touch the wound; the ungloved hand is used to manipulate the equipment.
9. Direct the fluid onto all parts of the wound, paying particular attention to areas with exudate or drainage.
10. Irrigate until no exudate is present, until solution returns clear, or until ordered volume has been used.
11. Use a sterile gauze square to dry the area.
12. Redress the wound, using sterile technique (see Module 37, Wound Care).

LONG-TERM CARE

Performing irrigations is a common procedure in the long-term care facility. Older people may have a decrease in lacrimal or tearing ability *so that small foreign bodies such as dust particles can enter the eye or other secretions can build up.* Eye irrigations with normal saline can remove the cause of any irritation and be very soothing.

The older adult *may produce an increased amount of cerumen (earwax), which can cause pain, hearing loss, or infection.* Patients who wear canal-fitting hearing aids tend to build up more wax than those who do not wear aids *because of the close contact of the aid with the auditory canal.* This wax must be removed *so that it does not interfere with the reception of sounds.*

Perhaps the most common irrigation you might perform in the long-term care facility is the bladder or catheter irrigation because many residents have an indwelling catheter in place and any blockage of the catheter *can place that person at risk for infection.* Knowledge and understanding of the irrigation procedure is essential for the nurse involved in long-term care.

Home Care

Irrigations have long been performed in the home by either the home care nurse or a family member. Removing foreign bodies in the eye and simple ear infections have required soothing irrigation. The family may have an older member residing in the home who either has a hearing deficit or wears a hearing aid. Inspection for wax buildup should take place regularly and ear irrigation performed, if appropriate, *to remove the wax.*

A common irrigation procedure done in the home is the vaginal douche. Although this procedure is unnecessary for the healthy woman with normal flora of the vaginal tract, some commercial businesses have promoted the douche as an important part of feminine hygiene. The antiseptic powders used in some commercial douche products *are irritating to some individuals* and should be used with caution.

Performance Checklist

General Procedure for Irrigation	Unsat	Needs More Practice	Sat	Comments
Assessment				
1. Verify: a. Type of irrigation ordered.				
b. Correct solution: amount, type, temperature, concentration.				
Planning				
2. Decide whether irrigation is clean or sterile.				
3. Wash your hands.				
4. Identify and gather the equipment needed for the specific irrigation. a. Solution				
b. Irrigating device				
c. Receptacle for used fluid				
d. Protective padding				
e. Clean gloves				
Implementation				
5. Identify the patient.				
6. Explain procedure to patient.				
7. Provide privacy.				
8. Position the patient.				
9. Place protective padding where needed.				
10. Put on clean gloves and carry out irrigation according to specific procedure below.				
11. Make sure patient is dry and comfortable.				
12. Dispose of used equipment correctly.				
13. Wash your hands.				
Evaluation				
14. Evaluate using the following criteria: a. Area of irrigation was thoroughly cleaned.				

General Procedure for Irrigation (Continued)	Unsat	Needs More Practice	Sat	Comments
b. Medication contacted desired area.				
c. Patient resting comfortably.				
Documentation				
15. Document the following: a. Type of irrigation.				
b. Type, concentration, and amount of fluid used.				
c. Appearance and odor of any secretions.				
d. Results of procedure.				
e. Patient's response.				

Bladder and Catheter Irrigation: Closed Technique Y Connector and Fluid Reservoir

Assessment				
1. Follow Checklist step 1 of the General Procedure for Irrigation (verify type of irrigation and solution amount, type, concentration, and temperature).				
Planning				
2. Use sterile technique.				
3. Wash your hands.				
4. Gather necessary equipment. a. Container of sterile irrigating solution				
b. Tubing to connect the solution bottle to catheter				
Implementation				
5. Follow Checklist steps 5–9 of the General Procedure (identify patient, explain procedure, provide privacy, position patient, place protective padding).				
6. Set up the irrigating system. a. Open sterile packages.				
b. Connect fluid tubing to fluid container and hang on IV pole.				
c. Expel air from tubing and clamp it closed.				

Bladder and Catheter Irrigation: Closed Technique Y Connector and Fluid Reservoir
(Continued)

	Unsat	Needs More Practice	Sat	Comments
d. Put on clean gloves and wipe the connector site with alcohol.				
e. Disconnect catheter.				
f. Insert Y connector into catheter and attach to drainage tubing.				
g. Attach fluid tubing to third arm of Y connector.				
7. Irrigate catheter. a. Clamp drainage tubing.				
b. Unclamp fluid tubing and allow appropriate volume to flow into catheter.				
c. Clamp off fluid tubing.				
d. Unclamp drainage tube and allow fluid to flow out of bladder.				
e. Observe returning fluid.				
f. Keep a record of the amount instilled so that you can deduct it from the total in the collection bag later.				

Evaluation

	Unsat	Needs More Practice	Sat	Comments
8. Follow Checklist step 14 of the General Procedure (check for fatigue and identify adequacy of cleansing).				

Documentation

	Unsat	Needs More Practice	Sat	Comments
9. Follow Checklist step 15 of the General Procedure (include type of irrigation, concentration, amount, and type of fluid used, appearance and odor of any secretions, results of procedure, and patient's response).				

Bladder and Catheter Irrigation: Syringe-and-Needle Method

Assessment

	Unsat	Needs More Practice	Sat	Comments
1. Follow Checklist step 1 of the General Procedure for Irrigation (verify type of irrigation and solution amount, type, concentration, and temperature).				

Bladder and Catheter Irrigation: Syringe-and-Needle Method (Continued)	Unsat	Needs More Practice	Sat	Comments
Planning				
2. Use sterile technique.				
3. Wash your hands.				
4. Gather necessary equipment. a. 20- to 30-ml syringe				
b. Alcohol wipe				
c. Solution ordered				
Implementation				
5. Follow Checklist steps 5–9 of the General Procedure (identify patient, explain procedure, provide privacy, position patient, place protective padding).				
6. Draw up solution into syringe.				
7. Clean entry port or distal portion of catheter with alcohol wipe.				
8. Insert needle into entry port or catheter wall.				
9. Clamp drainage tubing distal to needle.				
10. Inject fluid.				
11. Remove needle.				
12. Release catheter.				
13. Observe fluid return.				
14. Repeat as necessary.				
15. Follow Checklist steps 11–13 of the General Procedure (make patient dry and comfortable, dispose of equipment, wash your hands).				
Evaluation				
16. Follow Checklist step 14 of the General Procedure (check for fatigue and identify adequacy of cleansing).				
Documentation				
17. Follow Checklist step 15 of the General Procedure (include type of irrigation and type, concentration, and amount of fluid used).				

Bladder and Catheter Irrigation: Open Technique	Unsat	Needs More Practice	Sat	Comments
Assessment				
1. Follow Checklist step 1 of the General Procedure for Irrigation (verify type of irrigation and solution amount, type, concentration, and temperature).				
Planning				
2. Use sterile technique.				
3. Wash your hands.				
4. Gather necessary equipment. a. Sterile irrigation set				
b. Solution				
c. Clean gloves				
Implementation				
5. Follow Checklist steps 5–9 of the General Procedure (identify patient, explain procedure, provide privacy, position patient, place protective padding).				
6. Open set.				
7. Pour solution into irrigating bottle.				
8. Clean juncture of catheter and drainage tubing.				
9. Put on gloves and separate tubing, not allowing catheter to touch anything.				
10. Cover end of drainage tubing to preserve sterility.				
11. Instill fluid slowly. a. For a catheter irrigation:				
(1) Fill syringe with 30–60 ml solution.				
(2) Insert syringe tip into catheter and exert gentle pressure to instill fluid.				
(3) Pinch catheter closed.				
(4) Allow fluid to drain.				
(5) Observe drainage for sediment.				
(6) Repeat until fluid is clear.				
b. For a bladder irrigation:				

Bladder and Catheter Irrigation: Open Technique *(Continued)*

	Unsat	Needs More Practice	Sat	Comments
(1) Instill ordered fluid.				
(2) Clamp tubing, holding solution in bladder for several minutes.				
(3) Allow fluid to drain.				
12. Reconnect catheter to drainage tubing.				
13. Follow Checklist steps 11–13 of the General Procedure (make patient dry and comfortable, dispose of equipment, wash your hands).				

Evaluation

14. Follow Checklist step 14 of the General Procedure (check for fatigue and identify adequacy of cleansing).				

Documentation

15. Follow Checklist step 15 of the General Procedure (include type of irrigation, type, concentration, amount of fluid used).				

Bladder and Catheter Irrigation: Three-Way Irrigation (Continuous Drip and Cleaning)

Assessment

1. Follow Checklist step 1 of the General Procedure for Irrigation (verify type of irrigation and solution amount, type, concentration, and temperature).				

Planning

2. Use sterile technique.				
3. Wash your hands.				
4. Gather necessary equipment. a. IV standard				
b. Solution				
c. Tubing				

Implementation

5. Follow Checklist steps 5–9 of the General Procedure (identify patient, explain procedure, provide privacy, position patient, place protective padding).				

Bladder and Catheter Irrigation: Three-Way Irrigation (Continuous Drip and Cleaning) *(Continued)*	Unsat	Needs More Practice	Sat	Comments
6. Set up pole, fluid container, and tubing.				
7. Clear air from tubing by filling with fluid.				
8. Attach tubing to inflow tube on three-way catheter.				
9. Make sure outflow tube is open.				
10. Regulate flow: a. For continuous drip, regulate drip rate.				
b. For cleaning:				
(1) Open inflow tubing to continuous stream.				
(2) Continue flow until outflow is free of clots and sediment.				
(3) Reclamp tubing.				
11. Follow Checklist steps 11–13 of the General Procedure (make patient dry and comfortable, dispose of equipment, wash your hands).				
Evaluation				
12. Follow Checklist step 14 of the General Procedure (check for fatigue and identify adequacy of cleansing).				
Documentation				
13. Follow Checklist step 15 of the General Procedure (include type of irrigation and type, concentration, and amount of fluid used).				
Irrigating the Ear				
Assessment				
1. Follow Checklist step 1 of the General Procedure for Irrigation (verify type of irrigation and solution amount, type, concentration, and temperature).				
2. Check to see that ear has been examined.				
Planning				
3. Use clean technique.				

© 1992 by J.B. Lippincott Company

Irrigating the Ear (Continued)	Unsat	Needs More Practice	Sat	Comments
4. Wash your hands.				
5. Gather necessary equipment. a. Ear syringe or water pressure device				
b. Emesis basin				
c. Clean towels				
d. Solution				
e. Clean gloves				

Implementation

6. Follow Checklist steps 5–9 of the General Procedure (identify patient, explain procedure, provide privacy, position patient, place protective padding).				
7. Tilt patient's head to side.				
8. Place receptacle under ear.				
9. Place towel across shoulder.				
10. Fill syringe and straighten the ear canal.				
11. Direct tip of syringe against top of ear canal.				
12. Continue irrigation until ear is clean.				
13. Dry ear.				
14. Position the patient comfortably for drainage.				

Evaluation

15. Follow Checklist step 14 of the General Procedure (check for fatigue and identify adequacy of cleansing).				

Documentation

16. Follow Checklist step 15 of the General Procedure (include type of irrigation and type, concentration, and amount of fluid used).				

Small-Volume Eye Irrigation

Assessment

1. Follow Checklist step 1 of the General Procedure for Irrigation (verify type of irrigation and solution amount, type, concentration, and temperature).				

Small-Volume Eye Irrigation *(Continued)*	Unsat	Needs More Practice	Sat	Comments
Planning				
2. Use sterile technique. Do not touch irrigator to eye.				
3. Wash your hands.				
4. Gather necessary equipment. a. Sterile syringe				
b. Sterile solution				
c. Emesis basin				
d. Sterile cotton balls				
e. Sterile gloves				
Implementation				
5. Follow Checklist steps 5–9 of the General Procedure (identify patient, explain procedure, provide privacy, position patient, place protective padding).				
6. Position patient in supine position, with head turned toward eye to be irrigated.				
7. Place emesis basin.				
8. Put on gloves and hold eye open.				
9. Fill syringe with fluid.				
10. Release fluid with gentle pressure, from inner to outer canthus.				
11. Continue irrigation until eye is clear or all solution is used.				
12. Dry eye from inner to outer aspect.				
Note: If both eyes are to be irrigated, treat each separately.				
13. Follow Checklist steps 11–13 of the General Procedure (make patient dry and comfortable, dispose of equipment, wash your hands).				
Evaluation				
14. Follow Checklist step 14 of the General Procedure (check for fatigue and identify adequacy of cleansing).				

Small-Volume Eye Irrigation (Continued)	Unsat	Needs More Practice	Sat	Comments
Documentation				
15. Follow Checklist step 15 of the General Procedure (include type of irrigation and type, concentration, and amount of fluid used).				
Large-volume Eye Irrigation				
Assessment				
1. Follow Checklist step 1 of the General Procedure for Irrigation (verify type of irrigation and solution amount, type, concentration, and temperature).				
Planning				
2. Use sterile technique. Do not touch end of tubing to eye.				
3. Wash your hands.				
4. Gather necessary equipment. a. 1000 ml sterile IV solution				
b. IV tubing				
c. Emesis basin				
d. Bath basin				
e. Sterile cotton balls				
Implementation				
5. Follow Checklist steps 5–9 of the General Procedure (identify patient, explain procedure, provide privacy, position patient, place protective padding).				
6. Adjust IV standard to its lowest height.				
7. Hang solution on IV standard.				
8. Fill tubing with fluid.				
9. Position patient in supine position, with head turned toward eye to be irrigated.				
10. Position emesis basin by eye, with bath basin close.				
11. Open the control valve and allow fluid to flow across eye.				

Large-volume Eye Irrigation (Continued)	Unsat	Needs More Practice	Sat	Comments
12. Continue until eye is clear or all solution has been used.				
13. Dry eye from inner to outer aspect.				
Note: If both eyes are to be irrigated, treat each separately.				
14. Follow Checklist steps 11–13 of the General Procedure (make patient dry and comfortable, dispose of equipment, wash your hands).				
Evaluation				
15. Follow Checklist step 14 of the General Procedure (check for fatigue and identify adequacy of cleansing).				
Documentation				
16. Follow Checklist step 15 of the General Procedure (include type of irrigation and type, concentration, and amount of fluid used).				
Nasogastric Tube Irrigation				
Assessment				
1. Follow Checklist step 1 of the General Procedure for Irrigation (verify type of irrigation and solution amount, type, concentration, and temperature).				
Planning				
2. Use clean technique. Use sterile technique if patient has had stomach surgery.				
3. Wash your hands.				
4. Obtain necessary equipment. a. Irrigation set or syringe				
b. Solution				
c. Emesis basin				
Implementation				
5. Follow Checklist steps 5–9 of the General Procedure (identify patient, explain procedure, provide privacy, position patient, place protective padding).				

Nasogastric Tube Irrigation (Continued)	Unsat	Needs More Practice	Sat	Comments
6. Disconnect nasogastric tube from suction machine.				
7. Fill syringe.				
8. Gently instill approximately 30 ml.				
9. Aspirate fluid back and discard or reconnect to suction machine.				
10. Repeat as necessary.				
11. Reconnect to suction.				
12. Follow Checklist steps 11–13 of the General Procedure (make patient dry and comfortable, dispose of equipment, wash your hands).				

Evaluation

13. Follow Checklist step 14 of the General Procedure (check for fatigue and identify adequacy of cleansing).				

Documentation

14. Follow Checklist step 15 of the General Procedure (include type of irrigation and type, concentration, and amount of fluid used).				

Vaginal Irrigation (Douche)

Assessment

1. Follow Checklist step 1 of the General Procedure for Irrigation (verify type of irrigation and solution amount, type, concentration, and temperature).				

Planning

2. Use clean technique.				
3. Wash your hands.				
4. Gather necessary equipment. a. Douche set with douche tip				
b. Solution (1000 ml at body temperature)				
c. IV standard				
d. Waterproof pad				
e. Bedpan				

Vaginal Irrigation (Douche) *(Continued)*	Unsat	Needs More Practice	Sat	Comments
f. Tissues				
g. Clean gloves				
Implementation				
5. Follow Checklist steps 5–7 of the General Procedure (identify patient, explain procedure, provide privacy).				
6. Have patient void.				
7. Position patient flat on back.				
8. Place waterproof pad.				
9. Place bedpan under patient.				
10. Drape in dorsal recumbent position.				
11. Put on clean gloves and wash perineal area if needed.				
12. Fill fluid container.				
13. Hang on IV pole 18–24 inches above vagina.				
14. Fill tubing with fluid, clearing air.				
15. Moisten tip to lubricate.				
16. Insert tip 3–4 inches, angled toward base of spine.				
17. Unclamp tubing and allow fluid to flow.				
18. Rotate tip.				
19. Remove tip.				
20. Help patient to sit on bedpan.				
21. Provide tissue for drying perineum.				
22. Follow Checklist steps 11–13 of the General Procedure (make patient dry and comfortable, dispose of equipment, wash your hands).				
Evaluation				
23. Follow Checklist step 14 of the General Procedure (check for fatigue and identify adequacy of cleansing).				

Vaginal Irrigation (Douche) *(Continued)*	Unsat	Needs More Practice	Sat	Comments
Documentation				
24. Follow Checklist step 15 of the General Procedure (include type of irrigation and type, concentration, and amount of fluid used).				
Irrigating Wounds				
Assessment				
1. Follow Checklist step 1 of the General Procedure for Irrigation (verify type of irrigation and solution amount, type, concentration, and temperature).				
Planning				
2. Use sterile technique.				
3. Wash your hands.				
4. Gather necessary equipment. a. Irrigating set				
b. Sterile gloves				
c. Dressing materials				
d. Solution				
e. Padding				
Implementation				
5. Follow Checklist steps 5–9 of the General Procedure (identify patient, explain procedure, provide privacy, position patient, place protective padding).				
6. Open sterile set and pour sterile fluid.				
7. Remove sterile dressing, using gloves if necessary.				
8. Position patient.				
9. Position receptacle.				
10. Place padding.				
11. Fill syringe.				
12. Put on sterile gloves if wound must be touched.				
13. Direct fluid onto all parts of wound.				

Irrigating Wounds (Continued)	Unsat	Needs More Practice	Sat	Comments
14. Continue irrigation until clean or ordered volume is used.				
15. Dry area.				
16. Redress wound using sterile technique.				
17. Follow Checklist steps 11–13 of the General Procedure (make patient dry and comfortable, dispose of equipment, wash your hands).				
Evaluation				
18. Follow Checklist step 14 of the General Procedure (check for fatigue and identify adequacy of cleansing).				
Documentation				
19. Follow Checklist step 15 of the General Procedure (include type of irrigation and type, concentration, and amount of fluid used).				

Quiz

Short-Answer Questions

1. List two major purposes of irrigation.

   a. _____

   b. _____

2. Mrs. Jones has had bladder surgery. An irrigation with an antibacterial medication, nitrofurantoin, has been ordered. This irrigation is probably for which of the above purposes? _____

3. Name a type of irrigation in which sterile technique is essential.

   _____

4. Name a type of irrigation in which clean technique is safe.

   _____

5. List three factors in an irrigation that can cause irritation or damage tissue.

   a. _____

   b. _____

   c. _____

6. After prostate surgery, Mr. Jefferson has a continuous three-way irrigation setup. What is the most critical safety concern with this irrigation?

   _____

7. Under what circumstances should an ear not be irrigated? _____

   _____

8. Why is it not appropriate to administer a vaginal douche while the patient sits on a toilet? _____

   _____

9. Why must each eye be treated as a separate irrigation?

   _____

   _____

10. When might a water pressure device be used to irrigate wounds? _____

11. List three types of irrigations commonly performed in the long-term care facility for the older adult resident and the main reason each is done. _____

   _____

   _____

12. Why should healthy females be cautioned in the use of vaginal douches at home? _____

   _____

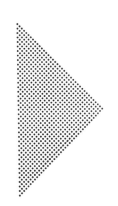

Unit 11

PROVIDING MEDICATION AND INTRAVENOUS THERAPY

MODULE 49
Administering Oral Medications

MODULE 50
Administering Medications by Alternative Routes

MODULE 51
Giving Injections

MODULE 52
Administering Medications to Infants and Children

MODULE 53
Preparing and Maintaining Intravenous Infusions

MODULE 54
Administering Intravenous Medications

MODULE 55
Caring for Central Intravenous Catheters

MODULE 56
Starting Intravenous Infusions

MODULE 57
Administering Blood and Blood Products

MODULE 58
Parenteral Nutrition

MODULE 59
Giving Epidural Medications

317

Module 49
Administering Oral Medications

Module Contents

Rationale for the Use of This Skill
Nursing Diagnoses
Systems of Administration
 Medication Cards
 Central Medication Records
 Unit-Dose Systems
Safety and Accuracy
 The Three Checks
 The Five Rights
Measuring Doses
Medication Orders

Procedure for Administering Oral Medications
 Assessment
 Planning
 Implementation
 Evaluation
 Documentation
Narcotics
Medication Errors
Giving Medications Through a Nasogastric Tube
Long-Term Care
Home Care

Prerequisites

1. *Successful completion of the following modules:*[1]

VOLUME 1

Module 1 An Approach to Nursing Skills
Module 2 Basic Infection Control
Module 3 Safety
Module 5 General Assessment Overview
Module 6 Documentation

2. *Before giving medications, you must have a satisfactory level of proficiency in the mathematics of dosages and solutions. A math quiz is included on the next pages. If you cannot answer at least 16 of the 20 problems correctly (or the number designated by your instructor), plan to complete one of the many programmed instruction units available on the mathematics of dosages and solutions. Consult your instructor for guidance.*

---

[1] For techniques related to giving medications to children, see Module 52, Administering Medications to Infants and Children. For information related to administering medications by ophthalmic, otic, nasal, skin/mucous membranes, vaginal, rectal, and inhalation routes, see Module 50, Administering Medications by Alternative Routes. For information related to parenteral medications, see Module 51, Giving Injections, and Module 54, Administering Intravenous Medications.

319

Self-Test: Mathematics of Dosages and Solutions

Directions: Read each problem carefully. Show your work beneath the questions and place your answers in the right-hand column.

1. Pronestyl 500 mg is ordered qid for Mr. Jones. Available are 250-mg tablets of Pronestyl. How many tablets will he receive each day? _____

2. The order reads: "Codeine phosphate gr 1/2." Tablets marked "codeine phosphate gr 1/4" are available. How many tablets will you need for one dose? _____

3. The order for the dosage of a drug reads: ".25 g." The only tablets available are in milligrams. How many milligrams is .25 g? _____

4. The order reads: "Milk of magnesia 1 oz." How many milliliters will you give? _____

5. You are to prepare streptomycin sulfate for injection. On hand is a vial containing 1.0 g dry drug. The label reads: "Add 9.2 ml diluent to yield 10.0 ml solution." Each milliliter will contain how many milligrams of the drug? _____

6. You are to administer insulin. The vial reads: "U-100." What does this mean? _____

7. The order reads: "meperidine 75 mg IM." The meperidine available is 100 mg/ml. How many milliliters will you give? _____

8. The order for IV fluid reads: "1000 ml 5% glucose in water to run 10 h." Determine the number of drops per minute the IV should run if the administration set delivers 15 gtt/ml. _____

9. If the centigrade temperature is 40°, what is the Fahrenheit reading? _____

10. If the adult dose of a medication is 500 mg, is the pediatric dose more likely to be 200 mg or 800 mg? _____

11. Name three factors that are commonly used to calculate pediatric dosage.

a. _____
b. _____
c. _____

12. A patient is ordered to have 1000 ml of 5% dextrose in normal saline to run over 8 h. A volume-controlled pump is to be used to deliver the IV fluid. How many milliliters per hour must you set the pump for? _____

13. How much morphine sulfate should a 6-year-old weighing 45 lb receive if the adult dosage is 10 mg? _____

14. The usual dosage of a certain drug for a child is 20 mg/kg. The child weighs 68 lb. What would the dosage be for this child? _____

15. The order reads: "Pentobarbital gr 3/4 at hs." The only drug available is marked in milligrams. How many milligrams do you need for the correct dosage? _____

16. The order reads: "Digoxin 0.25 mg daily." The drug is available in liquid form for this patient. The label reads: "Digoxin 0.05 mg/ml." How many milliliters will you give? _____

17. The order reads: "Aluminum hydroxide 1 dram as needed for indigestion." How many milliliters will you give? How many teaspoons is this? _____

18. The order reads: "Micro K .25 mg." The bottle is labeled "Micro K 250 mcg/tablet." How many tablets will you give? _____

19. The order reads: "Metronidazole 500 mg IV q6h." You have a small IV infusion bag with a label that reads: "Metronidazole 500 mg/100 ml, give over 1 h." The equipment available delivers 15 gtts/ml. How many drops per minute should the infusion run?

_____

20. The order reads: "Solu-cortef 25 mg IV." The label reads: "Solu-cortef 100 mg/2 ml." How many milliliters will you give?

_____

K e y

1. 8 tablets
2. 2 tablets
3. 250 mg
4. 30 ml
5. 100 mg
6. 100 units/ml
7. .75 ml
8. 25 gtts/min
9. 104°F
10. 200 mg
11. **a.** age
    b. weight
    c. body surface area

12. 125 ml/h
13. 3 mg
14. 618 mg
15. 45 mg
16. 5 ml
17. 4 ml; 1 tsp
18. 1 tablet
19. 25 gtts/min
20. 0.5 ml

Overall Objective

To prepare and administer oral medications to patients.

Specific Learning Objectives

	Know Facts and Principles	Apply Facts and Principles	Demonstrate Ability	Evaluate Performance
1. *Abbreviations*	Know meanings of abbreviations listed in Table 49–1.	Correctly interpret medication orders that include abbreviations.	Correctly use and interpret abbreviations used in preparation and administration of medications.	Evaluate own performance with instructor.
2. *Equivalencies*	Know equivalencies listed in Table 49–2.	Given problems, work out equivalencies in apothecary, metric, and household systems.	In the clinical setting (under supervision), correctly work out problems involving equivalencies.	Evaluate own performance with instructor.
3. *Administration methods*	State two broad methods of administering medication. Discuss at least two different methods of administering medications using individual medication supplies.	Outline medication administration procedure used in assigned facility.	Correctly carry out medication administration procedure used in assigned facility with supervision.	Evaluate own performance with instructor using Performance Checklist and facility procedure.
4. *Safety and accuracy*	State three checks and five rights.		Use three checks and five rights consistently.	Evaluate own performance with instructor.
5. *Giving oral medications*	Know procedure for preparation and administration of oral medication.	Adapt steps of procedures to those used in assigned facility.	Prepare and administer oral medication according to procedures in assigned facility.	Evaluate own performance with instructor.
6. *Documentation*	Know information to be recorded regarding medications administered.	Identify documentation method used in assigned facility.	Correctly document medications administered according to method used in assigned facility.	Evaluate own performance with instructor.

Learning Activities

1. Review the Specific Learning Objectives.
2. Read the section on administering medications in Ellis and Nowlis, *Nursing: A Human Needs Approach,* or comparable material in another textbook.
3. Look up the module vocabulary terms in the Glossary.
4. Read through the module and mentally practice the procedure.
5. Study the abbreviations and equivalencies in Tables 49–1 and 49–2.
6. In the practice setting:
   a. Identify
      (1) Paper soufflé cup
      (2) Calibrated medicine glass (usually made of glass or plastic but can be made of heavy waxed paper)
      (3) Mortar and pestle
      (4) Pill crusher, if available
      (5) Medicine tray or cart
   b. Review the medication administration method used in your facility.
   c. Go through the procedure step by step, referring to the Performance Checklist as necessary. Use the appropriate method for your facility.
   d. When you can remember the procedure, ask your instructor to check your performance.
7. In the clinical setting:
   a. Consult with your clinical instructor for an opportunity to give medications with supervision.

Vocabulary

capsule   suspension
dose   syrup
five rights   tablet
meniscus   three checks
route   unit dose
stock drugs

Administering Oral Medications

Rationale for the Use of This Skill

One of the nurse's most routine and yet most critical responsibilities is the preparation and administration of medications. Most medications are administered orally. The basic procedures to administer oral medications can be applied to the administration of medications by other routes as well.

The responsibility extends beyond preparation and administration. The nurse must know how medicines act, the usual dosage, the desired effects, and potential side effects, so that he or she can evaluate the effectiveness of the medication and recognize adverse effects when they occur. You will acquire this knowledge gradually as you study pharmacology and care for patients with varying problems.[2]

SYSTEMS OF ADMINISTRATION

In any health care facility, medications are administered according to a procedure defined by that facility. The procedure is usually based on one of two supply systems. *Stock supply* refers to drugs that are

[2] You will note that rationale for action is emphasized throughout the module by the use of italics.

▶ *Nursing Diagnoses*

> The major nursing diagnosis to keep in mind when giving medications is High Risk for Injury. Patients can be injured by medications given in the wrong dosage, at the wrong time, or by an incorrect route. They can also be injured by the omission of essential medications or the administration of an incorrect medication. Although this nursing diagnosis will not appear on the care plan, it applies to every situation in which a patient is being given medications.
>
> Another nursing diagnosis frequently appropriate when administering medications is Knowledge Deficit. In this case the knowledge deficit would be related to some aspect of the medication regimen; for example, the need to be aware of drug interactions when taking antacids.

Table 49–1 Common Abbreviations

PO	by mouth
ac	before meals
pc	after meals
qd	every day
qod	every other day
bid	twice a day
tid	three times a day
qid	four times a day
stat	immediately
$\bar{c}$	with
$\bar{s}$	without
$\overline{ss}$	one half
hs	at bedtime
prn	as needed
qh	every hour
q2h	every 2 hours

Also see Table 49–2, Equivalencies.

kept on the unit in fairly large containers and from which the medication orders for all patients on the unit are taken. *Individual patient supplies* are currently more common. These consist of enough medication for a single occasion, for one shift, for an entire day, or for an undefined period. Both supply systems have a method of recording and keeping track of the medications ordered and those that have or have not been given.

Medication Cards

Perhaps the oldest procedural method is that of using a card on which is recorded the patient's name and room number, the medication, dosage, and route. The nurse administering the medications checks the card against a permanent record of all medications ordered, such as a Kardex or a medication notebook. Then, using the cards as a guide, the nurse prepares and administers the medications. Documentation is done on the patient's chart. *Because it is so easy to misplace or lose medication cards*, this system is less commonly used than it once was.

Central Medication Records

In some health care facilities a large notebook or a Kardex containing a listing of the medications for each patient is used, both as a permanent record and

Table 49–2 Equivalencies

1. Metric doses and apothecaries' equivalents

Liquid

Metric	Approximate apothecaries' equivalents
1000 ml	1 quart
500 ml	1 pint
250 ml	8 fluidounces
30 ml	1 fluidounce
15 ml	4 fluidrams
5 ml	1 fluidram
1 ml	15 minims
0.06 ml	1 minim

Solid

130 g	1 ounce
15 g	4 drams
4 g	60 grains (1 dram)
1 g (1000 mg)	15 grains
0.5 g (500 mg)	$7\frac{1}{2}$ grains
60 mg	1 grain
30 mg	$\frac{1}{2}$ grain
15 mg	$\frac{1}{4}$ grain
10 mg	$\frac{1}{6}$ grain
8 mg	$\frac{1}{8}$ grain
1 mg (1000 mcg)	$\frac{1}{60}$ grain
0.6 mg (600 mcg)	$\frac{1}{100}$ grain
0.4 mg (400 mcg)	$\frac{1}{150}$ grain
0.3 mg (300 mcg)	$\frac{1}{200}$ grain
0.2 mg (200 mcg)	$\frac{1}{300}$ grain
0.1 mg (100 mcg)	$\frac{1}{600}$ grain

2. Approximate household measures

1 teaspoonful	1 fl dr	4–5 ml
1 tablespoonful	$\frac{1}{2}$ fl oz	15 or 16 ml
1 jigger	$1\frac{1}{2}$ fl oz	45 ml
1 cup	8 fl oz	240 ml

3. Prescription abbreviations

gr	grain or grains
gtt[1]	drops
ℨ	dram
℥	ounce
$\overline{aa}$	equal parts
$\overline{ss}$	one half
cc[2]	cubic centimeter
g	gram
mg	milligram
mcg	microgram
ml	milliliter
mEq	millequivalent
min	minim

[1] Gutta(e)
[2] Although technically not exactly equivalent, ml and cc are often used interchangeably.

as a guide as the medications are prepared and administered. The notebook or Kardex is often used for documenting the administration as well. In such cases the physician's order sheet is used as a safety check.

Unit-Dose Systems

Recently, pharmacy personnel have begun to play a larger role in the administration of medications to patients, which has resulted in the formulation of the *unit-dose system.* This system is widely used, especially in large health care facilities. Although it can vary substantially in procedure from one facility to another, basically the unit-dose system consists of the provision by pharmacy personnel of prepackaged and prelabeled *individual doses* of medications for pa-

tients. Medications are administered by nursing personnel on the nursing unit or by nursing or pharmacy personnel from the pharmacy. Studies have shown that the unit-dose system affords greater accuracy and convenience (especially in terms of time saved).

SAFETY AND ACCURACY

The Three Checks

Whichever system is used, certain basic considerations always apply. One of these considerations is the *three checks.* The name and dosage of the medication are checked (from the label) against that ordered (1) as the medication is taken off the shelf or out of the drawer, (2) before it is opened, and (3) before it is replaced on the shelf or in the drawer. Under the unit-dose system, the nurse checks first as he or she finds the dose in the patient's drawer. The second check is done when the dose is in hand and can be compared with the record. The nurse performs the final check before leaving the medication area to go to the patient's room. When several medications are to be given, you can do the first two checks on each medication; then, when all medications are ready, you can do the third check by going through the entire list again and comparing it with each dosage package. Leave the medications in their individually labeled packages until you are ready to give them to the patient. *When discussing a medication with a patient, you are then able to point out the labeled name of the drug as the patient observes its appearance. If the patient is not in the room or is unable to take the medication for some reason, you can return the medication, which is still in a labeled package, to the medication drawer for later administration because there is no chance of error in identification.* This is one of the extra safeguards that the unit-dose method provides.

The Five Rights

Another consideration basic to the administration of medication is the *five rights*. These rights serve as a guide for remembering (1) the right drug, (2) in the right dose, (3) by the right route, (4) to the right patient, and (5) at the right time. This is not *all* the nurse has to know, but fewer medication errors would be made if the five rights were consistently considered.

The right drug, the right dose, the right route, and the right time are ensured by following the three checks. To ensure you have the right patient, carefully identify the patient. Some type of identification card that lists the patient's name and other identifying information must be taken to the bedside *for accurate patient identification*. In systems using medication cards, the card itself is used for identifying the patient. In systems using a central medication record, you can take this record into the patient's room for identification. If you do not take the original medication record to the room, you must prepare a separate identification card. Compare this card with the medication administration record *to ensure that it correctly identifies the patient*. Once in the patient's room, you can compare the identification card with the patient's wrist identification bracelet, or ask the patient to state or spell his or her name while you check the identification record. With confused or unconscious patients, the use of the wristband is essential.

The patient should not be left alone until all medications have been swallowed. It is not appropriate to leave medications at the bedside for patients to take on their own unless so ordered by the physician or unless it is a policy for certain medications on the particular unit. Among the medications commonly left at the bedside are antacids and eye medications. Medications that patients have been taking regularly at home may also be their responsibility.

The nurse who prepares a given medication should administer it. Stated another way, you should administer only those drugs that you prepare. *Only the person who prepared the drug knows what it is and what strength or dosage it is, unless it is still in the unit-dose packaging.*

MEASURING DOSES

Measuring liquid medications is a special procedure. *To ensure accuracy,* you must read the medicine glass or cup at eye level, with the thumbnail placed at the bottom of the meniscus at the correct level on the medicine container.

MEDICATION ORDERS

Medications that are given on a regular basis until the order is cancelled are called *routine orders*. They may be given once a day (qd), several times a day (bid, tid, qid), every other day (qod), or on certain days of the week only (Tuesday, Thursday, and Saturday, for example). Medications that are given when needed or requested only (a laxative for constipation, a narcotic for pain) are ordered on a *prn* (as needed) basis. *One-time only* medications are those ordered to be given on one occasion only at a specified time. Medications given prior to surgery or a diagnostic test are examples of one-time only orders. Some physicians have developed a set of orders that they use for all of their hospitalized patients, adding individualized orders as necessary. These are termed *standing orders*. These various types of orders are transcribed onto different parts of the medication record in some facilities (see Figures 49–5 and 49–6).

PROCEDURE FOR ADMINISTERING ORAL MEDICATIONS

The general approach used to administer medications to a single patient can be modified as needed for a specific patient or for a group of patients.

Assessment

1. Assess the medication record used in your facility *to identify whether any medications are to be given to an individual patient on your shift.*

2. Check the medications listed against the physician's or nurse's orders (in some facilities nurses can write orders for certain medications, such as laxatives). The procedure in your facility may include a double-check system, in which case it may not always be necessary to check against the order sheet. In this procedure, as well as in all others, know the policy at your facility. Check the patient's name and room number, the name of the medication, the dosage, the route of administration, and the time(s) to be given.

3. Review information about the medication to be administered. When you are an experienced nurse, you may have committed this information to memory for some drugs. As a student, you will probably be expected to have written notes on each medication you are to administer. These notes should include the generic name of the drug and common trade names; the usual dosage range; the actions, side effects, and contraindications for the drug; and the nursing implications, such as the need to administer on an empty stomach, the need to take vital signs before giving, and appropriate health teaching.

   You may be permitted to use commercially prepared medication cards. If so, you will need to individualize the information to your specific patient(s).

4. Assess the status of the patient *to ascertain whether the patient can take the medications as ordered* (e.g., ability to swallow, level of consciousness).

5. Assess the patient *to identify a need for any prn medications ordered.*

Planning

6. Determine what equipment you will need.

7. Wash your hands *for infection control.*

8. Gather the equipment. You will need small paper cups for tablets and capsules, and calibrated plastic medicine cups for liquids. In some facilities the calibrated medicine cups are used for tablets and capsules as well as liquids.

Implementation

9. Read the name of the medication to be given from the record.

10. Check the label on the medication and take that medication from the shelf or drawer. (This is the first of the three checks.)

11. Check the label again, before removing the medication from the container. (This is the second of the three checks.)

12. Remove the correct amount of medication for the individual dose to be given at this time.

   a. For a tablet or capsule (not prepackaged):
      (1) Pour from the bottle into the bottle cap until you have the correct dosage.
      (2) Transfer to the medication cup. Generally, all pills to be given to the same patient at the same time can be placed in one container. *If the administration of a medication is contingent on a pulse or blood pressure measurement,* keep that medication separate from the others, and make the measurement immediately after identifying the patient.

   b. For a liquid:
      (1) Place the bottle cap upside down on the countertop, so as not to contaminate it.
      (2) With the medicine cup at eye level, pour the liquid to the desired level in the cup, using the bottom of the concave meniscus as your guide (Figure 49–1).
      (3) Pour with the label facing up *to prevent medication from running onto and distorting the label.*
      (4) Wipe the neck of the bottle with a clean paper towel before replacing the cap.

   c. For a unit-dose medication, place packages containing the correct number of tablets or capsules in the medication cup. Do not open the packages at this time.

13. Return the bottle to the shelf or drawer. Check the label one last time, being sure to read it carefully. (This is the third of the three checks.) For unit-dose medications, you can do this last check after all medications are prepared; check each medication once again.

14. Place the medication on the cart.

15. Place a medication card or label on the prepared medication *for identification of the patient.*

16. Approach and identify the patient *to be sure you are administering medication to the correct patient.* By identifying the patient before you begin the rest of the procedure, *you avoid causing distress by mistakenly offering medication that is intended for someone else.* Although you prevent an error

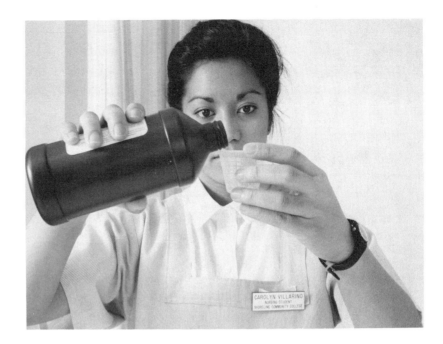

Figure 49–1 Measuring a liquid medication. The nurse holds the medicine cup at eye level using the bottom of the concave meniscus as guide for measurement.

if you check the identification after offering the medication, the patient may feel that a mistake was almost made and thus feel anxious. You can walk into the room and simply say, "Hello, may I check your wristband?" Another approach is to look at your identification record and say, "Hello, would you please spell your last name for me?" or "Hello, would you please state your full name for me?"

17. Explain what you are going to do and, if appropriate, what the medication is for and how it works. The information should be presented simply, in language easily understood by the patient. Explain any specific requirements related to the drug, such as increased fluid intake. For example, you might say, "I have your Lasix for you. This is the medicine that helps to remove the extra fluid that is causing your swollen ankles." Or you could say, "This is the aspirin that has been ordered for your sore shoulder. It is important for you to drink a full glass of water with it. The water helps to prevent irritation of your stomach." If assessment is needed before you give the medication, you might say something like, "This is your blood pressure medicine. I want to take your blood pressure before you take it." If the patient expresses doubts or confusion about a medication, such as "This doesn't look the same as what I take at home," or "I've never taken THIS medication before,"

recheck the order before administering the drug.

18. Give the patient a glass of fresh water. (You may have to change the water in the bedside pitcher.) If the medication has an unpleasant flavor, you can give juice with it instead of water, as long as this is not contrary to the patient's diet order or the drug manufacturer's directions. If the patient has a favorite juice, indicate it on the record, *so other nurses who administer the medication will know and will not have to ask the patient again.*

19. Watch the patient take the medication. *If you are not certain it has been swallowed, or if there seems to be a problem with swallowing,* have the patient open his or her mouth and look inside to see if the medication is still there. *If the patient cannot swallow a tablet or capsule,* give it in a vehicle, such as applesauce or jelly. It is common practice to crush tablets (except those with enteric coating) and to empty the contents from capsules to mix with the vehicle. Pills may be crushed in their unit-dose packaging or in a closed paper medication cup to avoid contaminating them with the pestle (Figure 49–2). Pill crushers are also available (Figure 49–3). Whole pills or capsules are sometimes given in a teaspoon of jelly. Unsweetened applesauce is a better vehicle for the patient with diabetes.

    Sometimes a patient will ask you to leave a medication to be taken later. This is not

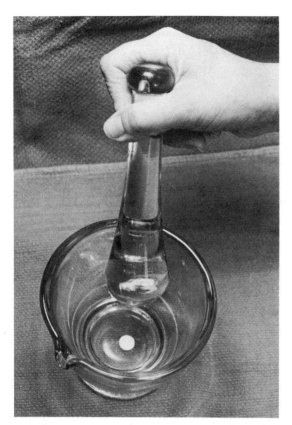

Figure 49–2 Pill being crushed with mortar and pestle. Pills may also be crushed in their unit-dose packaging to avoid contaminating them with the pestle. (*Courtesy Ivan Ellis*)

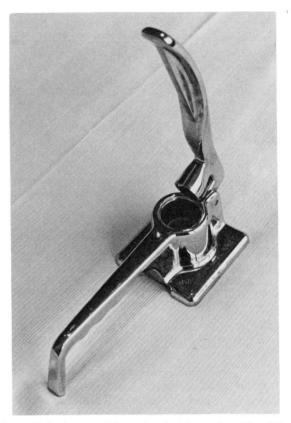

Figure 49–3 Commercially produced tablet crusher. The pill is placed in the circular area and crushed when the handle is pulled down. (*Courtesy Ivan Ellis*)

appropriate, *because you would not be able to record that the patient actually took the medication.* When you refuse the request, you might say, "No, I am responsible for it, so I don't want to leave it. If you can't take it now, I will come back with it later." If the medication is needed immediately, explain why it should be taken promptly. If a tablet or a capsule falls to the floor, it is considered contaminated and you will need to discard it and obtain a replacement.

20. Leave the patient in a comfortable position.

21. Discard the medication container *if it is disposable.* If it is not, rinse it out and replace it on the cart for reprocessing.

22. Wash your hands.

Evaluation

23. Evaluate, using the following criteria:
  a. The right patient received the right medication in the right dosage by the right route at the right time.

  b. The criteria established for ascertaining the effectiveness of a specific drug were used (e.g., for a given pain medication this might be "Pain relief obtained within 30 minutes").
  c. Side effects, if present, were promptly identified.

Documentation

24. Indicate on the medication record that the medication was given. Again, the exact method for doing this varies with the facility. Usually, the name of the medication, the dosage, the route of administration, the time, and your signature (with abbreviation indicating your position) are included. Initials are often used *to indicate that an individual medication has been given,* but a full signature is usually required on the medication record at least once during each shift (Figure 49–4).

Generally, medications should be given within 30 minutes of the time ordered.

(*text continues on page 334*)

Figure 49–4 Charting examples. **A:** Medication given. **B:** Medication omitted. **C:** Medication given with pulse recorded.

© **1992 by J.B. Lippincott Company**

NORTHWEST HOSPITAL MEDICATION RECORD - (ROUTINES)

Order Date	Exp. Date	Initial	ROUTINE MEDICATIONS MED - DOSE - ROUTE - FREQ	Schd Hrs	1/3/94 Init / Site	1/4 Init / Site	1/5 Init / Site	1/6 Init / Site	1/7 Init / Site	1/8 Init / Site	1/9 Init / Site
1/3/94		JE	Digoxin 0.125 mg p.o. daily	09	X	KT PO					
				AP	X	92					
1/4/94		KT	Lasix 40 mg. p.o. daily	09	X	X					
1/4/94		KT	Micro K 0.25 mg p.o. b.i.d.	09	X	KT PO					
				21	X	SM PO					
1/4/94		KT	Docusate Ca ÷ b.i.d.	09	X	KT PO					
				21	X	(SM) *					

DATE – TIME	1/4/94 (21)						
REFERENCE BOXES →	Refused due to loose stools. SM						

SIGNATURE AND TITLE BELOW TO IDENTIFY INITIALS			INJECTION SITE	CODE
JE Janice Ellis RN			DELTOID	RD/LD
KT Kay Taylor RN			ABDOMEN	RA/LA
SM Sue Morton RN			VENTROGLUTEAL	RV/LV
			GLUTEAL	RG/LG
			THIGH	RT/LT

M134A REV. 1/79

ADDRESSOGRAPH

Rogers, William F. M-76

09657321

Dr. J. L. Jepson

DIAGNOSIS: Congestive heart failure

ALLERGIES: Penicillin

DIET

RECOPIED BY:

PAGE:

Figure 49-5 Charting example—routine medications. Note documentation of medication that was held.

NORTHWEST HOSPITAL MEDICATION RECORD (P.R.N.'S)

(WRITE IN BELOW THE NEW P.R.N. MEDS AS ORDERED)

#	Order Date	Exp. Date	Initial	MED - DOSE - ROUTE - FREQ	#	Order Date	Exp. Date	Initial	MED - DOSE - ROUTE - FREQ
1	1/3/94		JE	M.O.M. 30 cc. q.d. prn	5				
2	1/3/94		JE	Halcion 25 mg. p.o. h.s.	6				
3	1/3/94		JE	A.S.A. gr X q 4 h prn pain	7				
4					8				

#	Date / Time	Dose	Site	REASON	EFFECT	INIT	#	Date / Time	Dose	Site	REASON	EFFECT	INIT
2	1/3/94 2100	25 mg	p.o.	for sleep	slept	RV							
3	1/4/94 08	gr X	p o	for shoulder pain	relief	SM							
2	1/4 2100	25 mg	p o	sleep	slept	KT							

Order Date	INIT	STATS MED / SINGLES DOSE / PRE-OPS ROUTE	To Be Given Date	To Be Given Time	INIT	(ONLY ON STATS & SINGLES) REASON	EFFECT
1/4/94	KT	Lasix 80 mg this a.m.	1/4	0900	KT	Fluid Retention	See Daily wt.

SIGNATURE AND TITLE BELOW TO IDENTIFY INITIALS			INJECTION SITE	CODE
RV Ronald Vaughn SN	JE Janice Ellis RN		DELTOID	RD/LD
SM Sue Morton RN			ABDOMEN	RA/LA
KT Kay Taylor RN			VENTROGLUTEAL	RV/LV
			GLUTEAL	RG/LG
			THIGH	RT/LT

M134A REV. 1/79

Rogers, William F. M-76
09657321
Dr. J. L. Jepson

ADDRESSOGRAPH

DIAGNOSIS: Congestive heart failure

DIET: Low Na

ALLERGIES: Penicillin

RECOPIED BY:

PAGE: 1 of 1

Figure 49–6 Charting example—prn and one-time dose medications.

Exceptions to this include preoperative medications and medications given every 2 hours or more frequently. These medications must be given precisely on time (Figures 49–5 and 49–6).

If for some reason the medication is not given (for example, it may be held at the nurse's discretion or refused by the patient), indicate this on the medication record. In many facilities this is indicated by a circle around the time that it should have been given along with an explanation in the nurses' notes. When the physician is notified regarding a medication not given, this should also be noted on the chart.

NARCOTICS

Narcotics are kept in a locked drawer or cupboard and must be signed out by the nurse administering the drug. The record indicates how many pills or capsules remain in the supply. Narcotics are routinely counted at change of shift and anytime the supply is replenished. If the amount of medication in the drawer does not check out with the record, the situation must be reported immediately. If you need to discard part or all of a narcotic that is prepared and ready to give to a patient, have another nurse witness your action and sign the narcotic record also. Follow the policy in your facility.

MEDICATION ERRORS

If a medication error occurs, it must be reported as soon as it is discovered, *so any necessary actions can be taken immediately.* In most cases an unusual-incident form is completed by the nurse who makes or discovers the error, and the physician is notified. Check the policy in your facility.

GIVING MEDICATIONS THROUGH A NASOGASTRIC TUBE

Patients with a nasogastric tube in place for feeding purposes are often given oral medications through the tube. The procedure is the same as for giving other oral medications, except that the medications must all be in a liquid or suspension form to be put down the tube. Tablets are crushed and dissolved as much as possible in water. Capsules are emptied into water. Because they often do not dissolve thoroughly, it is important to follow them by water *to flush the suspended medication completely out of the tube; otherwise the medication can occlude the tube.* Some medications are provided by the pharmacy as liquids or suspensions. The nurse can measure these medications in a syringe and then administer them directly from the syringe.

When giving the medications, follow the procedure in Module 29, Tube Feeding, for checking the placement of the tube and putting the medication in the tube. Do not put medications in the tube feeding itself, *because it is impossible to know whether the entire dosage is administered at the appropriate time.* If a continuous feeding is being administered, stop the feeding, give the medications, flush the tubing, and resume the feeding.

Home Care

Individuals of all ages need to take medications at home. Some patients are able to manage this task on their own and others need varying amounts of assistance. Written instructions must be individualized to the patient. Home medication schedules must be worked out around schedules that already exist for the patient and family. For example, a medication that is to be taken three times a day could logically be given with meals, if it can be taken with food and if the meals are somewhat evenly spaced. Many dispensers have been designed to assist patients to take the right medication in the right amount at the right time. Some of these, however, are difficult for patients to handle. As a result, some rather ingenious devices have been designed by patients for their own use. If you are responsible for teaching patients to take medications at home, be sure to include checking for expiration dates on medication packages. In addition, teach safe and appropriate storage, especially when small children are in the environment.

LONG-TERM CARE

The five rights and the three checks are used to ensure safety and accuracy in long-term care facilities as well as in acute care settings. The ability of the resident to swallow may be an additional consideration. It may be necessary to secure medication in liquid form or to crush pills before administering them. Many nursing homes use a "punch card" system for medication administration. The various medications are housed in "bubbles" on cards and punched out as they are given. This system helps to prevent medication errors in that the cards themselves serve as a check as to whether the medications have been given.

Performance Checklist

Administering Oral Medications	Unsat	Needs More Practice	Sat	Comments
Assessment				
1. Assess medication record to identify whether any medications are to be given to an individual patient.				
2. Check medications listed against physician's or nurse's orders.				
3. Review information regarding the medications.				
4. Assess patient's ability to swallow medications.				
5. Assess patient for need for prn medications.				
Planning				
6. Determine what equipment you will need.				
7. Wash your hands.				
8. Gather equipment.				
Implementation				
9. Read name of medication to be given from record.				
10. Check label on medication and take from shelf or drawer.				
11. Check label again, before removing the medication from the container.				
12. Remove correct amount of medication: a. Tablet or capsule				
(1) Pour from bottle into bottle cap until you have correct dosage.				
(2) Transfer to the medication cup unless prepackaged.				
b. Liquid				
(1) Remove bottle cap and place it upside down on the countertop.				
(2) Holding cup at eye level, pour liquid to desired level.				
(3) Pour with label facing up.				

Administering Oral Medications *(Continued)*	Unsat	Needs More Practice	Sat	Comments
(4) Wipe neck of bottle before replacing cap.				
c. Unit-dose medication				
(1) Place package containing medication in medication cup.				
13. Return bottle to shelf or drawer, checking label a third time.				
14. Place medication on cart.				
15. Place patient identification card with medication.				
16. Approach and identify patient.				
17. Explain what you are going to do and any specifics related to drug.				
18. Give patient a glass of water.				
19. Watch to be sure patient has swallowed medication.				
20. Leave patient in comfortable position.				
21. Discard medication container as appropriate.				
22. Wash your hands.				
Evaluation				
23. Evaluate, using the following criteria: a. The right patient received the right medication in the right dosage by the right route at the right time.				
b. The criteria established for ascertaining the effectiveness of a specific drug were used.				
c. Side effects, if present, were promptly identified.				
Documentation				
24. Record accurately according to the policy of the facility. Include: a. Name of medication				
b. Dosage				
c. Route				
d. Time of administration				
e. Signature				

Quiz

Short-Answer Questions

1. Medication procedures are usually based on the use of one of two general supply methods. Name these two methods.

   a. _____

   b. _____

2. At what times does the nurse check the name and dosages of the medication against that ordered when using the three checks?

   a. _____

   b. _____

   c. _____

3. List the five rights.

   a. _____

   b. _____

   c. _____

   d. _____

   e. _____

4. Name two methods of identifying the patient before giving medications.

   a. _____

   b. _____

5. 1 mg = _____ grains

6. 1 $\mathfrak{z}$ = _____ ml

7. 1 ml = _____ min

8. 5 ml = _____ $\mathfrak{z}$

9. The medication ordered is gr v; the tablets are marked in milligrams. How many milligrams are equivalent to 5 grains? _____

10. The order is 10 ml liquid medication. The patient must take this medication at home. How many teaspoons will this be? _____

Multiple-Choice Questions

_____ 11. Mrs. Brown is to receive a medication PO qid. This means

   a. by mouth every other day.
   b. before meals every day.
   c. after meals every day.
   d. by mouth four times a day.

_____ **12.** Mr. Green is to receive medication c̄ meals. This means

    a. before meals.
    b. after meals.
    c. with meals.
    d. none of the above.

_____ **13.** When pouring a liquid medication, you should measure from

    a. the top edge of the meniscus.
    b. the bottom of the meniscus.
    c. neither of these.
    d. It makes no difference.

Module 50

Administering Medications by Alternative Routes

Module Contents[1]

Rationale for the Use of This Skill
Nursing Diagnoses
Instilling Ophthalmic Medications
Implementation
Documentation
Instilling Otic Medications
Implementation
Documentation
Instilling Nasal Medications
Implementation
Documentation

Applying Medications to the Skin or Mucous Membranes
Dermal Medications
Implementation
Documentation
Transdermal Medication
Sublingual and Buccal Medication
Inserting Vaginal Medications
Implementation
Documentation
Administering Rectal Medications
Implementation
Documentation
Administering Medications by Inhalation

Prerequisites

1. *Successful completion of the following modules:*

VOLUME 1

Module 1 An Approach to Nursing Skills
Module 2 Basic Infection Control
Module 3 Safety
Module 5 General Assessment Overview
Module 6 Documentation

VOLUME 2

Module 35 Sterile Technique
Module 48 Irrigations
Module 49 Administering Oral Medications

2. *Satisfactory completion of the self-test on mathematics of dosages and solutions in Module 49, Administering Oral Medications. If you cannot meet this level of proficiency, you need additional practice in the mathematics of dosages and solutions. Many programmed texts are available for independent study.*

3. *Review of the anatomy and physiology of the eye, ear, nose, skin, vagina, and rectum.*

[1] See Module 49, Administering Oral Medications, for general steps using the Nursing Process.

340

Overall Objective

To prepare and administer medications safely, using ophthalmic, otic, nasal, skin and mucous membranes, vaginal, rectal, and inhalation routes.

Specific Learning Objectives

	Know Facts and Principles	Apply Facts and Principles	Demonstrate Ability	Evaluate Performance
1. *Ophthalmic medications*				
a. *Technique*	State whether sterile or clean technique is used.		Use sterile technique when instilling eye medication.	Evaluate own performance with instructor.
b. *Rationale*	Describe four reasons why patient might be receiving eye medication.	Given a patient situation, identify why patient might be receiving eye medication.	In the clinical setting, identify reason for eye medication.	Evaluate own performance with instructor.
c. *Positioning*	Describe positioning of patient for instillation of eye medication.		In the clinical setting, correctly position patient.	Evaluate own performance with instructor.
d. *Procedure*	Describe how to instill eye drops and ointments.		Correctly instill eye drops and ointments.	Evaluate with instructor using Performance Checklist.
2. *Otic medications*				
a. *Technique*	State when sterile technique is used and when clean technique is appropriate.	Given a patient situation, identify whether to use sterile or clean technique.	Use correct technique when instilling otic medications.	Evaluate own performance with instructor.
b. *Positioning*	Describe positioning of adult and pediatric patients for instillation of ear drops, including position of auricle.	Given a patient situation, select appropriate positioning for patient.	In the clinical setting, correctly position adult and pediatric patients to receive ear drops.	Evaluate own performance with instructor.
c. *Procedure*	Describe how to instill ear drops.		Correctly instill ear drops.	Evaluate with instructor using Performance Checklist.
	State how long patient should remain on his or her side after instillation of ear drops.		Instruct patients to remain on side 5–10 minutes after instillation of ear drops.	
3. *Nasal medications*				
a. *Technique*	State whether sterile or clean technique is used.	Given a patient situation and medication order, deter-	In the clinical setting, use careful asepsis when instill-	Evaluate own performance with instructor.

(continued)

© **1992 by J.B. Lippincott Company**

Specific Learning Objectives (Continued)

	Know Facts and Principles	Apply Facts and Principles	Demonstrate Ability	Evaluate Performance
		mine whether sterile technique is required.	ing nasal medications.	
b. Rationale	Know most common reason for instilling nasal medication. State rationale for instillation of water-soluble nasal medications.		In the clinical setting, check to be sure nasal medications are water soluble.	
c. Positioning	Describe positioning of patients to receive nasal medications, including Proetz and Parkinson positions.	Given a patient situation, identify appropriate position for patient.	In the clinical setting, correctly position patient.	Evaluate own performance with instructor.
d. Procedure	Describe how to instill nose drops and nasal sprays. State how long patient should remain in position after nose drops have been instilled.		Correctly instill nose drops and nasal sprays. In the clinical setting, instruct patients to remain as positioned for 5 minutes after instillation of nose drops.	Evaluate with instructor using Performance Checklist.
4. *Skin medications*				
a. Rationale	State rationale for use of lotions, ointments, liniments, and powders.	Given a patient situation, state preparation that might be used.		
b. Procedure	State how to apply medications to skin.	Given a patient situation, describe method of applying medication to skin.	Correctly apply medication to patient's skin.	Evaluate own performance with instructor.
5. *Mucous membrane medications*	State where to place sublingual and buccal medications.		Correctly place medications ordered by the sublingual or buccal route. In the clinical setting, instruct patients to hold the medication in place until completely dissolved.	Evaluate own performance with instructor.

(continued)

Specific Learning Objectives *(Continued)*

	Know Facts and Principles	Apply Facts and Principles	Demonstrate Ability	Evaluate Performance
6. *Vaginal medications*				
a. *Positioning*	Describe positioning of patient for insertion of vaginal medications.		In the clinical setting, correctly position patient.	Evaluate own performance with instructor.
b. *Procedure*	List methods of instilling vaginal medications.		Correctly administer vaginal medications.	Evaluate with instructor using Performance Checklist.
	State how long patient should remain quiet after medicated douche.		Instruct patient to remain quiet for 20 minutes following douche.	
7. *Rectal medications*				
a. *Positioning*	Describe positioning of patient for administration of rectal medications.		In the clinical setting, correctly position patient.	Evaluate own performance with instructor.
b. *Rationale*	State rationale for administration of retention enema after bowel movement.			Evaluate with instructor using Performance Checklist.
c. *Procedure*	State most common form of rectal medication.		Correctly administer rectal medication by suppository.	Evaluate own performance with instructor.
	Describe how to insert rectal suppository.			
	State how long patient should remain quiet after suppository insertion.		Instruct patient to remain quiet for 20 minutes following insertion of suppository.	
			Administer retention enema after patient has had bowel movement.	
8. *Documentation*	State items to be included in documentation for each route discussed.	Given a patient situation, do sample recording for medication discussed.	In the clinical setting, correctly document ophthalmic, otic, nasal, skin, sublingual, buccal, vaginal, rectal, and inhaled medications.	Evaluate own performance with instructor.

Learning Activities

1. Review the Specific Learning Objectives.
2. Read the section on administering drug therapy in Ellis and Nowlis, *Nursing: A Human Needs Approach,* or comparable material in another textbook.
3. Look up the module vocabulary terms in the Glossary.
4. Read through the module and mentally practice the specific techniques.
5. Using a partner for a patient, in the practice setting:
   a. Simulate the instillation of eye drops. If artificial tears are available, your instructor may want you to use these or a similar solution.
   b. Simulate the instillation of ear drops in an adult's ear. Do not use any actual drops.
   c. Simulate the instillation of nose drops and nasal sprays. Do not use any actual drops or sprays. Position your partner appropriately for the administration of a nasal spray and in the three positions described for nose drops.
   d. Practice the explanation necessary for administration of medications to be given by the sublingual and buccal routes.
   e. Practice the explanation and positioning for administration of a vaginal cream. Teach your "patient" self-administration.
   f. Practice the explanation and positioning for insertion of a rectal suppository.
   g. Change roles with your partner and repeat steps a–f.
   h. Evaluate each other's performance.
6. In the clinical setting:
   a. Seek opportunities to administer medications given by alternative routes.

Vocabulary

aspiration pneumonia	douche	ophthalmic	sphenoid sinus
auricle	ethmoid sinus	OS	sublingual
buccal	instillation	otic	suppository
canthus	liniment	OU	systemic
conjunctival sac	local	Parkinson's position	topical
dermatologic	lotion	Proetz position	tympanic membrane
dorsal recumbent position	ocular	rectal	vaginal
	OD	Sims' position	
	ointment		

Administering Medications by Alternative Routes

Rationale for the Use of This Skill

Drugs can be administered by various routes, depending on the patient's condition, the drug itself, and the desired effect. The nurse must be able to prepare and administer drugs correctly using these various routes, keeping in mind the basic concepts of safe administration as well as those related to these special routes. The nurse's knowledge of the anatomy and physiology related to the particular organ being treated and of the actions, usual dosage, desired effects, and potential side effects of the particular drug being administered are imperative for safe practice.

All types of medications discussed in this module should be administered using appropriate aspects of the steps of the procedure for Administering Oral Medications in Module 49. Substitute the steps given here for steps 18 and 19 of the Implementation section. The complete procedures, including all steps of the general procedure, are found in the Performance Checklist. Equipment needed and exact method of administration vary according to the medication. Directions are usually given by the physician or can be found in a package insert.[2]

▶ Nursing Diagnoses

The major nursing diagnosis to keep in mind when giving medications is High Risk for Injury. Patients can be injured by medications given in the wrong dosage, at the wrong time, or by an incorrect route. They can also be injured by the omission of essential medications or the administration of an incorrect medication. Although this nursing diagnosis will not appear on the care plan, it applies to every situation in which a patient is being given medications.

Another nursing diagnosis frequently appropriate when administering medications is Knowledge Deficit. In this case the knowledge deficit would be related to some aspect of the medication regimen; for example, the need for specific information related to the use of topical nitroglycerin.

[2] You will note that rationale for action is emphasized throughout the module by the use of italics.

INSTILLING OPHTHALMIC MEDICATIONS

Ophthalmic medications are used to soothe irritated tissue, to dilate or constrict the pupil, to treat eye disease, or to provide anesthesia. The administration of such medications is a sterile procedure. In addition to the five rights discussed in Module 49, you must be certain you are medicating the "right" (correct) eye. OS indicates the left eye, OD is the right eye, and OU indicates both eyes.

Implementation

18. Administer the eye medication.
    a. Wash your hands just before administering the eye medication.
    b. Clean the eyelids and lashes if necessary. Use a sterile cotton ball soaked in sterile normal saline. Move from inner canthus to outer canthus, using each cotton ball for only one wipe.
    c. Have the patient turn his or her head slightly to the side (away from the eye being medicated), and tip the head slightly backward. This can be done with the patient lying in bed or sitting in a chair.
    d. Have the patient look up.
    e. Rest your dominant hand (holding the eyedropper, container with dropper top, or ointment tube) on the patient's forehead *to avoid poking the patient in the eye*. Use your other hand to pull down on the lower lid of the eye to be medicated, *exposing the lower conjunctival sac*. Exert gentle pressure with the hand resting on the patient's face. Hold a cotton ball or 2×2 gauze *to catch any excess medication if necessary* (Figure 50–1).
    f. Instill medication.
       (1) Eye drops
           (a) Draw only as much solution into the dropper as you will need, *because unused solution is never returned to the medication bottle.*
           (b) Once you have the medication in the dropper, hold the bulb end up, *so the medication cannot run up into the bulb. The solution may become contaminated with particulate matter from the rubber bulb.* Many eye medications are now packaged in a flexible plastic container with an opening designed to deliver the drops.

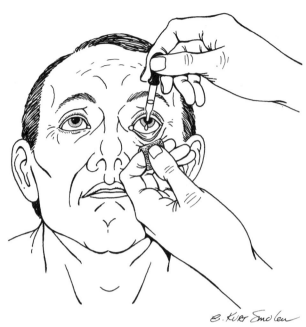

Figure 50–1 Instilling eye drops. Drop the ordered number of drops into the middle of the lowered conjunctival sac.

(c) Holding the eyedropper close to but not touching the eye, drop the ordered number of drops into the middle of the exposed conjunctival sac.
(2) Ointment
  (a) Squeeze out a ribbon of medication long enough for the entire lower conjunctival sac, moving from inner canthus to outer canthus.
  (b) Discontinue the ribbon by twisting the tube.
  (c) Wipe any excess ointment from the tube with sterile gauze.
g. Ask the patient to close the eye gently. *If the eye is squeezed tightly shut, the ointment or drops are pushed out.* If eye drops were instilled, have the patient move the eyeball around while it is closed *to help disperse the medication.* If ointment was used, have the patient keep the eye closed a full minute following the instillation, *to allow the medication to melt.* Use tissue or gauze to wipe away excess medication.
h. *Some medications (among them atropine) have systemic effects if allowed to pass into the lacrimal system and from there to be absorbed into the general circulatory system. To prevent this,* gently press the inner angle of the eye against the nose.

Documentation
Document as you would for oral medication, step 24, adding which eye was treated.

INSTILLING OTIC MEDICATIONS

Medication can be introduced into the ear to soften wax, to relieve pain, or to treat disease. The instillation of medication to the ear is a clean procedure, *except when the tympanic membrane is not intact,* in which case sterile technique is used. It is imperative that you have the correct ear in addition to the other five rights.

Implementation
18. Administer the ear medication.
  a. Warm the medication to body temperature by holding the container in your hand for a short time or by placing the container in warm water.
  b. If you are using a glass dropper, check to be sure it is not rough on the end. In the case of an uncooperative adult patient or a pediatric patient, you may want to attach a flexible rubber tip *to prevent injury to the patient in the event of sudden movement.* Fill the dropper.
  c. Have the patient lie on the opposite side of the ear being medicated.
  d. Gently pull the ear auricle upward and backward (Figure 50–2) *to straighten the canal. This allows the medication to reach all parts of the canal. In the infant and small child (under age 3), the canal is almost straight,* so pull the top of the ear downward and backward.
  e. Instill the correct number of drops, directing them toward the side of the ear canal.
  f. Have the patient remain on the side for 5–10 minutes after the drops have been instilled *to allow maximum contact with the canal.*
  g. Insert cotton loosely into the canal only if ordered. (This action is occasionally ordered *to keep the medication in contact with the canal and to prevent its running out.*) Never pack the ear tightly.

Documentation
Document as you would for oral medication, step 24, including which ear was treated.

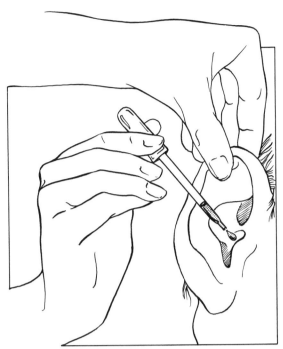

Figure 50-2 Administering ear drops to an adult. Gently pull the auricle upward and backward to straighten the canal.

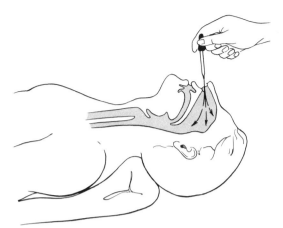

Figure 50-3 Proetz position for instilling nose drops. The patient is flat on the back with the head hanging straight back over the edge of the bed.

INSTILLING NASAL MEDICATIONS

Nasal medication is normally ordered *to relieve nasal and/or sinus congestion* and is often given in the form of nose drops. Nose drops and nasal sprays are usually water soluble *because of the danger of aspiration pneumonia with oil-based solutions.* The administration of nasal medication is not a sterile procedure, but careful clean technique should be practiced *because of the close and direct connection between the nose and the sinuses.*

Implementation

18. Administer the nasal medication.

    a. Have the patient clear the nasal passages, using a tissue and blowing gently.

    b. Position the patient according to the area you want to medicate.

        (1) Dropper

            (a) *Opening of the eustachian tube* Place the patient flat on the back.

            (b) *Ethmoidal and sphenoidal sinuses* Place the patient in the Proetz position, with the head hanging straight back over the edge of the bed (Figure 50–3).

            (c) *Frontal and maxillary sinuses* Place the patient in Parkinson's position, with the head slightly over the edge of the bed and turned toward the affected side (Figure 50–4). When the patient is positioned with the head hanging over the edge of the bed, you should help support the head with one hand *to prevent strain on the neck muscles.*

        (2) Nasal spray: position the patient in a chair, with the head tilted back.

    c. Instill the medication.

        (1) Dropper

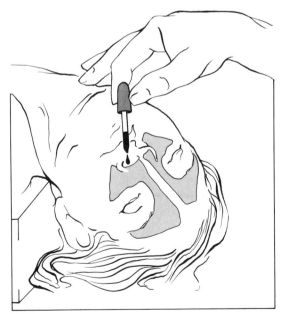

Figure 50-4 Parkinson's position for instilling nose drops. The head is slightly over the edge of the bed and turned toward the affected side.

(a) Draw in sufficient medication for both nostrils.

(b) With the tip of the dropper about ⅓ inch inside the nostril, instill the ordered number of drops into each side. Be careful not to touch the side of the nostrils, *which could cause the patient to sneeze.*

(c) Have the patient remain as positioned for 5 minutes after the medication has been instilled.

(2) Nasal spray

(a) Have the patient hold one nostril shut as you spray the medication into the other nostril.

(b) Ask the patient to inhale as the spray is being administered.

(c) Repeat on the other nostril.

(d) Keep the patient's head back for 1 or 2 minutes.

Patients often administer their own nasal sprays.

Documentation

Document as you would for oral medication, step 24, adding that the medication was administered nasally.

APPLYING MEDICATIONS TO THE SKIN OR MUCOUS MEMBRANES

Dermal Medications

Medications applied to the skin are commonly in the form of lotions, ointments, or liniments, and occasionally powders. *Lotions* protect, soften, soothe, and provide relief from itching. *Ointments* have an oil base, and body heat causes them to melt after application. Medications that fight infection or soothe inflamed tissues are usually available in ointment form. If obtained from a stock jar, remove the ointment with a sterile tongue blade. Discard any excess. Do not return it to the jar. *Liniments,* which are applied by rubbing, provide relief from tight aching muscles. *Powders* are applied for their soothing, drying action. The procedure requires sterile technique *if the application is on an open or infected area.* In some situations patients can be taught to apply the medication to their own skin, especially when the area to be treated is in easy view and reach.

Implementation

18. Apply the dermal medication.

a. Provide for the patient's privacy if necessary.

b. Provide adequate lighting.

c. Position the patient *so the area to be treated is accessible.* In some cases you may need assistance—for example, with the support of an arm or leg.

d. Be sure the area to be treated is clean *so the medication contacts the skin.* Skin medications are often applied immediately after a bath or shower.

e. Apply the medication to the area to be treated. *Using gloves wastes less medication and is less irritating than using gauze.* You should wear clean gloves *to apply any topical medication that can be absorbed through the skin, like a steroid cream, to protect yourself from the medication.* You may also wish to wear gloves when applying a medication that will stain your skin. *In situations in which sterile technique must be maintained,* for example, when applying ointment to an open wound, wear sterile gloves or apply the material with a sterile tongue blade or applicator. Apply the medication in thin even layers unless otherwise ordered.

To apply powder, instruct the patient to turn his or her head away *to prevent inhalation.* Spread it lightly and evenly, taking care not to let it accumulate between skin folds. Avoid shaking the powder directly over the patient. Put it in your own hand first, and then apply it to the patient.

f. Use a light dressing to cover the area only if ordered by the physician. *Some medications should not be covered.*

Documentation

Document as you would for oral medication, step 24, including the area treated and the appearance of the area before treatment.

Transdermal Medications

Some medications are now available in a form that is readily absorbed from the skin to provide systemic effects. They are called transdermal medications. Among these are nitroglycerin given for cardiac problems and scopolamine given for vertigo and nausea. The dosage of these medications must be as precise as the dosage of any other medication given for systemic effect. The correct dose may be impregnated in a small patch-type bandage. The backing is removed from the tape surface and the patch is then applied to clean skin. The medication is gradually absorbed. The patch is removed when the next dose is applied to the skin, and a new site is used for application *to avoid skin irritation from the tape or the medication.*

When the medication is an ointment, the order may call for a certain number of inches of ointment. A special pad of paper in which each sheet is marked in inches comes with the tube of ointment, so the nurse can carefully measure a line of ointment the diameter of the mouth of the tube and the ordered length onto the piece of paper. The paper is then placed on the skin, ointment side down, and secured around the edges with tape.

Sublingual and Buccal Medications

Some medications are ordered to be given by the sublingual route (placed under the tongue) or by the buccal route (placed between the cheek and gum). These medications are absorbed through the oral mucous membranes for rapid systemic effects. Instruct the patient not to swallow these medications but instead to hold them in place until they dissolve completely. An alert and capable patient may place the sublingual or buccal tablet or you may place it for the patient. If you place the medication, wear clean gloves *to protect yourself from body secretions.*

INSERTING VAGINAL MEDICATIONS

Vehicles used for the administration of vaginal medications include creams, gels, suppositories, and douches. Vaginal medications may be needed to treat infection, to relieve discomfort, or to alter pH. Use clean technique when inserting vaginal medications. Be especially alert to the patient's feelings of embarrassment.

Implementation
18. Insert the vaginal medication.
   a. Provide for the patient's privacy. Close the bed curtains.
   b. Provide adequate lighting.
   c. Place the patient in the dorsal recumbent position, with knees flexed and spread as for catheterization (see Module 39, Catheterization). Sims' position can also be used.
   d. Drape the patient.
   e. Put on clean gloves.
   f. Instill the medication.
      (1) Vaginal creams: introduce creams with

a narrow, tubular applicator that has a plunger attached.
      (2) Suppositories: introduce suppositories with a gloved and lubricated finger.
      (3) Douche
         (a) Obtain the equipment, and follow the procedure for vaginal irrigation in Module 48, Irrigations.
   g. Have the patient lie quietly for 20 minutes after the medication is inserted *to allow the medication to reach all surfaces.*

In some instances a hospitalized patient can be taught to administer vaginal medications to herself.

Documentation
Document as you would for oral medication, step 24. In some facilities, a douche is recorded on the treatment record. Follow the policy in your facility.

ADMINISTERING RECTAL MEDICATIONS

Rectal medications are usually given for their local effect, but some—for example, aspirin suppositories—are given for systemic effect. Suppositories are the most commonly used rectal medication, although creams and retention enemas can also be used. Clean technique is appropriate for all.

Implementation
18. Administer the rectal medication.
   a. Provide for the patient's privacy.
   b. Provide adequate lighting.
   c. Place the patient in the side-lying position. If for some reason this position is difficult for the patient, have him or her assume the dorsal recumbent position, with the knees flexed.
   d. Drape the patient.
   e. Put on clean gloves.
   f. Instill the medication.
      (1) Suppository
         (a) Open the package and lubricate the suppository.
         (b) Using a gloved, lubricated finger, insert the suppository beyond the internal sphincter.
         (c) Ask the patient to breathe in and out through the mouth while you are inserting the suppository, *to help relax the sphincter muscles.*
         (d) Have the patient lie quietly for 20 minutes after the insertion of a suppository.

(2) Rectal cream
  (a) Introduce the cream with the special tip attached directly to the tube of cream.
  (b) Remove the tip and clean after each use.
(3) Retention enema: administer the enema after a bowel movement *for maximum absorption of the medication.* See Module 28, Administering Enemas, for the necessary equipment and the procedure.

g. Clean the anal area with tissue *to remove the lubricant.*

Documentation

Document as you would for oral medications, step 24. In some facilities a retention enema is recorded on the treatment record. Follow the policy in your facility.

ADMINISTERING MEDICATIONS BY INHALATION

Medications are ordered by inhalation *for their local effect in the lungs.* They may be administered with an atomizer or nebulizer attached to oxygen or air under pressure. In this situation, the medication is placed in the device and the patient simply breathes in the mist through the device until all of the medication is gone. Alternatively, these same medications can be administered using hand nebulizers or atomizers. Some of these deliver a precise amount of medication with each puff. A specific number of puffs is ordered. The patient is instructed to start inhaling the puff of medication and to continue to breathe around the device, which acts to push the mist deeper into the lungs. Some nebulizers are equipped with spacer devices that deliver the medication followed by air, again *to push the medication deeper into the lungs. Because misuse of any of these devices can result in a wrong dosage of medication or in the medication not getting into the lower respiratory tract,* you must carefully follow the directions provided with each device.

Performance Checklist

Instilling Ophthalmic Medications	Unsat	Needs More Practice	Sat	Comments
1. Prepare yourself.				
Assessment				
1. Follow Checklist steps 1–3 in Module 49, Administering Oral Medications (check medication record, compare with physician's order, review medication information).				
Planning				
2. Follow Checklist steps 6–8 in Module 49 (determine equipment needed, wash hands, gather equipment).				
Implementation				
3. Follow Checklist steps 9–17 in Module 49 (read medication record, check label, take medication from storage, check label, prepare medication, return container, check label, place medication on cart, place patient identification on cart, approach and identify patient, explain to patient).				
4. Administer the eye medication. a. Wash your hands.				
b. Clean eyelids and lashes.				
c. Position patient with head slightly to affected side and tipped back.				
d. Have patient look up.				
e. Rest dominant hand on patient's forehead and pull down on lower lid to open eye wide with other hand.				
f. Administer medication.				
(1) Eye drops				
(a) Draw solution into eyedropper.				
(b) Hold bulb end up.				
(c) Without touching eye, instill drops.				
(2) Ointment				

Instilling Ophthalmic Medications (*Continued*)	Unsat	Needs More Practice	Sat	Comments
(a) Squeeze out medication.				
(b) Discontinue ribbon by twisting tube.				
(c) Wipe excess off tube.				
g. Ask patient to close the eye gently and move eyeball or keep eye closed as appropriate.				
h. Press inner angle of eye against nose if necessary.				
5. Follow Checklist steps 20–22 of Module 49 (make patient comfortable, dispose of equipment, wash your hands).				
Evaluation				
6. Evaluate as in Checklist step 23 of oral medication procedure (five rights, desired effects, and side effects). Add that correct eye was treated.				
Documentation				
7. Document as in Checklist step 24 of oral medication procedure (name of medication, dosage, route, time, and signature), plus which eye was treated.				
Instilling Otic Medications				
Assessment				
1. Follow Checklist steps 1–3 in Module 49, Administering Oral Medications (check medication record, compare with physician's order, review medication information).				
Planning				
2. Follow Checklist steps 6–8 in Module 49 (determine equipment needed, wash hands, gather equipment).				
Implementation				
3. Follow Checklist steps 9–17 in Module 49 (read medication record, check label, take medication from storage, check label, prepare medication, return container, check label, place medication on cart, place patient identification on cart, approach and identify patient, explain to patient).				

Instilling Otic Medications *(Continued)*	Unsat	Needs More Practice	Sat	Comments
4. Administer the ear medication. a. Warm medication to body temperature.				
b. Examine and fill glass dropper.				
c. Have patient lie on opposite side of ear being medicated.				
d. Pull auricle of ear to straighten canal.				
e. Instill drops.				
f. Have patient remain as positioned for 5–10 minutes.				
g. Insert cotton loosely in canal if ordered.				
5. Follow Checklist steps 20–22 of Module 49 (make patient comfortable, dispose of equipment, wash your hands).				
Evaluation				
6. Evaluate as in Checklist step 23 of oral medication procedure (five rights, desired effects, and side effects). Add that correct ear was treated.				
Documentation				
7. Document as in Checklist step 24 of oral medication procedure (name of medication, dosage, route, time, and signature), plus which ear was treated.				
Instilling Nasal Medications				
Assessment				
1. Follow Checklist steps 1–3 in Module 49, Administering Oral Medications (check medication record, compare with physician's order, review medication information).				
Planning				
2. Follow Checklist steps 6–8 in Module 49 (determine equipment needed, wash hands, gather equipment).				

Instilling Nasal Medications (*Continued*)	Unsat	Needs More Practice	Sat	Comments
Implementation				
3. Follow Checklist steps 9–17 in Module 49 (read medication record, check label, take medication from storage, check label, prepare medication, return container, check label, place medication on cart, place patient identification on cart, approach and identify patient, explain to patient).				
4. Administer the nasal medication. a. Have patient clear nasal passages.				
b. Position patient.				
(1) Dropper: according to area you want to reach				
(2) Nasal spray: in chair with head tilted back				
c. Administer medication.				
(1) Dropper				
(a) Draw sufficient medication for both nostrils.				
(b) Insert tip and instill drops.				
(c) Have patient remain in position for 5 minutes.				
(2) Nasal spray				
(a) Spray medication into nostril with patient holding the other closed.				
(b) Have patient inhale.				
(c) Repeat on other nostril.				
(d) Keep patient's head back for 1 or 2 minutes.				
5. Follow Checklist steps 20–22 of Module 49 (make patient comfortable, dispose of equipment, wash your hands).				
Evaluation				
6. Evaluate as in Checklist step 23 of oral medication procedure (five rights, desired effects, and side effects).				

Instilling Nasal Medications *(Continued)*	Unsat	Needs More Practice	Sat	Comments
Documentation				
7. Document as in Checklist step 24 of oral medication procedure (name of medication, dosage, route, time, and signature).				

Applying Medications to the Skin or Mucous Membranes

	Unsat	Needs More Practice	Sat	Comments
Assessment				
1. Follow Checklist steps 1–3 in Module 49, Administering Oral Medications (check medication record, compare with physician's order, review medication information).				
Planning				
2. Follow Checklist steps 6–8 in Module 49 (determine equipment needed, wash hands, gather equipment).				
Implementation				
3. Follow Checklist steps 9–17 in Module 49 (read medication record, check label, take medication from storage, check label, prepare medication, return container, check label, place medication on cart, place patient identification on cart, approach and identify patient, explain to patient).				
4. Apply the dermal medication. a. Provide for patient's privacy.				
b. Provide adequate lighting.				
c. Position patient appropriately.				
d. Be sure area being treated is clean.				
e. Apply medication appropriately.				
f. Use light dressing if ordered.				
g. Follow Checklist steps 20–22 of Module 49 (make patient comfortable, dispose of equipment, wash your hands).				

Applying Medications to the Skin or Mucous Membranes *(Continued)*	Unsat	Needs More Practice	Sat	Comments
Evaluation				
5. Evaluate as in Checklist step 23 of oral medication procedure (five rights, desired effects, and side effects). Add correct area.				
Documentation				
6. Document as in Checklist step 24 of oral medication procedure (name of medication, dosage, route, time, and signature). Include also the area treated and the appearance of the area before treatment.				
Inserting Vaginal Medications				
Assessment				
1. Follow Checklist steps 1–3 in Module 49, Administering Oral Medications (check medication record, compare with physician's order, review medication information).				
Planning				
2. Follow Checklist steps 6–8 in Module 49 (determine equipment needed, wash hands, gather equipment).				
Implementation				
3. Follow Checklist steps 9–17 in Module 49 (read medication record, check label, take medication from storage, check label, prepare medication, return container, check label, place medication on cart, place patient identification on cart, approach and identify patient, explain to patient).				
4. Insert the vaginal medication. a. Provide for patient's privacy.				
b. Provide adequate lighting.				
c. Place patient in dorsal recumbent position with knees flexed. (Sims' position can also be used.)				
d. Drape patient.				
e. Put on clean gloves.				
f. Instill medication.				

Inserting Vaginal Medications *(Continued)*	Unsat	Needs More Practice	Sat	Comments
5. Follow Checklist steps 20–22 of Module 49 (make patient comfortable, dispose of equipment, wash your hands).				
Evaluation				
6. Evaluate as in Checklist step 23 of oral medication procedure (five rights, desired effects, and side effects).				
Documentation				
7. Document as in Checklist step 24 of oral medication procedure (name of medication, dosage, route, time, and signature).				
Inserting Rectal Medications				
Assessment				
1. Follow Checklist steps 1–3 in Module 49, Administering Oral Medications (check medication record, compare with physician's order, review medication information).				
Planning				
2. Follow Checklist steps 6–8 in Module 49 (determine equipment needed, wash hands, gather equipment).				
Implementation				
3. Follow Checklist steps 9–17 in Module 49 (read medication record, check label, take medication from storage, check label, prepare medication, return container, check label, place medication on cart, place patient identification on cart, approach and identify patient, explain to patient).				
4. Administer the rectal medication. a. Provide for patient's privacy.				
b. Provide adequate lighting.				
c. Place patient in side-lying position.				
d. Drape patient.				
e. Put on clean gloves.				

Inserting Rectal Medications (Continued)	Unsat	Needs More Practice	Sat	Comments
f. Instill medication.				
g. Clean anal area.				
5. Follow Checklist steps 20–22 of Module 49 (make patient comfortable, dispose of equipment, wash your hands).				
Evaluation				
6. Evaluate as in Checklist step 23 of oral medication procedure (five rights, desired effects, and side effects).				
Documentation				
7. Document as in Checklist step 24 of oral medication procedure (name of medication, dosage, route, time, and signature).				

Quiz

Multiple-Choice Questions

_____ 1. Administration of which of the following requires the use of sterile technique? (1) ophthalmic medications; (2) nasal medications; (3) vaginal medications; (4) rectal medications

    a. 1 only
    b. 1, 2, and 3
    c. 1 and 3
    d. 2, 3, and 4

_____ 2. Eye drops are instilled into which part of the eye?

    a. Cornea
    b. Inner canthus
    c. Conjunctival sac
    d. Outer canthus

_____ 3. When administering ear drops to an infant, how do you straighten the ear canal?

    a. By pulling the auricle upward and backward
    b. By pulling the auricle downward and backward
    c. By pulling the auricle upward and forward
    d. By pulling the auricle downward and forward

Short-Answer Questions

4. Why are nose drops and nasal sprays usually water soluble?

_____

5. The Proetz position is used to reach which sinuses?

_____

6. List three reasons for the administration of lotions.

    a. _____

    b. _____

    c. _____

7. List two patient positions that can be used for the insertion of vaginal medication.

    a. _____

    b. _____

8. How long should the patient remain in bed after the administration of a medicated douche? _____

9. How far should a rectal suppository be inserted? _____

10. Why is it helpful to have the patient breathe in and out through the mouth when you are inserting a rectal suppository?

_____

Module 51
Giving Injections

Module Contents

Rationale for the Use of This Skill
Nursing Diagnoses
Equipment
  Syringes
    Glass Syringes
    Disposable Plastic Syringes
    Prefilled Syringes and Cartridges
    Insulin Syringes
    Tuberculin Syringes
  Needles
Medication Containers
Withdrawing Solutions from Containers
  Vials
  Ampules
Ensuring Accurate Dosages
Drawing Up Medication with an Air Lock
Mixing Powdered Medication for Injection
Mixing Medications in a Syringe
**Mixing Medications from Prefilled Syringes
    and Cartridges**
General Procedure for Giving Injections
  Assessment
  Planning
  Implementation
  Evaluation
  Documentation

Subcutaneous Administration
  Advantages and Disadvantages
  Selecting the Equipment
  Selecting the Site and Angle
  Procedure for Giving Subcutaneous
    Injections
  Special Concerns for Heparin Injections
Intramuscular Administration
  Advantages and Disadvantages
  Selecting the Equipment
  Selecting the Site
    Dorsogluteal Site
    Ventrogluteal Site
    Vastus Lateralis Site
    Rectus Femoris Site
    Deltoid Site
  Procedure for Giving Intramuscular
    Injections
  Z-Track Technique
Intradermal Administration
  Uses
  Selecting the Equipment
  Selecting the Site
  Procedure for Giving Intradermal
    Injections
Home Care

Prerequisites

1. *Successful completion of the following modules:*

VOLUME 1

Module 1   An Approach to Nursing Skills
Module 2   Basic Infection Control
Module 3   Safety

Module 5   General Assessment Overview
Module 6   Documentation

VOLUME 2

Module 35   Sterile Technique
Module 49   Administering Oral Medications

2. *Satisfactory completion of the self-test on mathematics of dosages and solutions in Module 49, Administering Oral Medications. If you cannot meet this level of proficiency, you need additional practice in the mathematics of dosages and solutions. Many programmed texts are available for independent study.*

3. *Review of anatomy as it relates to site selection for subcutaneous, intramuscular, and intradermal injections.*

360

Overall Objective

To prepare and administer subcutaneous, intramuscular, and intradermal medications safely to patients.

Specific Learning Objectives

	Know Facts and Principles	Apply Facts and Principles	Demonstrate Ability	Evaluate Performance
1. *Equipment* a. *Syringes*	Name five types of syringes available. Identify parts of syringe.	Given a patient situation, identify type of syringe appropriate for use. State which parts of syringe are kept sterile.	In the clinical setting, use correct type of syringe for injection. Handle syringe without contaminating sterile parts.	Evaluate with instructor.
b. *Needles*	Identify two methods used to size needles. Identify parts of needle.	Explain system used to size gauge of needle. State which parts of needle are kept sterile for injection.	Select needle appropriate to viscosity of medication to be injected, route to be used, and size of patient. Handle needle without contaminating sterile parts.	Evaluate with instructor.
c. *Medication containers*	Name two types of containers commonly used for injectable medications.	Differentiate between vial and ampule.	Correctly demonstrate removal of solution from vial and ampule.	Evaluate own performance using Performance Checklist.
2. *Subcutaneous administration* a. *Advantages and disadvantages*	Name three advantages of subcutaneous medication administration over oral medication administration. Name primary disadvantage of subcutaneous medication administration.	Given a patient situation, identify advantage of giving medication subcutaneously. State implications for nurse based on disadvantage.	In the clinical setting, identify advantages of giving medication subcutaneously.	
b. *Equipment selection*	State needle and syringe size most commonly used for subcutaneous injections.	Given a patient situation, select needle and syringe appropriate for subcutaneous injection.	In the clinical setting, select needle and syringe appropriate for patient.	Evaluate own performance with instructor.

(continued)

Specific Learning Objectives *(Continued)*

	Know Facts and Principles	Apply Facts and Principles	Demonstrate Ability	Evaluate Performance
c. Site selection	State angle at which needle is inserted for subcutaneous injections.	Given patient situation, identify appropriate angle for injection.	In the clinical setting, select appropriate angle for injection for patient.	Evaluate angle selection with instructor.
	State three areas acceptable for subcutaneous injections.	Given a patient situation, describe which site(s) is appropriate for subcutaneous injection.	In the clinical setting, select appropriate site for injection.	Evaluate site selection with instructor.
d. Injection technique	List steps in preparation and injection of subcutaneous medications.	Adapt steps to procedures in assigned clinical facility.	Prepare and inject sterile IV saline in practice setting under supervision.	Evaluate own performance with instructor, using Performance Checklist.
			Prepare and inject medication under supervision.	
3. Intramuscular administration				
a. Advantages and disadvantages	Describe speed of absorption of medication given intramuscularly as compared to subcutaneous administration.	Given a patient situation, select type of injection to be given in terms of absorption speed.	In the clinical setting, identify absorption speed of injection to be given.	
	Name five disadvantages of intramuscular injections.	State implications for nurse based on disadvantages.		
b. Equipment selection	State needle and syringe size most commonly used for intramuscular injections.	Given a patient situation, select needle and syringe appropriate for intramuscular injection.	In the clinical setting, select needle and syringe appropriate for patient.	Evaluate selection with instructor.
c. Site selection	State angle at which needle is usually inserted for intramuscular injections.	Given a patient situation, identify appropriate angle for injection.	In the clinical setting, select appropriate angle for injection for patient.	Evaluate angle selection with instructor.
	State four sites acceptable for intramuscular injections.	Given a patient situation, describe which site(s) is appropriate for intramuscular injection.	In the clinical setting, select appropriate site for injection.	Evaluate site selection with instructor.
d. Injection technique	List steps in preparation and injection	Identify critical way in which procedure	In the practice setting, under supervi-	Evaluate own performance with in-

(continued)

Specific Learning Objectives *(Continued)*

	Know Facts and Principles	Apply Facts and Principles	Demonstrate Ability	Evaluate Performance
	of medications intramuscularly, including Z-track technique.	differs from subcutaneous injection.	sion, prepare and inject sterile IV saline in one or more sites. In the clinical setting, under supervision, prepare and inject medication.	structor using Performance Checklist.
4. *Intradermal administration*				
a. Uses	State two reasons for use of intradermal injection technique.	Given patient situations, identify appropriate situation for use of intradermal technique.	In the clinical setting, correctly identify situation for which intradermal injection would be used.	Evaluate with instructor.
b. Equipment selection	State needle and syringe size most commonly used for intradermal injections.		In the clinical setting, select appropriate needle and syringe for intradermal injection.	Evaluate own performance with instructor.
c. Site selection	State angle at which needle is inserted for intradermal injection. State two commonly used sites for intradermal injections.	Given a patient situation, select area appropriate for intradermal injection.	In the clinical setting, select site appropriate for intradermal injection.	Evaluate own performance with instructor.
d. Injection technique	List steps in preparation and injection of intradermal medications.	Adapt steps to procedure in assigned clinical facility.	In the practice setting, under supervision, prepare and inject sterile IV saline intradermally. In the clinical setting, under supervision, prepare and inject intradermal medication.	Evaluate own performance with instructor using Performance Checklist.
5. *Documentation*	Know information to be documented.	Identify documentation method used in assigned facility.	Correctly document injections given according to method used in assigned facility.	Evaluate own performance with instructor.

Learning Activities

1. Review the Specific Learning Objectives.
2. Read the chapter on medication administration in Ellis and Nowlis, *Nursing: A Human Needs Approach,* or a comparable chapter in another textbook.
3. Look up the module vocabulary terms in the Glossary.
4. Read through the module and mentally practice the specific techniques.
5. In the practice setting:
   a. Observe and handle the assortment of needles and syringes available at your school and in your facility.
      (1) Using a 2- or 3-ml syringe and a 1½-inch needle, draw 1 ml solution from a multiple-dose vial.
      (2) Using the same equipment, draw all the solution from an ampule containing 1 or 2 ml solution.
      (3) Demonstrate changing a needle as you would if the first one had been contaminated.
      (4) Demonstrate drawing up the equivalent of 65 units of U-100 insulin in an insulin syringe.
   b. Read the procedures.
      (1) Using the Performance Checklist as a guide, give 1 ml solution to a simulated injection site as though you were giving it subcutaneously.
      (2) Using the Performance Checklist as a guide, give 1 ml solution to a simulated injection site as though you were giving it intramuscularly.
         To increase your manual dexterity before actually giving an injection, you might want to practice the sequence of movements involved in finding the site, taking the needle cover off the needle, cleansing the site, inserting, aspirating, injecting, and withdrawing the needle. You may practice this using a syringe or simply using a pen with a cap and an alcohol swab over a table. Although this does not simulate an actual injection, it will help you to feel more comfortable with handling the equipment and more able to remember what comes next when you are actually giving the injection.
      (3) Using the Performance Checklist as a guide, give a subcutaneous injection to a simulation pad or a partner, under supervision.
      (4) Using the Performance Checklist as a guide, give two intramuscular injections to a simulation pad or a partner, under supervision. Give one in the dorsogluteal site and one in the ventrogluteal site.
      (5) Using the Performance Checklist as a guide, give an intramuscular injection to a simulation pad or a partner, under supervision, using the Z-track technique.
      (6) Using the Performance Checklist as a guide, give an intradermal injection to a simulation pad or a partner under supervision.
6. In the clinical setting, when your instructor approves your practice performance, give subcutaneous, intramuscular, and intradermal injections in your facility under supervision.

Vocabulary

ampule	intradermal	plunger	Tubex
aspirate	intramuscular	point	vial
barrel	Luer-Lok	shaft	viscosity
bevel	lumen	subcutaneous	wheal
gauge	needle	syringe	Z-track
hub			

Giving Injections

Rationale for the Use of This Skill

The safe preparation and administration of subcutaneous, intramuscular, and intradermal medications is a routine nursing responsibility that requires dexterity; sterile technique; a knowledge of the actions, usual dosage, desired effects, and potential side effects of the drug being given; and a knowledge of how and where to give the drug. The latter requirement necessitates knowledge of human anatomy. Because drugs given by these routes not only are absorbed more quickly than by mouth but are irretrievable once injected, a firm mathematics foundation and routine practice of the three checks and the five rights are mandatory.[1]

▶ *Nursing Diagnoses*

The major nursing diagnosis to keep in mind when giving medications is High Risk for Injury. Patients can be injured by medications given in the wrong dosage, at the wrong time, by an incorrect route, or in an incorrect site. They can also be injured by the omission of essential medications or the administration of an incorrect medication. Although this nursing diagnosis will not appear on the Nursing Care Plan, it applies to every situation in which a patient is being given medications.

Another nursing diagnosis frequently appropriate when administering medications is Knowledge Deficit. In this case the knowledge deficit would be related to some aspect of the medication regimen; for example, the need to learn how to safely administer injections to oneself or to a family member.

EQUIPMENT

To give any injection, a syringe, a needle, a swab and disinfectant *to clean the skin,* and, of course, a medication are needed.

[1] You will note that rationale for action is emphasized throughout the module by the use of italics.

Syringes

Syringes are available in various sizes, shapes, and materials. Several commercially made syringes are designed for use with specific prefilled cartridges.

Glass Syringes. Once the mainstay of every hospital's syringe supply, glass syringes (Figure 51–1) are less widely used now that plastic disposable syringes are available. Glass syringes are still used, however, because they can be sterilized and included in surgical, obstetric, and treatment setups and because they adapt to the special tips (Luer-Lok) that are necessary for attachment to some irrigation devices.

Glass syringes are available in 2-ml, 5-ml, 10-ml, 20-ml, and 50-ml sizes. They can be secured with special control handles, which are sometimes used to administer local and regional anesthetics. The Luer-Lok is a specialized tip on the syringe that attaches the needle to the syringe by a threaded seal. This makes the connection more secure than the friction connection of a standard syringe.

Disposable Plastic Syringes. Disposable plastic syringes (Figure 51–2) are widely used and are available in various sizes, with or without needles attached. They are usually packaged either in a paper or cellophane wrapper or in a rigid plastic container.

Syringes with needles already attached are convenient and time-saving if the needles are the correct size and length. The needle fits on the syringe by friction. It is designed to be secure as long as it is pushed straight on and its cover is pulled straight off. When the hub of the needle is twisted, it releases and

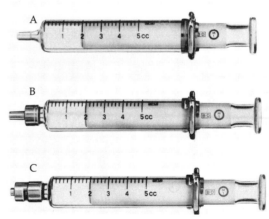

Figure 51–1 Glass syringes. **A:** Glass Luer. **B:** Metal Luer. **C:** Luer-Lok.
(Courtesy American Hospital Supply Corp., McGaw Park, Illinois)

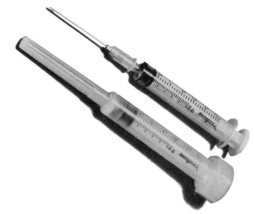

Figure 51-2 Disposable plastic syringe. This syringe is packaged in a rigid plastic container.
(Courtesy Monoject Division of Sherwood Medical)

comes off the syringe. There are also plastic syringes that have a threaded seal to attach the needle to the syringe hub, like the Luer-Lok on glass syringes.

Prefilled Syringes and Cartridges. Prefilled syringes usually come with appropriate needles attached and with directions for use. Especially helpful are syringes prefilled with drugs for emergency use. Prefilled syringes are disposable.

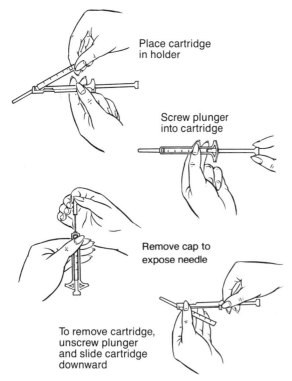

Place cartridge in holder

Screw plunger into cartridge

Remove cap to expose needle

To remove cartridge, unscrew plunger and slide cartridge downward

Figure 51-3 Prefilled cartridges and holder.

Prefilled cartridges contain medication and have appropriate needles attached. The disposable cartridge and needle are designed to fit into a nondisposable metal or plastic cartridge holder. The cartridge must be screwed into the holder *to secure it in place,* and the plunger of the holder must be screwed into the stopper of the cartridge *so that you can aspirate.* Although drawing up the medication is eliminated, which does make the procedure less difficult, mixing medications can be more difficult (Figure 51–3).

Insulin Syringes. Insulin syringes are marked in units specifically to measure dosages of insulin. They are available in both plastic (disposable) and glass (reusable) versions (Figure 51–4). U-100 insulin means that there are 100 units of insulin in 1 ml. The syringe holds 1 ml and is marked directly in units. A small size, which holds 0.5 ml or 50 units, is also available.

Tuberculin Syringes. Tuberculin syringes are usually chosen for the administration of very small amounts of medication, *because they are marked in 0.01-ml increments.* They are called tuberculin syringes because they were originally used to administer very small amounts of test material to check for exposure to tuberculosis. They are often marked in minims as well. The accuracy of the syringe allows you to measure small quantities precisely and makes them ideal for infant and pediatric use. These syringes are also available in disposable plastic (Figure 51–5) and reusable glass forms.

An insulin syringe is the safest to use when administering insulin, but insulin can also be measured accurately in a tuberculin syringe.

Needles

Needles for use with syringes come in standardized lengths (⅜–5 inches) and gauges (13–27). The needles most commonly used are ½–2 inches in length and 18–25 gauge. Both disposable and reusable versions are available. Most needles currently used are disposable. Reusable needles are found in special situations or for special procedures. They have metal hubs and metal shafts, and usually the lumen size is indicated on the hub. (Figure 51–6 shows the parts of a needle.) Disposable needles have plastic hubs and metal shafts, and the length and gauge are indicated on the outside of the packaging. *Sometimes color coding is used to indicate a needle's size. Because this practice is not standardized from one company to another,* you must be cautious when moving from one facility to another.

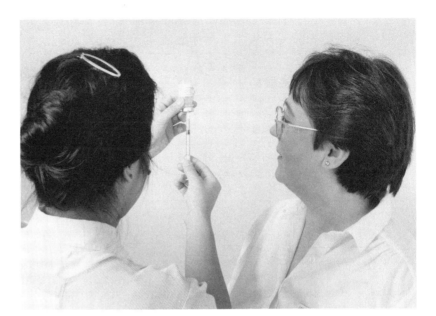

Figure 51-4 Disposable insulin syringe in use. The nurse checks the dosage of insulin with another nurse.

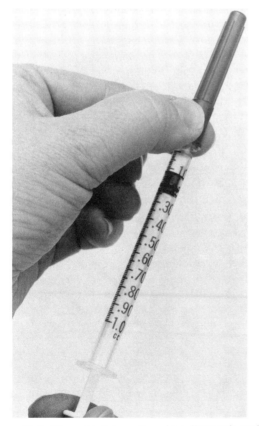

Figure 51-5 Disposable tuberculin syringe. Extremely small amounts of medication can be measured accurately in these syringes.

The larger the gauge number of a needle, the smaller the lumen. A needle with a small lumen is less painful to the patient when it is inserted. The choice of a needle is based on the relative viscosity or thickness of the medication. For example, most clear fluid solutions can be given intramuscularly with a 22- or 23-gauge needle. Subcutaneous injections of these kinds of fluids can be given with a 25- or 26-gauge needle. Thicker opaque medications given intramuscularly may require a 20- or 21-gauge needle. Larger needles are used primarily for blood transfusion and for injecting special intravenous fluids.

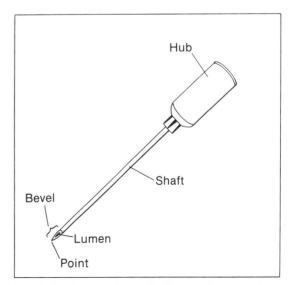

Figure 51-6 The parts of a needle. Most needles currently used are disposable.

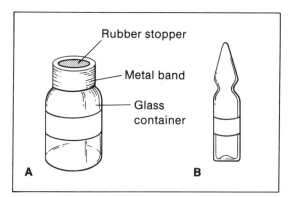

Figure 51–7 Medication containers. **A:** Vial. **B:** Ampule.

MEDICATION CONTAINERS

Two types of containers for injectable medications encountered frequently are the *vial* (either multiple dose or single dose) and the *ampule* (Figure 51–7). The vial is a small glass jar with an airtight rubber stopper sealed to the glass by a metal rim. The ampule is an all-glass container that has a narrow neck. The ampule must be broken open to remove medication.

WITHDRAWING SOLUTIONS FROM CONTAINERS

The procedure for drawing up the medication into the syringe is the same for all types of injections. It is presented here as a separate skill that you will integrate into the overall procedure.

Vials

1. Wash your hands *for infection control.*
2. Using an alcohol or other type of antiseptic swab, clean the rubber top of the vial with a firm circular motion. Allow the alcohol to dry *to obtain maximum antibacterial action.*
3. Discard the swab.

4. Prepare the syringe and needle, selecting the type of syringe used in your facility. Be careful to keep the needle, the syringe tip, the inside of the barrel, and the side of the plunger sterile *to prevent contamination of the medication* (Figure 51–8).
5. Draw as much air into the syringe as the volume of solution you have calculated you will need.
6. With the vial resting on the countertop, remove the needle guard and insert the needle through the rubber top of the vial.
7. Inject the air into the vial by pushing the plunger of the syringe into the barrel. *This prevents a vacuum when you withdraw the medication.*
8. Pick up the vial in your nondominant hand and hold the vial upside down at eye level. Many persons find it easiest to do this between the index and middle fingers. (Practice various techniques until you feel comfortable with one.) Pull the plunger down to withdraw the necessary amount of medication. Make sure the tip of the needle is beneath the level of the fluid in the inverted vial and that you do not touch the sides of the plunger as you withdraw medication. *The sides of the plunger will touch the inside of the barrel as you manipulate to expel air and get the exact dosage. If you have touched them, they can then contaminate the inside of the barrel.*
9. Examine the medication for air bubbles and remove any that are present. To do this, keep the syringe vertical and flick your index finger (or a pen) against the side of the syringe over the air bubble. *The vibration will usually cause the bubble to break loose and rise in the fluid to the top.* Once the bubble has risen to the top, you can push up on the plunger and expel the air into the vial. If the bubble does not rise when the syringe is tapped, you may have to push all medication back into the vial and draw up the medication again.

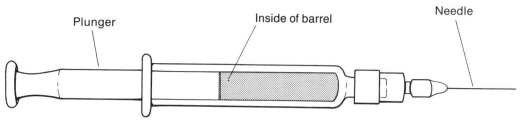

Figure 51–8 Parts of a syringe to be kept sterile. If your fingers touch the sides of the plunger, they can then contaminate the inside of the barrel.

10. Once all air is removed from the syringe, make sure that you have the exact volume needed. *Needles and syringes are marked so that the volume in the needle and hub is considered dead space. This means that this space is full of medication when you begin to give the injection and it is still full when the injection is completed. Therefore, the exact dosage measured in the syringe is given* (Wong, 1982). *The practice of drawing an air bubble into the syringe to clear the medication from the needle actually creates an error in dosage by expelling the medication that is in the dead space, unless you use the air-lock technique* (see pages 370–371).

11. Remove the needle from the vial.

12. Change the needle if the medication is one that is irritating to tissue.

13. Replace the needle guard, being careful to touch the needle to the inside of the needle guard only. *If the needle touches the outside of the needle guard, it has been contaminated and must be replaced. To protect yourself from needle sticks,* never place the needle guard over the needle with your hand. Get in the habit of keeping the hand that is not holding the syringe completely away from the needle guard. Some nurses simply place the needle guard in a convenient place on the counter or medicine cart and "scoop" it on. Some facilities use syringes that come housed in a case that becomes a vertical holder for the needle guard after the syringe is removed.

Ampules

1. Wash your hands *for infection control.*

2. If the medication is in the upper part of the ampule, move it down into the lower part by flicking the tip of the ampule with your index finger. Another method is to grasp the ampule by the tip and shake it firmly downward, as you would shake down a thermometer (Figure 51–9).

3. Using an alcohol or other type of antiseptic swab, clean the narrowest part of the ampule with a firm circular (twisting) motion.

4. Prepare the syringe and needle, using the procedure appropriate to the type of syringe used in your facility. Be careful to keep the appropriate parts sterile. Many facilities provide special filter needles to withdraw medications from ampules. *The filter needle prevents the aspiration of particulate matter into*

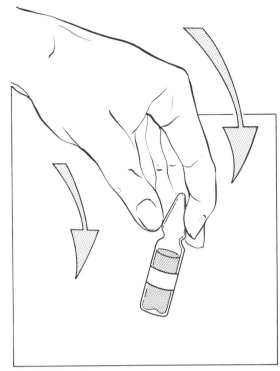

Figure 51–9 Shaking fluid to the bottom of an ampule. Grasp the ampule by the tip and shake it firmly downward, as you would a thermometer.

the syringe. The filter needle must not be used for injection and must be replaced with an appropriate needle after the medication has been drawn up.

5. Wrap a swab or gauze square around the neck of the ampule *to protect your hand from cuts.* Break off the top of the ampule away from yourself. To do this, hold the base of the ampule in one hand, grasp the top firmly with the other hand, and exert pressure (Figure 51–10). Discard the top in the disposal container for "sharps." *The sharp glass edges could cut through a plastic wastebasket liner and injure a housekeeping person.*

6. Remove the needle guard.

7. Hold the ampule firmly in your nondominant hand, either resting on the counter or supported in your hand, between your index and middle fingers. Insert the needle into the open end of the ampule, being careful to touch the ampule on the inside only (Figure 51–11).

8. Pull the plunger of the syringe back, being careful to keep the needle in the solution to avoid drawing air into the syringe.

9. Withdraw the needle from the ampule when

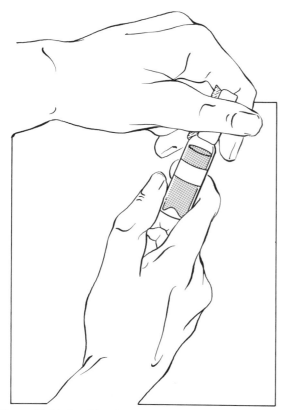

Figure 51–10 Breaking the neck of an ampule. Cover the neck of the ampule with a swab or gauze square to protect yourself from cuts. Then hold the ampule away from yourself with one hand and break the top off with the other.

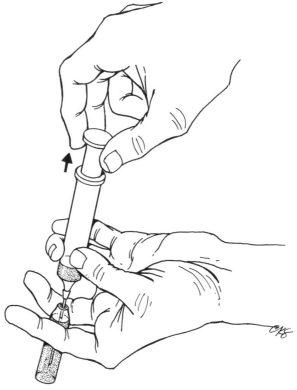

Figure 51–11 Withdrawing fluid from an ampule. Hold the ampule in your nondominant hand and insert the needle in the ampule. Pull back the plunger, keeping the needle in the solution, and withdraw the solution.

you have drawn slightly more than the amount of solution needed. Most ampules are slightly overfilled *so that you will be sure to have enough medication.*

10. With the needle pointing vertically, pull back slightly to aspirate the fluid from the needle into the syringe.

11. Push the plunger gently into the barrel until 1 drop of medication appears at the point of the needle. This drop can be removed with a gentle shake of the syringe and needle. *This prevents the medication from being on the outside of the needle and irritating the tissues as the needle is inserted.* If extra fluid must be ejected, the syringe can now be pointed downward over a sink or receptacle, *so excess medication does not flow back over the needle.*

12. Make sure you have the exact volume needed.

13. Change the needle if the medication is one that is irritating to tissue or if you used a filter needle when drawing up the medication.

14. Replace the needle guard, being careful to touch the needle to the inside of the needle

guard only. *If the outside of the guard is touched, the needle has been contaminated and must be replaced.* Use a one-hand technique to replace the needle guard as previously discussed.

ENSURING ACCURATE DOSAGES

When the exact measurement of a medication is critical—for example, a dosage of insulin or heparin—it is common practice to have two qualified individuals check the dosage together. The medication record and the filled syringe, still attached to the medication container if possible, are presented to the person who is doing the checking.

DRAWING UP MEDICATION WITH AN AIR LOCK

Some medications are irritating to subcutaneous tissue. These medications are given intramuscularly, but they could leak back into the subcutaneous tissue.

Injecting deep IM, injecting slowly so the medication can disperse, and using the Z-track technique, all of which are discussed later in this module, help to prevent this. Another technique to decrease the possibility that medication will leak back into the subcutaneous tissue is the use of an *air lock*—a bubble of air which is injected after the medication and *tends to block the needle track.* No research data support the value of using the air lock, and some researchers are concerned that errors in dosage occur if a nurse uses the air lock without understanding that there is dead space in the needle and syringe hub (Chaplin, Shull, & Welk, 1985).

The key concepts in drawing up medication with an air lock are the needs to have an accurate dosage of medication and to give the injection so that the air enters the tissue last. Follow these steps.

1. Draw air into the syringe equal to the volume of medication needed plus 0.4 ml.
2. When injecting air into a vial, leave 0.4 ml of air in the syringe.
3. Holding the syringe vertically with the needle pointing up, draw the medication into the syringe. The air will remain at the top of the fluid. Measure the dosage by subtracting the amount of air from the total volume. Obtain the exact dosage.
4. Withdraw the syringe from the vial.
5. Still holding the syringe vertically, with the needle pointing up, expel 0.2 ml of air to clear the needle of medication. This will leave 0.2 ml of air in the syringe, and the needle will be filled with air. *The dead space in the needle is filled with air at the beginning of the injection and will be filled with air at the end, so the correct dosage will be given.* Although needles and syringes differ as to the volume of dead space, it never exceeds 0.2 ml (Wong, 1982).
6. Give the injection with the syringe perpendicular to the floor *so that the air enters the tissue last.*

MIXING POWDERED MEDICATION FOR INJECTION

Some injectable medications come as a powder in a vial. The appropriate diluent, in the correct volume, must be injected into the vial, the contents mixed, and the medication then withdrawn. Follow these steps.

1. Read the label to determine:
   a. The appropriate diluent
   b. The quantity of diluent to be used
   c. The resulting strength of the prepared medication
2. Obtain the needed equipment:
   a. Alcohol swab
   b. Diluent
   c. Appropriate syringe
3. Cleanse the top of both the vial of diluent and the vial of powder *to decrease the potential for contamination of the needle and solution.*
4. Remove the appropriate volume of diluent from the vial using the directions given for withdrawing solution from a container.
5. Insert the needle through the rubber stopper of the medication vial and instill the diluent.
6. Withdraw the needle and recap it, using a one-hand technique.
7. Mix the medication by rotating the vial between your hands. *Shaking will create bubbles, which will be difficult to remove from the syringe.*
8. Draw up the appropriate dose of medication from the vial using the directions given above.
9. If sufficient medication remains in the vial to warrant saving it, label the vial with the date and the strength of the prepared solution and store it appropriately.

MIXING MEDICATIONS IN A SYRINGE

Frequently, physicians prescribe that injectable medications be given at the same time. It is possible to combine medications in order to give one injection. The important point is not to contaminate the medication in one vial with the medication from the other. Follow these steps.

1. Determine whether these two medications are compatible when mixed. This information can be found in many drug reference books or can be obtained from the pharmacy.
2. Determine the total volume of fluid that you will give if the drugs are mixed and given together. *If the volume is too large, you will need to plan for separate injections.*
3. Determine which medication you will draw up first. If one medication is in a vial and the other is in an ampule, draw up from the vial first, *because it will be used again.* If both are from ampules or one-dose vials, or both are from multiple-dose vials, then the order in which you draw up the medication is not important.

4. Obtain equipment:
   a. Appropriate syringe and needle
   b. Alcohol swabs
5. Clean the tops of both vials or open the ampules.
6. Draw up an amount of air equal to the combined volume needed.
7. Inject the correct amount of air into each vial, first injecting air into the last medication you plan to draw up.
8. After injecting the air into the medication to be drawn up first, withdraw the exact volume of that medication needed, as described above. Be sure all air is out of the syringe.
9. Withdraw the needle from the vial.
10. Insert the needle into the vial of the second medication.
11. Turn the vial upside down and make sure that the needle is under the surface of the fluid before aspirating. *You will not be able to push bubbles out of the syringe without contaminating the first medication with the second one,* so you must be careful not to draw up air.
12. Aspirate back until you have the precise volume needed for the combined medications, *because the medications will mix in the syringe immediately and you cannot expel any excess without making the dosage incorrect.*
13. Withdraw the needle from the vial.

MIXING MEDICATIONS FROM PREFILLED SYRINGES AND CARTRIDGES

When the injectable medications ordered to be given at the same time both come in prefilled syringes or cartridges, keep the following points in mind:
1. Determine whether these two medications are compatible when mixed.
2. Determine the total volume of fluid that you will give if the drugs are mixed and given together in the same syringe. *If the volume is too large, you will need to plan for separate injections.*
3. Measure accurate dosages of medication in each of the prefilled syringes or cartridges.
4. Obtain a syringe and needle appropriate for the amount and type of medication to be given. Do not attach the needle to the syringe. If the syringe comes packaged with the needle attached, remove the needle from the syringe. Be careful not to contaminate the needle.
5. Pull back on the plunger of the syringe until

there is adequate space for the total amount of medication to be given.
6. Inject the medication from each of the prefilled syringes or cartridges into the barrel of the syringe through the syringe tip.

GENERAL PROCEDURE FOR GIVING INJECTIONS

Use the general procedure for giving oral medications as the basis for giving injections. Alter the steps as indicated below. The complete procedure, including the steps of the general procedure, is found in the Performance Checklist.

Assessment
4. Assess the size and general build of the patient *in order to choose the correct size of needle for the injection.*
5. Assess whether you will need assistance to turn or restrain the patient during the injection.

Planning
6. Include in the equipment the appropriate needle and syringe and alcohol wipes to use in preparing the medication and in giving the injection.

Implementation
10. After checking the medication label the second time, calculate the volume of medication needed. *Most medication orders are written in terms of milligrams of the drug. You will need to read the label to determine how many milligrams are found in each milliliter, in order to calculate how many milliliters you are to give.*
12. Draw up the correct dosage, using the techniques described for drawing up from a vial or an ampule or for mixing medication in a syringe.
13. Recheck your calculation of dosage when you do your third check on the medication.
14. Carry the syringe and alcohol swab to the bedside. When giving an injection to a child, you may wish to conceal the syringe with your hand *to avoid frightening the child as you enter the room.* In all cases verbally prepare a child who is old enough to understand before giving the injection.
17. When explaining the injection to the patient, check which site was used for the previous

injection, if there was one, *in order to rotate to a different site and avoid excessive use of one area.*

18. Prepare the patient by pulling the curtains *for privacy*, making sure there is adequate lighting, and positioning the patient *for access to the injection site.*

19. Put a clean glove on your nondominant hand *to protect yourself from the potential of a blood spill* if you desire this added protection. You would then use this hand to massage the site after the injection is given. Wearing a glove is not necessary to safe practice according to the CDC.

20. Select the appropriate injection site and give the injection.
    a. Clean the site with a swab, using a circular motion and moving from the middle of the site outward.
    b. Allow the skin to air-dry.
    c. Place the swab between the third and fourth fingers of your nondominant hand.
    d. Remove the needle guard, being careful to pull it straight off and away from the needle. Again, the needle should touch only the inside of the guard.
    e. Using your nondominant hand, make the skin taut in an appropriate manner for the injection route chosen. *An injection is less painful if the skin is taut when pierced. Also, tautness allows the needle to enter the skin more easily.*
    f. Hold the syringe like a dart (the barrel between the thumb and index finger of your dominant hand) and insert the needle through the skin with a quick dartlike thrust. The needle should be at an angle appropriate for the patient and the injection route.
    g. As soon as the needle is inserted, transfer your nondominant hand to the barrel of the syringe to steady it, and transfer your dominant hand to the plunger.
    h. Pull back gently on the plunger (aspiration) *to be sure the needle is not in a blood vessel. Injection of a medication into a blood vessel can injure the vessel (the medication may not be appropriate for intravenous administration) and can produce a more immediate and considerably stronger effect than desired, possibly leading to serious complications.* If blood appears in the syringe, the needle is in a blood vessel. Withdraw the needle, discard the

medication, needle, and syringe, and start over. You would not use the blood-tinged medication, *because it would almost certainly lead to a discolored and sore area.*

    i. If no blood appears in the syringe, inject the medication by pushing the plunger into the barrel with slow, even pressure. *Slow infusion allows the medication to move into intracellular spaces, making room for additional fluid and reducing pain from pressure on the tissue.*
    j. Using your nondominant hand, steady the tissue immediately adjacent to the puncture site and quickly remove the needle. *This prevents the skin from dragging on the needle as it is removed, which causes pain.*
    k. Gently massage the injection site with the alcohol swab and discard it.

21. Discard the syringe and needle in the "sharps" container in the patient's room without replacing the needle guard. If the "sharps" container is centrally located, replace the needle guard using the one-hand technique previously discussed *in order to transport the needle and syringe safely.* Some facilities use a cup with a clay material inside to facilitate safe transport. The uncovered needle, with syringe still attached, is placed into the clay material and safely transported to the "sharps" container for disposal.

22. Remove the glove from your nondominant hand, if necessary.

Evaluation

23. Evaluate, using the following criteria:
    a. The right patient received the right medication in the right dosage by the right route at the right time.
    b. The correct site was used.
    c. The criteria established for ascertaining the effectiveness of a specific drug were used. For example, for a given pain medication this might be "Pain relief obtained within 30 minutes."
    d. Side effects, if present, were promptly identified.

Documentation

24. In addition to documenting the standard items, record the site of the injection. *This practice allows nurses to plan site rotation* (Figure 51–12).

DIAGNOSIS *Left lower lobe Pneumonia* Page *1* of *1*

ALLERGIES *NKA*

↓ CHART ROUTINES

DRUG & STRENGTH / ROUTE & DIRECTIONS	SHIFT	DATE 1/4/94	DATE 1/5/94	DATE 1/6	DATE 1/7	DATE 1/8
1/4 Staphcillin 800 mg IM q6h	23/07	24 (A) CS 06 (B) CS	24 (A) CS 06 (B) CS			
06 12 18 24	07/15	12 (G) PB	12 (G) PB			
JE	15/23	18 (H) EN	18 (H) HW			
1/5 Heparin 10,000 U	23/07	X				
sub cut. b.i.d.	07/15	X	09 (L) abd. CS			
09 21 CS	15/23	X	21 (R) abd. H			
1/5 Demerol 50 mg IM	23/07	X	X			
q4h PRN	07/15	X	08 (G) CS 12 (H) CS			
CS	15/23	X	16 (A) HW 20 (B) HW			
	23/07					
	07/15					
	15/23					
	23/07					
	07/15					
	15/23					
	23/07					
	07/15					
	15/23					
	23/07					
	07/15					
	15/23					
	23/07					
	07/15					
	15/23					
	23/07					
	07/15					
	15/23					

A = RIGHT UPPER OUTER QUAD C = RIGHT DELTOID E = RIGHT ANTERIOR THIGH G = RIGHT VENTROGLUTEAL
B = LEFT UPPER OUTER QUAD D = LEFT DELTOID F = LEFT ANTERIOR THIGH H = LEFT VENTROGLUTEAL

INITIAL	NAME	INITIAL	NAME	INITIAL	NAME
CS	C. Smith, RN	HW	H. Williams, RN		
PB	P. Benitez, RN				
EN	E. Norton, RN				

Cynthia Grant F-40
539-26-4967
Dr. John Torres

SWEDISH HOSPITAL MEDICAL CENTER

P-346 (R. 4/84) STOCK #5630 SEATTLE, WASHINGTON 98104

Figure 51–12 Documentation of injections. In addition to the standard items, document the site of the injection. **A:** Standard record. **B:** Subcutaneous injection flow sheet.

(continued)

This medication record and flow sheet is to be used for the documentation of all subcutaneous injections.
Label the columns with the parameters to be monitored. For example: INSULIN – Chemstrip blood glucose, lab blood glucose, type(s) of insulin. HEPARIN – Lab value (PT/PTT), heparin.

Parameters		Injection Site	Chemstrip Blood glucose	Lab Blood glucose	Regular Insulin U-100	NPH Iletin U-100	Comments	Int.
Date	Time							
1/4/94	0700			130				CS
	0730	E1			15 u	45 u		PB
	1130		120					PB
	1700		125					EN
	1730	E2			10 u	35 u	"hungry"	EN
	2100		210					
	2130	E3			4 u			EN
1/5/94	0710			140				CS
	0730	E4			15 u	45 u		PB

SUBCUTANEOUS INJECTION SITE CODES

C = Rt. deltoid   D = Lt. deltoid
I = Rt. abdomen   J = Lt. abdomen
E = Rt. thigh   F = Lt. thigh

This diagram shows the areas for subcutaneous injections. **For heparin the abdomen is preferred.** For insulin all sites may be used. When an injection site is used, chart the site under the Injection Site column (e.g., J4). The site may be marked off with an "X" on the diagram to facilitate the rotation plan. Each injection should be about one inch away from the other. Begin with one area and stay with that area until all the sites there have been used.

Identify Initials with Signature:	4.	8.
1. PB P. Benitez, RN	5.	9.
2. EN E. Norton, RN	6.	10.
3. CS C. Smith, RN	7.	11.

ADDRESSOGRAPH:

Cynthia Grant F-40
539-26-4967
Dr. John Torres

SWEDISH HOSPITAL MEDICAL CENTER
SEATTLE, WASHINGTON

NU-32 2/90 FC/SHMC

Figure 51–12 *(Continued)*

SUBCUTANEOUS ADMINISTRATION

Advantages and Disadvantages

Subcutaneous (SC) injections of medication have several advantages over the oral method of administration. First, if the patient has adequate circulatory status, you can depend on rapid, almost complete absorption of the medication. Second, gastric disturbances do not affect the medication given subcutaneously. And third, the patient does not have to be conscious or rational to receive the medication.

The greatest disadvantage of subcutaneous administration is that it penetrates the body's first line of defense, the skin. Thus, it is imperative that sterile technique be used *for the patient's safety.* Another disadvantage is the amount of patient teaching that is necessary for the patient who must continue subcutaneous administration at home.

Selecting the Equipment

In most instances a 25-gauge, ⅝-inch needle is used for subcutaneous injections. An extremely thin or especially obese patient may need individual consideration.

Because the maximum amount of solution that can be comfortably given subcutaneously is from 1½ ml to 2 ml, a 2-ml syringe is generally sufficient. In some facilities the smallest regular syringe available is 3 ml. Insulin and tuberculin syringes can also be used for lesser amounts.

Selecting the Site and Angle

Subcutaneous tissue lies directly below the skin. In many cases there is sufficient subcutaneous tissue present to use a 90° angle. In very thin patients you may need to use a 45°–60° angle. The angle of insertion depends on the size of the individual patient and on the length of the needle. In all cases the end of the needle must lie in the subcutaneous tissue (Figure 51–13).

The site you select varies with individual patients and circumstances. Generally, areas in the upper arms, anterior aspects of the thighs, and the lower abdominal wall are acceptable sites (see Figure 51–12, **B**). The upper back can also be used for patients who receive subcutaneous injections frequently (Figure 51–14).

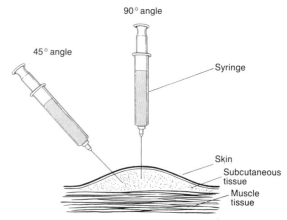

Figure 51–13 Subcutaneous injection. Either a 90° angle or a 45° angle may be used for subcutaneous injection if adequate subcutaneous tissue is present.

Procedure for Giving Subcutaneous Injections

20. Modify step 20 as follows:
   e. Using your nondominant hand, gently pinch the skin at the site selected between the thumb and index finger to elevate the subcutaneous tissue. If the patient is obese, you may have to spread the skin apart firmly to make the skin taut. Use a 45°–90° angle as selected for the individual patient (see above). Omit steps g, h, and i.

Special Concerns for Heparin Injections

The preferred sites for injection of heparin are those on the abdomen. When giving this drug, do not aspirate or massage the site afterward. *These actions might increase the capillary damage and contribute to bruising.* In addition, you should apply firm pressure to the injection site until all blood has stopped oozing *to help prevent bruising.* Sometimes ice is applied to the site for 15–30 minutes, for patients who bleed or bruise easily. *This causes vasoconstriction and hastens clotting.*

INTRAMUSCULAR ADMINISTRATION

Advantages and Disadvantages

Some of the advantages in using the intramuscular (IM) route for medications are the same as for the subcutaneous route: (1) medication is almost completely absorbed, (2) gastric disturbances do not affect

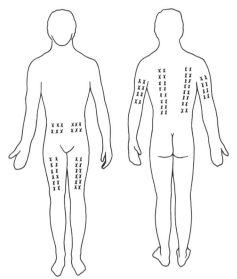

Figure 51–14 Sites used in rotating insulin injections. Record the site of the injection in order to accurately plan site rotation.

the medication, and (3) the patient does not need to be conscious or rational to receive the medication. Absorption occurs even more rapidly than with the subcutaneous route *because of the greater vascularity of muscle tissue.* Irritating drugs are commonly given intramuscularly, *because very few nerve endings are in deep muscle tissue.*

Disadvantages include the penetration of the skin, the possibility of nerve damage, pain that lingers long after the injection, and the potential for abscesses. More involved patient teaching is necessary for the individual being discharged on an IM medication.

Selecting the Equipment

A 19- to 22-gauge needle is used for intramuscular injections. The choice should depend on the medication's viscosity. The length of the needle depends on the size of the patient but is usually 1–2 inches long. A 22-gauge, 1½-inch needle is the one most commonly used.

Syringe size varies, but generally either a 2-ml or 3-ml syringe is used. In most facilities no more than 3 ml medication is injected into any one intramuscular site at a time.

Selecting the Site

Dorsogluteal Site. This is perhaps the most common of the four intramuscular injection sites for

adults. The injection is given in the gluteus medius muscle.

The patient should be lying prone, with the toes pointed inward. *This position helps to locate the site accurately and relaxes the muscle,* but it can be difficult or impossible for many patients to assume. An alternative is the side-lying position. The area should be adequately exposed (that is, all clothing must be completely away) *to aid site identification.*

One of two methods may be used for locating this site. The first and most traditional is to divide the buttock into quadrants, and then give the injection in the upper outer quadrant (Figure 51–15).

The landmarks of the dorsogluteal site are the upper iliac crest, the inner crease of the buttocks, the outer lateral edge of the patient's body, and the lower edge of the buttock (inferior gluteal fold). These landmarks should be palpated, not merely located by sight. Errors can easily be made, particularly in the location of the iliac crest.

Once you have established the location of the upper outer quadrant, give the injection 2–3 inches below the crest of the ilium. *Observing these precautions lessens the risk of injecting into large blood vessels or the sciatic nerve.*

The second method for locating the same site is more accurate when the patient is in the side-lying position. Draw an imaginary line between the posterior superior iliac spine and the greater trochanter of the femur (see Figure 51–15). An injection given laterally and superiorly to this line is away from the sciatic nerve, *because the line runs lateral to the nerve.*

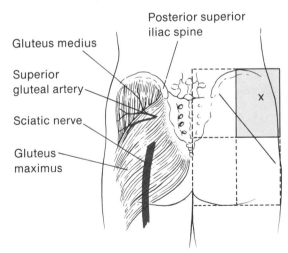

Figure 51–15 Dorsogluteal site for intramuscular injection. The quadrant outlined in solid lines surrounds the dorsogluteal site. The solid diagonal line provides another accurate way to locate this site.

Ventrogluteal Site. The ventrogluteal site has several advantages over the dorsogluteal site. No large nerves or blood vessels are in the area, it is generally less fatty, and it is cleaner, because there is less danger of fecal contamination. In addition, *because the gluteal muscle is not completely developed in small children,* the ventrogluteal site, rather than the dorsogluteal site, is preferred at least until a child is walking.

The patient can be placed in one of several positions: prone, side-lying, standing, or with the feet up in stirrups.

The landmarks of the ventrogluteal site are the greater trochanter, the crest of the ilium, and the anterior superior iliac spine. To identify the site, first locate these landmarks on the patient. Then place the heel of your palm on the greater trochanter. Point one finger toward the anterior superior iliac spine and an adjacent finger toward the crest of the ilium, forming a triangle with the iliac bone. (The size of your hand and the patient's bone structure may require small adjustments in hand position to form this triangle.) Use your nondominant hand to locate the site, *so that your dominant hand is free to manipulate the syringe.* The injection site is near the middle of this triangle, approximately 1 inch below the iliac bone (Figure 51–16).

Once the site is located, proceed as you would for a dorsogluteal injection, except point the needle slightly toward the iliac bone as you insert it.

Vastus Lateralis Site. The lateral thigh is relatively free from major nerves and blood vessels and is accessible in the dorsal recumbent or sitting position. This site is recommended particularly for infants and small children, *whose gluteal muscle is still undeveloped.*

In adults the superior boundary is a hand's breadth below the greater trochanter. The inferior boundary is a hand's breadth above the knee. On the front of the leg the midanterior thigh serves as a boundary. On the side of the leg the midlateral thigh is the boundary. The result is a narrow band (approximately 3 inches wide) that is suitable for intramuscular injection (Figure 51–17).

Insert the needle only to a depth of 1 inch and hold it parallel to the surface of the bed. This site is particularly well suited for large or obese patients. Small or slender persons have considerable pain when this site is used.

Rectus Femoris Site. The muscle that runs down the anterior surface of the midlateral thigh is called

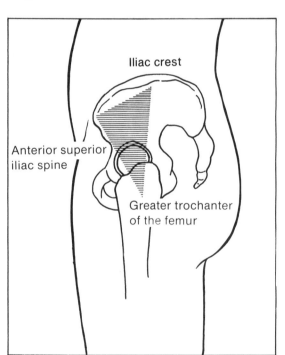

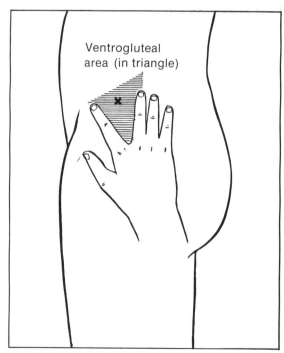

Figure 51–16 Ventrogluteal site for intramuscular injection. In this drawing the patient is lying on the right side with the left side up. The nurse's right hand is being used to locate the site. The site can be marked with the alcohol swab and the right hand removed to handle the syringe, or the left hand can be used to give the injection while the right hand remains in place, marking the site.

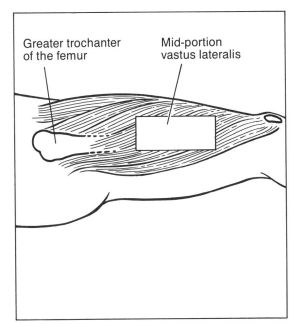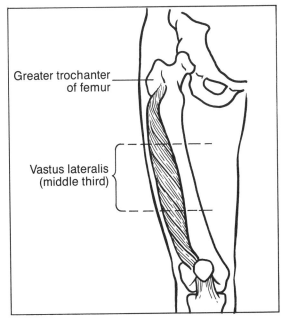

Figure 51–17 Vastus lateralis site for intramuscular injection. This site is recommended particularly for infants and small children whose gluteal muscle is still undeveloped.

the rectus femoris and is also available in the dorsal recumbent or sitting position. It is smaller than the vastus in the adult and is therefore used only for small injections. The rectus femoris is the site used for infants who are not yet walking and whose gluteal muscles are therefore not well developed. To concentrate the muscle mass and make the injection easier, compress the muscle tissue between your fingers. Place the injection straight down into the top of the thigh to a depth of 1 inch (Figure 51–18).

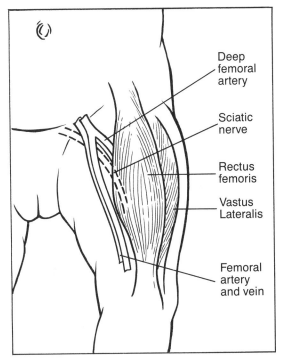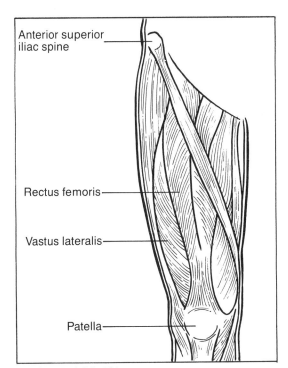

Figure 51–18 Rectus femorus site for intramuscular injection. **A:** Infant. **B:** Adult. This muscle is small and is therefore used only for small injections.

Deltoid Site. The deltoid muscle of the arm can also be used as a site for intramuscular injection. Although it is easily accessible, its use is limited, *because the small muscle is not capable of absorbing large amounts of medication.* Another, possibly more critical limitation on the use of this site *is the danger of injury to the radial nerve.*

The deltoid site is rectangularly shaped. The upper boundary is 2–3 fingerbreadths down from the acromion process on the outer aspect of the arm. The lower boundary is roughly opposite the axilla. Lines parallel to the arm, one third and two thirds of the way around the outer lateral aspect of the arm, form the side boundaries (Figure 51–19).

Although the size of the muscle varies with the size of the person, the amount of medication injected at this site should be limited to a maximum of 2 ml, preferably of nonirritating medication.

Procedure for Giving Intramuscular Injections

20. Modify step 20 as follows:
   e. Using your nondominant hand, spread the skin at the site selected between your thumb and index finger, making it taut. If the patient is very small or emaciated, you may have to pinch the tissue between the thumb and index finger to ensure sufficient muscle tissue. The needle should be at a 90° angle.

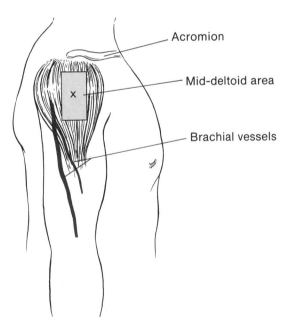

Figure 51–19 Deltoid site for intramuscular injection. The amount of medication injected at this site should be limited to a maximum of 2 ml.

Z-Track Technique

The Z-track technique of intramuscular injection is used when a drug stains the tissues, such as iron dextran (Imferon), or is extremely irritating, such as hydroxyzine hydrochloride (Vistaril). *Correct use of the Z-track technique prevents a drug from leaking back up through the needle track and staining or causing irritation.* The technique may be used for any intramuscular injection *to decrease discomfort and bruising.*

The equipment used for this procedure is generally the same as for routine intramuscular injections, except that a 2-inch needle is desirable. If a 2-inch needle is not available, a 1½-inch needle can be used.

The dorsogluteal area is the easiest site to use for a Z-track injection.

20. Modify step 20 as follows:
   e. Using the side of your nondominant hand, pull the skin and tissue laterally until it is taut (Figure 51–20).
   f. Holding the syringe like a dart, insert the needle at a 90° angle.
   g. As soon as the needle is inserted, use the thumb and index finger of your nondominant hand to steady the syringe, using your dominant hand to aspirate (Figure 51–21). Do not release the tissue that has been displaced laterally.
   h. Inject the medication slowly and wait several seconds (count to 10 silently).
   i. Remove the needle quickly, and immediately release the skin being held taut by your nondominant hand. The skin will

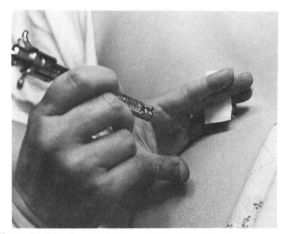

Figure 51–20 Z-track technique. Using the side of your nondominant hand, pull the skin laterally until it is taut. *(Courtesy Ivan Ellis)*

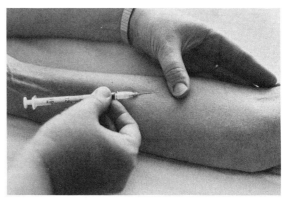

Figure 51–22 Intradermal injection technique. The syringe is held at a 10°–15° angle, with the bevel of the needle facing up. *(Courtesy Ivan Ellis)*

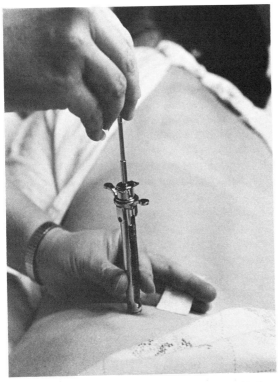

Figure 51–21 Z-track technique. Using the thumb and index finger of your nondominant hand to steady the syringe, use your dominant hand to aspirate. *(Courtesy Ivan Ellis)*

cover the needle opening, *preventing leakage.*

j. Do not massage the injection site.

According to Keen (1986), the Z-track technique, when compared with standard IM injection technique, significantly decreases discomfort and the severity of postinjection lesions.

INTRADERMAL ADMINISTRATION

Uses

The intradermal route is commonly used for diagnostic purposes, usually for diagnosing allergies and sensitivities, and for administering the tuberculin test. It has the longest absorption time of all the parenteral routes.

Selecting the Equipment

Because a very small amount of drug is used, a 1-ml, or tuberculin, syringe is used, with a short (¼–⅝ inch), fine-gauge (25–27) needle.

Selecting the Site

Intradermal literally means "between the skin layers," and the injection is administered just under the epidermis. The inner surface of the forearm is the most common site, although the subscapular region of the back can be used as well.

🏠 *Home Care*

Those caring for patients in the home setting, whether professionals or lay persons, must dispose of syringes and needles safely in that setting just as they do in an acute or long-term care setting. An alternative to purchasing the type of container used in a professional setting is to use a disposable container commonly found in the home. A plastic, disposable soft drink bottle resists puncture, can be capped tightly, and does not burst under pressure. Syringes and needles can be placed there as they would be placed in the "sharps" container in the hospital. The container must be stored where children cannot reach it and capped before disposal.

Lay persons caring for patients at home often need to administer medication by injection. It may be your responsibility to teach them this skill. Areas for emphasis include sterile technique and accurate dosage measurement.

Procedure for Giving Intradermal Injections

Because intradermal injections are often given in outpatient settings, you may have to adapt this procedure accordingly.

20. Modify step 20 as follows:

    e. Using your nondominant hand, stretch the skin at the selected site, making it taut.

    f. Hold the syringe at a $10°–15°$ angle, with the bevel of the needle facing up.

    g. Insert the needle just until the bevel is no longer visible (Figure 51–22).

    h. Inject the medication slowly.

    i. Withdraw the needle.

    j. Do not massage. A small wheal (raised area) is left at the point of injection.

    k. Circle area of injection with a skin-marking pen if the site must be assessed for reaction.

    l. Assess the site at the appropriate time interval for redness and swelling.

References

Centers for Disease Control. (1986). Recommendations for preventing transmission of infection with HTLV-III/LAV. *Morbidity and Mortality Weekly Report, 35,* 681–695.

Chaplin, G., Shull, H., & Welk, P. (1985). How safe is the air-bubble technique for injections? *Nursing 85, 15*(9), 59.

Keen, M. (1986). Comparison of I.M. injection techniques to reduce site discomfort and lesions. *Nursing Research, 35*(4), 207–210.

Wong, D. (1982). Significance of dead space in syringes. *American Journal of Nursing, 82*(8), 1236–1237.

Performance Checklist

General Procedure for Giving Injections	Unsat	Needs More Practice	Sat	Comments
Assessment				
1. Assess medication record to identify whether any medications are to be given to an individual patient.				
2. Check medications listed against physician's or nurse's orders.				
3. Review information regarding the medication.				
4. Assess size and general build of patient.				
5. Assess need for assistance.				
Planning				
6. Determine appropriate needle and syringe to be used.				
7. Wash your hands.				
8. Gather equipment.				
Implementation				
9. Read name of medication to be given from record.				
10. Check label on medication and take from shelf or drawer.				
11. Check label again, before calculating and preparing dosage.				
12. Draw up correct dosage of medication. a. From vial				
(1) Clean top of vial and allow to dry.				
(2) Discard alcohol swab.				
(3) Prepare syringe and needle.				
(4) Draw appropriate volume of air into syringe.				
(5) Insert needle into vial through rubber stopper.				
(6) Inject air into vial.				

General Procedure for Giving Injections (Continued)	Unsat	Needs More Practice	Sat	Comments
(7) Pick up vial with nondominant hand and withdraw correct volume of medication.				
(8) Examine for air bubbles and expel them.				
(9) Recheck volume of medication for accuracy.				
(10) Remove needle from vial.				
(11) Replace needle guard.				
b. From ampule				
(1) Get all medication into lower part of ampule.				
(2) Clean neck of ampule with alcohol swab.				
(3) Prepare syringe and needle.				
(4) Wrap neck of ampule and break off the top, away from yourself.				
(5) Remove needle guard.				
(6) Hold ampule in nondominant hand and insert needle into ampule.				
(7) Aspirate medication into syringe.				
(8) Withdraw needle from ampule.				
(9) Point needle vertically and pull back slightly.				
(10) Expel air from syringe.				
(11) Make sure that you have the exact volume of medication needed.				
(12) Replace needle guard.				
13. Reexamine vial or ampule to check the label a third time and recalculate the dosage.				
14. Place syringe, needle, and alcohol swab on cart.				
15. Place patient identification card with medication.				
16. Approach and identify patient.				
17. Explain to the patient and verify appropriate site.				

General Procedure for Giving Injections
(Continued)

	Unsat	Needs More Practice	Sat	Comments
18. Provide privacy.				
19. Put a clean glove on your nondominant hand if desired.				
20. Select the appropriate site for the injection and give the injection. a. Clean site, using circular motion.				
b. Allow site to dry.				
c. Place swab between fingers of nondominant hand.				
d. Remove needle guard.				
e. Pinch or spread tissue as indicated.				

Documentation

21. Follow Module 49, Checklist step 25 (name of medication, dosage, route and site, time, signature).				

Drawing Up Medication With an Air Lock

1. Draw air into syringe equal to volume of medication plus 0.4 ml.				
2. Inject air into vial leaving 0.4 ml of air in syringe.				
3. Hold syringe vertically to draw up medication. Measure dosage by subtracting the amount of air from the total volume.				
4. Withdraw syringe from vial.				
5. With syringe vertical, expel medication from needle, leaving air in the needle and 0.2 ml of air in the syringe.				
6. Give injection with syringe perpendicular to floor.				

Mixing Powdered Medication for Injection

1. Read label to determine diluent, quantity of diluent, resulting strength of solution.				
2. Obtain equipment: alcohol swab, diluent, syringe.				
3. Clean tops of both vials.				

Mixing Powdered Medication for Injection
(Continued)

	Unsat	Needs More Practice	Sat	Comments
4. Remove appropriate volume of diluent from vial.				
5. Insert needle into vial of drug and instill diluent.				
6. Withdraw needle.				
7. Mix medication by rotating.				
8. Draw up appropriate dose.				

Mixing Medications in a Syringe

	Unsat	Needs More Practice	Sat	Comments
1. Determine compatibility of two medications.				
2. Determine total volume of drugs to be administered.				
3. Determine medication to draw up first.				
4. Obtain equipment: alcohol swabs, syringe, and needle.				
5. Clean tops of both vials or open ampules.				
6. Draw up amount of air equal to combined volumes.				
7. Inject air into both vials: last to be drawn up receives air first.				
8. Withdraw exact volume of medication #1. Be sure all air is removed from syringe.				
9. Withdraw needle from vial.				
10. Insert needle into vial of medication #2.				
11. With vial upside down, make sure that the needle is under the surface of the liquid.				
12. Draw up the exact volume of medication #2 needed.				
13. Withdraw needle from vial.				

Mixing Medications From Prefilled Syringes and Cartridges

	Unsat	Needs More Practice	Sat	Comments
1. Determine compatibility of medications.				
2. Determine total volume of drugs to be given.				
3. Measure accurate dosage of each medication to be given.				

Mixing Medications From Prefilled Syringes and Cartridges *(Continued)*	Unsat	Needs More Practice	Sat	Comments
4. Obtain an appropriate needle and syringe. If syringe has needle attached, remove it.				
5. Pull back on plunger until there is room in syringe for total amount of medication.				
6. Inject medication from each prefilled syringe or cartridge into barrel of syringe through syringe tip.				

Quiz

Short-Answer Questions

1. Name four types of available syringes.

   a. _____

   b. _____

   c. _____

   d. _____

2. What does U-100 insulin mean? _____

3. Needles are sized according to _____ and _____ .

4. Name two types of containers that are commonly used for injectable solutions.

   a. _____

   b. _____

5. Air is injected before removing the solution when which type of container is used? _____

6. List three advantages of subcutaneous medication administration over oral medication administration.

   a. _____

   b. _____

   c. _____

7. What needle size is most commonly used for subcutaneous injections?

   _____

8. Name three areas that are acceptable for subcutaneous injections.

   a. _____

   b. _____

   c. _____

9. Absorption is most rapid in which of the three routes discussed?

   _____

10. What needle size is most commonly used for intramuscular injections?

    _____

11. Name four landmarks that are used to identify the dorsogluteal site.

    a. _____

    b. _____

    c. _____

    d. _____

12. Name three advantages of the ventrogluteal site over the dorsogluteal.

a. _____

b. _____

c. _____

13. What are two disadvantages of using the deltoid site for intramuscular injection?

a. _____

b. _____

14. In intramuscular injection, what is done immediately following the insertion of the needle? _____

_____

15. Why is the above action taken? _____

_____

Multiple-Choice Questions

_____ **16.** In a very slim person, which of the following angles would be most appropriate for subcutaneous injection?

a. 45° angle
b. 60° angle
c. 90° angle

_____ **17.** After which of the following injection techniques is massage *not* indicated? (1) intradermal; (2) subcutaneous; (3) intramuscular; (4) Z-track technique

a. 1 and 2
b. 1 and 4
c. 2 and 3
d. 3 and 4

Module 52

Administering Medications to Infants and Children

Module Contents

Rationale for the Use of This Skill
Nursing Diagnosis
Safety and Accuracy
Calculating Pediatric Dosage
Dosage Forms for Children
Parent Involvement
Vehicles for Administration of Oral
    Medications
Measuring Pediatric Dosages
    Tablets
    Liquids
General Approaches to Administering
    Medications to a Child

Gaining the Child's Cooperation
Techniques for Administering Medications
    to Children
Restraining Children for Injections
General Procedure for Pediatric Medication
    Administration
    Assessment
    Planning
    Implementation
    Evaluation
    Documentation
Home Care

Prerequisites

1. *Successful completion of the following modules:*

VOLUME 1

Module 1   An Approach to Nursing Skills
Module 2   Basic Infection Control
Module 3   Safety

Module 4   Basic Body Mechanics
Module 6   Documentation

VOLUME 2

Module 49 Administering Oral Medications

If you are giving medications by routes other than the oral route, you will need to complete the appropriate additional module.

Module 50 Administering Medications by Alternative Routes
Module 51 Giving Injections
Module 54 Administering Intravenous Medications

2. *Proficiency in mathematics of dosages and solutions is also essential to safe medication administration. This is especially critical with regard to medications for children because dosages are small. Even small numerical errors can have serious consequences. See Module 49, Administering Oral Medications, for a self-test on the mathematics of dosage and solutions.*

390

Overall Objective

To adapt medication-administering procedures to the special needs of children.

Specific Learning Objectives

	Know Facts and Principles	Apply Facts and Principles	Demonstrate Ability	Evaluate Performance
1. *Safety and accuracy*	State the nurse's responsibility for safe dosage.			
2. *Calculating pediatric dosages*	State the formula for obtaining a safe child's dose when the reference provides a dose per kilogram. State the formula for obtaining a safe child's dose when an adult dose is given and the child's weight is known. State the formula for obtaining a safe child's dose when an adult dose is given and a chart is available for determining child's body surface area.	Select correct formula to calculate a safe child's dosage, using the information available.	Calculate safe child's dosage when the reference provides a dose per kilogram. Calculate a safe child's dosage when the child's weight is known. Calculate a safe child's dosage when both weight and height are known.	Check accuracy of calculation with instructor.
3. *Dosage forms for children*	State the age at which a child can usually swallow tablets and capsules.			
4. *Parent involvement*	Discuss appropriate ways parents may be involved in giving medications.	Give an example of how you might involve a parent in giving an oral medication.	Include parents when giving medication to a child.	Evaluate interaction with instructor.
5. *Vehicles for the administration of oral medications*	List five vehicles commonly used to administer oral medications. State four factors to be considered when deciding which vehicle to use for mixing with a medication.	Given a specific situation, identify an appropriate vehicle to administer a medication.	Use an appropriate vehicle to administer a medication to a child.	Evaluate choice with instructor.

(continued)

Specific Learning Objectives *(Continued)*

	Know Facts and Principles	Apply Facts and Principles	Demonstrate Ability	Evaluate Performance
6. *Measuring pediatric dosages*	Identify which tablets can be divided. List methods of measuring liquids for children.	Given a situation, choose a method of measuring a liquid medication.	Measure a liquid medication in a syringe.	Evaluate choice with instructor.
7. *General approaches to giving medications to children*	Identify seven general approaches to giving medications to children.	Give an example of how each approach might affect nursing action.	In the clinical setting, choose an approach to be used for a specific child.	Evaluate choice with instructor.
8. *Techniques for gaining the child's cooperation*	List three techniques for gaining a child's cooperation.	Give examples of situations in which each technique might be used.	In the clinical setting, choose a technique for gaining a child's cooperation.	Evaluate choice with instructor.
9. *Restraining children for injections*	Describe three methods of restraining an infant or child.	Give examples of situations in which each method of restraining an infant or child for an injection might be used.	In the clinical setting, choose a method for restraining a specific child for an injection.	Evaluate choice with instructor.
10. *Procedure for administering pediatric medications*	List additional steps that must be taken when assessing a child for medication administration. List the various factors that affect planning of medication administration to children.	Adapt steps to individual patient situation.	Under supervision, give medication to a child or infant.	Evaluate own performance with instructor.
11. *Documentation*	Known information to be documented.	Identify documentation method used in assigning facility.	Correctly document medication given to child.	Evaluate own performance with instructor.

Learning Activities

1. Review the Specific Learning Objectives.
2. Read through the module and mentally practice the techniques.
3. For the list of medications below, calculate the safe dosage for the child described. Answers appear at the end of Learning Activities.
   a. Meperidine (Demerol), adult dose 50 mg, child's weight 44 lb
   b. Penicillin G, adult dose 600,000 units, child's height 4 feet 1 inch and child's weight 68 lb. Find body surface area and calculate safe dosage.
   c. Tetracycline, child's dosage 25–50 mg/kg/day divided into four doses. What is the safe individual dose for a 20-kg child?
4. In the practice setting:
   a. Examine various scored tablets. Practice breaking a scored tablet.
   b. Examine a 3-ml, a 5-ml, and a 1-ml (tuberculin) syringe. Compare the accuracy with which you could draw up 0.2 ml in each.
   c. Examine various liquid medications. Practice drawing up a correct dosage of oral medication in a syringe.
   d. Practice positioning a child for topical medications.
   e. Practice different methods of restraining a child for an injection.
5. In the clinical setting, arrange with your instructor to give medications to a child. Include an oral medication, an injection, and a topical medication.

Answers for Practice Problems:

   a. 14.67 mg
   b. 352,941 units
   c. 250 mg dose (1000 mg/day)

Administering Medications to Infants and Children

Rationale for the Use of This Skill

When children require medications, it is often necessary to use special techniques to administer the medication safely and successfully. Knowledge of physical growth and development is essential to enable you to make informed decisions regarding the necessary technique.[1]

▶ **Nursing Diagnosis**

The major nursing diagnosis to keep in mind when giving medications to children is High Risk for Injury. Children can be injured by medications given in the wrong dosage, at the wrong time, or by an incorrect route. They can also be injured by the omission of essential medications or the administration of an incorrect medication. Although this nursing diagnosis will not appear on the Nursing Care Plan, it applies to every situation in which a child is being given medications.

SAFETY AND ACCURACY

Safety and accuracy take on special meaning when you are giving medications to infants and children. Besides observing the three checks and the five rights, you must pay special attention when computing dosage. Although the physician computes the dosage when ordering the medication, the nurse should also compute the dosages *as a double check for safety*. If the nurse's computation indicates that the ordered dosage exceeds the safe dose level, it is the nurse's responsibility to consult with the physician, pharmacist, or nursing supervisor *to clarify the correct dosage before proceeding.*

Safety enters into each action taken. *Children are dependent on the adults around them for protection from the hazards of modern health care.* The nurse's judgment and discretion are crucial. Safety must be considered when deciding how to administer the medication, whether to restrain the child, how to restrain the child, and in every aspect of care.

[1] You will note that rationale for action is emphasized throughout the module by the use of italics.

CALCULATING PEDIATRIC DOSAGE

Many standard references provide the recommended dosage for children as a dosage *per kilogram of body weight.* When this is the case, the correct dosage is easily figured, using this formula:

$$\begin{matrix} \text{Recommended} \\ \text{dosage} \\ \text{per kilogram} \end{matrix} \times \begin{matrix} \text{Child's} \\ \text{weight in} \\ \text{kilograms} \end{matrix} = \begin{matrix} \text{Safe} \\ \text{child's} \\ \text{dosage} \end{matrix}$$

If the scales available do not weigh in kilograms, you can first figure the weight in kilograms by dividing the weight in pounds by 2.2.

Other commonly used formulas for calculating a safe pediatric dosage are based on weight and body surface area. The formula based on body surface area is considered the most accurate, *because it reflects several parameters related to metabolism and size.* The body surface area is found by plotting weight and height on a nomogram such as that found in Figure 52–1.

To find body surface area:

1. Locate the child's height on the scale to the left.
2. Locate the child's weight on the scale to the right.
3. Draw a straight line between the two and read the surface area in square meters from the scale labeled SA.

The line on the chart shows that for a child 116 cm tall and weighing 19 kg the body surface area is 0.78 m^2. In the center of the chart is a simple scale for using weight only for the child of normal height and weight.

$$\frac{\begin{matrix}\text{Body surface area of} \\ \text{child in square meters}\end{matrix}}{\begin{matrix}1.7 \\ \text{(Average adult body} \\ \text{surface in} \\ \text{square meters)}\end{matrix}} \times \begin{matrix}\text{Average} \\ \text{adult} \\ \text{dose}\end{matrix} = \begin{matrix}\text{Safe} \\ \text{child's} \\ \text{dose}\end{matrix}$$

The formula based on weight is commonly used, *because it is not necessary to have a nomogram available.* This formula is considered to have a fair degree of accuracy and is called *Clark's Rule.*

$$\frac{\begin{matrix}\text{Weight of child} \\ \text{in pounds}\end{matrix}}{\begin{matrix}150 \\ \text{(Average adult weight} \\ \text{in pounds)}\end{matrix}} \times \begin{matrix}\text{Average} \\ \text{adult} \\ \text{dose}\end{matrix} = \begin{matrix}\text{Safe} \\ \text{child's} \\ \text{dose}\end{matrix}$$

No formula for determining pediatric dosage is totally correct, *because children respond to drugs differ-*

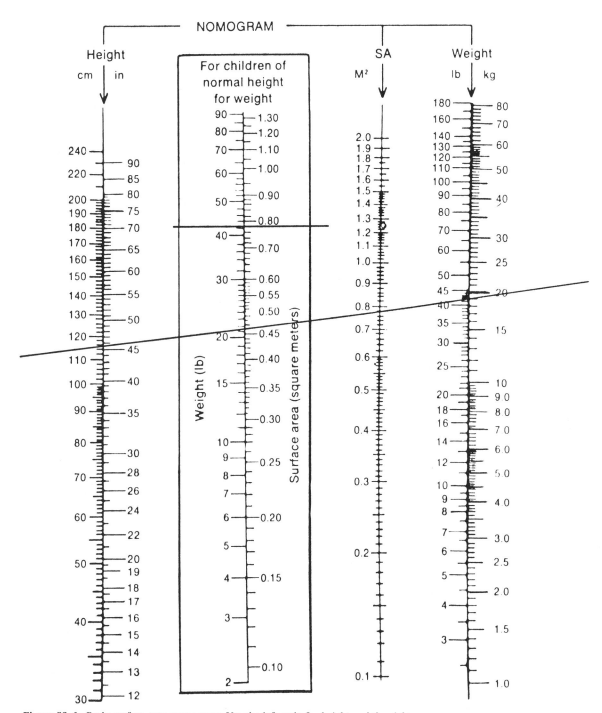

Figure 52–1 Body surface area nomogram. Use the left scale for height and the right scale for weight to locate the surface area on the scale labeled SA. Use the scale in the rectangle to determine surface area using weight only for the child of normal height and weight.
(From Nelson's Textbook of Pediatrics, 12th ed., 1983, Figure 29–1, page 814, by R. E. Behrman and V. C. Vaughan, III)

ently from adults. When an ordered dosage is larger than that identified as safe through calculation, consult with the pharmacist and the physician. The dosage may be appropriate based on the individual drug action, but an error in dosage is possible and must be checked out.

DOSAGE FORMS FOR CHILDREN

Most children can easily learn to swallow tablets and capsules by the time they are 4 or 5 years of age. Some children may be taught to take tablets as early as age 2, but this is unusual. Other children still cannot swallow tablets at age 6 or 7. Knowing the abilities of the individual child is important. Many medications are available in a liquid form that is suitable for children. It is always appropriate to consult with the pharmacist with regard to whether a liquid form is available. Sometimes tablets may be crushed and mixed with a soft food, such as applesauce or ice cream, *to facilitate the child's taking them.*

PARENT INVOLVEMENT

In many hospitals parents and other family members are encouraged to spend as much time as possible with the child. When giving medications to a child whose parent is present, include the parent as well as the child in your planning.

Explain to the parent what the medicine is. If the medicine produces any special care needs, such as a need for increased fluid intake, share that information *so the parent can participate effectively in the child's care.*

Often a child will take an oral medication with minimal fuss if it is given by the parent. This procedure is perfectly acceptable *as long as you stay to see that the medication is swallowed.* If you are giving an injection that is painful, do not ask the parent to restrain the child unless no other options are available. *This way the parent maintains the role of comforter and protector and is not associated with causing pain.* It is usually most helpful to the child if the parent stays and offers reassurance that the procedure will soon be over, *so the child does not feel abandoned.*

VEHICLES FOR ADMINISTRATION OF ORAL MEDICATIONS

Some foods and fluids are used *to make oral medications more palatable.* Honey, syrup, jelly, custard, applesauce, and other fruits may be mixed with crushed tablets *to make them easier for the child to swallow.* A puréed food or viscous liquid, such as syrup, holds particles in suspension. The medication should be mixed with the smallest amount of food possible, *so the child is more likely to take the entire amount.* Liquid medication may be mixed with juice or soda. Again, a small amount is used. The vehicle chosen is determined by the child's preferences, the taste of the medication (a strong taste is more effectively masked by a food with a distinct flavor), the diet prescribed for the child, and the nature of the medications. For example, one would not choose a sugared food for a diabetic child, or if the medication cannot be given with foods containing calcium, one would not give it with ice cream or custard.

It is unwise to mix a medication with the child's regular food or bottle, because two problems may arise. *First, if the child fails to eat all the food or finish the bottle, he or she has not received the complete dose, yet it is impossible to tell exactly what amount has been omitted. Second, the child may transfer dislike of the medication to dislike of the food, and this may interfere with adequate nutrition.*

MEASURING PEDIATRIC DOSAGES

Tablets

Whole tablets are used when possible, *because this makes dosage more accurate.* Tablets are broken only if they are scored by the manufacturer. *Scoring allows for a fairly clean break and accurate dosage. It is almost impossible to break an unscored tablet accurately.* Sometimes a tablet can be dissolved in a carefully measured amount of water, and then a portion of the solution given at a time. This method is accurate if the medication dissolves completely.

One effective way of crushing a tablet to mix with a vehicle is by using a mortar and pestle (see Figure 49–1). On some units a commercial pill crusher (see Figure 49–2) may be available. If neither of these is available, the tablet may be crushed between two spoons (Figure 52–2, **A**). Whichever method you choose, leave the tablet in the unit-dose package while it is being crushed, if possible (Figure 52–2, **B**). *The packaging keeps the medication clean and keeps the full amount contained so no part of the dose is lost.* If the tablet does not come in a unit-dose package, you can place it inside a paper medicine cup before crushing.

Liquids

Liquids can be measured in a medicine cup. *For accuracy,* a syringe (without a needle) should be used

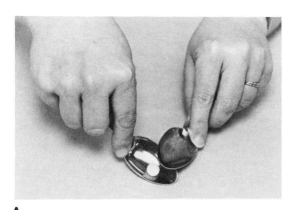
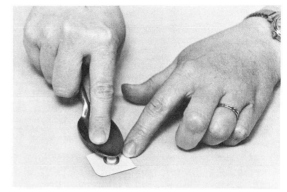

A　　　　　　　　　　　　　　　　　　　**B**

Figure 52-2 A: Crushing a tablet between two spoons. **B:** Crushing a tablet in a unit-dose package.
(Courtesy Ivan Ellis)

to measure very small amounts of liquid medication (Figure 52–3). *The smallest syringe that will measure the correct amount will give the most accurate dosage.* Some liquid medicine comes with a medicine dropper, with measuring gradations marked on the dropper. The dropper is used to measure the medication but not to give the medication orally, *because the dropper must be kept clean, so it can be returned to the bottle.* A dropper without calibrations will not provide an accurate drug measurement. Avoid transferring a liquid medication among containers unnecessarily, *because some of the medication will cling to the container each time it is transferred, and an inaccurate dose may result.*

GENERAL APPROACHES TO ADMINISTERING MEDICATIONS TO A CHILD

1. Be honest and direct with both the child and the parents. It is important to establish and maintain trust with children. *If trust is established, the child will cooperate more effectively in care.*
2. Accept the child's feelings and behavior. The child may be angry or upset. Telling the child that he or she should feel positive or cooperative is setting an unrealistic expectation. *Acceptance of the child's feelings enhances the child's feelings of self-worth.* If the child rejects you because you have caused discomfort, continue to be warm and positive toward the child, but do not press for a positive response.
3. Praise the child freely. *Praise is an effective reinforcer* and should be used at every opportunity. *The child who receives a lot of praise feels good about himself or herself and is better able to withstand adverse events.*

4. Offer only appropriate choices. *Whenever a choice is offered to a child, either alternative must be acceptable.* If no alternative is acceptable, do not offer one. Do not say, "Do you want to take your medicine now?" "No" is an unacceptable alternative. Instead, say, "It is time for your medicine. Do you want orange juice or grape juice to take it with?"
5. Be quick and positive in your actions. *If you hesitate or delay the process, you offer more*

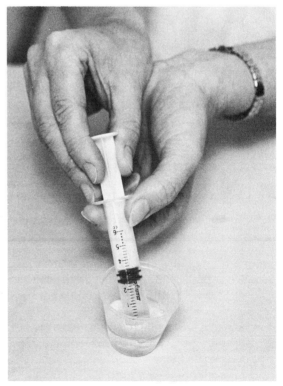

Figure 52-3 Measuring an oral liquid in a syringe.
(Courtesy Ivan Ellis)

opportunity for the child to respond negatively. The child will perceive your hesitancy and become more anxious and reluctant.

6. Offer all explanations in terms appropriate for the child's age. For a toddler, this may mean you say only, "O.K., take this." For a 5-year-old, you might say, "Here is some medicine to help you feel better." For a 10-year-old, you might say, "This medicine is to cure your throat infection." *A child's need for information is directly related to the ability to understand that information.*

7. Expect cooperation, but be prepared for noncooperation. *Expectations are transmitted to the child in various ways. In most instances the child will respond to your expectations.* If you expect cooperation, the child will cooperate. If you expect the child to resist, he or she often will. *Some children will not cooperate whatever the situation.* You should be prepared for this. If you are giving an injection, this means having everything ready and arranging ahead of time for others to help restrain the child. Those assisting should be unobtrusively present and should be called on to help the child "hold still" until the procedure is finished. Restraining should be regarded as a safety measure and not as punishment.

GAINING THE CHILD'S COOPERATION

Diverting the young child's or infant's attention with a toy or a game may *decrease concern about the medication.* This is not to imply that you sneak up on a child or lie, but simply give the child another interest on which to focus.

Role playing is sometimes successful in gaining a child's cooperation. The child first gives "pretend" medication to a doll or stuffed toy, and then the nurse gives the medication to the child. In the case of an injection it is more appropriate to give the medication to the child first, and then let the child pretend to give an injection.

For a toddler, making a game of taking medications, such as pretending a spoon is an airplane heading for the "hangar" (the open mouth), *can encourage participation by a reluctant child and make the process almost enjoyable.* In turning medicine time into a fun time, be careful not to give the impression that medicine is not really being given (honesty) or that not taking the medication is a choice. Do not pretend the medicine is candy, *because this presents an unsafe situ-*

ation. *A child may seek to have additional "candy" when at home and may take medication inappropriately.*

Forcing a child to take oral medication is not wise. *A child who is crying and upset may aspirate a medication. Medication forced into a child's mouth may be spit out. A child who is very upset may even vomit the medication.*

TECHNIQUES FOR ADMINISTERING MEDICATIONS TO CHILDREN

Take care to prevent aspiration when administering liquid medications to infants. Elevate the infant's head and use your thumb to depress the infant's chin to open the mouth. Then, using the dropper included with the medication or the plastic syringe in which the medication was measured, slowly drop the medication onto the middle of the tongue. The nurse can also insert a disposable dropper or syringe into the side of the mouth parallel to the nipple while the infant is being fed, or put the medication into an empty nipple for the infant to suck. Medications are never added to a bottle of formula.

To help older children who have difficulty swallowing tablets or pills, have them place the pill near the back of their tongue and then drink liquid to wash it down. Some facilities have special glasses that have a shelf that holds the pill. As the child drinks the liquid in the glass, the pill is carried to the back of the throat and swallowed.

RESTRAINING CHILDREN FOR INJECTIONS

When an injection is ordered, you will have to plan ahead for restraining a child who is younger than school age. For a child aged 5–10, you may still need another person to help the child "hold still." When choosing a restraining technique, you must first identify the injection site you intend to use (see Module 51, Giving Injections). Discuss the intended site with the person who will assist you in restraining the child. *The goal of restraining a child for an injection is to keep the body still, so the needle does not cause tissue damage.* Also make sure the child's hands cannot reach the syringe and that both hands and arms are positioned so they cannot hit the hands of the person giving the injection.

You may be able to restrain an infant effectively while you give the injection by using your dominant arm to stabilize the baby's body and your other hand

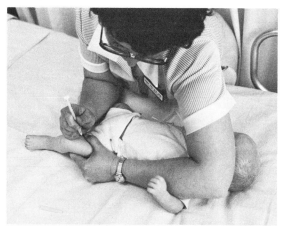

Figure 52–4 Restraining an infant while giving an injection. *(Courtesy Ivan Ellis)*

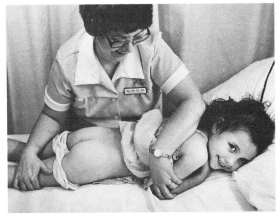

Figure 52–5 Restraining a child for someone else to give an injection. *(Courtesy Ivan Ellis)*

to hold the leg firmly (Figure 52–4). Holding a child on his or her side, with head and arms tucked under one arm and legs tucked under the other, works well (Figure 52–5).

For a small child who does not resist, you may be able to do this yourself, using the arms to hold the child and having your hands free to give the injection. If the child resists, it is safest to have a second person devote all his or her attention to restraining while you devote your attention to giving the injection.

On occasion, a larger child will resist injections. When this happens and the injection is essential (such as a preoperative sedation), it may be necessary to have two adults to help restrain—one restraining the upper body and arms and one restraining the legs (Figure 52–6).

Restraining a small child for nose drops or ear drops can usually be done by the person giving the medication. If you place the child across the crib, bed, or lap, with the head toward you extended over the edge, you can hold the head still as you give the drops (Figure 52–7).

GENERAL PROCEDURE FOR PEDIATRIC MEDICATION ADMINISTRATION

Assessment

1. Assess the medication record used in your facility *to identify whether any medications are to be given to a child on your shift.*
2. Check the medications listed against the physician's or nurse's orders (in some facilities nurses can write orders for certain

medications, such as laxatives). The procedure in your facility may include a double-check system, in which case it may not always be necessary to check against the order sheet. Check the child's name and room number, the name of the medication, the dosage, the route of administration, and the time(s) to be given.
3. If a medication is to be given, review information regarding the medication. Check for the recommended dosage of the drug, action, absorption, detoxification, and excretion as they relate to the diagnosis and maturity of the child.
4. Identify any special equipment you will need to prepare the medications and whether any vital signs need to be measured.
5. Assess the child to identify a need for any prn medications ordered.
6. Identify the child's physical growth and

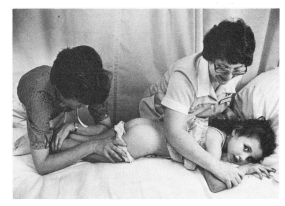

Figure 52–6 Two persons restraining a child for an injection. *(Courtesy Ivan Ellis)*

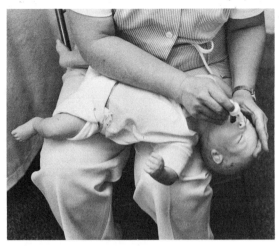

Figure 52–7 Holding a young child to give nose drops. (*Courtesy Ivan Ellis*)

development level, with special concern for swallowing ability, weight, age, and height.

7. Check a reference for a safe child's dosage. If a specific safe child's dosage is not given, compute a safe dosage using one of the formulas given. If any discrepancy occurs, consult with the physician or pharmacist before proceeding.
8. Check the medication forms available.
9. Check which vehicles are available for mixing with the medications.
10. Identify the child's psychosocial growth and developmental stage.

Planning
11. Plan a method of measuring the medication accurately.
12. Plan a method of making the medication acceptable to the child.
13. Plan an approach to the child that is appropriate to child's age and developmental level.
14. Plan for a method of restraint if necessary. Include asking for help if more than one person will be needed to restrain.
15. Determine what equipment you will need.
16. Wash your hands *for infection control.*
17. Gather the equipment. You will need cups for tablets and capsules, and medicine cups (calibrated) for liquids.

Implementation
18. Read the name of the medication to be given from the record.
19. Check the label on the medication and take that medication from the shelf or drawer.

20. Check the label again, before pouring.
21. Remove the correct amount of medication for the child's dose to be given at this time (See step 12 of the General Procedure for Administering Oral Medications, in Module 49). Use your planned method for measuring accurate dosage. The facility may have a policy requiring that a second nurse verify dosage on some medications such as insulin.
22. Return the bottle to the shelf or drawer. Check the label one last time, being sure to read it carefully.
23. Place the medication on the cart.
24. Place a medication card or label on the poured medication for identification if it is not a unit dose.
25. Approach and identify the patient *to be sure you are administering medication to the correct patient.* Always check the identification band. You may also verify with a parent that you have the right child in addition to checking the name band.
26. Explain what you are going to do and, if appropriate, what the medication is for and how it works.
27. Add appropriate planned actions related to:
    a. Making the medication acceptable to the child.
    b. Approaching the child.
    c. Restraining as needed.
28. Watch the child take the medication. If you are not certain it has been swallowed, or if there seems to be a problem with swallowing, have the child open the mouth and look inside to see if the medication is still there.
29. Leave the child in a comfortable position.
30. Discard the medication container if it is disposable. If it is not, rinse it out and replace it on the cart for reprocessing.
31. Wash your hands.

Evaluation
32. Evaluate, using the following criteria:
    a. The right patient received the right medication in the right dosage by the right route at the right time.
    b. If appropriate for the medication given, medication had desired effects, side effects were noted.

Documentation
33. Indicate on the medication record that the medication was given. Include:
    a. Name of medication.
    b. Dosage.

c. Route.

d. Time of administration.

e. Signature.

34. Successful methods of administering medications should be added to the Nursing Care Plan.

🔳 *Home Care*

When parents must give medications to children at home, they are faced with the same problems and concerns that nurses encounter in the hospital. The major concern is safety and a secondary concern is the technique for medication administration.

Nurses should counsel parents in regard to safe storage of medications so that they are out of reach of children. The importance of clearly differentiating medicine from food or candy should be emphasized because children may enjoy the taste of flavored medications and try to take more as they would a desired snack food. Teaching parents to read labels carefully is critical to medication safety. Some medications must be scheduled with meals and others given on an empty stomach. These scheduling details are important for medication effectiveness. Sometimes parents will benefit from hints for ways to remember medication administration times in a busy family. Scheduling medications in relationship to a meal, nap or bed time, or some other regular activity may help. A chart for checking off dosages may be of assistance. Plans need to be individualized to the situation in each home.

Measuring dosages accurately is another important aspect of safety. Household spoons vary in size and are not reliable for administering most children's medications. Many children's medications come with measuring droppers, which should be used for measuring. Most pharmacies also stock special measuring spoons and droppers designed to be used with infants and children. These provide accurate measurement as well as a device that is not easily spilled when a liquid is being given to a child.

Families may also need help with techniques of administering medications to children. Any of the techniques presented in this modules might be useful in some home situations. You might demonstrate how to give a medication while the child is in the hospital or clinic and if possible give the parent a chance to give it with you there as support before being expected to manage this task at home. When this is not possible, you can describe techniques and answer questions raised by the parents.

Performance Checklist

Administering Medications to Infants and Children	Unsat	Needs More Practice	Sat	Comments
Assessment				
1. Assess medication record to see whether any medications are to be given to a child on your shift.				
2. Check medications listed against physician's or nurse's orders.				
3. Review information regarding the medication.				
4. Identify any special equipment needed.				
5. Assess child's need for any prn medications ordered.				
6. Identify child's physical growth and development level, including swallowing ability, weight, age, and height.				
7. Check reference for safe child's dosage or compute a safe dosage.				
8. Check medication form available.				
9. Check which vehicles are available for mixing with medications.				
10. Identify child's psychosocial growth and developmental stage.				
Planning				
11. Plan a method of measuring medication accurately.				
12. Plan a method of making medication acceptable to child.				
13. Plan an approach to child that is appropriate to child's age and developmental level.				
14. Plan for a method of restraint if necessary. Include asking for help if more than one person will be needed to restrain.				
15. Determine what equipment will be needed.				
16. Wash your hands.				
17. Gather the equipment.				

Administering Medications to Infants and Children *(Continued)*	Unsat	Needs More Practice	Sat	Comments
Implementation				
18. Read the name of the medication to be given from record.				
19. Check the label on medication and take that medication from the shelf or drawer.				
20. Check label again, before pouring.				
21. Remove correct amount of medication for child's dosage.				
22. Check label again and return bottle to shelf or drawer.				
23. Place medication on cart.				
24. Place medication card or label on poured medication if not a unit dose.				
25. Approach and identify patient.				
26. Explain what you are going to do.				
27. Add appropriate planned actions related to: a. Making medication acceptable to child.				
b. Approaching child.				
c. Restraining as needed.				
28. Watch child take medication.				
29. Leave child in a comfortable position.				
30. Discard medication container.				
31. Wash your hands.				
Evaluation				
32. Evaluate according to the following criteria: a. Five rights maintained.				
b. Effects and side effects noted.				
Documentation				
33. Record accurately according to the policy of the facility. Include: a. Name of medication.				
b. Dosage.				
c. Route.				

Administering Medications to Infants and Children (Continued)	Unsat	Needs More Practice	Sat	Comments
d. Time of administration.				
e. Signature.				
34. Note successful methods of administration on Nursing Care Plan.				

Quiz

Short-Answer Questions

In questions 1 and 2, calculate the dosages.

1. Meperidine (Demerol) is ordered for a child who is 3 feet 11 inches tall and weighs 52 lb. The usual adult dosage is 50 mg. Find the body surface area and then calculate the safe dosage. _____

2. Penicillin G is ordered for a child of 48 lb. The usual adult dose is 600,000 units. Calculate the safe dose. _____

3. At what age can a child usually swallow a capsule or tablet? _____

4. Why is safety of dosage a particular concern for the pediatric patient?

   _____

5. Why is it unwise to ask the parent to restrain a child for a painful injection? _____

6. Why is it inappropriate to offer a 6-year-old child a choice of whether or not to take a medication? _____

7. What would you use to measure 0.4 ml of a liquid oral medication?

   _____

8. Tetracycline is ordered. The reference states that the usual dose is 25–50 mg/kg/day divided into four doses. The child weighs 32 kg. What is the safe dosage for 24 hours? What is the safe individual dose?

   a. _____

   b. _____

9. List four factors to be considered when deciding on a vehicle to mix with an oral medication.

   a. _____

   b. _____

   c. _____

   d. _____

10. Why would it be unwise to put a medication in an infant's bottle?

    a. _____

    b. _____

Module 53

Preparing and Maintaining Intravenous Infusions

Module Contents

Rationale for the Use of This Skill
Nursing Diagnoses
Equipment
  Fluid Containers
  Administration Sets
    Secondary Sets
    Safety Needles
    Extension Tubing
    In-Line Filters
    Controlled-Volume Sets
  IV Standards
  Extension Hanger
  Armboards
  Infusion Control Devices (ICDs)
    Controllers
    Pumps
Monitoring and Maintaining an Infusion
Procedure for Monitoring and Maintaining
    an Infusion
  Assessment
  Planning

  Implementation
  Evaluation
  Documentation
Regulating the Intravenous Infusion
Changing the Fluid Container and Tubing
  Assessment
  Planning
  Implementation
  Evaluation
  Documentation
Changing the Container Only
Changing a Gown over an IV
Discontinuing an IV
  Assessment
  Planning
  Implementation
  Evaluation
  Documentation
Troubleshooting IV Problems

Prerequisites

1. *Successful completion of the following modules:*

VOLUME 1

Module 1   An Approach to Nursing Skills
Module 2   Basic Infection Control
Module 3   Safety
Module 5   General Assessment Overview

406

Module 6   Documentation
Module 15 Intake and Output

VOLUME 2

Module 35 Sterile Technique
Module 49 Administering Oral Medications

2. *Satisfactory completion of the self-test on mathematics of dosages and solutions in Module 49, Administering Oral Medications. If you cannot meet this level of proficiency, you need additional practice in the mathematics of dosages and solutions. Many programmed texts are available for independent study.*

3. *Review of the anatomy and physiology of the vascular system*

Overall Objective

To maintain intravenous infusions correctly, with comfort and safety for patients.

Specific Learning Objectives

	Know Facts and Principles	Apply Facts and Principles	Demonstrate Ability	Evaluate Performance
1. *Equipment* *a. Fluid containers*	Describe two types of fluid containers. State rationale for checking fluid for clarity and sterility.		In the clinical setting, select correct fluid container and check for clarity and sterility.	Verify selection with instructor.
b. Administration sets	State purpose of each type of administration set.	Given a patient situation, identify type of administration set needed.	In the clinical setting, select correct administration set.	Verify selection with instructor.
2. *Monitoring and maintaining an infusion*	Describe phlebitis. Describe infiltration. List causes of obstruction of flow. List appropriate checks to be made when assessing IV.	Given a patient situation, differentiate between phlebitis and infiltration. Given a patient situation, identify problem that exists with IV.	In the clinical setting, make complete assessment of IV. In the clinical setting, determine correct action for problems identified. Chart assessment.	Verify adequacy of assessment with instructor. Verify decision with instructor.
3. *Regulating the flow*	State two methods of calculating correct drip rate.	Given a patient situation, identify whether IV must be regulated.	Calculate drip rate correctly. Regulate IV correctly.	Verify calculation with instructor.
4. *Removing and replacing gown*	Describe method for removing and replacing gown with IV in place.		In the practice or clinical setting, remove and replace gown with IV in place.	Check IV to be sure it is infusing properly when finished.
5. *Changing fluid containers and tubing*	State frequency for changing fluid container and tubing. State appropriate procedure for dressing IV site.		In the practice setting, change IV tubing, fluid container, and dressing correctly.	Evaluate own performance using Performance Checklist.
6. *Discontinuing intravenous infusion*	Describe procedure for discontinuing IV.		In the clinical setting, discontinue IV.	Check site for bleeding and inflammation. Evaluate performance with instructor.
7. *Documentation*	State what should be recorded regarding IV.		In the clinical setting, chart correctly regarding IVs.	Use Performance Checklist to check charting.

Learning Activities

1. Review the Specific Learning Objectives.
2. Read the section on intravenous fluid in Ellis and Nowlis, *Nursing: A Human Needs Approach,* or comparable material in another textbook.
3. Look up the module vocabulary terms in the Glossary.
4. Read through the module and mentally practice the skills.
5. In the practice setting:
   a. Examine the IV equipment. Identify each of the following:
      (1) Regular venosets
      (2) Microdrip (pediatric sets) and macrodrip sets. Differentiate between the two.
      (3) Secondary administration sets (piggybacks)
      (4) Extension tubing
      (5) In-line filters
      (6) Controlled-volume sets (Peditrol, Soluset, Volutrol)
      (7) IV standards
      (8) Fluid containers (bottles, plastic bags)
      (9) Any infusion control devices available
      (10) Armboards
   b. Read the directions on the package regarding how to set up the brand of equipment you will be using.
   c. Set up an IV line as if it were to be started. Pay particular attention to maintaining sterility.
   d. Attach the end of the IV line to another fluid container, so the fluid will run from the first container to the second. This will simulate an ongoing IV line.
   e. Regulate the drip rate by manual control or using an ICD.
      (1) To 32 drops/minute
      (2) To whatever rate would be needed to deliver the fluid remaining in the container in 4 hours. You will have to figure the drip rate. Consult the equipment container to identify the drops per ml delivered by the tubing.
   f. Change the fluid container only.
   g. Change the bottle and IV tubing and redress.
   h. Using a mannequin, remove and replace a gown with the IV in place.[1]
   i. Remove the IV from the mannequin's arm as if you were discontinuing the IV.
6. Practice documentation for the following situations:
   a. You have hung an IV, 1000 ml D_5W, to be given over 8 hours from 4:00 PM to 12:00 midnight.
   b. You are maintaining an IV, and it is the end of your shift. On the previous shift, 1000 ml D_5W was started. When your shift began, 100 ml had been given; 50 ml fluid remain. (Make up any observation data that would be needed.)
   c. You are carrying out an order to discontinue an IV. The entire amount, 500 ml normal saline, has been given.

Vocabulary

embolus
fluid overload
infiltration
infusion
intravenous
phlebitis
thrombophlebitis

[1] If you do not have a mannequin, consult with your instructor on improvising a substitute.

Preparing and Maintaining Intravenous Infusions

Rationale for the Use of This Skill

Intravenous infusions are used when patients need fluids, electrolytes, or nutritional supplements that cannot be taken orally. Such infusions are also used when continuous administration of intravenous medications is necessary.

Because the infusion provides direct access to the bloodstream, many hazards are involved in the procedure: it provides an optimum entry for infectious organisms; it can allow foreign material, including air, to be introduced and to act as emboli; both the equipment and the solution can irritate the tissue; and it can cause bleeding. It is the nurse's responsibility to guard against these dangers. Also, the fluid's rate of flow is critical: too rapid a flow can create a fluid overload of the circulatory system, resulting in death if not corrected. A flow that is too slow may deprive the patient of needed fluid. The nurse must monitor and maintain the correct infusion rate. It is also the nurse's responsibility to ensure that the correct fluid is administered, using the appropriate equipment.[2]

EQUIPMENT

Fluid Containers

Some fluid containers are glass bottles. *For the fluid to flow out of the bottle, there must be some kind of mechanism to allow air to enter the bottle.* This can be a vent incorporated into the bottle (Figure 53–1). If no air vent is in the bottle, there must be an air vent in the administration set. The air vent usually has a filter *that removes contaminants from the air entering the bottle.* Bottles are available in 50-ml and 100-ml sizes partially filled and in 150-, 250-, 500-, and 1000-ml sizes. The most common size is 1000 ml. *Fluid in containers, regardless of size, is comparable in cost,* so it is not a great saving to the patient to supply fluid from a small-volume container as an interim if a larger container is ordered but has not arrived on the unit.

Many IV fluids are now supplied in plastic containers (Figure 53–2). *Because the plastic container collapses as fluid is removed, no air vent is needed. This prevents nonsterile air from coming in contact with the IV fluid.*

Two types of plastic containers are flexible bags and semirigid bottles. Plastic bags have advantages

[2] You will note that rationale for action is emphasized throughout the module by the use of italics.

▶ *Nursing Diagnoses*

The major nursing diagnosis to keep in mind when preparing and maintaining intravenous infusions is High Risk for Injury. Patients can be injured by an intravenous infusion given at an incorrect rate. They can also be injured by the omission of an additive or by the administration of an incorrect infusion or by an incorrect additive in the infusion.

Patients are also at high risk for injuries related to tissue irritation from the equipment and/or the solution. Although this nursing diagnosis will usually not appear on the Nursing Care Plan, it applies to every situation in which a patient is receiving an intravenous infusion.

A second nursing diagnosis related to preparing and maintaining intravenous infusions is High Risk for Infection. Patients are at risk for infection related to the disruption of skin integrity inherent in the presence of an intravenous infusion. Fluid Volume Excess is a third possibility, usually related to too much fluid over a brief period of time or perhaps related to an incorrect infusion rate.

in terms of storage and disposal. Semirigid bottles collapse more evenly and are easier to handle. *Plastic containers have a characteristic that is of special concern to nurses. They can absorb some types of ink and transport the ink to the fluid.* For this reason it is appropriate to do all marking on tapes that can be adhered to the container and not to use any type of ink marker on the plastic. *To minimize the potential for infection and possible complications,* the nurse should closely inspect all containers before administration. Check for leaks, cracks, damaged caps, particulate material, and expiration date (Intravenous Nurses Society, 1990).

Another concern is the fact that *some medications or additives in IV solutions adhere to the inner surface of a plastic container, so the patient does not receive an accurate amount of the additive.* For this reason, IV solutions with these substances arrive from the pharmacy in glass bottles.

Plastic containers come in the same variety of sizes as glass containers.

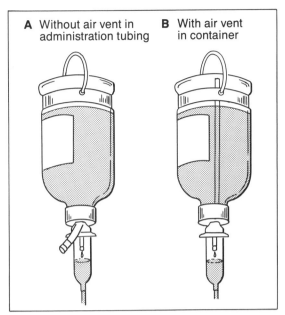

Figure 53–1 Glass IV fluid containers. If no air vent is in the bottle, there must be an air vent in the administration set.

Administration Sets

The conventional administration set consists of plastic tubing with a plastic spike that is inserted into the fluid container. The spike must be kept sterile. Below the spike is a drip chamber, *which allows the rate of fluid administration to be monitored by counting the drops falling into the chamber.* If an infusion control device (ICD) is used, the drop rate within the drip chamber may be monitored by a sensor. The pump cartridge serves as a volumeter, so that the device delivers a programmed volume within a specified period of time (see the section on ICDs, which follows).

Intravenous tubing with an integral air vent is shown in Figure 53–3. Nonvented tubing to be used with a plastic or glass container that has an airway looks much the same, except there is no air vent on the side of the drip chamber. Vented tubing may be used on a container that has an airway or on a plastic container. The fluid will still flow, although the plastic container may not collapse evenly *because of the air in the container.* A ventless glass bottle will not empty if nonvented tubing is used. Special tubing, some with an additional chamber which is like a cartridge, is used with volume-controlled infusion devices. Review the procedure for the type(s) used in your facility.

If the flow rate is not monitored by an ICD, it is usually controlled by a roller clamp. A screw clamp is also found on some types of tubing, but its primary purpose is to turn the flow on or off. *It does not provide an accurate way to control a flow rate manually.*

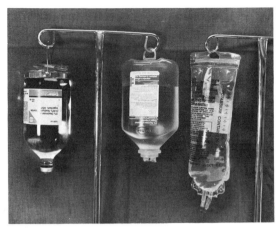

Figure 53–2 IV fluid containers. **A:** Glass bottle. **B:** Semirigid plastic bottle. **C:** Flexible plastic bag. (*Courtesy Ivan Ellis*)

The syringe tip (male adapter end of the tubing) fits into the hub of the needle in the vein. Most sets have one or more soft rubber entry ports that reseal after puncture by a needle. These ports are used to inject medications into the IV line. *If any other part of the plastic is punctured with a needle, a leak will result.*

Administration sets are constructed so the orifice in the drip chamber delivers a predictable number of drops for each milliliter of fluid. The most common sets are called *macrodrip sets.* These deliver 10–20 drops/ml (cc)[3] (see Figure 53–3). Sets vary, so consult the manufacturer's package for a correct figure for the delivery rate. Remember that this figure is correct for regular, water-type fluids. *When viscous fluids such as those containing amino acids and fats are given, the number of drops can vary. Because of this, most facilities use an infusion control device to deliver these solutions.* (The drop factor for an individual set is usually given on the box supplied with the product.)

Most manufacturers also supply *microdrip sets* (Figure 53–4). These sets deliver 60 drops/ml and can be identified by the fine metal orifice in the drip chamber.

Blood administration sets are characterized by a larger lumen, which delivers fewer drops per milliliter, and a large built-in filter in the drip chamber, which removes any clots or precipitates in the blood (see Module 57, Administering Blood and Blood Products).

Secondary Sets. These sets are designed to allow more than one fluid container to be hung at the same

[3] See Table 49–2, Equivalencies, in Module 49, Administering Oral Medications.

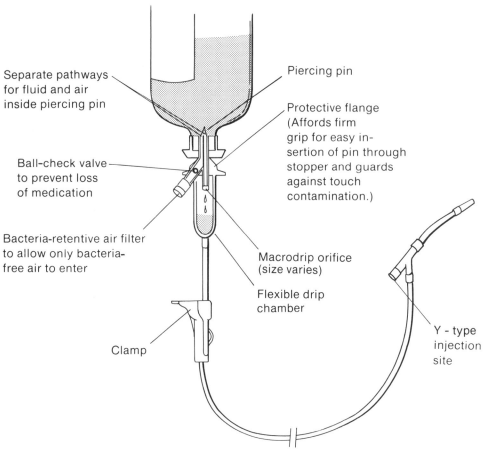

Separate pathways for fluid and air inside piercing pin

Ball-check valve to prevent loss of medication

Bacteria-retentive air filter to allow only bacteria-free air to enter

Clamp

Piercing pin

Protective flange (Affords firm grip for easy insertion of pin through stopper and guards against touch contamination.)

Macrodrip orifice (size varies)

Flexible drip chamber

Y - type injection site

Figure 53–3 Regular (macrodrip) IV administration set. Note that the airway is in the set.
(*Courtesy Abbott Laboratories, Chicago, Illinois*)

time, in one of three ways. Using a *tandem setup,* the second container is attached to the first by the secondary set. The fluid container on the secondary set (farthest from the patient) empties first, *because this is where the air enters and because it is higher.*

The second method is the *piggyback setup.* The secondary set is used to attach the second bottle to the primary set's tubing. Using the piggyback setup, either bottle can be made to run by shutting off the tubing to one container above the junction and keeping the tubing to the other container open (Figure 53–5).

The piggyback setup is most commonly used to deliver small volumes of fluid containing medications. In this situation, both lines are left open and the piggyback container is hung higher than the original container. The higher container runs in first. When that container is empty, a special valve at the piggy-

back entry port allows the lower container to start running, and the piggyback line no longer runs.

Two containers can also be hung at the same time by using a *Y-type administration set* (Figure 53–6). When both arms of the Y are open, the container with the fluid at a higher level empties first, and then the other container empties. The Y set can also be used to alternate solutions.

If the tubing does not contain a special stop valve for the container that empties first, the infusion must be closely monitored. The branch to the first-emptying container must be turned off while fluid still remains in the tube. *If air is allowed to enter one arm of the Y, it will be pulled into the fluid stream coming from the second bottle and could cause a significant air embolus.*

Safety Needles. Special needles that protect the staff from accidental sticks (''needle-lock'' devices)

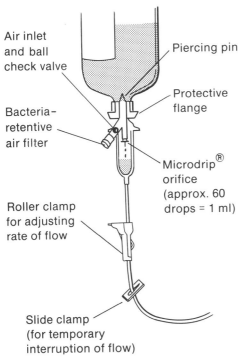

Air inlet and ball check valve

Piercing pin

Protective flange

Bacteria-retentive air filter

Microdrip® orifice (approx. 60 drops = 1 ml)

Roller clamp for adjusting rate of flow

Slide clamp (for temporary interruption of flow)

Figure 53–4 Microdrip® administration set. Note the fine metal orifice in the drip chamber.
(*Courtesy Abbott Laboratories, Chicago, Illinois*)

are available for use when attaching secondary lines. The needle is surrounded with rigid clear plastic which slides over the injection port, guides the needle into the injection port, and secures the needle in place (Figure 53–7).

Extension Tubing. Extension tubing (Figure 53–8) is a length of IV tubing with a male adapter on one end and a female adapter on the other, so it can be attached to the main set to create longer tubing. Some extension tubing has a clamp. Extension tubing is often added *to allow a patient greater mobility.*

In-Line Filters. In-Line filters (Figure 53–9) are sometimes used *to guard against particulate matter and bacteria entering IV fluids, and they also trap small air bubbles.* The filters are often an integral part of the tubing and are positioned near the end that connects the tubing and the needle. They look like they contain white cotton. When flushing the IV tubing, always thoroughly saturate the filter with solution *in order to obtain a steady flow of fluid.*

Controlled-Volume Sets. Controlled-volume administration sets (Figure 53–10) have a 100- to 250-ml chamber, which is attached just below the fluid container. The drip chamber is below this chamber.

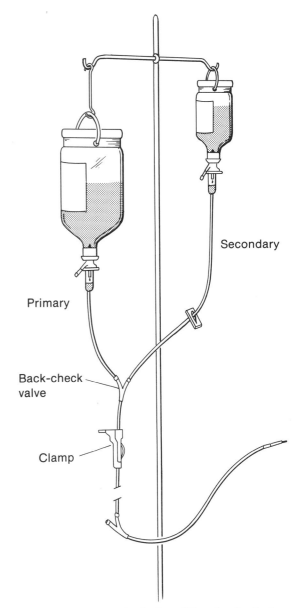

Secondary

Primary

Back-check valve

Clamp

Figure 53–5 Secondary piggyback set. When the piggyback container is empty, a special valve at the piggyback entry port allows the lower container to start running again.
(*Courtesy Abbott Laboratories, Chicago, Illinois*)

These sets usually deliver a microdrip, or 60 drops/ml. Some controlled-volume administration sets deliver a macrodrip, or regular drip, at 15 drops/ml. The package should be checked to make sure you know the correct drop factor. Controlled-volume sets are also used when medication must be added to a limited fluid volume. A newer device, primarily for pediatric use, is the Benzing retrograde set, which delivers a measured dosage of drug and at the same time displaces an equal amount of maintenance so-

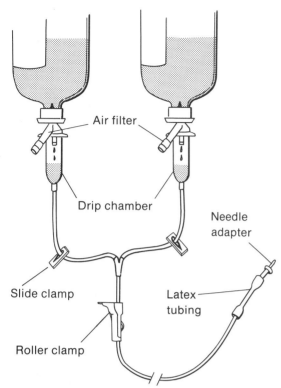

Figure 53–6 Y-type administration set. When both arms of the Y are open, the container with the fluid at a higher level empties first.
(*Courtesy Abbott Laboratories, Chicago, Illinois*)

lution from the IV line (Zenk, 1986). More common brands of controlled-volume sets are Peditrol, Soluset, and Volutrol.

IV Standards

IV standards (poles or stands) can be attached to a bed, placed on casters on the floor, or suspended from the ceiling with chains or hooks (Figure 53–11). *The height of the standard affects the flow rate. The higher the standard, the greater the pressure and the faster the rate.*

Extension Hanger

Various metal wires or plastic hooks may be used to hang one bottle on an IV standard lower than the other. The higher bottle then flows in first (see Figure 53–5).

Armboards

Commercially produced armboards often consist of a padded flat or molded board. Disposable armboards of heavy cardboard material are also available (Figure 53–12).

Armboards are used infrequently, *since they interfere with the motion of the wrist and/or elbow joint. Also, hand veins are preferred for the site of IV needles. The veins in the antecubital fossa are reserved for drawing blood and other essential tests.* Occasionally, however, *when a patient has hand veins that cannot be used or is extremely restless or confused,* an armboard is used to immobilize the needle site. Although armboards come in various lengths, it is best if you use the shortest board to accomplish the task, *so that maximum mobility can be maintained.* If the need for an armboard arises and none is available, you can improvise with cardboard padded with towels.

Infusion Control Devices (ICDs)

Hospitals are increasing their use of ICDs, *because these devices provide safer intravenous therapy for patients*

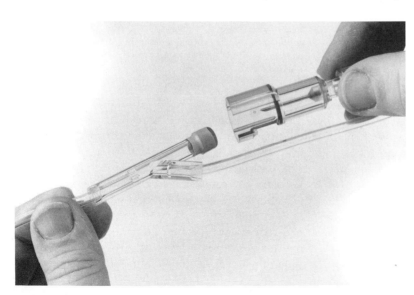

Figure 53–7 Safety needles. The needle is surrounded with rigid clear plastic, which slides over the injection port, guides the needle into the injection port, and secures the needle in place.

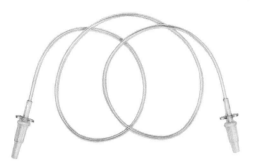

Figure 53–8 Extension tubing. Extension tubing is often added to allow patients greater mobility.
(*Courtesy C. R. Bard, Inc., Murray Hill, New Jersey*)

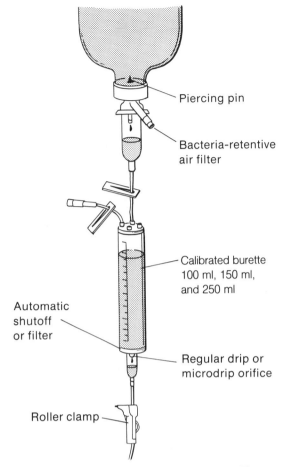

Figure 53–10 Controlled-volume administration set. These sets are often used when medication must be added to a limited fluid volume or for administering fluids to children.
(*Courtesy Abbott Laboratories, Chicago, Illinois*)

and save valuable staff time. Since more than two dozen manufacturers are producing ICDs, you will have to investigate the types used in your facility and follow the specific instructions for use (Koszuta, 1984). For purposes of this module, we will discuss these devices in general terms.

An infusion control device is most frequently used when the IV fluid contains a medication and a precise rate of administration is necessary to maintain a therapeutic blood level, when the fluid contains an additive that might have adverse effects if given too rapidly (such as a high concentration of glucose or amino acids), or when the patient is very sensitive to the volume administered. Two types of devices are used to regulate the flow rate of an intravenous infusion—controllers and pumps. Regardless of which is used, it is essential for the nurse to know that when the tubing is released from

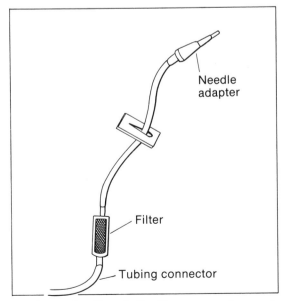

Figure 53–9 In-line filters. In-line filters are sometimes used to guard against particulate matter and bacteria entering IV fluids.

the machine, it must be manually regulated by using the clamp. The roller clamp is totally open when the machine is operating, and if it is not adjusted when the tubing is released, *the patient receives a bolus of solution.*

Both controllers and pumps can be either volumetric or nonvolumetric. *Volumetric* devices deliver a specific desired volume over a long period of time. An example is the administration of TPN (total parenteral nutrition). Devices that are *nonvolumetric* are designed to deliver a constant drop rate over a short period of time. One example is the administration of medications given to patients with heart irregularities or seriously low blood pressure. Studies show that nonvolumetric devices are less accurate than volumetric ones, *because the drop size of different solutions can vary* (Koszuta, 1984).

Controllers. The least complex type is one that regulates the rate in drops per minute. Many different

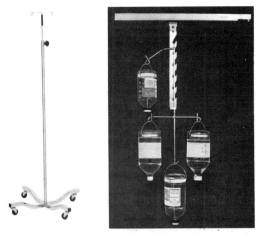

Figure 53–11 IV standards. IV poles and stands can be attached to a bed, placed on casters on the floor, or suspended from the ceiling with chains or hooks.
(*Courtesy American Hospital Supply Corp., McGaw Park, Illinois*)

brands of controllers are available (Figure 53–13). This type of device has a drop counter and a mechanism for applying pressure to the tubing. It is set for the desired number of drops per minute. Some models contain a calculator. With these models the amount of milliliters to be delivered per hour is set, and then the machine calculates and sets the correct number of drops per minute. After the device is set up, you should time the drops for a minute to make sure the number of drops delivered per minute is the same as what is set. If the device is inaccurate, it will need to be serviced. If this is impossible at the time, the setting will have to be adjusted *so the actual drop rate is correct even if the setting appears to be incorrect.*

In the controller, gravity is responsible for the pressure in the tubing. Changing the height of the fluid container changes the pressure and thus the flow. If the IV infil-

trates, the flow will stop, *because the pressure of gravity is less than the tissue pressure.* This feature makes the controller the preferred device when the fluid contains a medication that could cause tissue damage if infiltration occurred.

The controller can deliver a constant rate of flow but will not necessarily deliver a precise volume of flow, because variations in IV tubing and fluid viscosity affect the size of the drop. This feature makes it appropriate for situations where rate of flow is important for titrating medication dosage but the exact volume of fluid delivered is not critical.

Pumps. There are three types of pumps: syringe, peristaltic, and cassette. *Syringe pumps* are designed to deliver measured doses of medications and are discussed in Module 54, Administering Intravenous Medications. *Peristaltic pumps* deliver IV solutions by a squeezing action on the tubing. *Cassette pumps* collect a small, specified amount of solution in a reservoir and then deliver that volume. *Cassette pumps require special tubing,* which makes them more expensive to use than controllers. Pumps are set for milliliters per hour, and the fluid is then delivered at that rate. *Because of their high degree of accuracy in volume administered,* these devices are best suited to situations where the volume administered is critical, such as in the infant or for total parenteral nutrition (TPN).

Pressure is provided by a mechanism within the system rather than by gravity. This positive pressure allows the fluid to be administered into an arterial line where pressure is needed to overcome the arterial blood pressure. The same pressure is a disadvantage when infiltration occurs. *The machine can continue to pump fluid into the tissue, causing an extensive infiltration if the patient is not assessed frequently.*

All pumps have multiple alarm systems that notify you if the infusion is blocked, if air is in the system, or if the desired infusion volume has been reached. You should check the manufacturer's directions for specific information on operating the pumps in your facility (see Figure 53–13). Newer infusion control devices include one that is a combination pump and controller (the user chooses the function desired) and a pump that delivers infusions through two separate channels with separate controls for each line.

MONITORING AND MAINTAINING AN INFUSION

An important nursing responsibility is to monitor an IV infusion and to maintain its flow. When monitor-

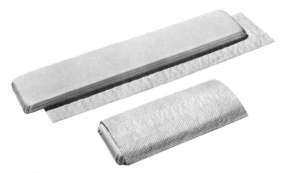

Figure 53–12 Armboards. It is best if you use the shortest board available to accomplish the task, so that maximum mobility can be maintained.
(*Courtesy American Hospital Supply Corp., McGaw Park, Illinois*)

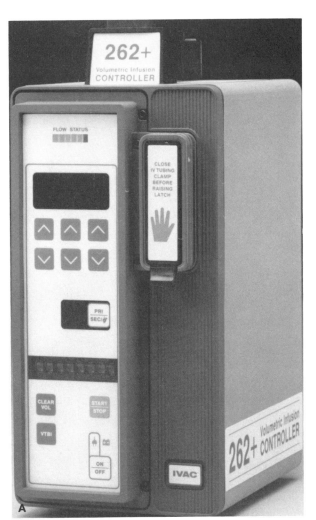
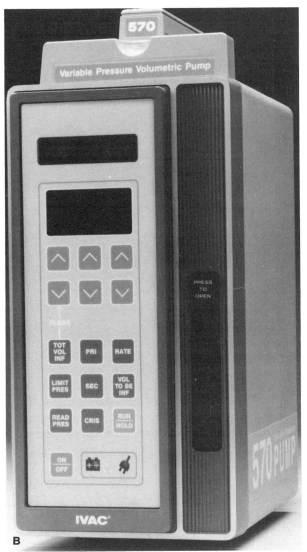

Figure 53–13 Infusion controller (**A**) and infusion pump. Hospitals are increasing their use of infusion control devices because these devices provide safer IV therapy for patients and save valuable staff time. (*Courtesy IVAC® Corporation, San Diego, California*)

ing, the nurse is looking for signs and symptoms of phlebitis (or thrombophlebitis), infiltration, and obstruction of flow. Maintaining the infusion includes taking actions to assure patency, adjusting the rate, changing the site dressing, and changing the fluid container and tubing.

Phlebitis—inflammation of the vein—can be present with or without a clot in the vein. When there is a clot, the condition is technically thrombophlebitis. In actual practice the two terms are used interchangeably. Phlebitis is characterized by redness, warmth, pain, and swelling at the IV site. It seems to occur more rapidly when plastic needles rather than metal needles

are used, when electrolytes (especially potassium) are in the solution, and when antibiotics are being administered through the IV, and results from direct irritation of the vessel. It has been shown that changing the dressing and tubing every 48 hours *decreases the incidence of phlebitis, which suggests that microorganisms play a role in the development of this condition* (Centers for Disease Control, 1983a). Some facilities have extended the use of tubing to 72 hours based on review of their own incidence of complications. Follow the policy in your facility.

When phlebitis occurs, the course of action is determined by the *degree* of the problem. Table 53–1

Table 53–1 Evaluation and Treatment of IV Phlebitis

Assessment Grading Criteria	Interventions
1+ Pain at site*	**1.** Assess severity of phlebitis.
2+ Pain at site and/or along vein Mild erythema localized at site	**2.** Discontinue IV catheter.* **3.** Apply warm pack to site assessed 3+ or greater.
3+ Pain at site and/or along vein Erythematous at site and streaking along vein	**4.** Determine if drug/fluid is causative factor of phlebitis. Arrange for drug dilution or rate change, if appropriate. **5.** 3+ and 4+: Initiate QA[1] Problem Record
4+ Pain and severe erythematous streak along vein Palpable cord or induration of vein area	**6.** 4+: Report problem to physician; obtain order for K-Pad® treatment. Notify unit RN if they are to be involved in treatment plan.

* 1+ Phlebitis—Intervention steps 3 and 4 may be initiated first to determine if mild pain relieved without removing IV catheter; reassess site in 1–2 h.
[1] Quality assurance
Courtesy Swedish Hospital Medical Center

shows one method of scaling degrees of phlebitis along with appropriate interventions.

Infiltration is caused by the leaking of IV fluid into the surrounding tissue. Pallor, swelling, coolness, pain at the site, and usually a diminished IV flow rate are all indications of infiltration. It occurs most often with metal needles that have become dislodged and have penetrated a vein wall. It can also occur around a plastic needle that has been in place for an extended period. An infiltrated IV must be discontinued. Degrees of infiltration can also be scaled. Table 53–2 shows a method of scaling infiltration along with corresponding interventions.

Decreased flow rate or cessation of fluid flow are indications of obstruction. Obstruction may be caused by a clot forming over the needle lumen, by particulate matter clogging the filters, by the lumen of the needle being positioned against the wall of the vein, by kinking or pressure on the tubing, or by a position of the arm that occludes the vessel proximal to the IV site. The source of the obstruction should be located and corrected (see Table 53–3).

The entire infusion should be checked systematically each time the nurse is at the patient's bedside. In addition, IVs should be routinely checked every 4 hours for rate of flow and level of fluid. Insertion sites should be routinely checked every 8 hours for redness, swelling, temperature changes, and patient comfort (Centers for Disease Control, 1983a).

PROCEDURE FOR MONITORING AND MAINTAINING AN INFUSION

Assessment

1. Identify the patient *to be sure you are performing the procedure for the correct patient.*
2. Review the entire system for obvious problems.

Table 53–2 Evaluation and Treatment of IV Infiltration

Assessment Criteria	Interventions
1+ Small area of swelling at or above IV site	**1.** Determine if infiltrated fluid/medication is a vesicant; refer to tx of extravazation.
2+ Area of swelling around IV site > 1" and < 2"	**2.** Assess severity of infiltrate; discontinue IV catheter.
3+ Area of swelling > 2"; involves one surface or extremity Skin cool over swollen area	**3.** Grade 3+ and 4+: Elevate extremity on two pillows. **4.** Grade 4+: Notify unit RN and initiate QA[1] Problem Record.
4+ Gross infiltrate involving circumference of extremity Skin very tight and cold to touch	

[1] Quality assurance
Courtesy Swedish Hospital Medical Center

Table 53–3 Troubleshooting IV Problems

Problem	Action	Rationale
1. IV Off Schedule	Calculate rate to finish IV over remaining time. If new rate is over 3 ml/min for adult or drastically changed (more than 20% increase), consider patient's condition and consult with physician before increasing rate.	a. Fluid is absorbed and utilized over time. Too rapid infusion will simply result in high urine output. If a patient's cardiovascular system is inadequate, fluid overload may occur. b. If fluid is behind schedule, infusing at original rate will result in inadequate fluid intake for 24-h period. c. Calculating new rate provides adequate fluids in an evenly distributed pattern. d. Exact rate may be critical to patient and should be determined by physician.
2. Incorrect Solution	Slow rate to minimum while initiating change to correct solution. Assess patient. Follow incident procedure for hospital. Notify physician.	You want to minimize amount of incorrect solution given without losing access to the vein. In some instances the type of solution is critical, and laboratory tests may be necessary to determine action.
3. Tubing Kinked	Straighten tubing and check flow rate again.	Kinked tubing slows flow rate. When kink is removed, rate may increase significantly.
4. Flow Stopped	Take the following steps to reestablish flow: a. Look for obstruction of tubing and correct if present. b. Open regulator completely, move to new position, and regulate again if flow begins. c. Reposition arm. d. Place bottle lower than needle to see if blood flows back, which would indicate tubing is patent. e. Gently raise needle hub. If this starts flow, support hub with cotton ball or gauze 2 × 2. f. Pinch off tubing close to arm above soft rubber section of tube. Then squeeze soft rubber firmly.	a. Pressure of arm, side rails, and other equipment can obstruct IV tubing. b. Changes in position or "fatigue" of plastic may alter flow rate. c. Flexing or twisting the forearm can obstruct vein proximal to IV site, stopping flow. d. Pressure in vein causes blood backflow when pressure in tubing is reduced. e. Bevel of needle may be against side of vein, obstructing flow. f. Slight pressure may force wall of vein away from needle. It may also release small clot. (A clot small enough to be dislodged in this manner is small enough not to be of danger as an embolus.)

(continued)

Table 53–3 *(Continued)*

Problem	Action	Rationale
	g. Obtain sterile needle and syringe. Insert into injection port closest to needle. Pinch off tubing above syringe and aspirate. Then open flow.	**g.** Aspiration can remove clot or clogged fluid. (Clot or clog moves into syringe and is removed, so it is not hazardous to patient.)
5. Bubbles in Tubing	**a.** For a few small bubbles high in tubing: (1) Turn off flow. (2) Stretch tubing taut downward. (3) Flick tubing with fingernail. Bubbles will flow up to drip chamber. (4) Start flow and regulate.	**a.** Air is lighter than fluid and therefore rises.
	b. For large amounts of air high in tubing: (1) Turn off flow. (2) Insert sterile open needle into injection port close to air. (3) Open flow slowly. When air reaches needle it will bubble out. (4) Start flow and regulate.	**b.** Because air is lighter than fluid, when it reaches opening it rises out of tubing.
	c. For air low in tubing, below last port: (1) Turn off flow. (2) Obtain sterile needle and syringe. (3) Insert into port closest to patient. (4) Pinch tubing distal to port to close it off. (5) Aspirate air into syringe. Blood will return into tubing. (6) Start flow rapidly to flush out blood. (7) Regulate flow.	**c.** Aspiration creates suction, pulling contents of tubing—including air—into syringe.
6. Drip Chamber Full of Fluid, so Drip is Not Visible	For flexible drip chamber: **a.** Pinch off tubing. **b.** Invert container. **c.** Squeeze fluid back into container. **d.** Hang up bottle. **e.** Release tubing.	With drip chamber full, it is not possible to monitor fluid rate. When fluid is squeezed into container, air at top of bottle can enter drip chamber.
7. Solution Falls Below Drip Chamber and Fluid Container is Empty	**a.** If tubing is scheduled to be changed: (1) Slow drip rate. (2) Follow directions for changing fluid container and tubing.	**a.** Prevent IV from clotting off.
	b. If tubing does not need to be changed: (1) Obtain next fluid container, syringe and needles. (2) Connect tubing in use to new container. (3) Fill drip chamber. (4) Aspirate column of air through port on tubing. (5) Regulate flow rate.	**b.** Aspiration creates suction, pulling contents of tubing—including air—into syringe.

3. Check the IV container.
   a. Note the date and time.
   b. Is it the correct solution?
   c. Which number bottle is it?
   d. What time will it be finished?

4. Check the drip chamber.
   a. Is the drip chamber filled to an appropriate level?
   b. Is it dripping?
   c. Is the rate correct?

5. Check the tubing over its entire length for kinks or obstructions.
6. Check the IV site for signs of phlebitis or infiltration:
   a. Skin color and temperature.
   b. Pain.
   c. Swelling.
7. If an armboard is being used, remove it periodically to move the arm or leg or *to examine for skin irritation and circulatory impairment.* Then replace the armboard.
8. Identify the specific problem present.

Planning
9. Using the chart on troubleshooting IV problems, determine which course of action you will take.

Implementation
10. Carry out the action planned.

Evaluation
11. Evaluate, using the following criteria:
    a. Any problem present is identified and corrected.
    b. The correct intravenous infusion is running at the correct rate.

Documentation
12. On the flow sheet, note that the IV is running on time, the rate at which it is running, and the appearance of the site.
13. If any problems were identified and corrected, note those on the nurses' notes or on the flow sheet, as prescribed by your facility.

REGULATING THE INTRAVENOUS INFUSION

The intravenous drip rate must be regulated in drops per minute to provide the ordered quantity of fluid over the ordered period. Many manufacturers provide tables that give this information, but the nurse should know how to figure the rate when tables are not available. Below we give two methods of calculation. Try both and determine which is easier for you.

To calculate the rate using either method, you need three items of information:

1. Volume of fluid to be infused
2. Length of time this volume of fluid is to run
3. "Drop factor" (number of drops per milliliter) for the administration set, which is commonly found on the package. (Most administration sets provide 10 gtt/ml, 15 gtt/ml, or 20 gtt/ml. Microdrip sets and most controlled-volume sets provide 60 gtt/ml.)

Method 1

Use the following formula:

$$\frac{\text{volume (in ml)} \times \text{drop factor}}{\text{time in minutes (hours} \times 60)} = \frac{\text{gtt}}{\text{min}}$$

The drops per minute is the correct drip rate.

Method 2

1. Divide the total volume by the number of hours to obtain the *milliliters per hour.*

$$\frac{\text{volume}}{\text{hours}} = \text{ml/h}$$

2. Divide the milliliters per hour by 60 to obtain the *milliliters per minute.*

$$\frac{\text{ml/h}}{60} = \text{ml/min}$$

3. Multiply the milliliters per minute by the drop factor to obtain the *drops per minute.*

$$\text{ml/min} \times \text{drop factor} = \text{gtt/min}$$

Note: The drop rate of microdrip sets, which deliver 60 drops/ml, is always equal to the number of milliliters per hour. Try a few examples using the methods above to check this.

If you are regulating an infusion that is being controlled with an ICD, consult the instructions for the specific device. Most ICDs have to be programmed in the reset mode. Then turn to "operate." If you are using an ICD set in ml/h, use step 1 of Method 2 above to calculate the rate.

CHANGING THE FLUID CONTAINER AND TUBING

Assessment
1. Check the physician's orders. Pay particular attention to the type of fluid and solution concentration and to the infusion rate. Many abbreviations are used; three of the most common are for concentrations of dextrose and/or saline.

5% dextrose in water = D_5W or 5% D/W

5% dextrose in normal saline = D_5N/S or 5% D/NS

half-strength normal saline = ½N/S

If you do not understand the orders, be sure to ask.

2. Check to see when the tubing was last changed. *The Centers for Disease Control currently recommend that all IV tubings be changed every 48–72 hours, to decrease the incidence of phlebitis at the site* (see Monitoring and Maintaining an Infusion, earlier in this module). *Containers are changed every 24 hours.*

Planning

3. Wash your hands *for infection control.*
4. Select the equipment. Obtain the correct fluid, using the three checks. Select an infusion set. Consider the amount of fluid to be administered and the rate. *If a very slow rate is needed, a microdrip set will provide more accurate regulation. If medications are to be given, a set with multiple injection ports may be needed. For an infant or child, the use of a controlled-volume set is usually routine.* Extension tubing may be needed *to give the patient more mobility.* Tape will be needed *to tape the line in place.* Gloves will be needed *to protect the nurse from exposure to blood.*

Implementation

5. Set up the equipment.
   a. Examine the fluid container against a light *to check for cracks (if glass), cloudiness, particulate matter, or other evidence of contamination.* If in doubt, do not use the fluid. Select another container and save the potentially contaminated container to be returned to the pharmacy or the central supply department. Check a plastic container for leakage by squeezing. Dampness on the outside of plastic bags is expected and is condensation from the sterilization procedure.
   b. Open the package containing the tubing. Be sure to maintain the sterility of the connectors. If the connectors are covered with plastic caps, leave the plastic caps in place until you are ready to connect the tubing. Check the drop factor of the tubing.

   c. Open the entry area of the fluid container according to the manufacturer's directions. There should be evidence that the container was sealed, which certifies sterility. Be careful not to contaminate the entry port.
   d. Follow the manufacturer's directions about cleaning the entry port with an alcohol swab. Most fluid containers are sealed, so the entry area is sterile and does not need to be cleaned if not touched.
   e. Close the regulator on the tubing, *so you do not inadvertently fill the tubing with air and spill fluid on the floor.*
   f. Insert the spike into the fluid container through the correct entry port.
   g. Invert the container with the tubing hanging down. It is convenient to be able to hang the container on a hook or standard at this time.
   h. For a flexible-plastic drip chamber, squeeze the chamber to fill it half full with fluid. A rigid drip chamber usually fills when the container is inverted.
   i. Hold the end of the tubing over a basin or a waste container. Open the regulator gradually and allow the tubing to fill. If the end of the tubing is tightly capped, the cap must be carefully removed *to allow the tubing to fill.* Allow a small amount of fluid to flow out of the line *to clear any particulate matter in the tubing.* Replace the cap when the tubing is full. Be sure all large bubbles are eliminated. *Very tiny bubbles that together do not constitute a large bubble cannot cause an embolus that is dangerous,* so don't be alarmed if a small bubble is inadvertently administered. But it is not wise practice knowingly to administer *any* air.
6. Identify the patient *to be sure you are performing the procedure for the correct patient.* Place a towel under the arm *to protect the linen.*
7. Hang the new container on the standard beside the current container.
8. Remove the tape and dressing on the IV site to expose the hub of the needle. Be gentle and careful. Do not pull at the needle *or you may dislodge it.*
9. Examine the needle site for signs of swelling or inflammation.
10. Put on gloves *to protect yourself from exposure to blood.*
11. When the hub is exposed, shut off the IV flow.

12. Hold the hub of the needle firmly and remove the tubing with a twisting motion.
13. Continue holding the hub of the needle with one hand while you remove the cap of the new tubing and insert it firmly into the hub with the other.
14. Immediately start the new IV infusion at a slow drip rate.
15. Redress the site according to your hospital's procedure. If your facility has no procedure, use the following:
    a. Clean the site with a povidone-iodine swab (acu-dyne, Betadine).
    b. Apply a small amount of water-soluble iodine ointment to the needle site. In some facilities an antibiotic ointment, such as Neosporin, is used.
    c. Some facilities place a folded 2×2 gauze square *under* the needle *so the site can be observed. This also protects the skin from the needle and stabilizes the needle at the correct angle.*
    d. Remove gloves.
    e. Make an occlusive, or airtight, seal over the dressing with tape or OpSite.
    f. Write the date and time dressed directly on the tape *to facilitate record keeping.* The date and time of *starting* the IV may also be recorded on the tape each time the dressing is changed. Initial the recording.

In some facilities a transparent plastic film is used to dress the IV insertion site. The film is applied so the needle hub is outside the dressing and does not have to be removed to change the tubing or examine the site. This type of dressing usually remains in place until it becomes loose, until the IV site needs to be changed, or for 1 week.

16. Regulate the IV to the ordered infusion rate.
17. Mark the container at the beginning level of the fluid with the time the IV was started. Note the time the fluid is to be completed at the bottom of the container. Mark appropriate intervals (such as the fluid level at 2-hour intervals). *This information facilitates checking the rate of the IV.* You may mark directly on glass bottles with a large marking pen. You may also place a piece of tape the length of the bottle and mark on that. Commercial tapes are made for this purpose. With a plastic container, remember that you must mark only on a tape *to prevent absorption of ink into the fluid.* This step may be completed when you first obtain the container.

18. Dispose of the used equipment.
19. Wash your hands.

Evaluation
20. Evaluate, using the following criteria:
    a. Tubing and fluid container are changed with no contamination.
    b. Dressing is replaced and dated.
    c. The correct intravenous infusion is running at the correct rate.

Documentation
21. For charting purposes, IVs can be treated like three other categories: (1) medications, (2) fluids, and (3) assessment.
    a. Like medications, the charting must include the exact time started and stopped and the exact contents in detail.
    b. Like fluids, careful records of fluid quantities must be recorded, often on the intake and output worksheet, to facilitate assessing the patient's fluid balance.
    c. Like assessment, the patient's response is noted.

Some charts contain a separate sheet on which IVs are recorded (Figure 53–14), but the fluid quantities are still entered on the intake and output sheet. Another option for hospitals is a parenteral therapy record (Figure 53–15). On other charts IVs are recorded with medications and treatments. Most hospitals number each bottle sequentially *to facilitate accuracy in administration and record keeping.*

When complete tubing is changed or when the IV site is redressed, a notation is made on a separate flow sheet, on the IV sheet, or on the nurses' notes.

CHANGING THE CONTAINER ONLY

1. Wash your hands *for infection control.*
2. Take the new fluid container to the bedside stand after using the three checks to verify the fluid.
3. Identify the patient *to be sure you are performing the procedure for the correct patient.*
4. Remove the cover from the entry port and place the container on the bedside stand.
5. Turn off the IV flow.
6. Invert the old fluid container.
7. Remove the tubing connector. Be sure not to touch the tubing end.
8. Insert the tubing into the new container.
9. Invert the new container and hang it on the IV standard.

(text continues on page 427)

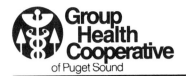
Group Health Cooperative of Puget Sound

PARENTERAL FLUID RECORD

DATE/ TIME INITIAL	BOTTLE NO.	VOLUME/SOLUTION/ADDITIVES	FLOW RATE	FLOW RATE CHANGE TIME/INIT	AMOUNT INFUSED			TIME BOTTLE COMPLETED/ INITIAL
					NITE	DAY	EVE.	
1/4/95 1100 PB	1	1000 ml LR	100 ml/ hr.			300	700	2100 EN
1/4/95 2100 EN	2	1000 ml D5NS	125 ml/ hr.				125	0500 CS
					875			
1/5/95 0500 CS	3	1000 ml LR	50 ml/ hr.		50	400	400	0100 CS
					150			
1/6/95 0100 CS	4	1000 ml D5NS	50 ml/ hr.	0800 100 ml PB	250	750		1400 PB

Initial/Signature

PB P. Benitez RN

EN E. Norton RN

CS C. Smith RN

Figure 53–14 Parenteral fluid record. Most facilities number each fluid container sequentially to facilitate accuracy in administration and record keeping.

424

Date and Time	TUBING	CHANGE			DEVICE		Initials	AMOUNT-SOLUTION-ADDITIVES (number consecutively)	Rate	SHIFT TOTALS		Solu' Time	DC'd Amount Absorb.
	MACRO SET	MICRO SET	PUMP SET	BLOOD SET	PUMP	CONTR-OLLER				Time	Total		
Date: 1/4/95 Time: 1100	✓						PB	#1 1000 ml LR	100 ml/ hr	1400	300	2100	1000
										2100	700		
Date: 1/4/95 Time: 2100							EN	#2 1000 ml D5NS	125 ml/ hr	2200	125	0500	1000
										0500	875		
Date: 1/5/95 Time: 0500	✓					✓	CS	#3 1000 ml LR	50 ml/ hr	0600	50		
										1400	400		
										2200	400		
Date: Time:										0100	150	0100	1000
Date: Time:													
Date: Time:													
Date: Time:													
Date: Time:													
Date: Time:													

Identify Initials with Signature:
1. PB *P. Benitez RN*   4.   7.
2. EN *E. Norton RN*   5.   8.
3. CS *C. Smith RN*   6.   9.

ADDRESSOGRAPH:

Bertha Johnson F-54
537-34-1409
Dr. James Gusher

CODE: ★ see Nurses Progress Notes

SWEDISH HOSPITAL MEDICAL CENTER

SEATTLE, WASHINGTON

NU-1547 Nursing Rev. 10/86 FC/SHMC
SN-6111

Figure 53–15 Parenteral therapy record. This form includes places to indicate control device and tubing change on one side and site assessment on the reverse side.

(continued)

Identify Initials with Signature:	4.	8.
1. PB P. Benitez RN	5.	9.
2. EN E. Norton RN	6.	10.
3. CS C. Smith RN	7.	11.

DATE TIME	IV CATHETER INSERTION TYPE/GAUGE/LENGTH OR RATIONALE FOR IV SITE EXTENSION > 72 HOURS	IV SITE LOCATION	IV OR H.L.	IV SITE OK	CV DSG. CHG.	IV CATHETER DC'D INTACT	SITE CONDITION WHEN DC'D				TREATMENTS	REFER TO NURSES NOTES	INITIALS
							SITE OK	PHLEBITIS	NONVESICANT INFILTRATE	OTHER (SPECIFY)			
1/4/95 1100	# 18 Angiocath inserted	RH	IV										PB
1600		RH	IV	✓									EN
2400		RH	IV	✓									CS
1/5/95 0800		RH	IV			✓		3+				✓	PB
	# 18 Angiocath inserted	LH	IV										PB
1600		LH	IV	✓									EN
2400		LH	IV	✓									CS
1/6/95 0100		LH	IV	✓		✓	✓						CS

SHADED COLUMNS DOCUMENT 08 HOURS

CODES:

LOCATION	Type of Catheter		
R - RIGHT	PAC - PORTACATH	IV - CONTINUOUS INFUSION	PHLEBITIS GRADE 1+ - 5+
L - LEFT	HK - HICKMAN	HL - INTERMITTENT TX	INFILTRATE GRADE 1+ - 4+
H - HAND	J - JUGULAR	HEPARIN LOCK	TREATMENT
W - WRIST	SC - SUBCLAVIAN	IV SITE: OK - W/O PLEBITIS OR	WP - WARM PACK TO SITE
FA - FOREARM		INFILTRATE , AND DRESSING	IP - ICE PACK TO SITE
UA - UPPERARM	CV DSG CHG-CENTRAL	INTACT	
F - FOOT	VENOUS DRESSING	C - IV NURSE CONSULTATION	
AC - ANTECUBITAL	CHANGE		

Figure 53–15 *(Continued)*

DATE/TIME	
1/10/95 8:15 AM	Tubing and dressing changed on IV site. Site Clear. S. Storm, NS

Example of Nursing Progress Notes Using Narrative Format

DATE/TIME		
2/3/95 1430		IV site inflammation:
	S	"When I move it, my hand hurts where the tube goes in."
	O	IV site slightly reddened. IV patent and infusing last 150 ml of ordered solution.
	A	Potential phlebitis at IV site.
	P	Observe IV site q h until completion of infusion.
		D. Myers, NS

Example of Nursing Progress Notes Using SOAP Format

10. Turn on the flow and regulate the rate.
11. Dispose of the old container.
12. Wash your hands.
13. Document.

CHANGING A GOWN OVER AN IV

In some facilities gowns with shoulder seams that open and close with snap fasteners are available for patients with IVs. If such gowns are not available, use the following procedure:

To Remove
1. Remove the gown from the free arm and chest.
2. Gather the sleeve on the IV arm until it forms a compact circle of fabric. Hold this circle firmly.
3. Move the sleeve down over the arm, being particularly careful as you pass over the IV site. The sleeve should now be around the tubing, not around the arm.
4. Move the gown up the tubing toward the fluid container.
5. Remove the fluid container from the standard.
6. Slip the gown over the fluid container.
7. Rehang the container.

To Replace
Proceed in the opposite direction.
1. Gather the appropriate sleeve of the gown into a firm circle.
2. Remove the fluid container from the standard.
3. Slip the gown over the fluid container (Figure 53–16).

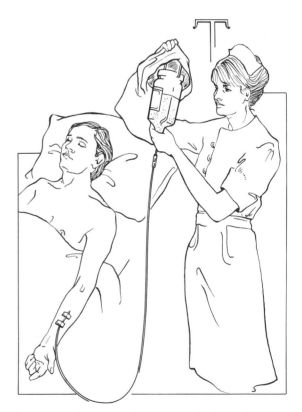

Figure 53–16 Changing patient's gown with IV in place. Slip the gown over the fluid container before moving the gown over the tubing and onto the arm.

DATE/TIME	
12/19/94 2038	*All fluid infused. IV DC'd with catheter intact. Catheter site without signs of infiltration or infection. ——— S. Juarez, NS*

Example of Nursing Progress Note Using Narrative Format

4. Rehang the fluid container.
5. Carefully move the gown over the tubing and onto the arm.
6. Adjust the gown on the IV arm.
7. Place the patient's other arm in the gown and fasten the gown.

DISCONTINUING AN IV

Assessment
1. Check the orders carefully. *It is painful as well as expensive for patients to have an IV restarted after being discontinued by mistake.*

Planning
2. Wash your hands *for infection control.*
3. Gather the necessary equipment.
   a. Sterile cotton ball or an alcohol swab (safe but uncomfortable) or a 2×2 sterile gauze square.
   b. Adhesive bandage (such as a Band-Aid)
   c. Clean gloves

Implementation
4. Identify the patient *to be sure you are performing the procedure for the correct patient.*
5. Explain to the patient that the procedure will not hurt.
6. Shut off the IV flow.
7. Carefully remove the tape and dressing.
8. Put on gloves *to protect yourself from exposure to blood.*
9. Hold the cotton ball or swab (according to your facility's policy) above the entry site. Be ready to exert pressure as soon as the needle is out, but do not exert pressure on the site while pulling the needle out. *The pressure compresses the vein wall between the needle and the swab and can damage the vein.*
10. Remove the needle by pulling straight out in line with the vein. Check the needle or catheter *to make sure no part of it has broken off and remains in the patient.*

11. Immediately put pressure on the site *to control bleeding.*
12. Elevate the patient's arm for about 1 minute. Keep pressure on the site until bleeding is controlled.
13. Remove gloves.
14. Put the adhesive bandage over the site.
15. Remove all the equipment. Be sure to note the volume of fluid remaining in the container, *in order to record intake accurately.*
16. Wash your hands.

Evaluation
17. Evaluate, using the following criteria:
    a. Intravenous infusion is discontinued.
    b. Bleeding is controlled.
    c. Needle or catheter is intact.

Documentation
18. Record the intake from the IV that has occurred on your shift on the intake and output sheet. To do this accurately, you will have to check whether any fluid was administered on the previous shift and subtract that amount from the total amount of fluid administered from the container.
19. Record that the IV was discontinued with needle or catheter intact, your assessment of the site, and the time on the flow sheet or on the nurses' notes.

References
Centers for Disease Control. (1983a). *Guidelines for prevention of intravascular infections.* Washington, DC: US Department of Health and Human Services.

Centers for Disease Control. (1983b). *Guidelines for control of nosocomial infections.* Washington, DC: US Department of Health and Human Services.

Intravenous Nurses Society. (1990) *Intravenous Nursing Standards of Practice.* Belmont, MA.

Koszuta, L. (1984). Choosing the right infusion control device for your patient. *Nursing 84, 14*(3), 55–56.

Lorenz, B. (1990). Are you using the right IV pump? *RN, 53*(5), 31–36.

Millam, D. (1990). Controlling the flow: Electronic infusion devices. *Nursing 90, 20*(8), 65–68.

Zenk, K. (1986). Administering I.V. antibiotics to children. *Nursing 86, 16*(12), 50–52.

Performance Checklist

Procedure for Monitoring and Maintaining an Infusion	Unsat	Needs More Practice	Sat	Comments
Assessment				
1. Identify patient.				
2. Review entire system for obvious problems.				
3. Check IV container. a. Date and time				
b. Correct solution				
c. Correct number of bottle				
d. Time to be finished				
4. Check drip chamber. a. Flow present				
b. Rate correct				
5. Check tubing for kinks or obstructions.				
6. Check site for phlebitis or infiltration. a. Skin color and temperature.				
b. Pain.				
c. Swelling.				
7. If armboard is used, remove and examine arm or leg for skin integrity and circulatory impairment. Replace armboard.				
8. Identify specific problem present.				
Planning				
9. Using the chart on troubleshooting IV problems, plan a course of action.				
Implementation				
10. Carry out action planned.				
Evaluation				
11. Evaluate, using the following criteria: a. Any problem present identified and corrected.				
b. Correct intravenous infusion running at correct rate.				

© 1992 by J.B. Lippincott Company

Procedure for Monitoring and Maintaining an Infusion *(Continued)*	Unsat	Needs More Practice	Sat	Comments
Documentation				
12. On flow sheet, note that IV is running on time, the current rate, and appearance of site.				
13. If problems were identified and corrected, note them on the nurses' notes or on flow sheet.				
Changing the Fluid Container and Tubing				
Assessment				
1. Check physician's order for type of fluid and infusion rate.				
2. Check date of last tubing change.				
Planning				
3. Wash your hands.				
4. Select correct fluid container and correct tubing and obtain tape and gloves.				
Implementation				
5. Set up equipment. a. Examine fluid container.				
b. Open package containing tubing and check drop factor of tubing.				
c. Open entry area of fluid container.				
d. Clean entry port if necessary.				
e. Close regulator on tubing.				
f. Insert spike of tubing into container.				
g. Invert container and hang it up.				
h. Fill drip chamber.				
i. Hold end of tubing over basin or waste container and fill tubing with fluid, expelling all air.				
6. Identify patient and protect linen.				
7. Hang new container on standard beside current container.				
8. Remove tape and dressing from IV site.				

Changing the Fluid Container and Tubing *(Continued)*	Unsat	Needs More Practice	Sat	Comments
9. Examine site.				
10. Put on gloves.				
11. Shut off flow of old IV tubing.				
12. Hold needle hub while removing old tubing.				
13. While holding hub, remove cap of new tubing and insert it into needle hub.				
14. Start new infusion at a slow rate.				
15. Redress site. a. Clean site with povidone-iodine swab.				
b. Apply ointment to site.				
c. Place sterile 2×2 gauze under needle at the entry site.				
d. Remove gloves.				
e. Use tape to make an airtight seal around the dressing.				
f. Write date and time of dressing change on tape.				
16. Regulate IV to ordered rate.				
17. Mark container with the times of beginning and ending and with intermediate times, to facilitate monitoring.				
18. Dispose of used equipment.				
19. Wash your hands.				
Evaluation				
20. Evaluate, using the following criteria: a. Tubing and fluid container changed with no contamination.				
b. Dressing replaced and dated.				
c. Correct intravenous infusion running at correct rate.				
Documentation				
21. Record information in correct location for your facility. a. Time started and stopped and exact contents of IV.				

Changing the Fluid Container and Tubing *(Continued)*	Unsat	Needs More Practice	Sat	Comments
b. Fluid intake from discontinued container.				
c. Assessment of IV line and site and patient's response.				

Changing the Container Only

Assessment

1. Check physician's order for type of fluid.				

Planning

2. Wash your hands.				
3. Select correct fluid container.				
4. Take new fluid container to bedside. (Use three checks to verify order.)				

Implementation

5. Check patient's identity.				
6. Remove cover from entry port of new container.				
7. Turn off IV flow.				
8. Invert old fluid container.				
9. Remove tubing without contamination.				
10. Insert tubing into new container.				
11. Invert and hang new container.				
12. Start and regulate flow rate.				
13. Dispose of old container.				
14. Wash your hands.				

Evaluation

15. Evaluate, using the following criteria: a. Fluid container changed with no contamination.				
b. Correct intravenous infusion running at correct rate.				

Documentation

16. Record in correct location for your facility.				

Removing Patient's Gown	Unsat	Needs More Practice	Sat	Comments
1. Remove gown from free arm and chest.				
2. Gather sleeve into circle.				
3. Move sleeve down over arm.				
4. Move gown up tubing, toward container.				
5. Remove fluid container from stand.				
6. Slip gown over container.				
7. Rehang container.				

Replacing Patient's Gown

	Unsat	Needs More Practice	Sat	Comments
1. Gather sleeve into circle.				
2. Remove fluid container from stand.				
3. Slip gown over container.				
4. Rehang container.				
5. Move gown over tubing and onto arm.				
6. Adjust gown on arm.				
7. Put gown on free arm and fasten.				

Discontinuing an IV

Assessment

	Unsat	Needs More Practice	Sat	Comments
1. Check orders.				

Planning

	Unsat	Needs More Practice	Sat	Comments
2. Wash your hands.				
3. Gather necessary equipment: a. Sterile cotton ball, alcohol swab, or sterile gauze square				
b. Adhesive bandage				
c. Clean gloves.				

Implementation

	Unsat	Needs More Practice	Sat	Comments
4. Identify patient.				
5. Explain procedure to patient.				
6. Shut off IV flow.				

Discontinuing an IV (*Continued*)	Unsat	Needs More Practice	Sat	Comments
7. Remove tape and dressing.				
8. Put on gloves.				
9. Hold swab above entry site.				
10. Remove needle by pulling straight out.				
11. Put pressure on site.				
12. Elevate patient's arm for 1 minute, keeping pressure on site until bleeding is controlled.				
13. Remove gloves.				
14. Put adhesive bandage over site.				
15. Remove all equipment.				
16. Wash your hands.				
Evaluation				
17. Evaluate, using the following criteria: a. Intravenous infusion discontinued.				
b. Bleeding controlled.				
c. Needle or catheter intact.				
Documentation				
18. Record intake on intake and output sheet.				
19. Record that IV was discontinued with needle or catheter intact, assessment of site, and time.				
Troubleshooting Problems				
1. IV off schedule a. Calculate rate.				
b. Reset flow.				
2. Incorrect solution a. Slow rate.				
b. Change to correct solution.				
c. Assess patient.				
d. Follow incident procedure.				
e. Notify physician.				
3. Tubing kinked a. Straighten tubing.				

Troubleshooting Problems *(Continued)*	Unsat	Needs More Practice	Sat	Comments
b. Check flow rate.				
4. Flow stopped a. Look for obstruction and correct.				
b. Open regulator completely, move to new position, regulate again if flow begins.				
c. Reposition arm.				
d. Place bottle lower than needle.				
e. Gently raise needle hub.				
f. Pinch off tubing close to arm above soft rubber section of tube and squeeze soft rubber firmly.				
g. Obtain sterile needle and syringe, insert needle into injection port closest to needle, pinch off tubing above syringe and aspirate. Open flow.				
5. Bubbles in tubing a. Stretch tube and flick with fingernail.				
b. Use sterile needle and syringe to aspirate from port.				
6. Drip chamber full of fluid a. Squeeze fluid back into container.				
7. Solution falls below drip chamber with fluid container empty a. If tubing schedule to be changed: slow drip rate, obtain new fluid container and tubing, insert new tubing into needle hub, regulate flow rate.				
b. If tubing does not need to be changed: obtain next fluid container, connect tubing to new container, fill drip chamber, aspirate column of air, regulate flow rate.				

Quiz

Short-Answer Questions

1. What type of administration set is best to use for administering fluids to a young child? _____

2. What type of set is used to administer a "piggyback" intravenous medication? _____

3. What is one advantage, in terms of sterility, of the plastic IV fluid container? _____

4. What is the proper action if the fluid in the container looks cloudy? _____

5. If two fluid containers are to be hung on a Y set, what are the two ways to make sure that the appropriate one empties first?

   a. _____

   b. _____

6. Calculate the drop rate for each of the following problems:

   a. 1000 ml to be given over 8 hours; the drop factor is 15 gtt/ml. _____
   b. 650 ml to be given over 4½ hours; the drop factor is 10 gtt/ml. _____
   c. 200 ml to be given over 2 hours; the drop factor is 20 gtt/ml. _____
   d. 100 ml to be given over 3 hours using a microdrip set, which delivers 60 gtt/ml. _____

7. How often should the entire intravenous setup be changed? _____

8. Why is it important to regulate the drip rate exactly? _____

9. What are two measures that will stop bleeding after an IV is discontinued?

   a. _____

   b. _____

10. Give five possible causes of obstruction in the IV flow.

    a. _____

    b. _____

    c. _____

    d. _____

    e. _____

11. What are the four common symptoms of phlebitis at the IV site?

    a. _____

    b. _____

    c. _____

    d. _____

12. What are the five common symptoms of infiltration of the IV?

a. _____

b. _____

c. _____

d. _____

e. _____

13. List six major elements that are part of a routine assessment of an IV.

a. _____

b. _____

c. _____

d. _____

e. _____

f. _____

Module 54

Administering Intravenous Medications

Module Contents

Rationale for the Use of This Skill
Nursing Diagnosis
Hazards of Administering IV Medication
Equipment
    Bolus or Push IV Medications
    Additive IV Medications
General Procedure for Administering IV
    Medications
    Assessment
    Planning
    Implementation
    Evaluation
    Documentation

Adding to a New Fluid Container
Adding to an Existing Fluid Container
Using a Controlled-Volume
    Administration Set
Using a Small-Volume Parenteral
Using a Syringe Infusion Pump
Using a Patient-Controlled Analgesia
    Infuser
Giving Medication by IV Push into an
    Existing IV
Giving Medication into an Intermittent
    Infusion Adapter (Heparin Lock)

Prerequisites

1. *Successful completion of the following modules:*

VOLUME 1

Module 1   An Approach to Nursing Skills
Module 2   Basic Infection Control
Module 3   Safety
Module 5   General Assessment Overview
Module 6   Documentation

VOLUME 2

Module 35 Sterile Technique
Module 49 Administering Oral Medications
Module 51 Giving Injections
Module 53 Preparing and Maintaining
    Intravenous Infusions

2. *Satisfactory completion of the self-test on mathematics of dosages and solutions in Module 49, Administering Oral Medications. If you cannot meet this level of proficiency, you need additional practice in the mathematics of dosages and solutions. Many programmed texts are available for independent study.*

3. *Review of the anatomy and physiology of the vascular system.*

438

Overall Objective

To prepare and administer intravenous medications using an intravenous line that is in place or a controlled-volume administration set, an intermittent infusion adapter (heparin trap or heparin lock), a small-volume container, an infusion pump, or a controller.

Specific Learning Objectives

	Know Facts and Principles	Apply Facts and Principles	Demonstrate Ability	Evaluate Performance
1. Hazards	State objective signs that can indicate adverse reaction to IV medication.		In the clinical setting, evaluate patient's response to IV medication.	Verify own evaluation with instructor.
2. Equipment	List various types of equipment available and purpose of each.	Given a specific situation, identify equipment needed.	In the clinical setting, choose correct equipment.	Validate choice with instructor.
3. Intravenous medication administration	Know where to find information on preparation of IV medication.		Read directions on package.	Double-check preparation and recheck with instructor.
a. Preparing the medication	Explain compatibility of IV fluids.		In the clinical setting, prepare IV medication correctly.	
b. Adding medications to IV fluid	State reason for injecting only at injection ports.	Identify entry port on fluid container into which medication should be injected.	Add medication to IV fluid container, maintaining sterility.	Evaluate own performance using Performance Checklist.
c. Using a controlled-volume administration set	Identify purpose of controlled-volume set. State amount of fluid to be used for diluting medication when using controlled-volume set.	Identify situations in which controlled-volume set is necessary.	Give medication using controlled-volume administration set.	Evaluate own performance using Performance Checklist.
d. Using a small-volume container and secondary administration set	Identify purpose of small-volume container.	Identify situations in which small-volume container and secondary administration set could be used.	Give medications correctly, using small-volume container and secondary administration set.	Evaluate own performance using Performance Checklist.
e. Using an infusion controller	Explain purpose of infusion controller.	Identify appropriate situations for using an infusion controller.	Give medications correctly using infusion controller.	Evaluate own performance using Performance Checklist.

(continued)

Specific Learning Objectives (Continued)

	Know Facts and Principles	Apply Facts and Principles	Demonstrate Ability	Evaluate Performance
f. *Using a syringe infusion pump*	Explain purpose of syringe infusion pump.	Identify appropriate situations for using a syringe infusion pump.	Give medications correctly using syringe infusion pump.	Evaluate own performance using Performance Checklist.
g. *IV push*	Explain reasons for differences in rate of injection. Explain how to decrease discomfort of IV push medications.	Identify entry port on IV tubing to be used for injection.	Maintain sterile technique while injecting medication at correct rate.	Evaluate own performance using Performance Checklist.
h. *Using an intermittent infusion adapter (heparin lock)*	List reasons for using a heparin lock. Explain purpose of heparin or saline solution in lock.	Identify situations in which heparin lock would be useful.	Give medication into heparin lock. Add heparin or saline solution to lock to maintain patency of heparin lock.	Evaluate own performance using Performance Checklist.

Learning Activities

1. Review the Specific Learning Objectives.
2. Read the section on intravenous infusions in Ellis and Nowlis, *Nursing: A Human Needs Approach,* or comparable material in another textbook.
3. Look up the module vocabulary terms in the Glossary.
4. Read through the module and mentally practice the skills.
5. In the practice setting:
   a. Draw up medication as you would for an IM injection, using a 21- or 22-gauge needle.
      (1) Inject the medication into an IV fluid container through the correct port, using sterile technique.
      (2) Invert the bottle, observe, and withdraw the needle.
   b. Draw up second dose of medication.
      (1) Inject this into the air vent of the IV bottle.
      (2) Withdraw the needle, invert the bottle, and observe the result.
   c. Draw up medication.
      (1) Set up a controlled-volume administration set (Peditrol, Soluset, Volutrol).
      (2) Fill the controlled-volume reservoir with 100 ml fluid.
      (3) Add the medication.
      (4) Start the flow rate.
      (5) Close both the airway and inlet to the reservoir. Observe the effect.
      (6) Close the airway and open the inlet to the reservoir. Observe the effect.
      (7) Close the exit to the reservoir, and open the airway and inlet. Observe the effect.
      (8) Regulate the flow to administer medication in 30 minutes. (Calculate the correct rate.)
   d. Draw up the medication using a small-gauge (25 or 26) needle. On an existing IV line, choose an entry port.
      (1) Inject the medication directly into the IV line.
      (2) Watch for air bubbles forced into the line.
      (3) Consider the speed with which the medication can be given.
   e. Draw up the medication using a large-gauge needle. On an existing IV line, choose an entry port. Repeat steps 1–3 in step d, above. Note the difference in effect of the large- and small-gauge needles.
   f. Draw up medication and heparin solution in separate syringes. Inject into the heparin lock.
   g. Set up a small-volume container, adding medication in the same way you added medication to the fluid container. Attach the secondary set to an ongoing IV, and regulate the rate.

Vocabulary

additive
anticoagulant
bolus
compatible
diluent

heparin trap (heparin lock)
intermittent infusion adapter
laminar airflow hood

piggyback
thrombophlebitis
transfer needle
venipuncture

Administering Intravenous Medications

Rationale for the Use of This Skill

Intravenous medications are being used with increasing frequency when rapid effect is necessary, when medications are too irritating to be given by another route, or when the discomfort of frequent intramuscular injections is to be avoided. IV medications are also commonly used for critically ill patients and when a constant blood level of a drug must be maintained.

The nurse must be aware of the potential hazards of intravenous medications. Sterile technique must be faultless to prevent infection, and all aspects of the procedure must be done correctly. Of course, careful attention to the three checks and five rights is always necessary for safety.[1]

▶ Nursing Diagnosis

The major nursing diagnosis to keep in mind when giving intravenous medications is High Risk for Injury. Patients can be injured by intravenous medications given in the wrong dose, at the wrong time, or at an incorrect rate of speed. They can also be injured by the omission of essential medications or the administration of an incorrect medication.

Patients are also at high risk for injuries related to tissue irritation from the equipment and/or the medication being administered. Although this nursing diagnosis will not appear on the Nursing Care Plan, it applies to every situation in which a patient is receiving an intravenous medication.

HAZARDS OF ADMINISTERING IV MEDICATION

Because an IV medication is immediately available to body tissue, any severe reaction to a medication may happen quickly. The major danger is from reactions that interfere with respiratory, circulatory, or neurologic function. Whenever a medication is given intravenously, watch for noisy respirations, changes in pulse rate, chills, nausea, or headache. *These can be early signs of severe*

---

[1] You will note that rationale for action is emphasized throughout the module by the use of italics.

reaction. If these occur, discontinue the medication and carefully assess the patient. Then notify the physician.

In addition to these general symptoms, you must be aware of the possible adverse reactions specific to the medication being given and of possible incompatibilities of different drugs that affect only certain people. Many IV medications are irritating to the vein and can cause local pain, redness, and swelling, a condition known as *thrombophlebitis.* This may involve the formation of a clot.

Drug incompatibilities can alter or negate the effects of the drug or, more seriously, cause the patient to experience untoward reactions. Factors that can affect incompatibility are concentration of the drug, length of time in contact, ionic or electrolyte strength, and pH level. Drug incompatibilities can be visual or chemical. A visual incompatibility may be evidenced by precipitation, color change, cloudiness, or the formation of gas bubbles. Chemical incompatibilities can cause the drugs to become inactive or toxic (Weiner & Pepper, 1985). An example is antibiotics, which often become unstable when the pH of a solution is very high or very low. *One of the most important ways to prevent incompatibilities is to become knowledgeable about the classifications of drugs that are likely to cause this problem.*

The literature accompanying medication is one of the best sources of information about incompatibilities as well as about the appropriate diluent, amount of diluent, and how slowly or rapidly to give the medication. (A rate of 1 ml/min is considered slow.) *The speed of instillation can be related to the desired effect of the medication.* For example, if the patient has suddenly become seriously ill, the physician may order a drug to be given as rapidly as possible. But the rate of instillation can also affect the degree of irritation to the vein, *which can cause patient discomfort.* Giving the medication slowly *allows the drug to become diluted by the flow of blood in the vein, which makes it less irritating and less painful.* Again, you should read the literature provided by the manufacturer carefully. If it does not answer your question, you should contact the pharmacist for assistance.

EQUIPMENT

Bolus or Push IV Medications

IV medications are sometimes ordered to be given as a *bolus* or *push,* which means that a measured amount of medication, diluted or undiluted, is manually instilled through some type of intravenous device or directly into the vein by venipuncture. When this is the case, the basic equipment is the same as for an intramuscular injection. To begin, select the size of syringe appropriate for the quantity of medication. A small-gauge needle (one with a high gauge number, 25 or 26) injects the medication more slowly; a large-gauge needle (one with a low gauge number, 19 or 20) injects medication rapidly. *The size selected depends on how fast the medication must be given in relation to its viscosity.*

Additive IV Medications

The fluid container has a special entry port for adding medications. In some facilities, medications are added to IV fluids only in the pharmacy, *where an area of minimal contamination from microorganisms is maintained through the use of a laminar airflow hood.* If IV additives are added on the nursing unit, it is the nurse's responsibility to add the medication to the container in an area as free from potential contamination as possible.

When adding medications to IV fluids, take precautions *to ensure that the medication and the fluid are thoroughly mixed.* One study showed that if a medication is lighter or heavier than the solution, it tends either to float or to fall to the bottom of the container, *which means that the patient receives a concentrated dosage of the added medication rather than the desired mixture* (Motz-Harding & Good, 1985). *To prevent this,* thoroughly agitate the intravenous bag or bottle before administering. If the added medication has a lipid or oil base, you should shake the container every 15–30 minutes during the infusion. It is a good idea to use a long needle when adding medications through the port of a container, *so the medication does not become trapped in the area around the port.*

A small-volume container (minibottle or partial-fill bag) holds 50–100 ml solution. *It is used to administer a small volume of medication that must be diluted.* The medication is added to the container, which is then hung as a secondary administration set.

A controlled-volume administration set (Peditrol, Soluset, Volutrol) is attached to a regular, large IV fluid container. *This set allows a measured volume of fluid to be withdrawn from the large container. The medication can then be added to the controlled-volume reservoir and given at the appropriate rate.* (For a complete discussion of the various types of infusion control devices, see Module 53, Preparing and Maintaining Intravenous Infusions.)

An intermittent infusion adapter, or heparin lock or heparin trap, is *designed to provide ready access to a vein without having an IV infusing continuously.* A needle is placed in the vein. Attached to the needle hub is a very short tubing with one or two IV entry ports at the end or a straight male adapter with a rubber cap. A dilute heparin solution (an anticoagulant) is injected through the port into the needle and tubing to fill them. *This solution prevents blood from coagulating and blocking the needle.* Whenever the trap is used, it must be refilled with fresh dilute heparin solution. Most facilities establish a routine for the strength of heparin solution and the amount needed to fill the particular intermittent infusion set in use. Usually, 1 ml containing 10 units or 100 units of heparin is used. (Prefilled cartridges are available for this purpose.)

Special needles that protect the staff from accidental needle sticks ("needle-lock" devices) are available for use when injecting medications into intravenous access devices. The needle is surrounded with rigid clear plastic which slides over the injection port, guides the needle into the injection port, and secures the needle into place (see Figure 53–7).

In some facilities it is the policy to flush peripheral intermittent infusion adapters with saline only (Dunn & Lenihan, 1987; Hale, 1990). These investigators have demonstrated that saline flushes are as effective as those containing heparin. They have also noted a lower incidence of phlebitis and infiltration than with heparin flushes. When saline only is used there is no need for concern regarding giving IV drugs incompatible with heparin or about the effect of heparin on systemic coagulation (Dunn & Lenihan, 1987).

An alcohol swab is needed *for cleaning* whenever a surface is punctured by a needle. Tape may be needed *to reinforce the point of attachment.*

GENERAL PROCEDURE FOR ADMINISTERING IV MEDICATIONS

Assessment

1. Check the physician's orders for the medication.
2. Gather information on the drug, including its effects, the dilution, the rate of administration, and any potential for incompatibility with other intravenous fluids or medications being given. Each IV medication has specific properties. It is essential that you know a medication's expected actions and potential adverse reactions when you administer IV

medication. *Because the system is affected so rapidly,* the patient must be observed closely for side effects or reactions while the medication is being given and in the period immediately after it is given. Be prepared to act swiftly should an emergency occur.

3. Check to see what type of intravenous access is present—that is, whether an existing intravenous infusion is running, whether a heparin lock is in place, or whether a venipuncture must be done to administer the medication.

Planning

4. Wash your hands *for infection control.*
5. Select the appropriate equipment based on the necessary method of administration. Often the physician's orders specify the method of IV administration. If an access to the vein is not present, the medication must be given by a nurse skilled in doing venipuncture. *When multiple IV push medications are needed,* the nurse may request an order for a heparin lock from the physician.

   "Add to the IV" indicates that the medication should be placed in the large-volume container and will be administered over the time period designated for the fluid. Medications given this way must be stable in solution for the length of time the infusion is to run.

   Currently many medications are administered intermittently. These are diluted and mixed in small volumes of solution and are usually prepared in the pharmacy and sent to the units clearly labeled for individual patients. If the medication comes in a small bottle or bag, it is hung piggyback, using a secondary administration set attached to an injection port of the primary IV. A second method for delivering small-volume medications is with a syringe infusion pump (Figure 54–1). This is a small battery-run device that can be carried by an ambulatory patient, hung on a stand, or placed on the bedside table. The medication-filled syringe, prepared either in the pharmacy or by the nurse, is attached to a small-diameter tubing and placed in the pump. *An alarm on the device alerts the nurse when all the medication has been infused.*

   Both of these small-volume methods cost less than other methods, *since tubing can be used for 48 hours with compatible medications.* Some

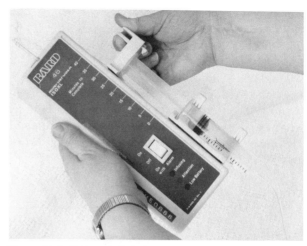

Figure 54–1 Syringe infusion pump. The syringe is placed into the pump so that the upper ridge on the syringe rests on the flange of the pump.

facilities have extended the use of tubing to 72 hours based on their own incidence of complications. Follow the policy in your facility.

The nurse must always use a sterile needle when starting medications through an existing line—that is, one within the 48–72 hour limit—and the delivery needle must be replaced with another sterile needle at the completion of the instillation. *A contaminated needle could spread microorganisms to the tubing. The cost of changing needles is minimal, and the procedure greatly reduces the chance of infection at the site.*

Implementation

6. Read the name of the medication to be given from the record.
7. Check the label to be sure you have the correct medication, time, and patient.
8. Compare the medication container with the record.
9. Prepare the medication, using sterile technique.
10. Prepare a syringe with 5 ml sterile normal saline, half of which is used to flush the intravenous line before administering the medication and half used after giving the medication *if the medication is incompatible with the solution already in the line. If you cannot find any information that tells you whether the medications are compatible, it is safer to proceed as if they are not.*
11. Explain the procedure to the patient. In

particular, focus on what the patient will experience.

12. Give the medication in the appropriate manner. See the next sections for specific procedures. Flush the line before and after giving the medication if necessary.

13. Observe the patient carefully while you are giving the medication *in order to identify any complications immediately.*

14. Dispose of the equipment correctly.

Evaluation

15. Evaluate, using the following criteria:
    a. The right patient received the right medication in the right dosage by the right route at the right time.
    b. The medication was given over the correct time period.
    c. The criteria established for ascertaining the effectiveness of a specific drug were used. For example, for a given pain medication this might be "Pain relief obtained within 10 minutes."
    d. Side effects, if present, were promptly identified.

Documentation

16. Record name of medication, dosage, intravenous route used, time, and your signature.

17. If 50 or 100 ml fluid is given, add this amount to the intake record if this is the policy. *The cumulative volume of fluid over 24 hours could be significant for the patient on measured intake and output.*

ADDING TO A NEW FLUID CONTAINER

Medications, vitamins, and electrolytes may be added to the main intravenous fluid container to be administered over many hours. *Medications given this way provide for a stable blood level. Vitamins and electrolytes given in this manner are available to the body as they are needed.*

1. Select the additive, using the five rights and three checks.

2. Select the appropriate equipment.
    a. You will need a large-volume fluid container that has the ordered intravenous fluid. Be careful when checking this fluid, *because all medications are not compatible with all intravenous fluids.*
    b. A syringe and needle are usually used to draw up the medication or additive to add it to the intravenous fluid. A transfer needle may also be used for this purpose. A transfer needle is a double-ended needle. One end of the needle is inserted into the small bottle containing the additive. The cover is then taken off the other end, exposing the second needle end. This needle end can be inserted directly into the large-volume fluid container. *The vacuum in the large container causes the additive to be drawn out of its container into the fluid container.* This can be used only if the entire small container is to be added to the large container.

3. Draw up the medication from the vial or ampule. If you are unsure of this procedure, review the section on Withdrawing Solutions from Containers in Module 51, Giving Injections.

4. Label the new fluid container with the name and amount of additive, the date and time, and your initials.

5. Open the top of the new fluid container and identify the injection port. This may be designated by the word *Add* or by a triangle on the rubber top. On a plastic bag the injection port usually appears as a conventional soft rubber injection port, which is self-sealing. If you inserted a needle through the plastic, *you would cause a leak.*

6. Clean the port with an alcohol swab *for infection control.*

7. Inject the medication. If the container has an air vent, be sure you do not inadvertently inject into it.

8. Tilt the container back and forth *to mix the additive thoroughly.*

9. Hang the new infusion container following the steps in Module 53, Preparing and Maintaining Intravenous Infusions. (Spike entry port of container with tubing, close roller clamp, invert container, and squeeze to fill drip chamber.)

10. Regulate the flow.
    a. If you are using an ICD, thread tubing through device according to manufacturer's instructions and set controls to desired milliliters per hour.
    b. If you are not using an ICD, slowly open the roller clamp and time flow to desired rate.

ADDING TO AN EXISTING FLUID CONTAINER

1. Prepare the medication, using the five rights and three checks.
2. Take the medication to the patient's room and identify the patient.
3. Turn off the IV flow.
4. Invert the fluid container.
5. Clean the medication port with an alcohol swab.
6. Inject the medication into the appropriate medication port on the container.
7. Tilt the container back and forth *to mix the additive thoroughly.*
8. Label the container appropriately.
9. Rehang the IV container.
10. Regulate the flow rate as ordered.

USING A CONTROLLED-VOLUME ADMINISTRATION SET

1. Prepare the medication, using the five rights and three checks.
2. Take the medication to the patient's room and identify the patient.
3. Label the chamber with the name and amount of medication, the date, time, and your initials.
4. Open the inlet to the controlled-volume chamber. Fill with 50–100 ml, depending on the dilution suggested by the drug manufacturer. (Usually 100 ml is used unless the patient has a fluid restriction.)
5. Tightly close the inlet to the chamber.
6. Check the chamber. If it is hard plastic, make sure the air vent is open.
7. Turn on the drip from the chamber to check that the system is functioning correctly before adding medication.
   a. *If the system does not work, the filters may be clogged,* and you will have to replace the set.
   b. If the system is functioning, turn off the drip again.
8. Clean the entry port of the fluid chamber with an alcohol swab.
9. Insert the needle through the entry port and inject the medication.
10. Calculate the drip rate and regulate the flow. Remember that the controlled-volume set usually has a microdrip orifice. In all sets that deliver 60 drops/ml, the drip rate is the same as the number of milliliters per hour.

USING A SMALL-VOLUME PARENTERAL

This method of administration is known as a partial-fill, a piggyback, a minibottle, or a small-volume parenteral.

1. Check to see whether the patient has an intravenous infusion running or whether a heparin lock is in place.
2. Select the correct equipment.
   a. For a heparin lock (intermittent infusion adapter), you will need regular long intravenous tubing *to give the patient enough line to move about comfortably.* You will also need a needle or "needle-lock" device to fasten to the end of the line and insert in the heparin lock. The needle should be 1 inch long. *A longer needle cannot enter the port completely, which means that the exposed portion could become contaminated with microorganisms. A longer needle can also damage the heparin lock itself or the catheter within the vein.* A 19-, 20-, or 21-gauge needle is preferred. *Larger needles put such large holes in the soft rubber cap that the lock may begin to leak. Smaller needles restrict the flow and make it difficult to administer a very viscous solution in the appropriate length of time.* You will also need tape *to fasten the tubing to the arm,* and an alcohol swab.
   b. For attaching to an existing infusion, you will need a secondary administration set. These sets usually come with a needle enclosed to allow you to insert the secondary set into the primary set. Most manufacturers include an extension hanger in the secondary set package. If the package you are using does not contain an extension hanger, check to find where one can be obtained on your unit. You also will need tape *to fasten the secondary set onto the primary set, or the needle to the heparin lock,* and an alcohol swab.
   c. For attaching a new container to an existing secondary or conventional line, you will need a new sterile needle. Although the needle on the line was sterile and was stored in a cover, *it is often impossible for you to know if the needle has become contaminated in any way. Because needles are inexpensive,* it is a prudent practice to change them. You will also need tape *to fasten the line,* and an alcohol swab.

3. If you must add the medication to the small container of fluid, follow the directions given above for adding to a fluid container.
4. If the container did not come from the pharmacy as a labeled, mixed medication, label the container with the medication, dosage, time, and your initials.

If you are using a new tubing set:

5. Close the regulator on the tubing.
6. Clean the top of the small container.
7. Attach the administration set to the container.
8. Place the needle on the end of the tubing.
9. Hang the small container (or hold it up), and fill the drip chamber half full of fluid.
10. Remove the needle cover and open the regulator *to allow the tubing to fill with fluid and the air to be expelled;* then re-cover the needle.
11. Identify the patient.
12. Hang the small container on the IV standard.
13. Place the main intravenous container on an extension hanger, *so it is lower than the small container. This allows the liquid in the small container to be instilled first.*
14. Clean the entry port near the top of the administration set.
15. Insert the needle from the secondary set into the high port.
16. Open the regulator on the secondary set.
17. Use the regulator on the primary line to set the drop rate. When the small container has emptied, the main IV will begin to drip again at the rate set for the small container. At that time you may need to return to the room to regulate the main IV.
18. Tape the connection where the needle enters the port. It is wise to tape the needle cover at the connection point also. *Then it is readily available to cover the needle when the secondary set must be removed. Covering a needle for removal from the secondary line is a safety precaution for the staff.* Anytime you place a needle cover on a needle, use the one-hand technique discussed in Module 51, Giving Injections.

If you are using an existing line:

5. Identify the patient.
6. Identify the correct used small container and tubing. If multiple medications are being given by secondary set and the drugs are incompatible, a different tubing is used for each. The tubings are changed every 48–72 hours, as are all intravenous tubings, *to guard against the possibility of infection from a contaminated line.*

7. Clean the top of the new small container.
8. Make sure the regulator is turned off.
9. Remove the old small container from the IV standard and detach the tubing.
10. Insert the spike of the used tubing into the new small container.
11. Hang the small container on the IV standard.
12. Hang the main IV container on the extension hanger.
13. If the needle for the secondary set is still attached to the primary set, you do not need to take the needle out of the port. If the needle was not attached but was hanging loose or in a used needle cover, change it *for sterility.* Then cleanse the port and reinsert the new needle.
14. Remove air in the secondary line by "back-filling." To do this, hold the small container lower than the main IV. Then open the regulator on the secondary line. Fluid will begin to flow from the main IV line into the secondary line. Allow the fluid to flow until the fluid has filled the drip chamber halfway.
15. When the fluid is at the appropriate level in the drip chamber, hang the small container on the IV standard.
16. Set the correct drip rate for the medication by using the regulator on the main IV. When the medication has finished running, the main IV will begin to drip at the same rate set for the small container. You may need to return to the room to regulate the IV to its previous rate.
17. Tape the connection, with the needle cover present, as discussed above.

USING A SYRINGE INFUSION PUMP

The infusion pump is used for volumes of 20 ml or less. Syringes containing the medication in a predetermined level of solution are prepared in the pharmacy. When the pump is activated, the medication is delivered at the correct rate.

1. Check the syringe from the pharmacy to make sure you have the right medication for your patient in the right dosage at the right time, or draw up drug in predetermined amount of solution.
2. Identify the patient and check to see whether the patient has an intravenous infusion or a heparin lock in place.
3. Select the correct equipment. You will need the infusion pump, which is usually requisitioned from the central supply department and charged to the patient, as well

as a special thin intravenous tubing designed for these sets. You will also need a sterile 1-inch needle or "needle-lock" device, an alcohol swab, and tape.

4. Attach the end of the tubing that has small "butterfly wings" to the syringe.

5. Attach the other end of the tubing to the needle.

6. Attach a label to the tubing with the date and time.

7. Remove the needle cover and manually flush the tubing and needle with solution. Replace the needle cover using the one-hand technique discussed in Module 51, Giving Injections.

8. Using the clips on the pump, place the syringe into the pump so that the upper ridge on the syringe rests on the flange of the pump. Secure the syringe into the pump by lowering the sliding clamp. *This clamp determines the rate of flow.*

9. Clean the port to be used and insert the needle.

10. Hang pump on IV stand or place it on table.

11. Turn the rocker switch of the pump on, with or without alarm as desired. When the pump is working properly, a green light will flash on and off.

12. Tape the hub of the needle in place.

13. When the medication has been infused, the pumping action will stop. Solution will remain in the tubing. Remove the needle and replace it with a covered sterile needle, which should be taped to the pump.

If you are using an existing infusion pump:

1. Check the tubing *to be sure it has not been used for more than 48–72 hours.* IV tubing should be replaced every 48–72 hours *to decrease the chances of infection* (Centers for Disease Control, 1983). If you are giving the same medication or one that is compatible, you can use the same tubing.

2. Remove the used syringe and discard it.

3. Attach the tubing to a new syringe.

4. Replace the existing needle with a 1-inch sterile needle.

5. Place the syringe in the pump.

6. Insert the needle into the port as before, and turn on the pump.

USING A PATIENT-CONTROLLED ANALGESIA INFUSER

Patient-controlled analgesia (PCA) is a system for administering intravenous pain medications. The pa-

tient is able to activate the system when the need for medication arises. PCA is currently available in two major types—electronic and mechanical.

The electronic version of PCA delivers pain medication through a computer-controlled infusion pump. The unit can be programmed to deliver a continuous infusion, an adjustable patient-controlled dose (sometimes called a *bolus*), or both. A lockout interval may also be specified. During that time the machine will not deliver another dose. In addition, a 4-hour limit may be set. The nurse programs the infuser according to the physician's orders.

The continuous infusion is ordered to provide the patient with a baseline amount of medication continuously *to prevent deep troughs in serum drug levels.* The patient-controlled dose is the number of milliliters of fluid that is to be given for each individual dose. The physician orders the number of milligrams of drug in each milliliter, or the pharmacy may provide a standardized solution. Morphine sulfate with 1 mg/ml and meperidine with 10 mg/ml are common solutions. The individual injection dose is then calculated to match the physician's prescription. The lockout interval is ordered *to prevent the patient from getting too much medication.* It can be adjusted to specify a period of from several minutes to several hours. The *4-hour limit* is set *to limit the total volume to be infused over any consecutive 4-hour period.*

The pump holds a syringe inside a locked case. This syringe is attached to a port on the patient's intravenous line by a microbore (small-diameter) tubing that has an antireflux valve *to prevent reverse pressure into the syringe.* The medication in the syringe is administered when the patient pushes a control button attached to the machine (Figure 54–2).

The computer contains a clock and a rechargeable battery *so that the device can be unplugged for transport or ambulation.* The computer records each attempt by the patient to receive medication and each dosage of medication given. By keying in a code on the machine, it is possible to get a complete history of the use of the pain medication, including the total number of milliliters used from the current syringe, the number of attempts and the number of injections given during each hour, and the dose and interval programmed into the machine.

The mechanical PCA is disposable and uses gravity rather than electricity to deliver the medication. While this device is much less expensive than the electronic version, it does have some limitations. The delivery rate is set at either 2 or 5 ml/h. The patient-controlled dose volume is 0.5 ml and cannot be adjusted. Lockout times are preset at 6 or 15 minutes. This means the strength of the medication solution

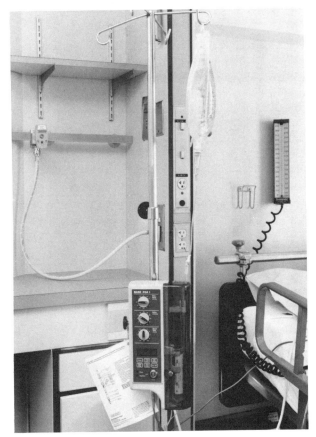

Figure 54–2 PCA infuser. The medication is administered when the patient pushes a control button attached to the machine.

must be adjusted accordingly. Since the device cannot be reset, if the patient should need a change in medication dosage, the patient will need a new infuser.

Because patients on either type of PCA are receiving narcotics via the IV route, careful assessment of respiratory status, sedation level, and analgesic effect is essential. Figure 54–3 gives an example of a flow sheet used to record the monitoring of a patient on a PCA.

For the PCA to be effective, the patient must be alert and oriented. Careful teaching is needed *for the patient to use the PCA effectively.* It is important to emphasize that the administration is safe *because the machine is programmed to give only the prescribed dose and cannot give the patient too much medication or too many injections.* It is also important to encourage the patient to use the medication *to maintain comfort* and not to wait a specified time to seek more medication.

In evaluating the effectiveness of a PCA, the nurse should consider whether the patient is frequently attempting to get injections unsuccessfully. This may indicate that the patient is not feeling adequate pain relief. Excessive sedation or respiratory depression may indicate that the individual dose is too large for the patient or that the interval between injections is too short.

To set up a PCA unit, refer to the specific directions for the brand used in your facility. Also refer to your facility's policy book for guidelines on managing the narcotics used in the machine and monitoring the patient.

GIVING MEDICATION BY IV PUSH INTO AN EXISTING IV

1. Prepare the medication, using the five rights and three checks.
2. Identify the patient.
3. Check to see that the existing IV is functioning properly.
4. Identify the injection port closest to the patient. (*An injection port must be used, because it is self-sealing. Puncturing the plastic tubing will create a leak.*)
5. Clean the port with an alcohol swab.
6. Insert the needle firmly into the port.
7. Pinch off the IV line between the port and the end of the bottle *to close it off. This prevents the medication from going up into the bottle.*
8. Inject the medication at the correct rate, taking into account the amount of tubing between the injection port and the intravenous insertion site. If the amount of medication to be injected is small and the distance to the IV insertion site large, you will need to recalculate the IV rate of flow *to ensure that the medication does not enter the patient's body at a rate too rapid to be safe.* Alternatively, you can flush the IV tubing with an amount of normal saline equal to the amount of fluid in the tubing between the injection port and the IV insertion site. If the normal saline is injected at the appropriate rate, the medication will enter the patient's circulation at the correct rate.
9. Observe the patient.
10. Release the tubing when the injection is completed.
11. Withdraw the needle.
12. Dispose of the equipment.

GIVING MEDICATION INTO AN INTERMITTENT INFUSION ADAPTER (HEPARIN LOCK)

This is a variation of giving an IV push medication.
1. Prepare the medication and the dilute heparin solution or saline solution in separate syringes.

MORPHINE SULFATE 1mg/ml ☒
MEPERIDINE 10mg/ml ☐

DATE	TIME	RESP RATE	ANALG. RATING	SYRINGE NUMBER	DOSE (ml)	LOCK OUT INTERVAL (min)	4 HR LIMIT (ml)	LOADING DOSE/BOLUS (ml)	8-HR (ml)	TOTAL (mg)	NALOXONE 0.2mg	REMARKS	INIT.
5/29/94	1000	22	4	1	1 ml	10 min	20 ml	2 ml				crying	PH
	1200	18	2	1	1.5 ml	10 min	24 ml					resting	PH
	1400	16	1	1	1.5 ml	10 min	24 ml		27 ml	30 mg		sleeping	PH
	1500	14	0	2	1.5 ml	10 min	24 ml					drowsy	PH
	1600	16	1	2	1.5 ml	10 min	24 ml					"comfortable"	ST

NOTIFY PHARMACY WHEN PCA IS DC'd

ASSESS AND RECORD:
Analgesic level q2hr X 8hr, then q4hr.
Respiratory rate q2hr X 8hr, then q4hr.
Pump settings — on initiation of therapy, then every 8 hrs (0600, 1400, 2200)
    and whenever new syringe added.
Total amount of narcotic infused q8hr (0600, 1400, 2200).

ANALGESIC RATING SCALE
0 – None
1 – Mild
2 – Discomforting
3 – Distressing
4 – Severe
5 – Excruciating

INIT.	SIGNATURE
PH	P. Hansen RN
ST	S. Trummell RN

Johnson, Bertha   F-54
537-34-1409
Dr. James Gusher

NORTHWEST HOSPITAL
Seattle, Washington

PCA DOCUMENTATION RECORD

M-432   (2/89)

Figure 54–3 Pain management flow sheet. Documentation requirements for PCA and continuous IV narcotic infusion are listed at the bottom of the form.

2. Identify the patient.
3. Locate the heparin lock. It is usually on the forearm or the back of the hand.
4. Inspect the site. Look for signs of phlebitis and check that the needle has not dislodged.
5. Clean the port of the heparin lock with an alcohol swab.
6. Insert the needle of the syringe with medication or the needle on an infusion pump tubing firmly through the soft rubber while stabilizing the lock with your nondominant hand.
   a. If saline is being used in the lock or if heparin is being used in the lock and the medication is compatible with heparin, proceed to step 7.
   b. If heparin is being used in the lock and the medication is *not* compatible with heparin, you will need to flush the heparin lock with 2–2½ ml normal saline before and after the injection of the medication.
7. Aspirate gently to see if blood returns, *to verify the lock's position in the vein.* In some facilities, it is no longer policy to aspirate, since blood may not return *because the vein collapses.*
8. If blood returns, inject the medication at the recommended rate.
9. If blood does not return, *the needle may be against the wall of the vein or it may be dislodged.* Inject a small amount of medication while feeling the tissue over the site with your fingertips.
   a. *If the fluid is being injected into the tissue,* you can feel a small swelling. Also, ask the patient whether he or she feels discomfort. *The dilute heparin solution usually produces burning when injected into the subcutaneous tissue.* If evidence indicates that the medication is going into the subcutaneous tissue, remove the heparin lock and replace it.
   b. If there is no evidence that fluid is moving

into the tissue, inject a bit more medication, continuing to check for burning and swelling. Continue to give the medication in this manner.
10. Withdraw the needle after all medication is given.
11. Clean the injection port again.
12. Insert the needle of the heparin- or saline-filled syringe.
    a. If saline is being used in the lock or if heparin is being used in the lock and the medication is compatible with heparin, proceed to step 13.
    b. If heparin is being used in the lock and the medication is *not* compatible with heparin, flush with 2–2½ ml normal saline before injecting the heparin.
13. Inject the solution slowly, no faster than 1 ml/min.
14. Remove the syringe and needle from the port.
15. Dispose of the equipment.

References

Centers for Disease Control. (1983). *Guidelines for control of nosocomial infection.* Washington, DC: US Department of Health and Human Services.

Cyganski, J., Donahue, J., & Heaton, J. (1987). The case for the heparin flush. *American Journal of Nursing, 87*(6), 796–797.

Dunn, D., & Lenihan, S. (1987). The case for the saline flush. *American Journal of Nursing, 87*(6), 798–799.

Hale, M. (1990). Heparin versus saline flushes—again. *American Journal of Nursing, 90*(5), 77–78.

Jones, L., & Brooks, J. (1990). The ABCs of PCA. *RN, 53*(5), 54–60.

Motz-Harding, E., & Good, F. (1985). The right solution: Mixing IV drugs thoroughly. *Nursing 85, 15*(2), 62–67.

Noah, V. (1990). Preop teaching is the key to PCA success. *RN, 53*(5), 60–63.

Weiner, M., & Pepper, G. (1985). *Clinical pharmacology and therapeutics in nursing.* New York: McGraw-Hill.

Performance Checklist

General Procedure for Administering Intravenous Medications	Unsat	Needs More Practice	Sat	Comments
Assessment				
1. Check the orders.				
2. Gather information on the drug, including effects, dilution, rate of administration, reactions, compatibility with other fluids and medications.				
3. Check type of intravenous access available.				
Planning				
4. Wash your hands.				
5. Select appropriate equipment based on the method to be used.				
Implementation				
6. Read name of medication from record.				
7. Check label to make sure it is for correct patient, time, and dosage.				
8. Compare medication container with record.				
9. Prepare the medication, using sterile technique.				
10. Prepare 5 ml normal saline in a syringe for flushing if necessary.				
11. Explain the procedure to the patient.				
12. Give medication, using the appropriate specific procedure.				
13. Observe patient for complications.				
14. Dispose of equipment correctly.				
Evaluation				
15. Evaluate, using the following criteria: a. The right patient received the right medication in the right dosage by the right route at the right time.				
b. The medication was given over the correct time period.				

General Procedure for Administering Intravenous Medications *(Continued)*	Unsat	Needs More Practice	Sat	Comments
c. The criteria established for ascertaining the effectiveness of a specific drug were used. (For example, for a given pain medication this right be "Pain relief obtained within 10 minutes.")				
d. Side effects, if present, were promptly identified.				
Documentation				
16. Record name of medication, dosage, intravenous route used, time, and signature.				
17. If 50 or 100 ml fluid given, add amount to intake record.				
The following are steps in the planning or implementation of the various methods for administering intravenous medications. They should be used appropriately with the other steps outlined in the General Procedure.				

Adding to a New Fluid Container

	Unsat	Needs More Practice	Sat	Comments
1. Select ordered additive.				
2. Select appropriate equipment: large-volume fluid container, syringe, and either a regular needle or a transfer needle.				
3. Draw up medication from vial or ampule.				
4. Label new fluid container with name, amount of additive, date, time, and your initials.				
5. Open new fluid container.				
6. Clean the port with alcohol swab.				
7. Inject the medication into the container.				
8. Tilt container back and forth to mix thoroughly.				
9. Hang new infusion container.				
10. Manually set desired flow rate or set ICD to desired rate.				

Adding to an Existing Fluid Container

	Unsat	Needs More Practice	Sat	Comments
1. Prepare medication, using sterile technique.				
2. Take medication to room and identify patient.				

Adding to an Existing Fluid Container
(Continued)

	Unsat	Needs More Practice	Sat	Comments
3. Turn off IV flow.				
4. Invert fluid container.				
5. Clean port with alcohol.				
6. Inject medication into port.				
7. Tilt container back and forth to mix additive thoroughly.				
8. Label container appropriately.				
9. Rehang IV container.				
10. Regulate flow as ordered.				

Using a Controlled-Volume Administration Set

1. Prepare medication using sterile technique.				
2. Take medication to room and identify patient.				
3. Label chamber with name, amount of solution, date, time, and your initials.				
4. Open and fill inlet with required 50 to 100 ml.				
5. Tightly close inlet.				
6. If chamber is hard plastic, make sure air vent is open.				
7. Turn on drip rate to test.				
8. Clean entry port with alcohol.				
9. Insert needle and inject medication.				
10. Regulate correct flow.				

Using a Small-Volume Parenteral

1. Check to see whether patient has an intravenous or a heparin lock.				
2. Select correct equipment. a. Heparin lock: regular long IV tubing, 1-inch needle or needle-lock device, tape, alcohol swab				
b. Existing infusion: secondary administration set, tape, alcohol swab				
c. Existing secondary set: new needle, tape, alcohol swab				

Using a Small-Volume Parenteral *(Continued)*	Unsat	Needs More Practice	Sat	Comments
3. If medication has to be added to the small container, follow directions above for adding to a fluid container.				
4. If you mixed container, label with name, dosage, time, and your initials.				
If using a new tubing set:				
5. Close regulator on tubing.				
6. Clean top of small container.				
7. Attach administration set to small container.				
8. Place needle on end of tubing.				
9. Hang container, and fill drip chamber half full.				
10. Remove needle cover, open regulator, fill the tubing with fluid, reclose regulator, and replace needle cover.				
11. Identify patient.				
12. Hang small container on IV standard.				
13. Place main intravenous bottle on an extension hanger.				
14. Clean entry port near top of main administration set.				
15. Insert needle or needle-lock device from secondary set into high port.				
16. Open regulator on secondary set.				
17. Regulate rate for secondary container using regulator on main set.				
18. Tape connection, including needle cover.				
If using an existing secondary line:				
5. Identify correct used container and tubing.				
6. Clean top of new small container.				
7. Make sure regulator is turned off.				
8. Remove old small container from IV standard and detach tubing.				
9. Insert spike of used tubing into new small container.				
10. Hang new small container on IV standard.				

Using a Small-Volume Parenteral (Continued)	Unsat	Needs More Practice	Sat	Comments
11. Hang main IV container on extension hanger.				
12. If needle was not in the port, change it.				
13. Remove air in secondary line by back-filling.				
14. When fluid is at appropriate level, rehang small container.				
15. Set correct drip rate, using regulator on main IV.				
16. Tape connection, including needle cover.				

Using a Syringe Infusion Pump

	Unsat	Needs More Practice	Sat	Comments
1. Check syringe to make sure it is correct drug and dosage for your patient.				
2. Identify patient and see whether patient has an intravenous or a heparin lock.				
3. Select correct equipment: infusion pump, special thin tubing, sterile 1-inch needle or needle-lock device, alcohol swab, and tape.				
4. Attach proper end of tubing to syringe.				
5. Attach other end of tubing to needle.				
6. Place label on tubing with date and time.				
7. Remove needle cover and flush tubing. Replace needle cover using one-hand technique.				
8. Attach syringe to pump, checking placement.				
9. Clean port and insert needle.				
10. Hang pump on stand or place on table.				
11. Turn on rocker switch, with or without alarm.				
12. Tape in place.				
13. When infusion is completed, replace used needle with a sterile one and tape to pump.				
If you are using an existing infusion pump:				
1. Check tubing to be sure it is not older than 48–72 hours.				
2. Remove used syringe and discard.				
3. Attach tubing to new syringe.				
4. Replace existing needle with new needle.				

Using a Syringe Infusion Pump *(Continued)*	Unsat	Needs More Practice	Sat	Comments
5. Place syringe in pump.				
6. Insert needle into port and turn on pump.				

Giving Medication by IV Push into an Existing IV

1. Prepare the medication, using sterile technique.				
2. Identify the patient.				
3. Check IV functioning.				
4. Select injection port.				
5. Clean port with swab.				
6. Insert needle through rubber.				
7. Pinch off tubing above port.				
8. Inject medication at appropriate rate.				
9. Observe patient.				
10. When all is injected, release tubing.				
11. Withdraw needle.				
12. Dispose of equipment.				

Giving Medication into an Intermittent Infusion Adapter (Heparin Lock)

1. Prepare the medication, using sterile technique.				
2. Identify the patient.				
3. Locate heparin lock.				
4. Inspect site.				
5. Clean port with swab.				
6. Insert needle of medication syringe. a. If saline is being used in lock or if heparin is being used and medication is compatible with heparin, proceed to step 7.				
b. If heparin is being used in lock and medication is *not* compatible with heparin, flush lock with 2–2½ ml normal saline before and after injection of medication.				
7. Aspirate.				

Giving Medication into an Intermittent Infusion Adapter (Heparin Lock) *(Continued)*	Unsat	Needs More Practice	Sat	Comments
8. If blood returns, give at appropriate rate.				
9. If blood does not return, give small amount while checking for swelling and discomfort.				
10. Withdraw needle.				
11. Clean port again.				
12. Insert needle of heparin- or saline-filled syringe. a. If saline is being used in lock or if heparin is being used in lock and medication is compatible with heparin, proceed to step 13.				
b. If heparin is being used in lock and medication is *not* compatible with heparin, flush with 2–2½ ml normal saline before injecting heparin.				
13. Slowly inject heparin or saline solution into lock.				
14. Remove needle from port.				
15. Dispose of equipment.				

Quiz

Short-Answer Questions

1. Why is a needle inserted into an IV line only at an injection port?

   _____

2. If there is no designated speed of injection for an IV push medication, how fast should it be injected and why? _____

   _____

3. When adding medications to a small- or large-volume container, why should you agitate the solution to mix it thoroughly?

   _____

4. What are two effects of drug incompatibilities? _____

   _____

5. What are two resources for determining the actions and possible incompatibilities of drugs? _____

   _____

6. What is the purpose of an intermittent infusion adapter? _____

   _____

7. Why must the premeasured syringe of medication be accurately placed in the infusion pump? _____

   _____

8. Why is heparin or saline solution left in the heparin lock? _____

   _____

9. How many milliliters of fluid are used to dilute the medication in a controlled-volume administration set? _____

Module 55
Caring for Central Intravenous Catheters

Module Contents

Rationale for the Use of This Skill
Nursing Diagnosis and Potential
    Complications
Types of Central Intravenous Catheters
Standard Central Intravenous Catheter
    Inserting the Standard Central Intravenous
        Catheter
        Assessment
        Planning
        Implementation
        Evaluation
        Documentation
    Changing the Central Intravenous Dressing
        Assessment
        Planning
        Implementation
        Evaluation
        Documentation
    Changing the Fluid Container and the
        Tubing
        Assessment
        Planning
        Implementation
        Evaluation
        Documentation
Peripherally Inserted Central Intravenous
    Catheters
Internal Jugular Catheters
Surgically Inserted Central Intravenous
    Catheters
    Subcutaneous Catheter Ports
    Hickman and Broviac Catheters
    Groshong Catheters
    Changing the Exit Site Dressing
        Assessment
        Planning
        Implementation

        Evaluation
        Documentation
Establishing a Heparin Lock on a Central
    Intravenous Catheter
    Assessment
    Planning
    Implementation
    Evaluation
    Documentation
Irrigating a Central Intravenous Catheter
    Assessment
    Planning
    Implementation
    Evaluation
    Documentation
Giving a Medication Through the Heparin
    Lock on a Central Intravenous
    Catheter
    Assessment
    Planning
    Implementation
    Evaluation
    Documentation
Drawing Blood Through a Central
    Intravenous Catheter
    Assessment
    Planning
    Implementation
    Evaluation
    Documentation
Accessing a Subcutaneous Catheter Port
    Assessment
    Planning
    Implementation
    Evaluation
    Documentation
Home Care

460

Prerequisites

1. *Successful completion of the following modules:*

VOLUME 1

Module 1   An Approach to Nursing Skills
Module 2   Basic Infection Control
Module 3   Safety
Module 5   General Assessment Overview
Module 6   Documentation

VOLUME 2

Module 35 Sterile Technique
Module 37 Wound Care
Module 49 Administering Oral Medications
Module 53 Preparing and Maintaining Intravenous Infusions
Module 54 Administering Intravenous Medications

2. *Review the anatomy of the large central veins in the neck and chest and of the right atrium.*

Overall Objective

To set up and maintain various types of central venous infusion catheters with comfort and safety for the patient.

Specific Learning Objectives

	Know Facts and Principles	Apply Facts and Principles	Demonstrate Ability	Evaluate Performance
1. General information				
a. Purposes	State two common reasons for using a central intravenous line.	When given an example of a patient with a central intravenous line, identify the purpose of the line.	In the clinical setting, identify the reason a specific patient has a central intravenous line.	Evaluate with your instructor.
b. Complications	State two major complications associated with central intravenous lines.	Given a patient situation with a complication of a central intravenous line occurring, identify the complication.	In the clinical setting, make appropriate observations to identify complications.	Evaluate with your instructor.
2. Standard central venous line	List common sites for insertion of the standard central venous line. Describe the procedure used for inserting a central intravenous line.		In the practice or clinical setting, select correct equipment for inserting a central intravenous line.	Evaluate selection with your instructor.
3. Changing the central intravenous dressing	State four purposes of changing the central intravenous dressing. List the supplies used in your facility for changing a central intravenous dressing. Explain the rationale for using various antiseptic agents for cleansing the skin when inserting a subclavian line or changing a subclavian dressing. Describe the procedure for changing the central intravenous dressing.	Select appropriate materials for a central intravenous dressing.	In the practice setting, change a central intravenous dressing.	Evaluate your own performance using the Performance Checklist and consultation with instructor.

(continued)

Specific Learning Objectives *(Continued)*

	Know Facts and Principles	Apply Facts and Principles	Demonstrate Ability	Evaluate Performance
4. *Changing the fluid container and the tubing*	State the special concern when changing the tubing on the central intravenous line. Describe the procedure for changing the fluid container and the tubing.		In the practice setting, change the fluid container and tubing on a central intravenous line safely.	Evaluate own performance using the Performance Checklist and consultation with your instructor.
5. *Right atrial catheter with a peripheral exit site*	Identify the special problems associated with the right atrial catheter with a peripheral exit site.	Outline actions that can prevent the development of problems related to the right atrial catheter with a peripheral exit site.		
6. *Surgically implanted central intravenous catheter*	Describe the Hickman, the Broviac, double-lumen Hickman catheters and subcutaneous catheter ports pointing out similarities and differences. List the uses of the above catheters.			
a. *Changing the exit site dressing*	List supplies needed for changing the exit site dressing.		In the practice setting, change an exit site dressing.	Evaluate own performance with instructor using the Performance Checklist.
b. *Establishing an intermittent line with a heparin lock*	List supplies needed to establish an intermittent line with a heparin lock. Describe the procedure for establishing the intermittent line.		In the practice setting, set up a central line as an intermittent line with a heparin lock.	Evaluate own performance with instructor using the Performance Checklist.
c. *Irrigating a central intravenous catheter*	List supplies and equipment needed to irrigate the line. Describe the procedure for irrigating a central intravenous line.		In the practice setting, irrigate a central line.	Evaluate own performance with instructor using the Performance Checklist.

(continued)

Specific Learning Objectives *(Continued)*

	Know Facts and Principles	Apply Facts and Principles	Demonstrate Ability	Evaluate Performance
d. *Giving a medication through an intermittent central intravenous catheter*	List supplies and equipment needed to give a medication through the catheter. Describe the procedure for giving a medication through the central intravenous line.		In the practice setting, give a medication through the central line.	Evaluate own performance with instructor using the Performance Checklist.
e. *Drawing blood through a central intravenous catheter*	List supplies needed for drawing blood through a central intravenous catheter.		In the practice setting, go through the procedure for drawing blood from a central intravenous catheter.	Evaluate own performance with instructor using the Performance Checklist.
f. *Accessing a subcutaneous catheter port*	List supplies and equipment needed to access a port.	Given a patient situation, identify what problem in accessing the port might be present and what nursing action is appropriate.	In the practice setting, access a subcutaneous catheter port.	Evaluate own performance with instructor using the Performance Checklist.

Learning Activities

1. Review the Specific Learning Objectives.
2. Look up the module vocabulary terms in the Glossary.
3. Read through the module and mentally practice the skills.
4. Examine samples of the various central intravenous catheters used in the facility in which you practice.
5. Review the following procedures in the procedure book for your facility:
   a. Central intravenous subclavian dressing change
   b. Hickman catheter care
   c. Broviac catheter care
   d. Subcutaneous catheter port (Port-a-cath, Infus-a-port) care
6. Arrange for time to practice handling central intravenous lines.
7. In the practice setting:
   a. Practice the procedures outlined in the Performance Checklist.
   b. When you have mastered these procedures, select a partner and critique each other's performance using the Performance Checklist.
   c. Arrange for your instructor to evaluate your performance.
8. In the clinical setting:
   a. Identify patients with central intravenous lines in place.
   b. Arrange an opportunity to observe care for these patients.
   c. Ask your instructor for an opportunity to carry out the specific care needed by the patient.

Vocabulary

air embolism	Hickman catheter	Port-a-cath	subcutaneous catheter port
Broviac catheter	inferior vena cava	right atrium	superior vena cava
cardiac output	Infus-a-port	sclerose	Trendelenburg's position
cephalic vein	Intrasil catheter	septicemia	
Groshong catheter	noncoring needle	subclavian vein	

Caring for Central Intravenous Catheters

Rationale for the Use of This Skill

In modern acute care settings, a large number of patients are receiving intravenous medications and nutritional solutions. Many of these products are irritating to small veins but are tolerated without local irritation in large vessels, which have a high-volume blood flow, allowing for rapid dilution of the product. With the increased use of all intravenous products we also see patients in whom all available small vessels have been used repeatedly and subsequently become irritated or sclerosed or in other ways are unusable. For these patients the central intravenous catheter offers an effective route for the administration of needed therapy. *Because of the direct access to the central circulation, the special dynamics of blood flow in the large central veins, and the difficulty in replacing central intravenous catheters, specialized care techniques are required.*[1]

TYPES OF CENTRAL INTRAVENOUS CATHETERS

Several types of central intravenous infusion catheters are in current use. Two major types—the standard central intravenous line and the surgically inserted

[1] You will note that rationale for action is emphasized throughout the module by the use of italics.

▶ **Nursing Diagnosis and Potential Complications**

High Risk for Infection is a major nursing diagnosis for patients with central lines. *Infection is a serious complication associated with the use of central intravenous lines. First, the solution is flowing directly into the central circulation. Any bacteria introduced with the fluid circulate freely, and generalized septicemia may result. Second, the catheter enters through the skin and provides a direct path that microbes may follow from the surface, along the outside of the catheter, and into the central circulation. Again, septicemia may easily result. Many of the steps in the procedures for care are designed to guard the patient against this high infection risk.* Careful observation of the entry site for redness, swelling, or exudate is necessary *to identify local infection.* Assessment for elevated temperature, malaise, and chills is necessary *to identify systemic infection.*

The Potential Complication: *Air embolism is another special risk for the patient with a central intravenous catheter. As a result of the dynamics of fluid flow and pressure changes within the thoracic cavity, negative pressure develops in the large central veins, facilitating their filling and returning blood to the heart and thus maintaining adequate cardiac output.* When a catheter is placed in one of these large veins, negative pressure occurs at the tip of the catheter, facilitating the movement of fluid from the catheter into the vein. *If the catheter is not filled with fluid and is open to the air, the* negative pressure at the tip draws air into the catheter, creating an air embolism. *Of course, the amount of air that actually enters the catheter depends on the amount of negative pressure and the length of time negative pressure is exerted against an open catheter.* The amount of air needed to create an air embolus large enough to be symptomatic is not known. Some authorities believe that as little as 50 ml of air may cause a fatal air embolus (Pederson & Hessov, 1978). No data are given to substantiate this. *Because an air embolus can interfere with effective emptying of the ventricles and diminish cardiac output even when not great enough to cause death,* it is wise to try to eliminate air entirely by careful technique. Care should be taken not to frighten the patient by overzealous behavior, because inadvertently allowing a single small air bubble to enter the line will certainly not cause problems to the patient. Symptoms that may indicate air embolus include shortness of breath, irregularities in the apical heartbeat, and chest discomfort. If the patient is being monitored, arrhythmias may be observed.

To prevent air embolism, many central venous catheters are produced with a clamp located near the external end that can be closed whenever the catheter is being opened to the air. If the catheter does not have a clamp, a 6-inch extension tubing with a clamp may be attached for the same purpose.

central intravenous line—are discussed here. The central intravenous line with a peripheral exit site is discussed briefly. Other types of central intravenous lines may be used in your facility. By analyzing the type of line in use, you should be able to adapt these procedures to your situation as necessary.

STANDARD CENTRAL INTRAVENOUS CATHETER

The standard central venous line is inserted by the physician in a sterile procedure. The catheter may be sutured to the skin at the exit site and may be short or long. The short length rests with the tip of the catheter in the vein. The long catheter is threaded farther into the vein until the tip rests in the right atrium. The most common insertion site is the right or left subclavian vein, but the right cephalic vein or the right or left internal jugular vein may also be used (Figure 55–1). Care for all is the same.

INSERTING THE STANDARD CENTRAL INTRAVENOUS CATHETER

Assessment
1. Check the order for insertion of a central intravenous line.
2. Assess the patient's ability to participate in and tolerate the procedure.
   a. Check whether the patient can be positioned flat or in Trendelenburg's position.
   b. Check the patient's ability to hold breath on command.
   c. Check the patient's ability to understand and follow directions in regard to the position of the head and remaining still.

Planning
3. Wash your hands *for infection control.*
4. Obtain the necessary equipment and supplies. In many facilities a standard disposable set is used for inserting central intravenous lines. If such a set is used, be sure to check the contents, *so you know which other items you will need.* The following supplies are commonly used:
   a. Masks for all those assisting with the procedure *to reduce the possibility of contamination from microbes from the nose and mouth.* In some facilities the procedure specifies that the patient also be masked.

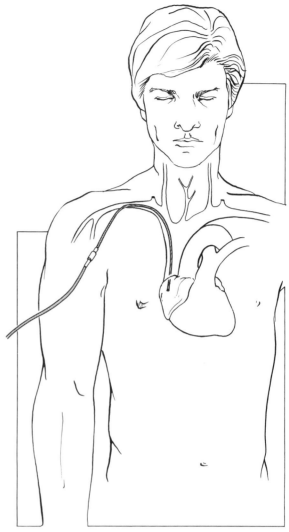

Figure 55–1 Subclavian IV line in place. Note the entry point and the position of the tip of the catheter in the right atrium.

Because this often creates anxiety, in most facilities the patient is positioned with the face away from the insertion site and the drapes are positioned to provide a screen between the patient's nose and mouth and the insertion site.
   b. Sterile gown for the physician inserting the catheter. In some facilities a sterile gown is not required, but a clean gown is used to cover the physician's clothes *to protect against contamination of the site and to protect the physician.*
   c. Two pairs of sterile gloves of the appropriate size for the physician.
   d. Skin preparation materials. Procedure in some facilities includes the use of acetone

to defat the skin. *Evidence has shown, however, that removing the normal protective coat increases skin irritation and local inflammation and does not lower the infection rate,* so it is not recommended (Stratton, 1981).

Povidone-iodine swabs or solution and sterile gauze swabs are an excellent skin antiseptic, but a potential for skin reaction exists. A large area is prepared and the solution allowed to dry. *This process liberates free iodine and is the basis for the effectiveness of this solution in lowering the bacterial count* (Stratton, 1981).

Tincture of iodine may be used as an antiseptic agent, but because it often causes skin reactions it is removed with 70% alcohol after it has dried. *This lessens the incidence of skin reaction and preserves the antiseptic effect* (Stratton, 1981).

Also 70% alcohol alone may be used as a skin antiseptic.

e. Razor to shave the skin, if necessary.

f. 1% lidocaine for use as a topical anesthetic.

g. Sterile drapes *to drape the site.* A fenestrated drape (one with a hole in the center) is commonly used, or four plain drapes may be used *to surround the area.* Towel clips to hold the plain drapes in place are useful but not essential.

h. Suitable intracatheter and a syringe. A 16-gauge, 20-cm intracatheter is a common size. The catheter may be either polyethylene or silicone rubber.

i. Suturing materials. 000 silk sutures with atraumatic needles attached are commonly used. A needle holder, a hemostat, and scissors are needed.

j. Intravenous fluid with tubing attached, ready to be connected to the catheter. A 6-inch extension tubing with a clamp is often used on central lines. This is treated as a part of the primary line and allows the line to be clamped when tubing is being changed or other procedures are performed.

k. Dressing materials *to dress the exit site.* Various techniques can be used for dressing the central intravenous site, each requiring slightly different materials.

(1) Transparent, moisture/vapor-permeable dressing material (OpSite, Tegaderm) is gaining favor as a dressing material. *It allows for easy inspection of the site, stays moist but does not allow excess moisture to accumulate beneath the dressing, due to its moisture/vapor-permeable nature, and forms an effective barrier to microbes. Because nurses can observe the site without removing the dressing,* this type of dressing is changed less frequently than others—in some facilities only once a week.

(2) Large adhesive bandages with water-repellent backing are included in many prepackaged kits. The adhesive surface extends on all sides of the bandage's gauze pad *so the dressing may be securely taped in place in an occlusive manner.*

(3) Plastic adhesive drape material may be used *to cover a gauze dressing* placed directly over the site. In this case two 3×3 gauze squares are used for the underneath dressing. Tape may also be used *to fasten the edges of the dressing more securely.*

(4) 3×3 gauze squares and impermeable plastic tape may be used *to form an occlusive dressing over the site. If the patient's skin is sensitive to this kind of tape,* use hypoallergenic paper tape instead.

Povidone-iodine ointment is used *to seal the opening through which the catheter passes into the body, regardless of the type of dressing used. This seal helps prevent microbes from entering.* Studies indicate that *using an antiseptic or antimicrobial ointment at an intravenous insertion site lessens the incidence of local infection* (Stratton, 1981). In some facilities an antimicrobial ointment is used. *Povidone-iodine ointment is more effective in preventing fungal infections, and antimicrobial ointment is more effective against bacterial infections. Either type of ointment may cause skin irritation* (Stratton, 1981).

l. Sterile towel *to provide a sterile field.* If a prepackaged set is used, the wrapper may serve as the sterile field.

Implementation

5. Check the patient's identification *to be sure you are performing the procedure for the correct patient.*

6. Explain the procedure to the patient. The patient who is responsive needs a careful, nonthreatening explanation of the procedure, *to reduce anxiety.* The explanation should focus on what the patient will personally experience. Briefly explain the advantage of this method of access to the vein: both arms may be free for movement and the arms may be spared further discomfort from intravenous lines. You might also point out that the patient may become aware that special care procedures will be used that were not used for the peripheral intravenous lines, such as a more elaborate procedure for the dressing change. Emphasize that these procedures are added safety measures. During the procedure the area will be anesthetized, *so the insertion will not be painful.* A sedative may be ordered by the physician. Explain that lying still is important *to facilitate the physician's task* and that the patient may be asked to inhale and then bear down briefly while the tubing is attached. (This is a Valsalva maneuver.) This is done to prevent air embolus, although you may not wish to explain this in detail, because it might frighten the patient unnecessarily.

If the patient cannot understand the explanations, you will want to make brief statements throughout the procedure, *to reduce anxiety.* Emphasize that you are there to help the patient. Extra assistants may be needed *if the patient must be restrained to maintain immobility.*

7. Prepare a clean table as a sterile field for all the supplies. If an overbed table is used, it is prudent to clean the surface thoroughly with a germicidal agent, such as 70% alcohol, or a phenol disinfectant, *because overbed tables may have been used to hold urinals, bedpans, or other contaminated items.*

8. Set up the equipment on the table. Using careful sterile technique, arrange a sterile towel or the wrapper of the package to form a sterile field. Then carefully place all sterile equipment within the field.

9. Place the patient in a supine position. If this is not possible for the entire procedure, be prepared to place the patient in a flat position for the time needed. A slight Trendelenburg's position is desirable when the vein is entered and when the tubing is being connected. *With the patient in Trendelenburg's position, slight positive pressure occurs in the central veins and protects against air embolism. This positioning also causes the vessels to dilate, facilitating insertion.* If the bed cannot easily be adjusted from flat to Trendelenburg's, the patient may have to be

placed in a slight Trendelenburg's position for the entire procedure. If the patient cannot tolerate this position, he or she remains lying flat during all parts of the procedure, and connections are made quickly *to lessen the opportunity for air to enter the catheter.* Place a rolled towel under the shoulder on the side being used for the insertion *to provide better access to the vein.*

10. Support the patient psychologically.
    a. Maintaining touch with the patient is important. Often this takes the form of holding the patient's hand.
    b. Help the patient maintain the proper position by supporting the head if necessary.
    c. Give positive reinforcement to the patient for cooperative efforts.
    d. Provide feedback to the patient *to reassure that the procedure is progressing satisfactorily.*
    e. If difficulties are encountered, try to reassure the patient, *so anxiety does not increase.*
    f. If necessary, remind others in the environment that the patient is alert even though the face is covered. Discourage inappropriate comments by staff.

11. Assist the physician if necessary. If the physician will need assistance with materials, have two persons present, *so one can focus on the patient and the other can take care of procedural needs.* An experienced nurse may be able to accomplish both tasks simultaneously.
    a. You may be asked to hold the vial of anesthetic while the physician withdraws the medication.
    b. Equipment or supply packages may need to be opened, *so the contents are accessible to the physician without risking contamination of the sterile gloves.*
    c. An assistant may need to connect the intravenous tubing to the catheter, start the flow rate, and prepare the tape for stabilizing the catheter on the skin.
    d. An assistant may be asked to complete the dressing.

12. After the line has been inserted, remove the drapes and position the patient comfortably. It is important that the patient be made as comfortable as possible as soon as the procedure is completed.

13. Regulate the intravenous flow rate as prescribed. Often the flow rate is set at a slow

DATE/TIME	
12/28/95 11:00 AM	*No. 16, 20 cm single-lumen subclavian intravenous catheter inserted by Dr. M. Sanchez at 10 AM. Position verified by x-ray. 1000 ml D₅W with 40 mEq KCl started at 30 ml/h. Pt. resting comfortably with all vitals stable. See graphic record. ——— R. Nichols, RN*

Example of Progress Note Using Narrative Format

drip when the line is first connected. An x-ray to verify correct placement may be done before the rate is increased. An alternative is to place a heparin lock on the line, fill it with heparinized saline, and start the fluid after the x-ray. You will want to begin providing the prescribed flow rate as quickly as possible, *so the patient is receiving all the fluid required at a rate that allows for appropriate utilization.*

14. Remove all used supplies and packaging materials. Most will be disposable. Care for nondisposable items according to your facility's procedure.
15. Wash your hands *for infection control.*

Evaluation
16. Evaluate the following:
    a. Patient comfort.
    b. The intravenous line *to be sure that the flow is not obstructed, the rate is correctly set, and all connections are securely taped.*
    c. The dressing *to be sure it is secure.*

Documentation
17. Record on the patient chart:
    a. Time the central intravenous line was inserted.
    b. Type and size of the catheter.
    c. Site used.
    d. Solution started and the rate of administration.
       In some facilities, this information may be recorded on an intravenous flow sheet. If it is recorded on the narrative, the same information is included.
    e. Patient's response.
    f. If an x-ray was used to verify the position of the catheter, note the time the x-ray was taken.

CHANGING THE CENTRAL INTRAVENOUS DRESSING

The same procedure may be used for changing dressings over subclavian lines, total parenteral nutrition (TPN) lines, and all other types of central lines.

The frequency with which these dressings are changed is not standardized. In some facilities in which standard gauze and tape dressings are used, the dressings are changed daily or every other day. In other hospitals such dressings are changed three times weekly on a prescribed schedule. In some hospitals where transparent, moisture-permeable dressings (OpSite and Tegaderm) are used, dressings are left in place until they begin to loosen or for 1 week, whichever comes first. These hospitals report no increase in infection rate and reduced incidence of irritation when dressings are changed less frequently. This method also saves nursing time. No specific recommendation is forthcoming from the Centers for Disease Control at this writing. It would be appropriate to watch the literature closely for research results and specific recommendations. Meanwhile, continue to follow the procedure designated in your facility. In addition to regularly scheduled changes, the dressing is changed if it pulls loose or becomes wet, *because this situation increases the potential for contamination of the entry site.*

The dressing change permits careful assessment of the insertion site, thorough cleansing of the area and removal of any debris that might foster microbial growth, application of antiseptic or antimicrobial agents to decrease future growth of microbes, and application of new sterile dressing materials to replace those that may have become contaminated.

Assessment
1. Check the date and time of the last dressing change.
2. Review the facility procedure *to identify the appropriate dressing materials to use.*

Planning
3. Wash your hands *for infection control.*
4. Obtain the necessary supplies, including the following:
   a. Mask for the nurse *to prevent contamination of the sterile field from microorganisms of the mouth, nose, and throat.* In some facilities a mask is used for both patient and nurse, and in others no masks are used. Follow the policy in your facility.

b. Disinfectant or germicidal cleansing agent *to prepare a clean surface to use as a base for the sterile field.*

c. Sterile gloves *to maintain the dressing's sterility.*

d. Cleansing materials. These vary from facility to facility, but those most commonly used are hydrogen peroxide, applied with cotton-tipped applicators *to cleanse any exudate from the site or to remove crusts around the catheter,* and povidone-iodine solution and gauze squares or povidone-iodine swabs *to cleanse and disinfect the skin.* When swabs are used, you do not need sterile gloves, because the hands are separated from contact with the wound. Some facilities use acetone, but this is not recommended, as discussed previously. Tincture of iodine may be used and then followed with 70% alcohol to remove the iodine in order *to decrease the incidence of skin reaction to the tincture of iodine. For patients with sensitivity to iodine,* 70% alcohol alone may be used.

e. Dressing supplies for the site vary, as discussed earlier. Select those used in your facility.

f. Antiseptic or antimicrobial ointment *to decrease microorganisms at the insertion site.*

g. Clean gloves to remove the soiled dressing.

Implementation

5. Check the patient's identification *to be sure you are performing the procedure for the correct patient.*

6. Explain the procedure to the patient.

7. Clean the overbed table with disinfectant and allow it to dry.

8. Place the patient in the supine position, with the head turned away from the insertion site.

9. Put on the mask if your facility procedure includes its use.

10. Set up your materials on the overbed table. Open sterile packages so the contents are accessible but remain protected. If a prepackaged set is used, open it so the outer wrap serves as a sterile field.

11. Put on clean gloves, remove the old dressing, and discard it. *Clean gloves protect your hands from possible contact with drainage from the wound.*

12. Take off the gloves and wash your hands.

13. Inspect the site carefully, especially noting any redness, swelling, or drainage, *to assess for infection and reaction to the materials used in cleansing. If irritation is noted without signs of*

infection, it is appropriate to change to an alternate cleansing material or to use only hydrogen peroxide.

14. Put on the sterile gloves.

15. Cleanse the area around the catheter with the hydrogen peroxide *to remove secretions, crusts, or exudate.*

16. Use the antiseptic solution *to cleanse the entire site and surrounding area.* Cleanse in a circular manner, starting at the catheter and moving outward in concentric circles. Do not go back over areas previously cleansed. Cleanse an area 3 inches from the site in all directions *to provide a wide area of antiseptic protection.* Cleanse for a total of 2 minutes. *This provides good contact with the antiseptic activity of the agent.*

17. Allow the antiseptic solution to dry. If you used tincture of iodine, you then use 70% alcohol to remove the iodine and allow the alcohol to dry. *This provides maximum antiseptic action.*

18. Obtain a small amount of antiseptic or antimicrobial ointment on an applicator and apply it to the insertion site, completely filling the space and occluding it. *This provides a mechanical and a chemical barrier to microbes.*

19. Apply the new dressing.

a. If using gauze squares and tape, place one gauze square under the catheter and one over the insertion site. Arrange the catheter so the connection end is outside the dressing. *This allows the tubing to be changed without disturbing the dressing.* Remove the sterile gloves, and tape the dressing down on all sides. To seal the edge under the catheter completely, cut a small slit in the tape and slide this onto each side of the catheter to secure the dressing (Figure 55–2).

b. If using a plastic adhesive drape material, place one gauze square under the catheter and one over the insertion site. Remove the gloves and pull the backing off the plastic. Place it over the gauze and begin pressing it down from one side to the other. When securing it at the catheter, mold the plastic around the catheter so it forms a seal (Figure 55–3).

c. If using a transparent, moisture/vapor-permeable dressing (OpSite or Tegaderm), do not use gauze squares. *Skin moisture will gradually escape through the dressing material.* Remove your gloves before handling the

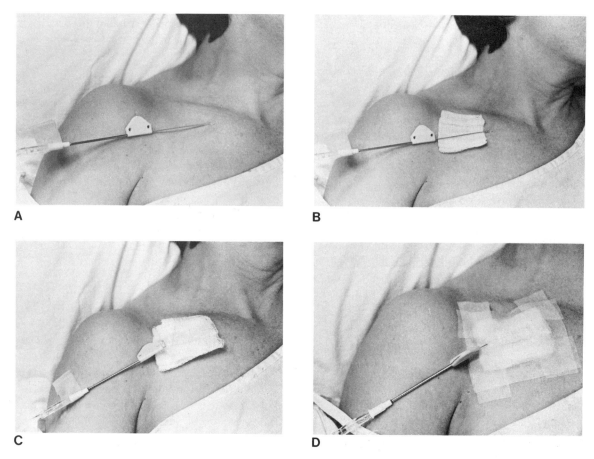

Figure 55-2 Using gauze squares as a dressing for a subclavian IV line. **A:** Catheter and insertion site. **B:** The first gauze square is placed under the catheter. **C:** The second gauze square is placed over the catheter exit site. **D:** The edges are taped down to form a seal on all sides. Note how the tape is placed around the catheter. (*Courtesy Ivan Ellis*)

materials. Peel off the backing gradually as you apply the material to the skin, *so it goes on smoothly.* Allow enough slack *so you can mold the dressing material around the catheter, forming a seal* (Figure 55–4). There are also

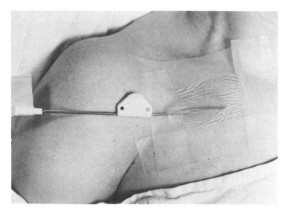

Figure 55-3 Using a clear plastic adhesive drape over the subclavian dressing. (*Courtesy Ivan Ellis*)

commercially produced transparent dressings designed for use with central lines (Figure 55–5).

20. Change the tape over the connection between the catheter and the intravenous tubing. Make tabs on each end of the tape *so it can be removed easily,* and then apply the tape around the connection securely (Figure 55–6).
21. Remove your mask, if you are wearing one.
22. Label the dressing with date and time of changing by writing on the dressing itself or by writing on a piece of tape placed on the dressing. Use a pen with ink that will not rub off.
23. Reposition the patient *for comfort.*
24. Dispose of all packages and materials used.
25. Wash your hands.

Evaluation
26. Evaluate the following:
    a. Patient comfort.
    b. The intravenous line *to be sure that the flow is*

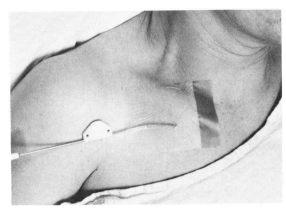

Figure 55–4 Dressing the subclavian IV line with transparent, moisture-permeable dressing (OpSite)
(*Courtesy Ivan Ellis*)

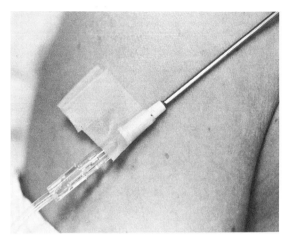

Figure 55–6 Taping the connection between the catheter and the IV tubing.
(*Courtesy Ivan Ellis*)

not obstructed, the rate is correctly set, and all connections are secure.

c. The dressing *to be sure it is secure.*

Documentation

27. Record the dressing change as prescribed in your facility either on a flow sheet or on the narrative progress notes. Be sure a description of the site is included.

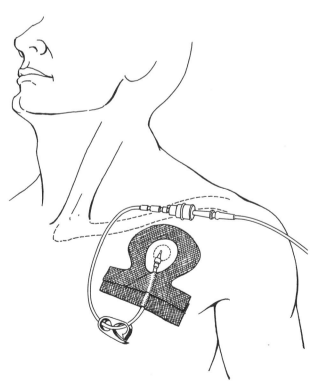

Figure 55–5 Commercial dressing for a central line.

CHANGING THE FLUID CONTAINER AND THE TUBING

When changing an intravenous fluid container connected to a central line, use the same technique as for changing a container on a conventional intravenous line (see Module 53, Preparing and Maintaining Intravenous Infusions).

When changing the tubing, *you must take special precautions to protect the patient against air embolism caused by the negative pressure at the catheter's tip.*

Assessment

1. Follow Assessment steps 1 and 2 of the procedure for changing an intravenous bottle and tubing as outlined in Module 53, Preparing and Maintaining Intravenous Infusions (check physician's order and date of last tubing change).

Planning

2. Follow the Planning steps of the procedure for changing an intravenous bottle and tubing as outlined in Module 53 (wash your hands and select the correct equipment).

Implementation

3. Proceed with Implementation steps 5–10 for changing tubing found in Module 53 (set up equipment, identify the patient, hang the new container on the IV standard, remove tape and dressing from old tubing, examine site, shut off IV flow).

4. Remove the tape from the connection between the catheter and the tubing.

5. Cleanse the junction between the catheter and

DATE/TIME	
12/30/95 9:30 AM	*Subclavian dressing changed at 10 AM. Site clean and dry with no drainage, redness, or swelling. Sutures remain intact.* — M. Washington, NS

Example of Progress Notes Using Narrative Format

the tubing with an alcohol swab and allow it to dry *to decrease the number of microbes in the area.*

6. Clamp the line if there is a clamp on the tubing. *This prevents air embolism. If there is no clamp, you must do one of three things to increase intrathoracic pressure and prevent air embolism:* pinch or fold the tubing, place the patient in Trendelenburg's position, which will slow the flow in the vein, *thus increasing venous pressure,* or have the patient take a deep breath and hold it while you change the tubing *to increase intrathoracic pressure.* This last method is called the Valsalva maneuver and should be done just at the time of the tubing change.

7. Loosen the old tubing from the connection by twisting it but do not disconnect it.

8. Remove cap from new tubing.

9. Remove the old tubing from the connector and insert the new tubing immediately (Figure 55–7).

10. Start the new fluid at a slow rate.

11. Tape the connection as previously described.

Evaluation

12. Evaluate the following:
   a. Patient comfort.
   b. Patency, correct flow, and secure connections.
   c. Dressing secure.

Documentation

13. Document as follows:
   a. Intravenous flow sheet: time, fluid discontinued, fluid added, tubing change.
   b. Intake and output record.

PERIPHERALLY INSERTED CENTRAL INTRAVENOUS CATHETER

This central intravenous catheter is inserted through a vein in the arm and threaded into the subclavian vein until its tip rests in the superior vena cava. It is referred to as a PIC (peripherally inserted central) catheter or as a central catheter with a peripheral

exit site. The catheter is inserted, and then fluoroscopy is used to verify its position. The catheter volume is 0.4 ml. *This catheter allows the administration of fluids and medications that can only be infused into the large central veins without the necessity of the more complex procedure necessary to insert a conventional central intravenous line or the surgical procedure to implant a catheter.* This type of line may also be used to measure pressures in the right atrium and to draw blood (Figure 55–8).

In most facilities care is identical to that given for the standard central intravenous line. In some facilities the care is the same as that given for other peripheral IVs unless nutrient solutions are being administered. Be sure to check the policy in your facility.

It is important that clear communication be established *so members of the health care team are aware that this is not a peripheral intravenous line.* In addition to recording this information in the permanent medical record and on the Kardex, it is wise to note the

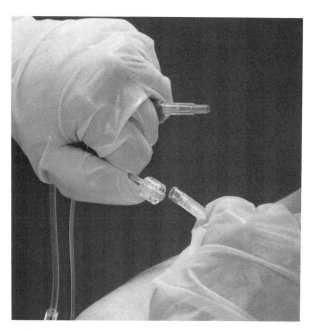

Figure 55–7 Hold the new IV line carefully to prevent its contamination while you separate the used tubing from the catheter.

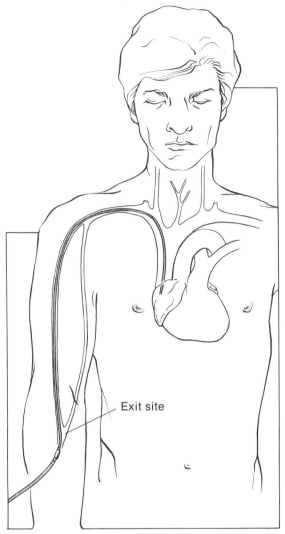

Exit site

Figure 55–8 The peripherally inserted central IV catheter (sometimes called a PIC catheter).

type of line being used by writing directly on the dressing or on a piece of tape placed over the dressing. Then, *even if someone has not thoroughly read the record, the information will be immediately apparent when the line is used or cared for.*

INTERNAL JUGULAR CATHETERS

A variety of catheters designed for insertion through the internal jugular vein, including the Arrow catheter, are available. The triple-lumen catheter has three color-coded ports, each going to a different lumen. Each lumen exits and opens separately from the other lumens *so that one can be designated for nutritional solutions, another for drawing blood, and the*

third for intermittent medications. Any one, any two, or all three may be capped and filled with heparin solution *for intermittent use.*

SURGICALLY INSERTED CENTRAL INTRAVENOUS CATHETERS

Subcutaneous Catheter Ports

The subcutaneous catheter port (Port-a-cath, Infuse-a-Port, or Hickman port) is a surgically inserted central intravenous line that does not have an exit site. The catheter ends in a reservoir that has a rubber diaphragm for a top and is implanted under the skin. To access it, the nurse uses a special needle inserted through the skin (see page 485). The subcutaneous port can be filled with heparinized saline and used intermittently or connected to intravenous fluids and medications. *Because it has no exit site, the potential for infection is decreased,* but a needle puncture is needed each time it is used. It is cared for as if it were a standard central intravenous line, except that a larger volume of heparinized saline (5 ml) is needed to fill it (Figure 55–9). *These devices appear to be more susceptible to clotting closed when used for blood drawing than other central lines.* Therefore, careful attention to thorough flushing after all blood drawing is needed.

Hickman and Broviac Catheters

The *Hickman catheter* is a right atrial catheter that is surgically inserted into the chest and into a central vein. As shown in Figure 55–10, it is tunneled under the chest tissue after it exits from the vein so that the exit site at the skin is a distance from the exit from the vein. In the subcutaneous tunnel the catheter is surrounded by a Dacron cuff, which *allows tissue to grow into the material, forming a seal against microbes. It takes approximately 3 weeks for the catheter to thoroughly heal into place.* (This time varies with the health and healing ability of the patient.)

The internal diameter of the Hickman catheter is 1.6 mm. This is large enough to allow withdrawal of blood and infusion of fluid into the vein. This type of catheter may be kept open with a continuous infusion or may be capped and filled with heparinized saline, to be used as an intermittent access to the vein. The Hickman catheter may have one, two, or three lumens.

The *Broviac catheter* is a similar single-lumen catheter that is inserted in the same way as the Hickman catheter. The major difference between the two

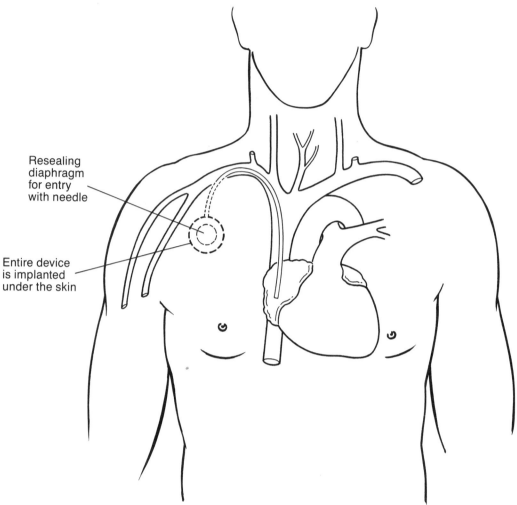

Resealing diaphragm for entry with needle

Entire device is implanted under the skin

Figure 55–9 The implanted central IV port. The IV catheter is threaded into the right atrium. The catheter exists the vein and attaches to the metal reservoir, which has a resealable rubber diaphragm on the top.

is that the Broviac catheter has an internal diameter of 1 mm and so cannot be used for drawing blood. It is used only for infusing fluids.

The double-lumen Hickman catheter is actually a fusion of two Hickman catheters or of a Broviac catheter and a single-lumen Hickman catheter (Figure 55–11). The double-lumen catheter is used principally to allow adequate nutrients to be infused without interruption while allowing medications to be given and blood to be drawn intermittently. A continuous infusion of a nutritional solution is administered through the smaller-lumen Broviac while the larger-lumen Hickman is used for drawing blood samples (with the Broviac temporarily clamped) and for infusing medications (may be done simultaneously with the infusion of the nutrient solution). When both lumens are the same size (Hickman diameter), either lumen may be used for all purposes.

Care is the same for all three catheters. The insertion site is dressed as any surgical site until it has healed (see Module 37, Wound Care). The exit site must be cared for and dressed and a special technique is necessary for drawing blood from the Hickman line. When the line is used intermittently, it must be filled with heparinized saline *to prevent coagulation at the tip, which would occlude the line. Because these lines are intended for long-term use,* the patient and the family must be taught to carry out the care at home. A clamp is kept on the catheter whenever fluid is not being infused *to guard against inadvertent separation of the cap and line, with the resulting chance of air embolism.* Plastic clamps are in place on many central catheters. When one is not already present, a bull dog clamp is placed on the line over a piece of tape. The tape protects the tubing from possible damage from the metal clamp.

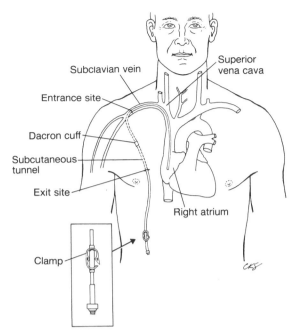

Figure 55-10 A surgically inserted central intravenous catheter. This is a Hickman catheter.

Groshong Catheters

The Groshong catheter is a surgically implanted central venous catheter made of silicone rubber. It is inserted through a tunnel in a manner similar to a Hickman catheter. It has a specially designed tip that allows the pressure of fluid being instilled to open the tip and administer fluid. The tip can also be opened by the negative pressure created by a syringe and therefore can be used for drawing blood. How-

ever, the tip will not open from the blood pressure in the central vein, *so no blood can get into the catheter and form a clot.* In addition, the patient is protected from air embolism *because the tip does not allow the negative pressure in the chest to be transmitted to the catheter lumen.* This catheter is filled with normal saline when not in use. *Because no heparin is administered to keep it open,* it is safer for the patient who should not receive heparin. However, some facilities do use heparin solution in Groshong catheters.

CHANGING THE EXIT SITE DRESSING

The dressing over the exit site is changed daily for the first 3 weeks after surgical insertion. When the exit site is thoroughly healed, the procedure may be different. In some facilities the dressing is changed only when soiled or loose or at specified intervals, such as three times a week. At the Fred Hutchinson Cancer Research Institute in Seattle, Washington, where the Hickman catheter was developed, the practice is to leave the exit site open without a dressing after it is fully healed. The exit site is cleaned as necessary with hydrogen peroxide. The tubing is clamped to the patient's underclothing *to prevent pulling,* or a small gauze square is taped over the site and the catheter is clamped to the dressing *to prevent pulling.*

Assessment

1. Check the date and time of the last dressing change.

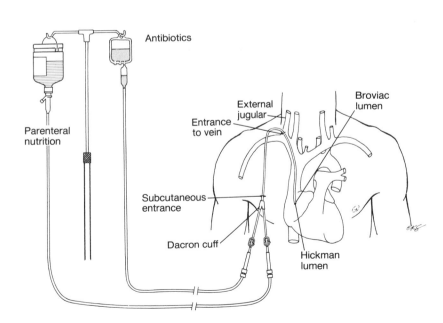

Figure 55-11 The double-lumen Hickman catheter.

© 1992 by J.B. Lippincott Company

2. Review the facility procedure *to identify the appropriate dressing material to use.*

Planning
3. Wash your hands *for infection control.*
4. Gather the necessary supplies.
   a. Hydrogen peroxide and sterile cotton-tipped applicators
   b. Povidone-iodine swabsticks or povidone-iodine solution and additional sterile cotton-tipped applicators. In some facilities you also need an alcohol wipe.
   c. Povidone-iodine ointment or triple antibiotic ointment.
   d. Sterile 2×2 gauze squares
   e. Paper tape
      You will notice that sterile gloves and mask are not needed. *Because the exit site is a distance from the entry into the vein, the infection danger is considerably lessened.* Sterile equipment is used, and the sterility of all items that touch the exit site is maintained. *This has been demonstrated to provide adequate protection against infection.*

Implementation
5. Identify the patient *to be sure you are performing the procedure on the correct patient.*
6. Explain the procedure to the patient.
7. Remove the old dressing and inspect the site for redness, exudate, and swelling, *which might indicate infection.* Wear clean gloves for handling the soiled dressing. Check also for skin reaction to the iodine products.
8. Using the sterile cotton-tipped applicators, cleanse the exit site with hydrogen peroxide. Remove any crusts that have formed. Use a new sterile applicator each time it is necessary to dip into the container of peroxide, *so you do not contaminate the supply.* Next cleanse outward for 3 inches in all directions from the catheter, using a spiral that starts at the catheter and progresses outward, *so microbes are moved away from the exit site.*
9. Cleanse the same area in the same way, using the povidone-iodine swabsticks or cotton-tipped applicators dipped in povidone-iodine solution.
10. Allow the iodine solution to dry on the skin for 2 or 3 minutes. *This frees the iodine and leaves an antiseptic film on the skin.* In some facilities the iodine cleansing is done first and the iodine is allowed to dry, and then the peroxide cleansing is done. This does not leave the antiseptic film on the skin, but *removal of the*

iodine may lessen the chance of skin reaction. Follow the procedure established in your facility.
11. Squeeze antibacterial ointment directly onto the exit site, completely occluding the opening around the catheter. *This provides both a mechanical and a chemical barrier against microbes.*
12. Lift the catheter up and use a povidone-iodine swabstick to cleanse it from the exit site to the connector. *This decreases the number of bacteria present and moves them away from the exit site.* In some facilities this step is done with an alcohol wipe.
13. Place one 2×2 gauze square under the catheter, and one over the exit site, *to provide an absorbent surface between the plastic of the catheter and the skin, and to act as a barrier between outside contaminants and the exit site.*
14. Tape the dressing in place *to secure it.*
15. Loop the catheter and tape it to the body. *Looping prevents direct pull on the catheter and lessens the chance of disturbing it. Taping the catheter down prevents it from twisting and being caught on clothing.*
16. Write the date and time of the change on the dressing itself. *This provides immediate reference for those caring for the patient.*
17. Dispose of used equipment and packaging materials.
18. Wash your hands.

Evaluation
19. Evaluate using the following criteria:
    a. Dressing is secure.
    b. Catheter is not under tension.

Documentation
20. Record the dressing change as appropriate in your facility, either on a flow sheet or on the narrative progress record. Include the appearance of the site in your recording.

ESTABLISHING A HEPARIN LOCK ON A CENTRAL INTRAVENOUS CATHETER

When a Hickman line or central intravenous catheter is being used for intermittent infusion and drawing of blood, it must be capped with a special type of injection cap that screws onto the line like a jar lid. This cap is used to make sure the cap does not become dislodged accidentally, providing an opportunity for air to enter. As in the regular heparin lock, the catheter must be filled with a heparinized saline solution *to prevent clots from forming at the tip of the catheter and occluding it.* A solution of 10–100 units heparin per milliliter of normal saline is the most common mixture. The heparin solution is injected at least twice a day *to maintain patency of the catheter.* Some facilities are experimenting with using a stronger heparin solution (100–500 units/ml) and allowing longer intervals between the times when new solution is added. Be sure you check the policy in your facility.

As another precaution against accidental opening of the Hickman line or catheter, a clamp without teeth, such as a shunt clamp—sometimes called a Scribner clamp, cannula clamp, or bulldog clamp, is used (Figure 55–12) if the line does not have an integral clamp. Even though the clamp has no teeth, *to prevent damage to the catheter* the clamp is placed over a piece of tape on the line. Remember that a Hickman line may be in place for months and that repairs and replacement are problems. Thus, careful handling is essential. When the line is being used, the bulldog clamp is kept attached to the dressing or a tape for safe keeping.

Assessment
1. Check the order for establishing a heparin lock on a central line.
2. Check the facility procedure for the type of solution to be used.
3. Check the type of central intravenous line in place and the number of milliliters of fluid necessary to fill it.

Planning
4. Wash your hands *for infection control.*
5. Gather the necessary equipment.

a. Sterile screw-type injection cap. (Some types of central intravenous lines do not use a screw cap. For these lines, a regular male adapter for an intravenous line is used.)
b. Syringe with heparinized saline and a 1-inch needle. *The Hickman catheter has an internal volume of 2 ml. An extra 0.5 ml (2.5 ml total) is usually added to make sure the tip of the catheter is free of clots.* Some facilities use a larger volume to irrigate the catheter. Surgically implanted ports require 5 ml of solution. Follow the procedure in your facility. *The 1-inch needle is used because it is less likely to penetrate beyond the tip and damage the catheter wall.* A 20-gauge or smaller needle is used *because repeated punctures with large needles can lead to leaks in the rubber diaphragm.*
c. Tape. Plastic tape is commonly used *because it is thick and protects the catheter from the clamp better than other tape does. Plastic tape does not usually leave adhesive residue when it is removed.*
d. Appropriate clamp if one is not already in use on the line. It is common practice to attach a clamp to the dressing of a Hickman line even when a continuous infusion is being administered. *This makes the clamp immediately available during tubing changes and if the line must be used for drawing blood.* An extension tubing within an integral clamp is often placed on a conventional central line.
e. Alcohol swab
f. Clean gloves

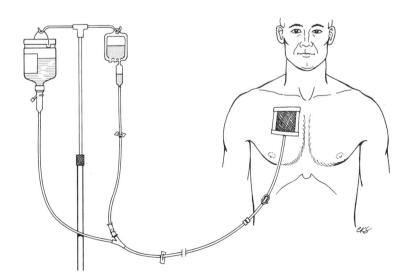

Figure 55–12 Administering medication through the Hickman catheter using a piggyback administration set.

Table 55–1 Example of Flow Sheet

Date	IV #	Content	Start	Stop	Amount	Signature
9/12/94	5	5%D/NS	1600	2210	500 ml	N. McGill, SN
9/12/94	Heparin lock to IV		2210			N. McGill, SN

Implementation

6. Identify the patient *to be sure you are performing the procedure for the correct patient.*
7. Explain the procedure to the patient.
8. Place the tape over the catheter. Make folded-over pull-tabs at each end of the tape *so it will be easy to remove for replacement.*
9. Turn off the intravenous infusion.
10. Put on gloves *to protect yourself from the possibility of any blood returning through the catheter,* although this is not likely.
11. Place the clamp on the catheter, over the tape.
12. Cleanse the junction of the catheter and the tubing with an alcohol swab *to decrease the number of microbes in the immediate area when the tubing is opened.* Allow the solution to dry before proceeding.
13. Open the package containing the sterile cap. Hold the cap carefully by the outside rim of the rubber injection cap. *To preserve sterility,* make sure you do not touch the end that will be placed in the central intravenous line.
14. Loosen the IV tubing connector by twisting it.
15. Remove the IV tubing and quickly insert the injection cap, being careful to maintain sterility of the ends of the catheter and the cap. Screw the cap in securely by hand. Do not use excessive force, *because this will make the cap difficult to remove.*

16. Insert the needle of the filled syringe into the center of the cap, *where the rubber is thinnest.*
17. Release the clamp.
18. Inject 2.5 ml heparinized saline into the catheter. In some facilities the following alternative is used.
    a. Inject 2 ml heparinized saline.
    b. Inject the remaining 0.5 ml heparinized saline as you are clamping the catheter. *This is done to provide a slight positive pressure in the tubing, thereby preventing backflow into the tip of the catheter.* No research data demonstrate that this step is necessary. Follow the procedure in your facility.
19. Replace the clamp on the catheter.
20. Remove the needle and syringe from the cap.

Evaluation

21. Evaluate using the following criteria:
    a. Catheter clamp secure.
    b. Catheter not caught in clothing.

Documentation

22. Discontinuing the continuous infusion and placing a heparin lock on the central line are often noted on the intravenous flow sheet. If this is not the case in your facility, make a brief note on the narrative progress record (Table 55–1).

DATE/TIME	
9/12/94 2210	IV number 5 discontinued with 500 ml infused. Heparin lock placed on Hickman catheter. ———— N. McGill, SN

Example of Progress Note Using Narrative Format

DATE/TIME	
7/28/94 9:30 AM	Drsg over Hickman catheter changed. Catheter entry site is clean and dry with no drainage or redness. Suture remains intact. ———— S. Garcia, NS

Example of Progress Note Using Narrative Format

IRRIGATING AN INTERMITTENT CENTRAL INTRAVENOUS CATHETER

If the catheter is being used for intermittent administration of drugs and for drawing blood, careful attention must be paid to maintaining the patency of the catheter through periodic irrigation with a heparinized saline solution. Use the schedule stipulated in the policy of your facility.

Assessment

1. Determine when medications are being administered or blood is being drawn. *If these two procedures are done regularly, the heparin injected after each procedure is adequate irrigation to maintain patency. If the catheter is not being used regularly,* a schedule for irrigation should be developed. Follow the policy in your facility for frequency of irrigation (every 12 hours is common).
2. Check your facility's policy on the strength of heparinized saline and the amount to be used. The two most common strengths and amounts are 2.5 ml of 10 units/ml and 2.5 ml of 100 units/ml. Some facilities flush with saline before using the heparin solution *to ensure that the line is patent.*

Planning

3. Wash your hands *for infection control.*
4. Gather the necessary equipment.
   a. Syringe with 2.5 ml heparinized saline, with a 1-inch needle
   b. Povidone-iodine or alcohol swab
   c. Clean gloves
   d. Normal saline solution 2.5 ml in a syringe with a 1-inch needle if prescribed by your facility

Implementation

5. Check the patient's identity *to be sure you are performing the procedure for the correct patient.*
6. Explain the procedure to the patient.
7. Put on gloves *to protect yourself from the possibility of accidental separation of the tubing and blood return that might contaminate your hands.*
8. Cleanse the cap by scrubbing for 1 minute with the antiseptic swab. *This provides mechanical cleansing as well as antiseptic action. For maximum antiseptic effect, allow the solution to dry.*
9. Insert the needle into the cap.
10. Remove the clamp from the catheter.

11. Inject 2.5 ml heparinized saline. If resistance is felt and the solution cannot be injected or the injection causes pain, pause and have the patient turn. Then try again. *If the catheter was resting against the wall of the vein, turning will cause the catheter to move and the solution can then be injected with ease. If you still cannot inject the solution with ease, notify the physician. The catheter may be occluded.*
    Optional steps:
    a. Inject the first 2 ml heparinized saline.
    b. Clamp the catheter while injecting the remaining 0.5 ml of solution.
12. Reclamp the catheter if not done as part of step 10.
13. Remove the needle and syringe from the cap and remove gloves.

Evaluation

14. Evaluate using the following criteria:
    a. Catheter clamp secure.
    b. Catheter not caught in clothing.

Documentation

15. Usually the heparin flush is recorded on the medication record. In some facilities, all procedures related to the central line are recorded on a special flow sheet (Table 55–2).

GIVING A MEDICATION THROUGH THE HEPARIN LOCK ON A CENTRAL INTRAVENOUS CATHETER

Assessment

1. Check the medication *to find out if it is compatible with the heparinized saline.* The pharmacist may be consulted if the information is not available in your unit references. *If the medication is not compatible with the heparinized saline,* you will have to

Table 55–2 Example of Flow Sheet

Medication	12/23/94	12/24/94	12/25/94
Ampicillin 500 mg IV 6-12-18-24	6KD 12RS 18MN 24KD	6KD	
Heparin Flush 10 U/ml, 2.5 ml 6-12-18-24	6KD 12RS 18MN 24KD	6KD	

incorporate the optional steps listed throughout the module.

2. Check your unit procedure for the strength of heparin solution to use.

Planning

3. Wash your hands *for infection control.*
4. Obtain the necessary supplies.
   a. Medication in a syringe with a 1-inch needle or in a small-volume parenteral container with tubing and a 1-inch needle attached. (See Module 54, Administering Intravenous Medications, for preparation instructions.)
   b. Povidone-iodine or alcohol swab
   c. Syringe containing 2.5 ml heparinized saline, with a 1-inch needle
   d. Clean gloves
   Optional:
   e. Syringe with 5 ml plain saline solution or two syringes with 2.5 ml saline in each if the medication is incompatible with the heparin. Check the policy in your facility.

Implementation

5. Identify the patient *to be sure you are performing the procedure for the correct patient.*
6. Explain the procedure to the patient.
7. Put on gloves *to protect yourself from the possibility of accidental separation of the tubing and blood return that might contaminate your hands.*
8. Cleanse the cap by scrubbing for 1 minute with the antiseptic swab, *for mechanical cleansing and antiseptic action.* Allow the solution to dry.
9. Optional steps if medication is not compatible with heparin:
   a. Insert needle of syringe with plain saline in the cap.
   b. Release the clamp.
   c. Inject 2.5 ml saline to flush the heparin from the line.
   d. Reclamp the line.
   e. Remove the syringe and needle.
10. Insert the needle for the medication into the cap.
11. Release the clamp.
12. Inject the medication at the rate ordered or as recommended by the manufacturer. If an infusion set is used, regulate the infusion set to the correct rate to deliver the medication as ordered or recommended by the manufacturer (see Figure 55–12).
13. When all the medication has been injected or infused, clamp the catheter over the tape.

14. Remove the needle from the cap.
15. Scrub the cap again for 1 minute *if the medication has been infusing over an extended period. If the medication was injected while you were there,* it is not necessary to rescrub the cap.
16. Optional steps if the medication is not compatible with heparin. Follow steps 9a through 9e above *to flush the medication out before the heparin is instilled.*
17. Insert the needle for the heparinized saline into the cap.
18. Open the clamp.
19. Inject 2.5 ml heparinized saline into the catheter.
   Optional steps:
   a. Inject the first 2 ml heparinized saline into the catheter.
   b. Clamp the catheter while injecting the remaining 0.5 ml of saline so the syringe is not emptied.
20. Clamp the catheter if not clamped in step 19.
21. Remove the needle and syringe and your gloves.
22. Dispose of the used equipment and gloves.
23. Wash your hands *for infection control.*

Evaluation

24. Evaluate using the following criteria:
   a. Catheter clamp secure.
   b. Catheter not caught in clothing.
   c. Medication given according to five rights.
   d. No adverse response to medication noted.

Documentation

25. Record the medication on the medication record. The heparin flush is usually noted with the medication and charted at the same time (Table 55–3).

Table 55–3 Example of Flow Sheet

			12/23 KD	12/24 KD
12/23/94	Ampicillin 500 mg IV followed by 2.5 ml heparin flush·q6h, 6-12-6-12	6	KD	KD
		12	RS	
		6	MN	
		12	KD	

DRAWING BLOOD THROUGH A CENTRAL INTRAVENOUS CATHETER

Some central catheters may be used for drawing blood as well as for administering fluids and medications. The criteria for determining suitability are usually the internal diameter of the catheter and the material of which it is made. Larger-diameter catheters are less likely to clot with blood and become unusable. Silicone rubber catheters are more flexible and are smoother, which decreases the likelihood that drawing blood through them will cause clotting.

Most surgically implanted central lines are routinely used for drawing blood. With many of the multiple-lumen catheters, one lumen is reserved for drawing blood. There is a great advantage to the patient in having all blood drawn through an existing line rather than having multiple needle sticks on already difficult veins. Follow the policy of your facility regarding which central catheters may be used for drawing blood.

The procedure presented here is for drawing blood through a Hickman line. The only difference for other catheters is that they may be shorter and need less solution to clear them. If a multiple-lumen catheter is in use, shut off the other lines temporarily while drawing the blood *to prevent erroneous laboratory test results based on large amounts of solution in the blood.*

Assessment

1. Determine the suitability of the central intravenous catheter for drawing blood. The policy or procedure book for your facility is usually the best resource for this information.
2. Determine which ordered laboratory tests require blood specimens.
3. Consult the laboratory or a reference *to identify the amount of blood needed and the type of laboratory specimen tube (heparinized, plain, etc.) that should be used to obtain blood for the planned tests.* These are often designated by the color of the test tube's rubber stopper, i.e., red top, green top, lavender top.

Planning

4. Wash your hands *for infection control.*
5. Gather the necessary equipment.
   a. One empty 5-ml syringe without a needle
   b. One syringe large enough to aspirate the amount of blood required for the laboratory test ordered
   c. One syringe with 20 ml saline *to flush blood from the line.* In some facilities two 10-ml syringes are used.
   d. One syringe with 2.5 ml heparinized saline *to reheparinize the line and prevent clotting*
   e. Sterile 2 × 2 gauze squares *to hold the cap* or a sterile needle in its cover *to place on the end of an intravenous tubing*
   f. Povidone-iodine or alcohol swab *to cleanse the cap*
   g. Test tubes appropriate for the type of specimen needed. It is wise to mark each tube *so you know the amount of blood needed for that particular test.*
   h. Tape *to secure all connections*
   i. Clean gloves *to protect your hands from possible contamination*
   j. Eye protection *to protect your eyes from the possibility of blood splashing from an accident with the syringe or the blood tube.* Face shields and goggles are the best eye protection *because they completely shield the eyes from all directions.* Regular eyeglasses may be considered adequate eye protection in some instances, but they do not protect from the side. Check the policy in your facility as to whether or not eyeglasses may be used for eye protection.

Implementation

6. Identify the patient *to be sure you are performing the procedure for the correct patient.*
7. Explain the procedure to the patient.
8. Remove the protective tape holding the cap or line firmly in place.
9. Put on clean gloves and eye protection.
10. Cleanse the junction of the catheter and the cap with the antiseptic swab for 1 minute and allow it to dry. *This decreases the number of microbes in the immediate area.*
11. Open the package of sterile 2 × 2 gauze squares.
12. Check to make sure the catheter is firmly clamped, over the tape.
13. Remove the cap or line from the catheter and place the cap between two sterile 2 × 2 gauze squares. Put a sterile capped needle on the intravenous line if one is currently in use. Hold the end of the catheter in your fingers *so it does not touch anything.* The cap is removed when blood is being drawn *so it does not become damaged from the large-diameter needles that are necessary to draw blood. The damaged cap will begin to leak and admit microbes. It must be*

discarded and replaced. Some facilities keep a supply of sterile caps, and a fresh cap is placed on the line each time the cap is removed.

14. Connect an empty 5-ml syringe to the catheter.
15. Release the clamp on the catheter.
16. Aspirate 5 ml fluid from the catheter. *This will completely remove the heparinized saline or IV fluid from the catheter and the catheter will be filled with undiluted blood.* If the syringe will not aspirate with ease, have the patient turn. *Turning will move the tip of the catheter in the vein* and, if it was against the wall of the vein, will allow it to move away. Gently aspirate again. If you still cannot aspirate, stop the procedure and notify the physician.
17. Reclamp the catheter. Remember, the catheter must always be clamped when the syringe is being attached or removed *so the patient is protected from air embolism.*
18. Remove the first syringe from the catheter and discard it, along with its contents.
19. Attach the empty syringe *to draw blood from the catheter.*
20. Unclamp the catheter.
21. Aspirate the amount of blood needed for the tests into the syringe (Figure 55–13).

22. Reclamp the catheter.
23. Remove the syringe of blood from the catheter. The blood should not be allowed to remain in the syringe, because it may clot. At this point you may wish to ask another person to assist you by putting the correct amount of blood into the correct test tubes while you are finishing with the catheter. As you become more experienced, the next steps will be done rapidly and then there will be no problem with the blood remaining in the syringe while you finish.
24. Attach the syringe with 20 ml saline. *This flushes all blood from the catheter.* Some facilities use less saline. The important point is to thoroughly flush *so no blood residue remains in the tubing.*
25. Unclamp the catheter.
26. Inject the saline.
27. Clamp the catheter.
28. Remove the empty syringe.
29. Attach the syringe with the heparinized saline solution to the catheter. *The heparin will prevent clotting in the catheter.*
30. Unclamp the catheter.
31. Inject 2.5 ml heparinized saline solution.

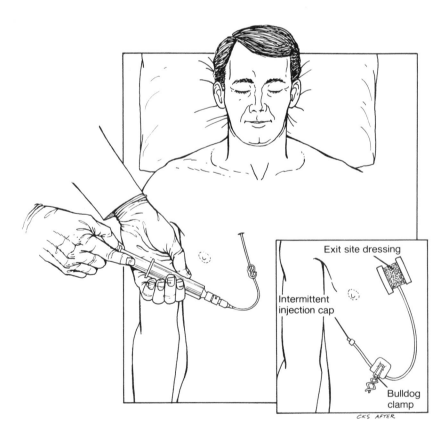

Figure 55–13 Drawing blood from a Hickman catheter. A bulldog clamp is shown on a catheter that does not have an integral clamp.

Optional step: Inject the last 0.5 ml while clamping the catheter.

32. Clamp the catheter.

33. Remove the empty syringe.

34. Replace the cap or IV line on the catheter, being careful to maintain sterility of the catheter and of the cap or IV line.

35. Inject the blood into the proper laboratory test tubes.

36. Tape the cap to the catheter *for extra security.* Be sure to make tabs at the ends of the tape *so that removal is easier.*

37. Discard used equipment and gloves.

38. Wash your hands.

39. Send the blood to the laboratory with the correct requisition forms and labeling. The laboratory specimens are usually enclosed in a plastic bag *for safe handling during transport.*

Evaluation

40. Evaluate using the following criteria:
   a. Catheter clamp secure.
   b. Catheter not caught in clothing.
   c. Appropriate blood sample obtained.

Documentation

41. Record on a flow sheet or on a narrative record that blood was drawn from the central line and sent to the laboratory.

ACCESSING A SUBCUTANEOUS CATHETER PORT

To administer intravenous fluids or medications or the heparinize an implanted infusion port, it must

first be accessed. This means that a special noncoring needle is inserted into the port. A noncoring needle has a tip constructed so that it opens a slit into the rubber diaphragm and does not create a hole from a segment "cored" out. The access needle can be a straight needle attached to a syringe to administer medication or draw blood or may be right-angle needle (sometimes called a Huber needle) that is used to connect to an intravenous line. Noncoring needles are shown in Figure 55–14.

Assessment

1. Check the physician's order to determine whether an ongoing access or simply temporary access is needed and medications that need to be given.

2. Identify the type and location of the patient's subcutaneous port.

Planning

3. Wash your hands *for infection control.*

4. Obtain the equipment you will need.
   a. Three povidone-iodine swabs
   b. Dry cotton swab or 2×2 gauze
   c. Sterile gloves
   d. Alcohol swabs in addition to the povidone iodine swabs if used in your facility
   e. An empty syringe with an extension tubing that has a clamp attached to a noncoring needle
   f. One of the following groups of supplies
   For temporary access:
   (1) Materials to draw blood or give medication
   (2) Syringe with heparinized saline in the dilution prescribed by your facility

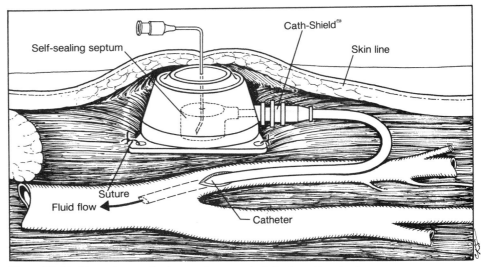

Figure 55–14 Noncoring needles leave only a smooth slit in the rubber diaphragm.

(frequently 100 units/ml) *to reheparinize the line when you have finished.* If you are only reheparinizing a port that is not being used, you may use a straight noncoring needle attached directly to the syringe of heparinized saline. If you must change syringes, you will need to use a right-angle needle attached to extension tubing listed above *in order to clamp the line closed while you are changing syringes.*

(3) Medication ordered. Remember to use the five rights and three checks when preparing any medication.

For ongoing access:

(1) Intravenous fluid with tubing set up and ready to attach (see Module 54, Preparing and Maintaining Intravenous Infusions).

g. In some facilities, ethyl chloride spray is used *to decrease discomfort.* If used in your facility, obtain spray.

Implementation

5. Check the patient's identification *for safety.*

6. Explain the procedure to the patient *to alleviate anxiety and elicit the patient's cooperation.*

7. Draw the curtains and close doors *to maintain the patient's privacy.*

8. Prepare a clean surface to set up your equipment *so that your materials will not become contaminated and they are convenient.*

9. Place the patient in a supine or semi-Fowler's position and expose the port site. *This makes the area easier to work on.*

10. Put on a mask *to reduce the chance of microorganisms from your mouth and nose contaminating the site.* In some facilities this is not a part of the procedure. In others, both patient and nurse wear a mask. There is no evidence to support one method over another. Follow the policy in your facility.

11. Set up your equipment on the table in the order you will use it. *This helps you to remember what you must do next and makes the procedure go more quickly.* Open sterile packages to have the contents ready to use.

12. Palpate the area over the port *to determine exactly where the port is located.*

13. Prepare the skin *to lessen the chance of infection at the site.* Swab the area with povidone-iodine

in concentric circles starting at the center and moving out to form a circle approximately 3–4 inches in diameter. Do this three times with separate swabs. Allow the solution to remain on the skin for a full minute. If your facility procedure calls for cleaning the iodine solution off with alcohol, do it at this time. Use a dry sterile swab to dry the skin site.

If your facility procedure calls for ethyl chloride spray, use it at this time. Spray the site until it appears frosted.

14. Put on sterile gloves. *Sterile gloves assure the patient that organisms are not introduced by your hands.*

15. Attach the extension tubing and syringe to the needle. (Some manufacturers make noncoring needles with tubing attached.) Leave the clamp on the tubing open at this time *so that you will be able to aspirate the syringe after you have accessed the port.*

16. Palpate the site with your nondominant hand *to determine the site of the diaphragm* and hold the edges of the port firmly in place *to prevent its shifting as you access it.*

17. Using your dominant hand, insert the needle firmly straight into the center of the diaphragm until you feel it touch the needle stop in the bottom.

18. Hold the needle firmly in place while you aspirate. *A blood return indicates that the port is functioning.* If blood does not return immediately, having the patient turn to either side, cough slightly, and take deep breaths *may move the catheter in the vessel enough that blood will return.* If you cannot get blood return, *the catheter may be plugged (the most likely cause) or the end may have migrated out of the vessel.* In this case remove the needle and notify the physician.

19. If the port is functioning, proceed to draw blood, administer medications, attach fluid set, or flush and heparinize the line as planned. Use the procedures previously outlined.

20. Complete procedure.
   a. For intermittent access: remove the needle after flushing and heparinizing.
   b. For ongoing access: tape connections, apply dressing as described previously.

Evaluation

21. Evaluate using the following criteria:
   a. Catheter dressing and tapes intact.

Home Care

Increasing numbers of individuals who need long-term intravenous therapy are being taught to care for central intravenous catheters. This includes people who need long-term antibiotic therapy for cardiac infections, people who need parenteral nutrition on an ongoing basis, and those who need pain medication or other therapies on an ongoing basis. In some instances the individual's catheter is maintained at home, but the person comes in for therapy. In other instances the patient is able to administer therapy at home as well. When the patient is not able to manage this care, a family member or friend may be the primary caregiver in the home.

To enable individuals to assume this highly technical care, a carefully planned instructional program is needed. While the individual is still in the hospital, instruction is begun. Then follow-up by a home care nurse is extremely important to help with problem-solving in the home environment.

b. Site clean and free of signs of infection.
c. Patient received correct medication or correct blood sample was obtained.

Documentation

22. Record that implanted port was accessed including date and time on the intravenous flow sheet or the progress notes.

23. Record any heparin or medication given on the medication record.

References

Pederson, N. T., & Hessov, I. (1978). Venous air embolism through infusion sets. *ACTA Anaesthesia Scandinavia, 22,* 117–122.

Stratton, C. (1981). Infection related to intravenous infusion. *Heart and Lung, 11*(2), 123–127.

Performance Checklist

Inserting the Standard Central Intravenous Catheter	Unsat	Needs More Practice	Sat	Comments
Assessment				
1. Check order.				
2. Assess patient's ability to participate in and tolerate the procedure. a. Position flat or in Trendelenburg's?				
b. Able to hold breath?				
c. Able to understand and follow directions?				
Planning				
3. Wash your hands.				
4. Obtain necessary equipment and supplies. a. Masks				
b. Sterile gown for physician				
c. Two pairs of sterile gloves				
d. Skin preparation materials				
e. Razor				
f. Topical anesthetic agent				
g. Sterile drapes				
h. Intracatheter and syringe				
i. Suturing materials				
j. Intravenous fluid with tubing attached				
k. Dressing materials				
l. Sterile towel				
Implementation				
5. Check patient's identification.				
6. Explain procedure to patient.				
7. Prepare a clean table.				
8. Set up equipment on table.				
9. Place patient in a supine position.				
10. Support patient. a. Maintain touch.				
b. Help patient maintain position.				

Inserting the Standard Central Intravenous Catheter *(Continued)*	Unsat	Needs More Practice	Sat	Comments
c. Give positive reinforcement to patient.				
d. Provide feedback to alleviate anxiety.				
e. Reassure patient.				
f. Remind others that patient is alert, if necessary.				
11. Assist physician as necessary. a. Hold anesthetic vial.				
b. Open equipment and supplies.				
c. Connect intravenous tubing.				
d. Complete dressing.				
12. Remove drapes and position patient comfortably.				
13. Regulate intravenous flow rate.				
14. Remove used supplies and packages.				
15. Wash your hands.				

Evaluation

	Unsat	Needs More Practice	Sat	Comments
16. Evaluate the following: a. Patient comfort.				
b. Intravenous line for patency and correct flow, secure connections.				
c. Dressing secure.				

Documentation

	Unsat	Needs More Practice	Sat	Comments
17. Record on patient's chart: a. Time the central intravenous line was inserted.				
b. Type and size of catheter.				
c. Site used.				
d. Solution and rate of administration.				
e. Patient's response.				

Changing the Central Intravenous Dressing	Unsat	Needs More Practice	Sat	Comments
Assessment				
1. Check date and time of last dressing change.				
2. Review facility procedure to identify appropriate dressing materials.				
Planning				
3. Wash your hands.				
4. Obtain necessary supplies. a. Masks, as directed by facility policy				
b. Disinfectant cleansing agent for table				
c. Sterile gloves				
d. Cleansing materials				
e. Dressing supplies				
f. Antiseptic ointment				
g. Clean gloves				
Implementation				
5. Check patient's identification.				
6. Explain procedure to patient.				
7. Clean overbed table and allow to dry.				
8. Place patient in supine position, with head turned away from site.				
9. Put on mask.				
10. Set up materials on overbed table.				
11. Put on clean gloves and remove old dressing.				
12. Remove gloves and wash your hands.				
13. Inspect site carefully.				
14. Put on sterile gloves.				
15. Cleanse area with hydrogen peroxide, moving in a spiral pattern beginning at the exit site.				
16. Cleanse area with antiseptic solution in a similar pattern for 2 minutes.				
17. Allow antiseptic solution to dry.				

Changing the Central Intravenous Dressing
(Continued)

	Unsat	Needs More Practice	Sat	Comments
18. Apply antiseptic ointment to exit site with cotton-tipped applicator.				
19. Apply new dressing.				
20. Change tape over connection between catheter and intravenous tubing.				
21. Remove mask.				
22. Label dressing with date and time.				
23. Reposition patient for comfort.				
24. Dispose of packages and materials.				
25. Wash your hands.				

Evaluation

	Unsat	Needs More Practice	Sat	Comments
26. Evaluate the following: a. Patient comfort.				
b. Intravenous line for patency and correct flow, connections secure.				
c. Dressing secure.				

Documentation

	Unsat	Needs More Practice	Sat	Comments
27. Record on flow sheet or on narrative record.				

Changing the Fluid Container and the Tubing

Assessment

	Unsat	Needs More Practice	Sat	Comments
1. Follow Checklist steps 1 and 2 of Changing the Fluid Container and Tubing, in Module 53, Preparing and Maintaining Intravenous Infusions (check physician's order and date of last tubing change).				

Planning

	Unsat	Needs More Practice	Sat	Comments
2. Follow Checklist steps 3 and 4 of Changing the Fluid Container and Tubing (wash your hands and select the correct tubing).				

Implementation

	Unsat	Needs More Practice	Sat	Comments
3. Follow Checklist steps 5–10 of Changing the Fluid Container and Tubing (set up equipment, identify the patient, hang the new container, remove old tape and dressing, examine site, shut off IV).				

Changing the Fluid Container and the Tubing *(Continued)*	Unsat	Needs More Practice	Sat	Comments
4. Remove tape from connection.				
5. Cleanse junction between catheter and tubing.				
6. Clamp line, place patient in Trendelenburg's position, or plan for patient to a Valsalva maneuver.				
7. Loosen old tubing by twisting it and leave connected.				
8. Remove cap from new tubing.				
9. Remove old tubing from connector and insert new tubing.				
10. Start new fluid at a slow rate.				
11. Tape connection.				
Evaluation				
12. Evaluate the following: a. Patient comfort.				
b. Patency, correct flow, and secure connections.				
c. Dressing secure.				
Documentation				
13. Document as follows: a. Intravenous flow sheet: time, fluid discontinued, fluid added, tubing change.				
b. Intake and output record.				

Changing the Exit Site Dressing

Assessment				
1. Check date and time of last dressing change.				
2. Review facility procedure to identify correct dressing materials.				
Planning				
3. Wash your hands.				
4. Gather necessary supplies. a. Hydrogen peroxide and sterile cotton-tipped applicators				

Changing the Exit Site Dressing *(Continued)*	Unsat	Needs More Practice	Sat	Comments
b. Povidone-iodine swabsticks or solution and applicators (in some facilities you also need an alcohol wipe)				
c. Antibacterial ointment				
d. Sterile 2×2 gauze squares				
e. Paper tape				
f. Clean gloves				
Implementation				
5. Identify patient.				
6. Explain procedure to patient.				
7. Put on clean gloves to remove old dressing and inspect site.				
8. Cleanse with hydrogen peroxide and applicators in a spiral fashion outward for 3 inches, removing any crusts.				
9. Cleanse with povidone-iodine swabs in the same way.				
10. Allow iodine solution to dry on skin.				
11. Apply antibacterial ointment to exit site.				
12. Cleanse catheter from exit site outward, using povidone-iodine or alcohol wipe.				
13. Place one gauze square under catheter and one over exit site, touching only outside of gauze.				
14. Tape dressing in place.				
15. Loop catheter and tape it to body.				
16. Write date and time on dressing.				
17. Dispose of used materials and packages.				
18. Wash your hands.				
Evaluation				
19. Evaluate using the following criteria: a. Dressing is secure.				
b. Catheter is not under tension.				

Changing the Exit Site Dressing (Continued)	Unsat	Needs More Practice	Sat	Comments
Documentation				
20. Record on a flow sheet or on the narrative record.				
Establishing a Heparin Lock on a Central Intravenous Catheter				
Assessment				
1. Check order.				
2. Check facility procedure for type of solution used.				
3. Check type of line in place and number of milliliters necessary to fill it.				
Planning				
4. Wash your hands.				
5. Gather necessary equipment. a. Sterile screw-type injection cap				
b. Syringe with 1-inch needle and heparinized saline				
c. Tape				
d. Clamp for line				
e. Alcohol swab				
f. Clean gloves				
Implementation				
6. Identify patient.				
7. Explain procedure to patient.				
8. Place tape over catheter, making folded tabs at ends.				
9. Turn off intravenous infusion.				
10. Put on gloves.				
11. Place clamp on catheter, over tape.				
12. Cleanse junction of catheter and tubing.				
13. Open package containing sterile cap.				
14. Loosen IV tubing by twisting it.				

Establishing a Heparin Lock on a Central Intravenous Catheter *(Continued)*

	Unsat	Needs More Practice	Sat	Comments
15. Remove IV tubing and insert injection cap.				
16. Insert needle of syringe into center of cap.				
17. Release clamp.				
18. Inject the heparinized saline. Alternative: Inject remaining 0.5 ml of solution while clamping catheter.				
19. Replace clamp.				
20. Remove needle and syringe and gloves.				
Evaluation				
21. Evaluate using the following criteria: a. Catheter clamp secure.				
b. Catheter not caught in clothing.				
Documentation				
22. Record on the intravenous flow sheet or on the narrative record.				

Irrigating an Intermittent Central Intravenous Catheter

	Unsat	Needs More Practice	Sat	Comments
Assessment				
1. Determine when medications are being administered or blood is being drawn.				
2. Check facility policy regarding strength and amount of heparinized saline to be used.				
Planning				
3. Wash your hands.				
4. Gather necessary equipment.				
a. Syringe with heparinized saline and 1-inch needle				
b. Povidone-iodine or alcohol swab				
c. Clean gloves				
Implementation				
5. Check patient's identity.				
6. Explain procedure to patient.				

Irrigating an Intermittent Central Intravenous Catheter *(Continued)*

	Unsat	Needs More Practice	Sat	Comments
7. Put on gloves.				
8. Cleanse cap by scrubbing for one minute.				
9. Insert needle into cap.				
10. Remove clamp from catheter.				
11. Inject heparinized saline into line. Optional steps:				
a. Inject first 2 ml into line.				
b. Inject remaining 0.5 ml while clamping line.				
12. Reclamp catheter.				
13. Remove needle and syringe from cap and remove gloves.				

Evaluation

	Unsat	Needs More Practice	Sat	Comments
14. Evaluate using the following criteria: a. Catheter clamp secure.				
b. Catheter not caught in clothing.				

Documentation

	Unsat	Needs More Practice	Sat	Comments
15. Record heparin flush on medication record or on special flow sheet for Hickman catheter.				

Giving a Medication Through the Heparin Lock on a Central Intravenous Catheter

Assessment

	Unsat	Needs More Practice	Sat	Comments
1. Check medication to find out if it is compatible with heparinized saline.				
2. Check unit procedure for strength of heparin solution to use.				

Planning

	Unsat	Needs More Practice	Sat	Comments
3. Wash your hands.				
4. Obtain necessary supplies. a. Medication in syringe with 1-inch needle (See Module 54, Administering Intravenous Medications, for preparation instructions.)				
b. Povidone-iodine or alcohol swab				
c. Syringe with heparinized saline and 1-inch needle				

Giving a Medication Through the Heparin Lock on a Central Intravenous Catheter
(Continued)

	Unsat	Needs More Practice	Sat	Comments
d. Clean gloves				
Optional:				
e. Syringe with 5 ml plain saline and 1-inch needle or two syringes with 2.5 ml saline in each if the medication is not compatible with heparin.				
Implementation				
5. Identify patient.				
6. Explain procedure to patient.				
7. Put on gloves.				
8. Cleanse cap by scrubbing for 1 minute with antiseptic swab. Allow solution to dry.				
9. Optional steps if medication is not compatible with heparin. a. Insert needle of syringe with plain saline.				
b. Release clamp.				
c. Inject 2.5 ml saline to flush out heparin.				
d. Reclamp line.				
e. Remove syringe and needle.				
10. Insert needle for medication into cap.				
11. Release clamp.				
12. Inject medication at rate ordered or recommended. If medication is to be infused over time, regulate the rate.				
13. When all medication has been infused or injected, reclamp catheter.				
14. Remove needle from cap.				
15. Scrub cap if medication has been infusing over extended period.				
16. Optional steps if medication is not compatible with heparin. Follow steps 9a–e above.				
17. Insert needle for heparinized saline.				
18. Open clamp.				

Giving a Medication Through the Heparin Lock on a Central Intravenous Catheter
(Continued)

	Unsat	Needs More Practice	Sat	Comments
19. Inject heparinized saline into catheter. Optional steps:				
a. Inject 2 ml heparinized saline into catheter.				
b. Clamp catheter while injecting remaining 0.5 ml heparinized saline.				
20. Clamp catheter.				
21. Remove needle and syringe and gloves.				
22. Dispose of used equipment and gloves.				
23. Wash your hands.				

Evaluation

	Unsat	Needs More Practice	Sat	Comments
24. Evaluate using the following criteria: a. Catheter clamp secure.				
b. Catheter not caught in clothing.				
c. Correct medication given according to five rights.				
d. No adverse response to medication noted.				

Documentation

	Unsat	Needs More Practice	Sat	Comments
25. Record medication on medication record.				

Drawing Blood Through a Central Intravenous Catheter

Assessment

	Unsat	Needs More Practice	Sat	Comments
1. Determine suitability of catheter for drawing blood.				
2. Determine which ordered laboratory tests require specimens.				
3. Consult laboratory or reference to identify amount of blood needed and type of tube to be used for sample.				

Planning

	Unsat	Needs More Practice	Sat	Comments
4. Wash your hands.				
5. Gather necessary equipment. a. One empty 5-ml syringe without needle				

Drawing Blood Through a Central Intravenous Catheter *(Continued)*	Unsat	Needs More Practice	Sat	Comments
b. One syringe large enough to aspirate amount of blood needed for tests				
c. One syringe with 20 ml saline				
d. One syringe with heparinized saline				
e. Sterile 2×2 gauze squares to hold cap or sterile capped needle				
f. Povidone-iodine or alcohol swab				
g. Test tubes appropriate to specimens needed				
h. Tape to retape connections				
i. Clean gloves				
j. Eye protection				

Implementation

	Unsat	Needs More Practice	Sat	Comments
6. Identify patient.				
7. Explain procedure to patient.				
8. Remove protective tape holding cap in place.				
9. Put on gloves and eye protection.				
10. Cleanse junction of catheter and cap.				
11. Open package of sterile 2×2 gauze squares.				
12. Check to make sure catheter is firmly clamped.				
13. Remove cap from catheter and place cap between two sterile 2×2 gauze squares or place sterile capped needle on IV line.				
14. Connect empty 5-ml syringe to catheter.				
15. Release clamp on catheter.				
16. Aspirate 5 ml fluid from catheter.				
17. Reclamp catheter.				
18. Remove first syringe from catheter and discard.				
19. Attach empty syringe.				
20. Unclamp catheter.				
21. Aspirate desired amount of blood.				
22. Reclamp catheter.				
23. Remove syringe of blood.				

Drawing Blood Through a Central Intravenous Catheter (Continued)	Unsat	Needs More Practice	Sat	Comments
24. Attach syringe with 20 ml saline.				
25. Unclamp catheter.				
26. Inject saline.				
27. Clamp catheter.				
28. Remove empty syringe.				
29. Attach syringe with heparinized saline.				
30. Unclamp catheter.				
31. Inject heparinized saline.				
Optional: Inject remaining 0.5 ml while clamping catheter.				
32. Clamp catheter.				
33. Remove empty syringe.				
34. Replace cap or line on catheter.				
35. Inject blood into proper laboratory test tubes.				
36. Tape cap to catheter.				
37. Discard used equipment and gloves.				
38. Wash your hands.				
39. Send labeled blood to laboratory with proper forms.				

Evaluation

	Unsat	Needs More Practice	Sat	Comments
40. Evaluate using the following criteria: a. Catheter clamp secure.				
b. Catheter not caught in clothing.				
c. Appropriate blood samples obtained.				

Documentation

	Unsat	Needs More Practice	Sat	Comments
41. Record on flow sheet or on narrative record that blood was drawn and sent to laboratory.				

Accessing a Subcutaneous Catheter Port

Assessment

	Unsat	Needs More Practice	Sat	Comments
1. Check the physician's order.				
2. Identify the type and location of the port.				

Accessing a Subcutaneous Catheter Port
(Continued)

	Unsat	Needs More Practice	Sat	Comments
Planning				
3. Wash your hands.				
4. Obtain needed equipment. a. Three iodine swabs				
b. Dry cotton swab				
c. Sterile gloves				
d. Mask, alcohol, and ethyl chloride if facility indicates.				
For temporary access: noncoring needle, extension tubing with clamp, and syringe. Other materials based on purpose.				
For ongoing access: right-angle noncoring needle with extension tubing, clamp and empty syringe and intravenous setup				
Implementation				
5. Check the patient's identification.				
6. Explain the procedure to the patient.				
7. Draw the curtains and close doors.				
8. Prepare a clean area for your equipment and supplies.				
9. Place the patient in a supine or semi-Fowler's position.				
10. Put on a mask, if required in your facility.				
11. Set up your equipment and open sterile packages.				
12. Palpate area over the port.				
13. Prepare the skin over the port. a. Use povidone-iodine swab in a concentric circle three times.				
b. Allow solution to remain on skin a full minute.				
c. Wipe off iodine solution with alcohol swab if prescribed by your facility.				
d. Dry area with sterile swab.				
e. Spray with ethyl chloride if indicated.				

Accessing a Subcutaneous Catheter Port
(Continued)

	Unsat	Needs More Practice	Sat	Comments
14. Put on sterile gloves.				
15. Attach noncoring needle, extension tubing with clamp, and syringe.				
16. Palpate site and hold the edges of port firmly with nondominant hand.				
17. Insert needle firmly straight in the center of the diaphragm until you feel needle stop.				
18. Hold needle firmly in place while aspirating.				
19. After blood return, draw blood, administer medications, attach fluid set, or flush and heparinize according to performance check lists.				
20. Complete procedure: a. For intermittent access: remove needle after flushing and heparinizing.				
b. For ongoing access: tape connections and apply dressing according to Performance Checklist.				
Evaluation				
21. Evaluate using the following criteria: a. Catheter dressing and tapes intact.				
b. Site clean and free of signs of infection.				
c. Patient received correct medication or fluids or correct blood sample was obtained.				
Documentation				
22. Record accessing of port including time and date on flow sheet or progress notes.				
23. Record medications or heparin on medication record.				

Quiz

Short-Answer Questions

1. What are two common reasons for the use of central intravenous catheters?

   a. _____

   b. _____

2. Name two major complications of central intravenous infusion catheters.

   a. _____

   b. _____

3. List four purposes for changing the dressing on a central intravenous catheter.

   a. _____

   b. _____

   c. _____

   d. _____

4. Why is acetone not recommended as an agent to prepare the skin when changing the dressing on a central intravenous catheter? _____

5. What is the purpose of applying an antiseptic or antimicrobial ointment to the insertion site? _____

6. Why should a right atrial catheter with a peripheral exit site be labeled as a central intravenous catheter directly on the dressing? _____

7. Why is the patient asked to perform a Valsalva maneuver when the tubing is being changed on a central intravenous catheter? _____

8. What is the difference between the Hickman catheter and the Broviac catheter? _____

9. Why is the cap removed from the Hickman line for drawing of blood? _____

10. Why are the Hickman and Broviac lines always clamped when not in use? _____

11. What type of needle is used to access an implanted subcutaneous central venous port such as a Port-a-cath and why?

_____

_____

12. What is used to prepare the skin before accessing a subcutaneous port?

_____

_____

Module 56

Starting Intravenous Infusions

Module Contents

Rationale for the Use of This Skill
Nursing Diagnoses
Psychological Implications
Indications for Intravenous Fluids/Access
Wearing Gloves
Equipment
Selecting a Vein
Procedure for Starting an Intravenous Infusion
  Assessment
  Planning
  Implementation
  Evaluation
  Documentation
Procedure for Converting an IV to a Heparin Lock
  Assessment
  Planning
  Implementation
  Evaluation
  Documentation

Prerequisites

1. *Successful completion of the following modules:*

VOLUME 1

Module 1   An Approach to Nursing Skills
Module 2   Basic Infection Control
Module 3   Safety
Module 5   General Assessment Overview
Module 6   Documentation

VOLUME 2

Module 35 Sterile Technique
Module 49 Administering Oral Medications
Module 51 Giving Injections
Module 53 Preparing and Maintaining Intravenous Infusions

2. *Review of the anatomy and physiology of the vascular system.*

505

Overall Objective

To start intravenous infusions safely and comfortably for patients, using the equipment correctly while maintaining safety for the nurse.

Specific Learning Objectives

	Know Facts and Principles	Apply Facts and Principles	Demonstrate Ability	Evaluate Performance
1. *Psychological implications*	State three reasons why patients become anxious about IV infusions.	Given a patient situation, assess and plan appropriate nursing intervention to decrease patient's anxiety about receiving IV infusion.	Prepare patient psychologically for IV therapy immediately before initiating. Bring equipment into room at time IV is to be started.	Evaluate own performance with instructor.
2. *Indications for intravenous fluids*	State four indications for intravenous fluids.	Given a patient situation, state why patient is receiving IV fluids.	In the clinical setting, discuss reason(s) for IV therapy for assigned patient(s).	Evaluate own performance with instructor.
3. *Equipment*	List four kinds of equipment generally available for starting IV infusions.	Correctly identify equipment for starting IVs.	Choose correct equipment for particular clinical situation.	Evaluate own performance with instructor.
4. *Setting up an intravenous infusion*	List steps for setting up IV.	Given a patient situation, discuss ways basic procedure might be modified.	In the practice setting, set up IV correctly.	Check entire setup using Performance Checklist.
5. *Locating a vein*	State usual sites for adult and infant IVs, and give rationale for their use. State four methods that can be used to distend veins.	Given a patient situation, state potential IV site. Given a patient situation, discuss which method of distending veins might be used.	In the practice or clinical setting, locate potential IV sites on peers or patients. In the practice or clinical setting, demonstrate how to cause vein to distend using peer or actual patient.	Evaluate own performance with instructor.
6. *Procedure for starting an intravenous infusion*	Describe steps in procedure.	Given a patient situation, describe how procedure might be adapted.	Start IV in practice or clinical setting.	Evaluate with instructor using Performance Checklist.
7. *Documentation*	State items of information to be included when recording insertion of IV infusion.	Given a patient situation, do sample charting for insertion of IV infusion.	In the clinical setting, correctly record insertion of IV infusion.	Evaluate with instructor.

Learning Activities

1. Review the Specific Learning Objectives.
2. Read the section on administering fluids intravenously in the chapter on nutrition and fluids in Ellis and Nowlis, *Nursing: A Human Needs Approach,* or a comparable chapter in another textbook.
3. Look up the module vocabulary terms in the Glossary.
4. Read through the module and mentally practice the skills included.
5. In the practice setting:
   a. Examine the various pieces of equipment available for starting an IV. Identify each of the following:
      (1) 18-, 19-, or 20-gauge, short-beveled needles. (Compare a short-beveled needle with a regular needle.)
      (2) A butterfly
      (3) An IV catheter inside a needle (Intracath, Venocath)
      (4) Any other available devices
   b. Read the package instructions accompanying each of the above devices. Handle the equipment and attempt to follow the instructions.
   c. Using a mannequin or IV "arm," start an IV with a 20-gauge, short-beveled needle. Do the complete procedure, including the explanation to the "patient," and taping and dressing. Review Module 53, Preparing and Maintaining Intravenous Infusions, and if time permits, set up the IV as well. When you have had sufficient practice, ask your instructor to evaluate your performance.
   d. If sterile equipment is available and school policy permits, practice starting an IV on another student. Perform the entire procedure and have the student evaluate your performance.
   e. Practice charting, using the form used in the facility to which you are assigned, as well as a narrative note.
6. In the clinical setting:
   a. Ask your instructor to arrange for you to observe an IV being started.
   b. Ask your instructor to arrange for you to start an IV under supervision in your facility, if the facility's policies permit. For your first experience, a patient with "good" veins (for example, a young male) is preferable.
   c. If your facility employs an IV nurse, ask your instructor if arrangements can be made for you to accompany him or her to observe. If time permits, ask if you can practice locating a suitable vein, and have the nurse evaluate your choice. If policy permits, ask if you can start an IV on a patient with good veins.

Vocabulary

antecubital space
armboard
bevel
bifurcation
butterfly
laminar airflow hood
NPO
Penrose drain
tortuous
tourniquet

Starting Intravenous Infusions

Rationale for the Use of This Skill

Depending on the facility's policies, unit nurses may or may not start intravenous infusions. If it is the unit nurse's responsibility to start intravenous infusions, the nurse must follow the five rights and three checks, as well as manipulate the required equipment skillfully, keeping the patient comfortable and safe. If specially trained IV nurses are responsible for starting intravenous infusions, the unit nurse must still be sufficiently familiar with the equipment and the procedure to be of assistance.[1]

▶ *Nursing Diagnoses*

Patients may require intravenous therapy when a wide variety of nursing diagnoses are present. The most common is High Risk for Fluid Volume Deficit. Patients with this nursing diagnosis are those who are not taking oral fluids and need fluids to avoid a problem. The actual problem of Fluid Volume Deficit may also be treated by intravenous therapy. Those receiving intravenous fluids are also at High Risk for Infection because normal defenses have been breached. The various potential complications of intravenous therapy such as phlebitis and infiltration will also be a concern.

PSYCHOLOGICAL IMPLICATIONS

To some patients, the knowledge that they are about to receive intravenous fluids is threatening. *Some patients feel the procedure implies serious illness. Others are frightened by the threat of pain, discomfort, and immobility. Still others fear contracting infections such as AIDS.* Previous experience can help make the patient less apprehensive, assuming the experience was a good one. For some patients the memories of problems related to the IV make the impending experience truly frightening.

Explain the procedure just a few minutes before the IV is to be started. *This prepares the patient without providing a long time for worry.* In addition, keep the

equipment out of the room until you are actually going to begin. In some facilities the policy is to use 0.1–0.2 ml local anesthetic intradermally before starting an IV, *to numb the skin and the vein. This makes it easier for the patient to cooperate and removes most of the pain and discomfort associated with the insertion.* However, the anesthetic sometimes makes it more difficult to identify the vein in difficult situations.

INDICATIONS FOR INTRAVENOUS FLUIDS/ACCESS

Intravenous fluids are ordered for various reasons. *They maintain the daily requirements for fluid (in the patient who is NPO or who is nauseated and vomiting); they replace lost fluid (in the postoperative patient); they provide large amounts of fluid rapidly (for a patient who has taken a drug overdose); and they serve as a vehicle for medications, most commonly antibiotics.*

The fluid is ordered by the physician specifically *to meet the needs of the individual patient.* Refer to Module 53, Preparing and Maintaining Intravenous Infusions, for a discussion of the variety of solutions available and of things to check before using a solution.

A heparin lock is inserted and maintained *when there is need for intravenous access without need for intravenous fluids.* Some examples of such situations are need for IV antibiotic therapy and need for access in terms of specific prn drug therapy. Advantages of a heparin lock include greater patient mobility and reduction in cost of care. Module 54, Administering Intravenous Medications, includes a discussion of heparin locks.

WEARING GLOVES

Gloves provide protection from the possibility of contamination of the caregiver's skin breaks by the patient's blood. Gloves do not protect from inadvertent needle sticks. Needle sticks present more of a risk for blood-borne infections than do blood spills. The Centers for Disease Control (CDC) do not specifically recommend that all individuals starting intravenous infusions wear gloves. The CDC recommendation is that the use of gloves be based on the individual situation and the potential for blood spills. Some hospitals, therefore, leave the decision of whether to wear gloves to the individual. Other hospitals have a policy that those doing any venipuncture wear gloves *for protection from blood spills.*

For students learning the technique, blood spills are

---

[1] You will note that rationale for action is emphasized throughout the module by the use of italics.

more likely than with a very experienced nurse. Therefore, we recommend that all students wear gloves when attempting any venipuncture. *If sensitivity for palpation of a vein becomes a problem*, it is possible to cut the end off of one glove index finger. This provides protection for hands that handle the needle, syringe, and tubing while allowing for sensitivity of touch.

EQUIPMENT

No single type of equipment is ideal. All have advantages and disadvantages. When choosing equipment, you must consider the age and mobility of the patient, the length of time the equipment will be in place, and the individual patient's vein condition and structure. Then compare these factors to the characteristics of the equipment and make your choice.

Most facilities select a single manufacturer of intravenous solutions and equipment as their supplier. You will become familiar with this equipment over time. Types of fluid containers and administration sets are discussed in Module 53, Preparing and Maintaining Intravenous Infusions. Similar equipment is available for starting infusions.

A *straight sterile needle* (usually 18, 19, or 20 gauge) with a short bevel can be used for short-term IVs (Figure 56–1). The short bevel prevents puncturing the posterior wall of the vein as the needle enters. A metal needle tends not to irritate the vein but may damage or puncture the vein if the patient moves about, which would cause an infiltration. The large gauge allows for administration of blood or rapid administration of fluids.

A *butterfly* (or scalp vein infusion set) comes with plastic "wings" that are attached to the needle's hub for easier manipulation during insertion (Figure 56–2). After the vein has been entered, the wings lie flat against the skin and provide a means for securing the needle and tubing. Available from 16 gauge to 25 gauge, the butterfly can be used in a variety of

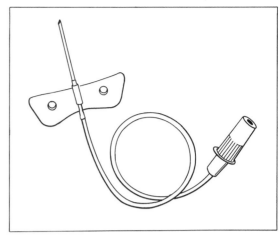

Figure 56–2 Butterfly infusion set. Hold the wings to stabilize the needle for insertion.

situations. The smaller sizes (25 and 23) are particularly useful for infant scalp veins and for patients with small, fragile, or rolling veins. A butterfly is also available for intermittent use (Figure 56–3), such as on a heparin lock.

An *intravenous catheter inside a needle* (Figure 56–4) (Intracath, Venocath) is threaded into the vein and is used when the intravenous is expected to remain in place for several days. After the needle is pulled back out of the skin, leaving the approximately 11-inch-long catheter in place, a guard is secured over the needle, covering it completely. *This device is usually quite stable and affords the patient maximum mobility.* It is available in several sizes. *The plastic is less likely to puncture or injure the vein* but may be a source of irritation, leading to phlebitis. These devices are not recommended for routine peripheral IV use (Intravenous Nurses Society, 1990).

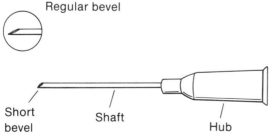

Figure 56–1 Straight needle with a short bevel.

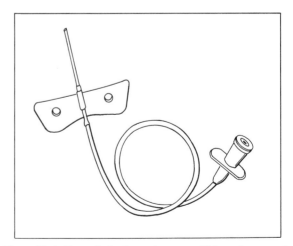

Figure 56–3 Butterfly for intermittent use. This set is accessed by a needle through the rubber port.

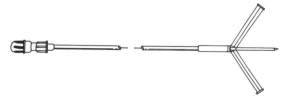

Figure 56–4 IV catheter inside a needle.

Still another device consists of an *intravenous catheter* about 2 inches long *over a needle* (Figure 56–5). The needle and catheter are inserted. When blood returns the needle is removed, leaving the catheter in place. This device is used when veins are tortuous and will not receive a long catheter. The over-the-needle catheter is more likely to be damaged by the needle's sharp edge, which can result in the plastic catheter breaking off in the vein and becoming an embolus.

SELECTING A VEIN

For the adult patient, intravenous infusions are usually started in an arm or a hand. Legs are avoided *because of the danger of thrombus formation and subsequent pulmonary emboli. Circulation is also less in lower extremities.* Selection depends on a number of factors, including the reason for the IV, the length of time it is expected to be needed, the condition of the patient's veins, and the comfort and safety of the patient.

Although it is usually easy to start an IV in the branches of either the cephalic or the basilic vein located near the antecubital space (inner aspect of the elbow), these veins are often not a good choice. *Insertion there limits the patient's mobility in that arm, laboratory technicians often rely on these veins for blood samples, and these veins are the preferred site for peripheral central line access.* They should be used as a last resort and in emergency situations.

Better sites in the adult patient are the lower branches of the basilic and the cephalic veins (Figure 56–6). The scalp veins are used in the infant *because there is less movement there and hence less chance of dislocation.*

It is best to start distal in the vein (in the hand or forearm). *Then, if you are unsuccessful or if the IV comes out later, you can choose a vein proximal to or higher*

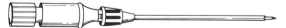

Figure 56–5 IV catheter over a needle.

than the first one. A site where there is bifurcation may be easier to enter if you can enter from below. Compare the length of the device you plan to use with the available vein. Given that you have a choice, it is preferable not to use the dominant hand or arm and also better to change sides with subsequent IVs. Your choices are often limited by the diagnosis, the condition of the patient's veins, the presence of additional equipment, and so forth. IVs are not started on the arm with a dialysis access nor on the side of a mastectomy.

Select the vein by looking, palpating, and attempting to distend any veins in the area. You want a clearly visible vein that can be palpated and that has a straight section for entry. If one is not visible, look for the faint outline of a blue vein under the skin *to determine where to begin.* If not even an outline is visible, you must begin to distend the veins, *to make them visible or palpable.* To distend the veins, place a tourniquet (using a length of Penrose drain) a few inches above the area where you want to start the IV, and ask the patient to "pump," opening and closing the fist. Generally, these maneuvers distend the vein, *making it easier to locate and enter.* If you still cannot locate a vein, place the arm in a dependent position for 5–10 minutes, or apply warm wet packs to the area (see Figure 56–7). Veins that are not visible but are palpable can be used.

Some veins can be entered without using a tourniquet, a procedure that is advisable when a patient's veins are particularly fragile or rolling. The extra distention produced by a tourniquet can cause a vein to burst or roll even more.

If you have tried two times and have been unable to enter a vein, it is best to get assistance. *The procedure is uncomfortable for the patient, and you do not want to use up all the available veins. If no member of the nursing staff can start the IV,* it may be necessary to ask the anesthesia department for assistance (depending on the policies in your facility), or the physician may elect to use the jugular vein. This site is often chosen when other veins cannot be used and is also used as a site for a central line.

PROCEDURE FOR STARTING AN INTRAVENOUS INFUSION

Assessment

1. Check the physician's orders. The orders include the type and amount of solution and the length of time over which the solution should run. The physician may also order

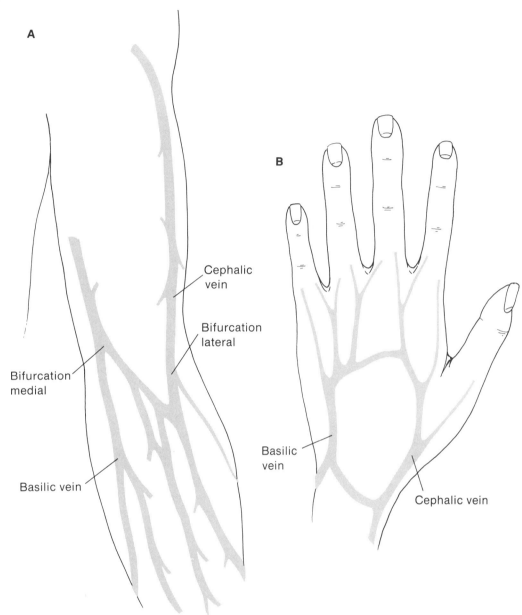

Figure 56–6 Suitable veins for starting IVs. **A:** Forearm. **B:** Hand.

additional medications to be added to the solution. Depending on the policies of the facility in which you work, you may add them yourself or they may be added in the pharmacy under a laminar airflow hood (see Module 54, Administering Intravenous Medications).

Planning

2. Wash your hands *for infection control.*
3. Choose equipment to set up the IV and to start the IV, including the following:
   a. Sterile intravenous solution as ordered with timing strip
   b. Administration set that contains tubing to deliver the fluid and a means of regulating the flow rate
   c. IV standard
   d. Tourniquet
   e. Antiseptic swab
   f. Means of entry into the vein (needle or catheter)
   g. Tape (tear four 6-inch strips and place them conveniently)
   h. Antiseptic or antibiotic ointment (if indicated by the hospital's procedure)

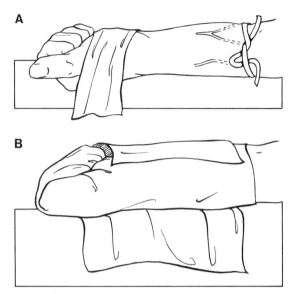

Figure 56–7 Ways to distend a vein. **A:** Tourniquet. **B:** Moist heat.

   i. Dressing materials
   j. Armboard
   Much of this equipment may be in an "IV Start" package or may be kept together in a box or on a cart. This is a convenient practice *because you often will not know which device you'll want to use until you have examined the patient.* Be sure that this box or cart is kept well stocked.
   k. Clean gloves

4. Set up the intravenous fluid and tubing as described in Module 53, Preparing and Maintaining Intravenous Infusions.

5. Take the equipment to the bedside.

Implementation

6. Identify the patient *to be sure you are performing the procedure for the correct patient. Starting an intravenous infusion should be handled with the same careful checking as the administration of any medication.*

7. Prepare the patient psychologically. Just a few minutes before you plan to start the IV, tell the patient that intravenous fluids have been ordered and for what reason. Do not take the equipment to the bedside until you are actually ready to start. (See Psychological Implications, above, and refer to Module 53, Preparing and Maintaining Intravenous Infusions.)

8. Adjust the lighting. Make sure you have adequate lighting, a factor that is extremely important and often overlooked. If the room

lights are not adequate, locate a portable lamp for temporary use.

9. Prepare the patient physically. First provide for the patient's privacy. Look at the gown or pajamas the patient is wearing, and help the patient to change to more convenient garb if necessary. *A pajama top with narrow sleeves or a long nightgown may be difficult if not impossible to remove once the IV is in place.* A hospital gown with a shoulder snap opening is often the easiest and best "clothing" for the patient to wear. Then position the patient as comfortably as possible. Place a towel under the arm *to protect the bed.* You may have to remove the patient's watch or change the position of the nameband *if either is in the way.*

10. Wash your hands and put on clean gloves. *Starting an IV is a sterile procedure, for which you use sterile equipment. Your hands must be clean. Gloves protect you from blood spills.*

11. Position yourself. To start an IV, you'll find that it is as important for you to be comfortable as it is for the patient. The position you choose must be comfortable for you and may not be as orthodox as a chair at the bedside. Some nurses put the bed in high position and stand. Others sit on the bed. Of course, the policy in your facility may somewhat limit your range of choices.

12. Locate a vein in which to start the IV. Examine both hands and forearms and select a site to begin. Place a tourniquet a few inches above the area where you want to start, and ask the patient to open and close the fist. If the vein does not distend, you may have to place the arm in a dependent position or apply warm, moist packs to the area. Remember not to use a tourniquet if the veins are extremely fragile or rolling *because the extra distention may cause the veins to burst or roll even more.*

13. Release the tourniquet.

14. Clean the area thoroughly. Start from the point at which you want to enter and move with a circular motion away from it, cleaning the skin thoroughly at and around the vein you have selected. If the area is especially hairy, shave it before you attempt to start the IV, *both for aseptic reasons and to prevent the tape from pulling.* Clean the area after it has been shaved. The antiseptic agent used for cleaning is usually indicated by unit or facility policy. Tincture of iodine is preferred, but 70% alcohol can be used (Centers for Disease

Control, 1987). Try not to touch the area after it has been cleaned.

If it is necessary to touch the area after it has been cleaned (e.g., to repalpate the vein), you may clean your fingers with the antiseptic as well, if hospital policy allows.

15. Anesthetize the area if policy allows. Use a local anesthetic sprayed or injected onto the skin *to decrease the sensitivity of the skin and vein.* Be sure to check whether the patient is allergic to local anesthetics.

16. Reapply the tourniquet.

17. If you are using a device with a catheter, inspect it for defects.

18. Insert the needle. Using the thumb of your nondominant hand, gently retract the skin away from the site. Holding the needle at about a 45° angle, with the bevel up, pierce the skin immediately beside the vein you have selected (Figure 56–8). When the needle is through the skin, decrease the angle until it is almost parallel with the skin, and enter the vein (Figure 56–9). When blood comes back into the tubing or syringe (depending on the device you are using), insert the needle almost the full 1½ inches. Follow the package instructions for the use of any other device.

19. Holding the needle or other device steady with your dominant hand, release the tourniquet with your other hand.

20. Connect the tubing and initiate the flow. Remove the protective cap from the IV tubing (maintaining sterile technique), connect it securely to the needle, and open the regulator *to initiate the flow.* This should be done quickly

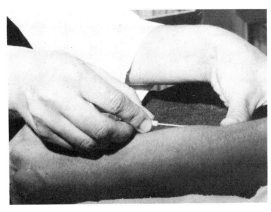

Figure 56–9 Needle at angle to enter vein. (*Courtesy Ivan Ellis*)

to prevent the patient's blood from clotting and occluding the needle.

21. Remove your gloves, tape the needle securely, and dress the site. This should be done according to unit or facility procedure. If you have no procedure, use one of the three following methods:

   a. Chevron tape with gauze dressing (Figure 56–10)

   (1) Place a sterile folded 3 × 3 or 2 × 2 gauze square under the needle (folded side toward the needle). *This protects the skin from the needle hub.*

   (2) Place a small amount of antiseptic ointment at the needle site. (Povidone-iodine ointment or a topical polyantibiotic ointment may be used.) *This decreases the incidence of infection.*

   (3) With ¼-inch adhesive tape (check for patient allergy), tape the needle in place, using a chevron configuration *to hold the needle securely in place.*

   (4) Place a sterile 3 × 3 or 2 × 2 gauze square open over the IV site.

   (5) Tape the needle and tubing in place, using paper tape (if available—*it is usually less traumatic to the patient's skin*), and make a loop of tubing near the point of entry. *This helps prevent the weight of the tubing from pulling the needle out of place.* A commercially produced firm plastic U-shaped connector is available for this purpose (see Figure 56–10).

   (6) Tape the armboard in place if necessary.

   (7) Write the date, time, type of device,

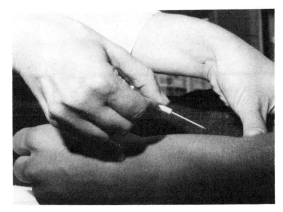

Figure 56–8 Skin retracted and needle at angle to pierce skin. (*Courtesy Ivan Ellis*)

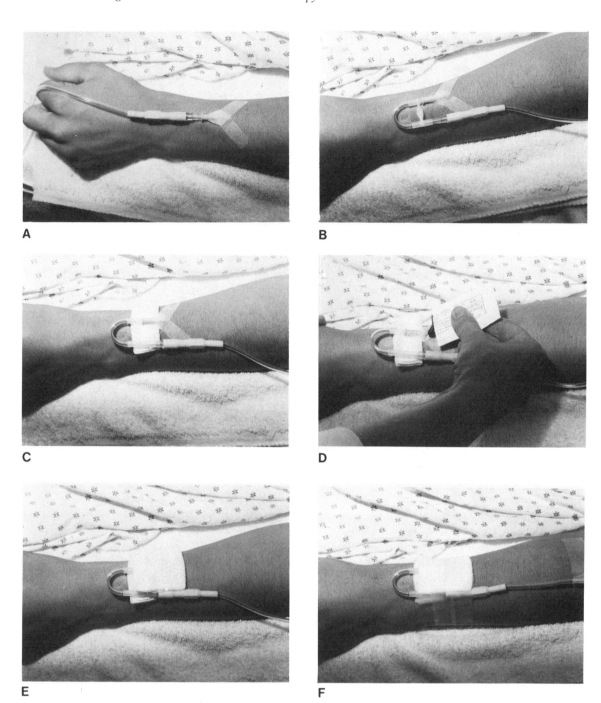

A B C D E F

Figure 56–10 Chevron tape with gauze dressing. **A:** Chevron tape in place, **B:** Tubing curved by using a U-shaped connector, **C:** Gauze square under hub to support position, **D:** Applying antiseptic ointment on needle entry site, **E:** 2 × 2 dressing, **F:** Dressing and tubing taped in place.
(*Courtesy Ivan Ellis*)

catheter gauge, and your initials on the tape.

b. U method of taping (Figure 56–11)

(1) Apply antiseptic ointment at the needle site according to your facility's procedure.

(2) Place the middle portion of a ½-inch tape strip, sticky side up, under the tubing.

(3) Fold each end of the tape down, so the sticky side is toward the skin and the tape is parallel to the needle.

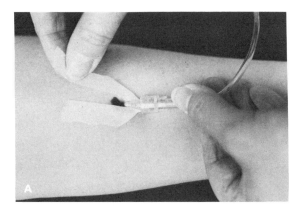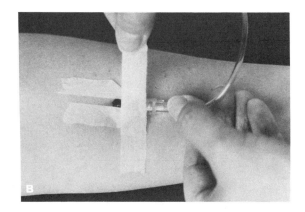
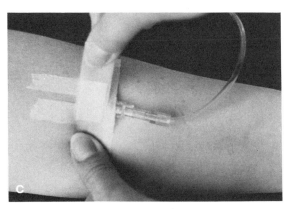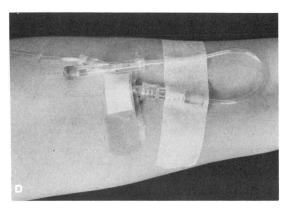

Figure 56–11 U method of taping. **A:** Apply antibacterial ointment and U-tape, **B:** Cross tape to secure needle hub, **C:** Bandage across insertion site. **D:** Tubing looped and taped in place.
(*Courtesy Ivan Ellis*)

(4) Place a piece of ½-inch tape over the hub of the needle, extending out on either side over the strips parallel to the needle.

(5) Cover the needle site with an adhesive strip.

(6) Make a loop in the tubing and secure it with 1-inch tape.

(7) Write the date, time, type of device, catheter gauge, and your initials on the tape.

c. Transparent dressing (Figure 56–12). Some facilities use transparent, moisture/vapor-permeable adhesive dressings (OpSite, Tegaderm) rather than the traditional IV site dressings described above. The dressing covers the IV site and seals snugly around the hub of the needle, leaving the hub out *for ease of tubing change.* Follow specific package directions. An advantage is that this dressing does not need to be removed in order to assess the needle site.

22. Adjust the flow rate. The physician will have ordered a specific amount of fluid to be administered over a certain period. In some facilities you will figure the rate of flow yourself, based on the number of drops per milliliter administered by the equipment you are using. In others the rate will be figured by pharmacy personnel, but you still must be able to check that rate and to figure it again in the event the IV gets "ahead" or "behind." Many facilities stock narrow strips of paper calibrated according to the number of hours the IV is to run (Figure 56–13). The nurse adds the specific times appropriate for the individual IV. *These forms make it easier for the nursing staff to assess the progress of the infusion.* You may also be using a controller or pump as described in Module 53, Preparing and Maintaining Intravenous Infusions.

23. Care for the equipment appropriately.

24. Wash your hands.

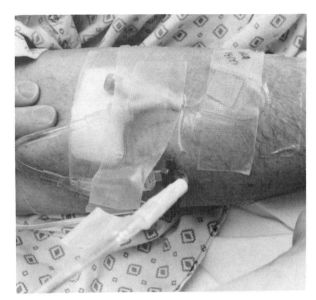

Figure 56–12 Transparent dressing is used to cover IV sites in many hospitals.

Evaluation

25. Evaluate, using the following criteria:
    a. Right patient, right solution, right amount, right rate, right time.
    b. Intravenous secure (on armboard if positional).
    c. Patient comfortable.

Documentation

26. Record the IV insertion. Usually a special form is used for this purpose (see Module 53, Figures 53–14 and 53–15). Include the time the IV was started, the type of fluid, any additives, where the IV was started, and by whom. When an IV is discontinued, include the time and the amount of fluid absorbed. A patient with an infusing IV is usually on intake and output as well.

PROCEDURE FOR CONVERTING AN IV TO A HEPARIN LOCK

When there is no longer a need for IV fluids but the need for intravenous access remains, you may be asked to convert an intravenous infusion to a heparin lock.

Assessment

1. Check the physician's orders.
2. Check the IV site for signs and symptoms of phlebitis, infiltration, and obstruction of flow.

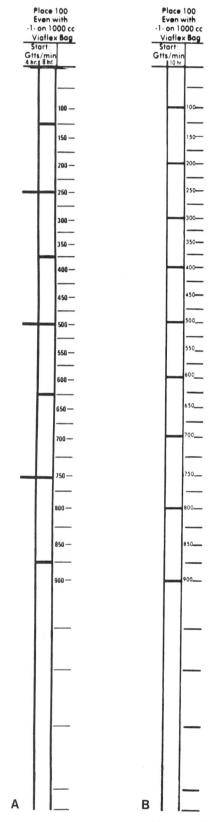

Figure 56–13 Calibration labels. **A:** 4- or 8-hour label, **B:** 10-hour label.

Planning

3. Wash your hands *for infection control.*
4. Take the equipment to the bedside. You will need the heparin lock adapter, 10 units/ml heparin solution, dressing and taping materials, and clean gloves.

Implementation

5. Identify the patient *to be sure you are performing the procedure for the correct patient.*
6. Instill the heparin lock adapter with the dilute heparin, using sterile technique.
7. Turn off the existing IV and disconnect it at the hub of the catheter or needle.
8. Attach the heparin lock adapter and instill the remainder of the heparin.
9. Dress and tape according to facility policy or refer to step 21 under Procedure for Starting an Intravenous Infusion, above.
10. Observe and document the amount remaining in the IV container and dispose of the tubing and the container.
11. Remove your gloves and wash your hands.

Evaluation

12. Evaluate, using the following criteria:
    a. Heparin lock securely in place.
    b. Patient comfortable.

Documentation

13. Record the conversion of the intravenous infusion to a heparin lock on the IV record or as appropriate in your facility.

References

Centers for Disease Control. (1987, August 21). Recommendations for prevention of HIV transmission in health care settings. *Morbidity and Mortality Weekly Report Supplement, 36,* 25–185.

Centers for Disease Control. (1988, June 24). Update: Universal precautions for prevention of transmission of human immunodeficiency virus, hepatitis B virus, and other blood borne pathogens in health care settings, *Morbidity and Mortality Weekly Report, 37,* 1–7.

Intravenous Nurses Society. (1990). *Intravenous Nursing Standards of Practice.* Belmont, MA: INS.

Performance Checklist

Starting an Intravenous Infusion	Unsat	Needs More Practice	Sat	Comments
Assessment				
1. Check physician's orders.				
Planning				
2. Wash your hands.				
3. Choose appropriate equipment: Fluid, administration set, IV standard, tourniquet, antiseptic swab, needle or catheter, tape, antiseptic ointment, dressing material, armboard, clean gloves				
4. Set up intravenous fluid and tubing.				
5. Take equipment to bedside.				
Implementation				
6. Identify patient.				
7. Prepare patient psychologically.				
8. Adjust lighting.				
9. Prepare patient physically.				
10. Wash your hands and put on gloves.				
11. Select position of comfort for yourself.				
12. Locate vein. Apply tourniquet.				
13. Release tourniquet.				
14. Clean area thoroughly.				
15. Anesthetize if policy allows.				
16. Reapply the tourniquet.				
17. If using a device with a catheter, inspect it for defects.				
18. Introduce needle.				
19. Release tourniquet.				
20. Connect tubing and initiate flow.				
21. Tape needle and dress site.				
22. Adjust flow rate.				

Starting an Intravenous Infusion *(Continued)*	Unsat	Needs More Practice	Sat	Comments
23. Care for equipment.				
24. Wash your hands.				
Evaluation				
25. Evaluate using the following criteria: a. Right patient, right solution, right amount, right rate, right time.				
b. Intravenous secure.				
c. Patient comfortable.				
Documentation				
26. Record IV on appropriate chart form.				

Converting an IV to a Heparin Lock

Assessment				
1. Check physician's orders.				
2. Check IV site.				
Planning				
3. Wash your hands and put on gloves.				
4. Take equipment to bedside.				
Implementation				
5. Identify patient.				
6. Instill dilute heparin into the heparin lock adapter.				
7. Turn off IV and disconnect it at needle/catheter hub.				
8. Attach heparin lock adapter and instill remainder of heparin.				
9. Dress and tape.				
10. Observe amount remaining in IV container and dispose of tubing and container.				
11. Dispose of gloves and wash your hands.				

Converting an IV to a Heparin Lock *(Continued)*	Unsat	Needs More Practice	Sat	Comments
Evaluation				
12. Evaluate using the following criteria: a. Heparin lock securely in place.				
b. Patient comfortable.				
Documentation				
13. Record appropriately.				

Quiz

Short-Answer Questions

1. List three reasons why patients often fear intravenous infusions.

   a. _____

   b. _____

   c. _____

2. List two reasons why a patient might be receiving IV fluids.

   a. _____

   b. _____

3. List the four pieces of equipment discussed in this module that can be used to start an IV.

   a. _____

   b. _____

   c. _____

   d. _____

4. a. Where is an IV usually started in an infant? _____

   b. Why? _____

5. List four methods that can be used to distend a vein.

   a. _____

   b. _____

   c. _____

   d. _____

6. Name two agents that can be used to cleanse the skin before starting an intravenous infusion.

   a. _____

   b. _____

7. List five items of documentation to include on the tape that secures the intravenous dressing in place.

   a. _____

   b. _____

   c. _____

   d. _____

   e. _____

Module 57
Administering Blood and Blood Products

Module Contents

Rationale for the Use of This Skill
Nursing Diagnoses
Use of Blood and Blood Products
  Blood Donated by an Unrelated Donor
  Autologous Transfusion
  Hemodilution
  Salvage During Surgery
Types of Blood Products
  Whole Blood
  Blood Products
    Packed Red Blood Cells
    Platelets
    Plasma
    Plasma Protein Fraction
    Human Serum Albumin
    Cryoprecipitate
Typing and Crossmatching
Reactions to Transfusions
Equipment
**General Guidelines for Administration of
    Blood and Blood Products**
**Procedure for Administering Blood and
    Blood Products**
  Whole Blood and Packed Red Cells
  Assessment
  Planning

  Implementation
  Evaluation
  Documentation
  Platelets
  Assessment
  Planning
  Implementation
  Evaluation
  Documentation
  Albumin
  Assessment
  Planning
  Implementation
  Evaluation
  Documentation
  Cryoprecipitate
  Assessment
  Planning
  Implementation
  Evaluation
  Documentation
Long-Term Care
Home Care

Prerequisites

Successful completion of the following modules:

VOLUME 1

Module 1   An Approach to Nursing Skills
Module 2   Basic Infection Control
Module 3   Safety
Module 5   General Assessment Overview
Module 6   Documentation
Module 13 Inspection, Palpation,
    Auscultation, and Percussion

Module 15 Intake and Output
Module 16 Temperature, Pulse, and
    Respiration
Module 17 Blood Pressure

VOLUME 2

Module 35 Sterile Technique
Module 53 Preparing and Maintaining
    Intravenous Infusions

522

Overall Objective

To prepare and administer blood and blood products with comfort, safety, and maximum effectiveness for patients and to recognize common complications and intervene appropriately.

Specific Learning Objectives

	Know Facts and Principles	Apply Facts and Principles	Demonstrate Ability	Evaluate Performance
1. *Rationale for administration of blood and blood products*	State three reasons for administration of blood and blood products.	Given a patient situation, identify the reason for the administration of blood or a blood product.	In the clinical setting, identify the reason for the administration of blood or a blood product to a specific patient.	Verify rationale with instructor.

2. *Use of blood and blood products*
  a. Whole blood
  b. Blood products
    (1) Packed red blood cells
    (2) Platelets
    (3) Plasma
    (4) Plasma protein fraction
    (5) Human serum albumin
    (6) Cryoprecipitate
	State rationale for the use of blood and blood products discussed.
	
	State two advantages of component therapy.
		Given a patient situation, identify appropriate type(s) of blood or component therapy.	In the clinical setting, identify rationale for the use of blood or a blood product in a specific patient situation.	Verify with instructor.

3. *Typing and crossmatching*	Name the four main blood groups in the ABO system of typing. State the major advantage of regular crossmatching over 10-minute crossmatching. State a valid reason for using a 10-minute crossmatch.	Given a patient situation, identify which type of crossmatching would be appropriate.	In the clinical setting, identify the appropriate type of crossmatching for a specific patient.	Verify with instructor.

4. *Potential reaction to transfusion*
  a. Hemolytic
  b. Febrile
  c. Allergic
  d. Transmission of disease
  e. Circulatory overload
	State signs and symptoms of each type of transfusion reaction discussed.
	
	State appropriate intervention for
		Given a patient situation, identify type of transfusion reaction from symptoms listed.
		
		Given a patient
			In the clinical setting, take appropriate preventive measures as the situation allows.	Evaluate with your instructor.

(continued)

Specific Learning Objectives *(Continued)*

	Know Facts and Principles	Apply Facts and Principles	Demonstrate Ability	Evaluate Performance
f. Hypothermia g. Hyperkalemia h. Hypocalcemia i. Air embolus	each type of transfusion reaction discussed. State appropriate measures to prevent various transfusion reactions.	situation, identify appropriate intervention for that particular type of transfusion reaction. Given a specific reaction, state appropriate preventive measures.		
5. Equipment	Identify special equipment needed for administering blood and blood products.		In the practice or clinical setting, select the correct equipment to administer blood or a blood product.	Verify selection with instructor.
6. General guidelines for administration of blood and blood products	Discuss the general guidelines for administration of blood and blood products.	Given a patient situation, state appropriate use of guidelines presented.	In the clinical setting, use guidelines appropriate to the specific patient situation.	Evaluate with your instructor.
7. Procedure for administering blood and blood products (whole blood, packed red cells, platelets, albumin, cryoprecipitate)	Describe procedure for administering whole blood, packed red cells, platelets, albumin, and cryoprecipitate.	Given a patient situation, identify whether correct procedure is being used for administering blood or blood product.	In the clinical setting, give whole blood, packed red cells, platelets, and cryoprecipitate safely.	Evaluate performance with instructor using Performance Checklist.

Learning Activities

1. Review the Specific Learning Objectives.
2. Read the section on blood transfusion in Ellis and Nowlis, *Nursing: A Human Needs Approach,* or comparable material in another textbook.
3. Look up the module vocabulary terms in the Glossary.
4. Read through the module and mentally practice the specific procedures.
5. In the practice setting:
   a. Examine the blood administration equipment. Identify each of the following:
      (1) Y blood administration sets
      (2) Primary blood administration sets
      (3) Secondary blood administration sets
      (4) Secondary intravenous administration sets
      (5) Forms for recording blood administration
   b. Read the directions on the package regarding how to set up the blood administration equipment you will be using.
   c. Set up a blood administration set as though you were going to administer blood. Attach a secondary administration set as a normal saline line if that is the policy in your facility.
   d. Regulate the drip rate so 500 ml blood will be delivered in 4 hours. Consult the blood administration set package to identify the drops per milliliter delivered by the tubing.
   e. Demonstrate what you would do if it were necessary to stop the transfusion.
   f. Practice recording:
      (1) The administration of a unit of whole blood, started at 1:00 PM and completed at 4:00 PM, as appropriate to your facility
      (2) As though the recipient of the blood had an allergic reaction. Make up appropriate observation data and indicate appropriate nursing intervention
6. In the clinical setting:
   a. Consult with your instructor regarding an opportunity to set up and administer blood or a blood product to an adult or pediatric patient.

Vocabulary

allergic reaction	donor	hyperkalemia	recipient
autologous transfusion	erythrocyte	hypocalcemia	salvaged blood transfusions
circulatory overload	febrile reaction	hypothermia	serum hepatitis
	hemolytic reaction	packed red blood cells	
citrated blood	hemodilution	plasma	type and crossmatch
compatibility	human serum albumin	platelets	whole blood
cryoprecipitate			

Administering Blood and Blood Products

Rationale for the Use of This Skill

Blood and blood products may be administered for various reasons, including restoration of circulating blood volume, replacement of clotting factors, and improvement of oxygen-carrying capacity. Whatever the situation, potential complications are involved. The nurse must be cognizant of these complications and work to prevent them as well as be able to intervene appropriately as necessary.[1]

▶ ***Nursing Diagnoses***

The patient's nursing diagnoses are often those that lead to the need for transfusion rather than ones centered around the procedure. These may involve activity intolerance or hemorrhage.

For example:

Activity Intolerance: Weakness related to too few red blood cells (anemia)

Impaired Physical Mobility: Fatigue related to low red blood cells (anemia)

Fluid Volume Deficit, Actual: Hemorrhage related to vascularity of surgical site

High Risk for Injury: Hemorrhage into joints and soft tissue

Fluid Volume Excess, Actual: Related to increase in vascular fluid volume.

Alteration in Emotional Integrity: Anxiety related to the fear of pending blood transfusion.

The nursing diagnoses related to the transfusion procedure itself are more collaborative. They are in response to the medical diagnosis rather than the nursing diagnosis. Here, the nurse identifies problems and reports those problems as well as responds to the physicians orders. For example:

High Risk for Injury, Transfusion Reaction: (type can be named, such as hemolytic, allergic) related to previous reaction to a transfusion

---

[1] You will note that rationale for action is emphasized throughout the module by the use of italics.

USE OF BLOOD AND BLOOD PRODUCTS

Commonly, patients receive packed red blood cells or whole blood, depending on the patient's medical need. Before a description on the various blood products, you should understand the five methods now in use to administer blood.

Blood Donated by an Unrelated Donor

The majority of blood needed by patients is obtained from an unrelated donor. The identity of the donor is not revealed to the recipient. Through an exposure process, the blood from each is "typed and cross-matched" *to make sure that the two are compatible and that a reaction will not occur.* In addition, the donor's blood is tested for a variety of blood-borne diseases such as hepatitis and AIDS. If tested positive, the blood is discarded.

Blood Donated by a Related Donor

In some states, blood may be donated by a relative of the patient and the blood designated only for use by the family member for whom the donation is given. Statistically, these donations are no safer from disease than is blood given by an unrelated donor *because of the unwillingness of family members to reveal life-style or medical history.* A special charge is assessed for blood donation by a related donor and the blood undergoes the same tests as blood given by an unrelated donor.

Autologous Transfusion

For patients anticipating elective surgery, the trend toward autologous transfusion is increasing. In some areas 5% to 10% of all blood transfusions are now autologous. This means that the patient goes to the community blood center 1–3 weeks before the scheduled surgery where a unit of blood is collected. The patient may go at designated intervals later to donate additional units. This method *eliminates the chances of transmission of hepatitis, AIDS, and other diseases transmitted by contaminated blood.* A written referral must have previously been sent by the surgeon to the blood center. The person may not have a hemoglobin value of less than 11 g/dl to be eligible for self-donation. (Butler, 1989). The donated blood or red blood cells are labeled for the patient and stored as fresh or frozen blood until ready for use. The patient may be placed on oral iron supplements *to aid in regenerating the hemoglobin.* There is a special charge to the patient for the autologous transfusion process.

Hemodilution

As the patient is prepared for surgery, 1–2 units of blood is withdrawn and this volume replaced with an intravenous infusion of a "plasma expander" or colloidal solution *to maintain blood volume.* During the surgery, the blood that was collected immediately prior to surgery is reinfused into the patient to replace blood loss.

Salvage During Surgery

When there is massive blood loss during surgeries, which sometimes occurs during vascular or cardiac surgeries, the blood may be recovered with a special suction device, filtered, and reinfused into the patient. The blood is mixed with an anticoagulant *to prevent clotting.*

TYPES OF BLOOD PRODUCTS

Whole blood may be ordered as a part of patient therapy or, because blood can be separated into its component parts, only the specific component needed in a patient's therapy may be used. Below is a discussion of indications and contraindications for using whole blood and some of its components.

Whole Blood

Whole blood transfusion is most commonly used in *instances of acute massive blood loss* or *for total blood exchange in neonates. Its use to increase the oxygen-carrying capacity and circulating volume of the blood* should be restricted to situations where both indications are present. A unit of blood equals approximately 500 ml (450 ml of blood from a donor and 60–70 ml of preservative/anticoagulant). Whole blood is not indicated *when blood volume is normal or increased.*

Blood Products

The use of blood products (or components) has increased in recent years, making it possible to give only the *needed* factor to the recipient. This practice also makes it possible *to serve more needs with fewer donations* and *to decrease the risk of complications, such*

as circulatory overload and blood-carried diseases, to the recipient.

Packed Red Blood Cells. Packed red blood cells make up the blood product remaining after up to 80% of the plasma is removed from whole blood. *Because red blood cells provide the same oxygen-carrying capacity as whole blood but in smaller volume,* they may be used in situations in which the patient is at risk for circulatory overload but has need of hemoglobin for its oxygen-carrying capacity. Red cells are usually infused over 2 or 3 hours and may be made less viscous by the addition of normal saline (50–100 ml) if the patient's condition permits. A unit of red cells equals approximately 250 ml. The use of red blood cells (also called packed cells) necessitates typing and crossmatching.

Platelets. Platelets (thrombocytes) are used *in cases of thrombocytopenia caused by lack of platelet production, resulting in increased bleeding time.* They are only indicated *for treatment of life-threatening hemorrhage.* A unit of platelets consists of a large number of platelets in a small amount of plasma (50–70 ml). The usual volume for a bleeding adult with thrombocytopenia is 6–10 units. Platelets should be type-compatible, but Rh antigens are not found on platelets. The risk for acquiring blood-carried diseases is the same as for whole blood.

Plasma. Plasma is the fluid portion of the blood remaining after the red blood cells, platelets, and leukocytes have been removed. Fresh frozen plasma can be stored for 12 months and *provides clotting factors, proteins, and fluid volume.* Such IV solutions as dextran and lactated Ringer's solution are recommended for volume expansion, and such plasma derivatives as albumin and plasma protein fraction are recommended for protein replacement, *because they do not expose the recipient to the risk of blood-carried diseases, as does fresh or fresh frozen plasma.*

Plasma Protein Fraction. Plasma protein fraction is the portion of the plasma remaining after fibrinogen and globulin have been removed. This component is used in situations where *the replacement of intravascular volume is necessary.* The risk of hepatitis is eliminated because of a pasteurizing process.

Human Serum Albumin. Human serum albumin *increases the colloidal osmotic pressure of the blood and is administered for shock, burns, and hypoproteinemia.* Typing and crossmatching is not required. It is heat-treated at 60°C for 10 hours to decrease hepatitis risk.

Cryoprecipitate. Cryoprecipitate is prepared from fresh frozen plasma and *contains clotting Factor VIII—the factor lacking in hemophiliacs. It contains a very small number of red cells,* which makes crossmatching unnecessary, but it is advisable to give ABO-compatible cryoprecipitate if the total volume is more than 100 ml. It may be stored frozen for 12 months, and the risk for blood-carried diseases is present.

Under investigation is a dried cryoprecipitate product that has an indefinite shelf life and must be reconstituted before infusing. At present, this is being used only with children. It is very costly and will be released for more general use when studies have been completed. See Table 57–1 for a list of commonly used blood products.

TYPING AND CROSSMATCHING

Basic to safe administration of blood and blood components is accurate typing and crossmatching of the blood. Four main blood groups are in the ABO system of blood typing: A, B, AB, and O. Blood is also classified as either Rh positive or Rh negative. In the laboratory the recipient's blood is first tested for type. Next, samples of the donor's and recipient's blood are mixed to determine compatibility. If they are *not* compatible, antibodies in the recipient's plasma will agglutinate the erythrocytes from the donor's blood and cause the most serious complication of blood transfusion therapy—hemolytic reaction (Table 57–2).

Crossmatching may be done in one of two ways. In an urgent situation the blood is tested for type, and a 10-minute crossmatch for blood compatibility may be done. *Because this crossmatch is incomplete,* the recipient of this blood must be watched closely for reactions. The regular crossmatch may take up to 2 hours but *includes more complete testing of compatibility, and thus potential for reactions is reduced.*

EQUIPMENT

Whole blood, packed red blood cells, and plasma should be administered using a standard (170-micron) blood filter. The filter should be entirely covered with blood or blood product before blood is run through the tubing *to remove the air* (Figures 57–1 and 57–2). Although a standard blood filter can be used for 2–3 units of blood before debris accumulates and slows

the rate of flow, the filter should not be left hanging for more than 6 hours *because of the hazard of bacterial contamination.*

Some facilities use a pump to infuse blood while others do not. You will have to check with the policy in your facility to determine this.

Platelets are administered using a component administration set with a standard 170-micron filter. A new filter should be used each time platelets are administered. Cryoprecipitate may be administered using either a primary set or a component set.

Plasma protein fraction and human serum albumin are commercially packaged, and tubing to be used for administration is enclosed in the package.

A secondary IV set (see Module 53, Preparing and Maintaining Intravenous Infusions) is used if saline is to be piggybacked into the blood administration setup. In some facilities, Y blood administration sets are used, in which case one administration set is used for both the blood or blood product and the saline. The Y set is convenient for diluting some blood products such as platelets or packed red blood cells. If the patient has a mild transfusion reaction, the blood flow can be shut off and the saline continued until an assessment can be made. If a serious reaction occurs, which is rare, the blood flow should be stopped immediately, someone called to assist, and the line heplocked to maintain access to a vein in case it is needed for treatment of the reaction. Some feel that with serious reactions, even though the blood is shut off and the saline started, the small amount of blood in the tubing that would be infused ahead of the saline flow could add to the danger and that inserting a heplock *prevents this from occurring.*

A size 19 or larger needle, butterfly, or other device is used to start an intravenous through which blood is to be infused. If the patient is an infant or young child, a size 20–23 needle may be used (see Module 56, Starting Intravenous Infusions).

GENERAL GUIDELINES FOR ADMINISTRATION OF BLOOD AND BLOOD PRODUCTS

1. An 18- or 19-gauge (or larger) needle is used for the administration of whole blood or packed red blood cells. A 20- to 23-gauge needle may be used for infants and other patients with small veins. Smaller needles may also be used for other blood products.
2. The transfusion should be started within 30 minutes of the time the blood is removed from

Table 57-1 Commonly Used Blood Products

Component	Major Indications	Special Points	Time Lapse Expected for Receipt of Blood Bank Items	Product Expiration Time After Arrival to Blood Bank	Rate of Infusion
Red blood cells	Symptomatic anemia		4–6 h (routine)	48 h	Usual rate 2–4 h
			1 h (10 min type and crossmatch)		For massive loss, fast as patient can tolerate
Whole blood	Symptomatic anemia with large volume deficit		4–6 h (routine)	48 h	Usual rate 4 h
			1 h (10 min type and crossmatch)		For massive loss, fast as patient can tolerate
Leukocyte poor RBCs	To prevent febrile reactions from leukocyte antibodies while treating symptomatic anemia	Leukocyte poor RBCs must be specifically prescribed by physician.	4 h	24–48 h check expiration time on bag	Usual rate 2–4 h
					For massive loss, fast as patient can tolerate
Leukocyte poor RBCs (obtained by washing)	Paroxysmal nocturnal hemoglobinuria and some types of immune globulin disorders	To order, physician must make special arrangement at blood bank.	4 h	24 h	Should be administered stat after arrival to blood bank.
					For massive blood loss, fast as patient can tolerate.
					Usual rate 2–4 h
Platelets	To decrease clotting times for platelet function abnormality, or for decreased platelets	Do not refrigerate. Give as soon as possible after arrival. The greater the delay of administration, the less value platelets are to the patient. Platelets are probably of some value for several hours.	1½ h	Check expiration time on bag	As rapidly as possible
Granulocytes	Neutropenia and infection	Increased risk of allergic reaction. Physician must order through the blood bank.	6–24 h depending on availability	Unknown— probably 24 h	Infuse over 2–4 h

(continued)

Table 57-1 Commonly Used Blood Products (Continued)

Component	Major Indications	Special Points	Time Lapse Expected for Receipt of Blood Bank Items	Product Expiration Time After Arrival to Blood Bank	Rate of Infusion
Plasma (fresh frozen)	Deficit of labile plasma coagulation factors		½ h + 45 min to thaw	1 h after thaw	Approximately 10 ml/min
Cryoprecipitate	1. Hemophilia A 2. Replacement of fibrinogen 3. Replacement of factor VIII	Do not refrigerate. To minimize trauma to vessels a new butterfly needle is inserted for each infusion and removed upon completion.	1 h	1. 6 h after thawing OR 2. 4 h after pooling	10 ml diluted component per min

Swedish Hospital Medical Center Nursing Policy/Procedure Committee Revised: July 1987

refrigerated storage in the facility's blood bank. It should not be stored in the refrigerator on the nursing unit, *because refrigerators used for blood storage are monitored to maintain the correct temperature.*

3. Stay with the patient for the first 15 minutes or first 50 ml of the transfusion *to observe for reactions and complications.* Blood should be infused slowly during this time. The rate of administration is determined by the blood product being used and the patient's age and clinical condition.

4. *Because red cells settle to the bottom and plasma rises to the top,* gentle mixing of whole blood is necessary before and during the transfusion. Packed cells should be mixed by squeezing the bag gently every 20–30 minutes *to prevent settling of red blood cells.*

5. Blood should not be allowed to hang at room temperature longer than 4–6 hours *because of the danger of bacteria proliferation and red blood cell hemolysis.* Each facility has a specific policy regarding time.

6. Medications should not be added directly to blood or a blood product. If the tubing being used to administer blood *must* be used to give medications, flush it with saline before and after.

7. An IV of normal saline may be piggybacked into the blood tubing *to maintain access to the line in case it is necessary to discontinue the blood.* Dextrose in water should not be used for this

purpose, because *it may hemolyze the red cells it contacts.*

8. In instances of massive transfusion, it may be necessary to warm the blood before transfusion *to prevent a severe temperature drop.* A blood-warming coil immersed in a water bath at a temperature of 37°C (98.6°F) is used for this purpose. Blood should not be warmed unless it is going to be given immediately. Blood that has been warmed may not be returned to the blood bank for future use.

9. *When blood volume and oxygen-carrying capacity need to be increased immediately,* a blood pump may be used *to increase flow rate.*

10. *Even though all blood is tested for hepatitis B virus and AIDS antibodies, infectious agents may still be present.* If needles have been used, they are removed with gloved hands and placed in the sharps container. All bags and transfusion equipment should be disposed of in the special plastic-lined containers kept in the soiled utility room and never in the wastebasket in the patient's room.

PROCEDURE FOR ADMINISTERING BLOOD AND BLOOD PRODUCTS

Whole Blood and Packed Red Cells

Assessment

1. Check the physician's orders. The orders include the type of blood product, the number

© 1992 by J.B. Lippincott Company

Table 57–2 Reactions to Transfusions

Reaction	Cause	Assessment	Nursing Intervention
Hemolytic Reaction	Incompatibility of types of red cells	Flank pain, dark urine, chest constriction, low back pain, hypotension, tachypnea, tachycardia, fever, chills, apprehension	Stop transfusion immediately and maintain IV line. Monitor vital signs. Notify physician. Monitor urine output. Collect blood and urine samples and send to lab. Prevention: Careful identification of patient and blood before transfusion. Careful observation of patient during first 15 min of transfusion.
Febrile Reaction	Sensitivity to white cells in the blood	Fever, chills, headache, nausea, and vomiting	Mild: Slow rate of transfusion. Notify physician. Administer antihistamine as ordered. Severe: Stop transfusion and maintain IV line. Monitor vital signs. Notify physician. Administer aspirin or acetaminophen to reduce fever as ordered.
Allergic Reaction	Antibody reaction to allergens in donor's blood	Mild: Hives, itching, flushing Severe: Shortness of breath, broncho-spasm, wheezing	Mild: Slow transfusion. Notify physician. Give antihistamine as ordered. Severe: Stop transfusion and maintain IV line. Notify physician. Give antihistamine, epinephrine, or adrenocorticosteroid as ordered. Prevention: If recipient is known to be allergic, reaction may be prevented by administration of antihistamine 1 h before transfusion.
Transmission of Disease (serum hepatitis most common)*	Presence of virus in donor's blood	May appear from 6 weeks to 6 months after transfusion	Prevention: Careful screening of blood donors
Circulatory Overload	Excessive volume, excessive rate (infants, elderly, and those with cardiac disease especially at risk)	Dyspnea, cough, rales in bases of lungs: distended neck veins; elevated central venous pressure	Slow or stop transfusion. Raise patient's head and place feet in dependent position. Notify physician. Give diuretics if ordered by the physician. Prevention: —Administer at slow rate. —Suggest packed cells for patients at risk.
Hypothermia	Rapid transfusion of large volume of cold blood (infants	Chills; may lead to cardiac arrhythmias, fibrillation, arrest	Slow transfusion. Keep patient covered. Prevention:

(continued)

Table 57–2 Reactions to Transfusions (Continued)

Reaction	Cause	Assessment	Nursing Intervention
	and children especially at risk)		—Give blood at room temperature. —Suggest warming coils for rapid transfusion (microwave warmers *not* recommended, *because they cause lysis of red cells*).
Hyperkalemia	Breakdown of red blood cells in stored blood—potassium released into plasma	Nausea, diarrhea, muscle weakness, slowed pulse rate, cardiac arrest	Stop transfusion. Notify physician. Prevention: Use of blood of a short-storage interval.
Hypocalcemia	Rapid rate of transfusion of large quantities of blood, possibly causing calcium deficit *from ability of citrate in stored blood to combine with serum calcium*	Tingling of fingers, circumoral tingling, muscle cramping, convulsion, laryngospasm	Stop transfusion. Notify physician. Administer intravenous calcium as ordered.
Air Embolus	Entry of air into vein	Cyanosis, dyspnea, shock, arrhythmias, cardiac arrest	Lower patient's head and turn patient on left side. Notify physician. Treat shock or cardiac arrest appropriately. Prevention: Cover blood filter *completely* with blood before infusing, and avoid giving blood under pressure.

* Licensed antibody tests detect 97% of AIDS-infected donors.

of units, and sometimes the period over which the product is to be infused.

2. Check the existing intravenous infusion or heparin lock for patency and needle size or initiate an intravenous infusion with a size 19 or larger needle or other means of entering the vein. A 20- to 23-gauge needle may be used for infants and other patients with small veins (see Module 56, Starting Intravenous Infusions).

Planning

3. Wash your hands *for infection control.*
4. Gather the necessary equipment. If it is necessary to start an intravenous infusion, you will need the equipment discussed in Module

56, Starting Intravenous Infusions, step 3), in addition to the following:

a. Primary blood administration set (see Figure 57–1) or Y blood administration set (see Figure 57–2), as facility policy indicates

b. Bottle or bag of normal saline with a secondary administration set, as facility policy indicates

c. Tape

5. Obtain the blood product from the facility blood bank immediately before using and check it out according to facility procedure. Careful identification is done with all blood and blood products, including autologous donations. *This prevents any chance that a mistake has been made.* This usually includes having the

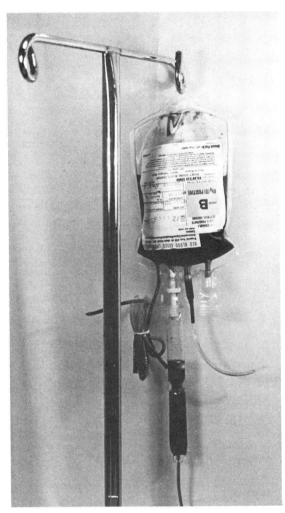

Figure 57-1 Blood administration set.
(*Courtesy Ivan Ellis*)

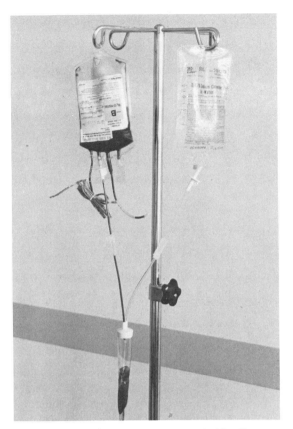

Figure 57-2 Y blood administration set used with saline.
(*Courtesy Ivan Ellis*)

hospital blood lab and unit personnel check the patient's name, hospital number, blood and Rh type, and blood unit identification number and sign the necessary release form.

6. With another nurse, check the following. *Any discrepancy* must be investigated before the blood is administered.
   a. Patient's name and spelling, hospital number, and physician's name as on face sheet with the blood bank invoice
   b. Blood product type, Rh, and blood unit administration number on blood bag with the blood bank invoice
   c. Expiration date on the blood bag
7. You and the other nurse sign your names, titles, date, and time on the blood bank invoice if all the above information checks out.
8. Prepare equipment as follows:

a. If blood is to be infused using a pump, obtain one. Select pump tubing and use either b or c blood administration set. Put on clean gloves.
b. Y blood administration set
   (1) Close all control clamps on the Y set.
   (2) Insert one administration set spike into the normal saline bag according to package directions.
   (3) Open the clamp closest to the normal saline bag and fill the drip chamber half full.
   (4) Open the lower control clamp and flush the air from the tubing; reclamp.
   (5) Insert the other spike of the administration set into the blood bag according to package directions.
   (6) Open the clamp closest to the blood and squeeze the filter chamber and release it until the filter is completely covered; reclamp.
   (7) Open the lower control clamp and flush the tubing with blood.
c. Primary blood administration set

(1) Turn the control on the blood tubing to the off position.

(2) Open the entry port on the blood bag.

(3) Insert the administration set into the blood bag according to package directions.

(4) Squeeze the drip chamber and release it, to allow blood to flow into the filter chamber. Repeat until the filter is completely covered with blood.

(5) Clear the tubing of air, and clamp and cap it with the sterile cap provided. (In some facilities the procedure includes the use of normal saline [NS]. The blood may be piggybacked into the NS or the NS piggybacked into the blood. The latter method is preferable, *because the red cells receive less trauma being infused directly into the patient than they do being forced through two needles, as they are when piggybacked.* It is always preferable to disconnect the existing IV tubing at the needle hub and connect the blood, but if it *is* piggybacked into the existing IV line, flush the tubing with normal saline first. The normal saline line should be *clamped* during the administration of the blood or blood product.)

Implementation

9. Identify the patient *to be sure you are performing the procedure for the correct patient.* Check the patient's identification band against the blood bank invoice.

10. Explain the procedure to the patient. Your explanation should include the product to be administered, the rationale for the therapy, and approximately how long it will take. Tell the patient that transfusion reactions are uncommon but that you should be called if he or she experiences any of the following: itching, headache, tightness in the chest, shortness of breath, chills, or sudden anxiety (see Table 57–2).

11. Measure and record the patient's blood pressure, temperature, pulse, and respirations for baseline data.

12. Wearing clean gloves, hang the blood bag (and normal saline if used) on the IV stand.

13. Remove the tape securing the intravenous tubing.

14. Clamp the tubing on the intravenous infusion that is running.

15. Remove the tubing from the needle and cap it with the sterile needle and cover.

16. Remove the sterile cap from the blood tubing and connect it to the needle hub.

17. Open the clamp on the tubing and check for patency.

18. Calculate the flow rate to run over 2–6 hours as indicated by the physician or patient condition.

19. Tape the blood tubing in place.

20. Adjust the flow rate to run at a TKO rate (or about half the rate you calculated) for the first 15 minutes.

21. Monitor vital signs 5 and 15 minutes after the blood product is started and compare them with baseline measurements. *Because most reactions start within the first 15 minutes,* it is desirable to stay with the patient during this time.

22. Regulate the rate to run as calculated.

23. Check periodically (at least every 20–30 minutes) *for the rate of infusion and symptoms of reaction.*

24. If a transfusion reaction occurs:

    a. Stop the blood. Keep the IV open with normal saline or the previous intravenous infusion.

    b. Recheck the vital signs.

    c. Notify the physician for further orders.

25. On completion of the transfusion:

    a. If the IV is to be resumed:

      (1) Remove the tape from the blood tubing.

      (2) Clamp the blood tubing and remove it from the needle.

      (3) Immediately connect the normal saline to flush the tubing and needle or catheter.

      (4) Clamp the normal saline tubing and remove it from the needle.

      (5) Connect the previous intravenous infusion.

      (6) Release the clamp on the IV tubing, adjust the flow rate, and secure the tubing with tape.

    b. If the IV is to be discontinued (see Module 53, Preparing and Maintaining Intravenous Infusions, for detailed directions):

      (1) Clamp the blood tubing and remove the needle or other intravenous device.

(2) Check to make sure that no part has broken off and remains in patient.

(3) Apply pressure and raise the patient's arm.

(4) Apply an adhesive bandage or pressure dressing.

c. If a heparin lock is to be applied (see Module 56, Starting Intravenous Infusions, for detailed directions):

(1) Clamp the blood tubing and remove it from the needle.

(2) Immediately connect the heparin solution-filled lock adapter.

(3) Flush the lock with the remaining heparin solution or saline, following the policy of your facility.

(4) Secure the heparin lock with tape.

26. Monitor vital signs and compare them with baseline measurements.

27. Discard the blood administration set in the special container in the soiled utility room.

28. Place the blood bag in a plastic bag and return it to facility blood bank if so indicated by policy, *so the blood samples connected to the bag are available in case of a delayed blood reaction.*

29. Remove gloves and wash your hands *for infection control.*

Evaluation

30. Evaluate, using the following criteria:
   a. Correct blood product at correct rate.
   b. TPR within normal limits and patient free of other signs of reaction.
   c. Patient comfortable.

Documentation

31. Record the following:
   a. Type and amount of blood product.
   b. Blood unit identification number.
   c. Time started and completed.
   d. Vital signs before, at 5 and 15 minutes after initiation of transfusion, and on completion of transfusion.
   e. Flow rate.
   f. Pertinent patient responses and clinical observations.

Some facilities have a special form on which to record information about blood administration (Figure 57–3). In other facilities the parenteral fluid sheet is used, along with flow sheets and nurses' notes, to record vital signs and other pertinent observations (Figures 57–4).

Unless contraindicated, 50–100 ml normal saline

may be added to packed red cells *to facilitate infusion,* if facility policy allows. A Y infusion set may be used for this purpose.

Platelets

Assessment

1. Check the physician's orders.
2. Check the existing intravenous infusion or heparin lock for patency and needle size or initiate an intravenous infusion with a 21-gauge needle (23-gauge needle for children).

Planning

3. Wash your hands *for infection control.*
4. Gather the equipment. If it is necessary to start an intravenous infusion, you will need the equipment discussed in Module 56, Starting Intravenous Infusions, step 3, in addition to the following:
   a. Blood administration set
   b. Bottle or bag of normal saline with a secondary administration set, as facility policy indicates. Normal saline is the only appropriate IV fluid to use with platelets.
   c. Tape
5. Obtain the platelets from the facility blood bank.
6. With another nurse, check the following:
   a. Patient's name and spelling, hospital number, and physician's name as on the face sheet with the blood bank invoice.
   b. Blood type of platelets with the blood type of the patient. If a discrepancy exists, look under remarks to see if the physician who ordered the platelets has accepted ABO-incompatible platelets. If the physician has accepted this risk, it is permissible to give unmatched platelets.
   c. Blood type and blood unit identification numbers listed on the platelet pack with the blood type and blood unit identification numbers on the blood bank invoice.
7. You and the other nurse sign your names, titles, date, and time on blood bank invoice(s) if all the above information checks out.

Implementation

8. Put on clean gloves and follow steps 9–17 of the procedure for administering whole blood and packed red cells (identify the patient, explain the procedure, measure and record vital signs, hang the platelet bag and normal

(text continues on p. 538)

DATE: *7-27-94* TIME: *0800*

Number: **MH 70530**	Previous Transfusion Yes No	Time Completed *1100*
	Previous Reaction Yes No	
Group: *O* RH: *+*	Starting TPR: *97^{8} 64 18* BP: *110/70*	Amount Received: *500 cc.*
Donor: *Timothy Benson*	TPR: 5" *98-66-18* BP: *114/76*	D/C'd by whom: *P. Jones, RN*
Whole Blood: *✓* Packed Cells: ____		
Platelets: ____ Plasma: ____	15" *98^{4}-66-18* BP: *114/78*	
Fibrinogen: ____ Gamulin D: ____	TPR	
Checked by: *P. Jones* RN	Completion *98^{8}-66-18* BP: *116/78*	Patient tolerated: *3 problems*

J. Russell RN	CLINICAL SYMPTOMS OF REACTION	If reaction, was Reaction Procedure followed? Yes No
Started by: *P. Jones, R.N.*	Low back pain Yes No	
	Chest discomfort Yes No	
Solution used: *Normal Saline*	Chilling Yes No	1. Urine specimen Yes No
	Drop in BP Yes No	
Amount: *250 cc*	Flushing of face Yes No	2. Blood samples drawn Yes No
	Distended neck veins Yes No	
Needle size: *19*	Headache Yes No	3. Blood samples to Blood Bank Yes No
	Dizziness Yes No	
Type: *Butterfly*	Respiratory discomfort Yes No	
Filter: New Yes No Changed Yes No	Nausea-vomiting Yes No	4. Transfusion: continued discontinued
	Urticarial Eruptions Yes No	
Location: *(L) forearm*	Urine output adequate Yes No	
Rate of flow: *25 gtts/min.*	Pt. observed by: *P. Jones, R.N.*	5. Antihistamine antipyretic therapy Yes No
	M.D. notified:	

DATE: ____ TIME: ____

Number: ____	Previous Transfusion Yes No	Time Completed ____
	Previous Reaction Yes No	
Group: ____ RH: ____	Starting TPR: ____ BP: ____	Amount Received: ____
Donor: ____	TPR: 5" ____ BP: ____	D/C's by whom: ____
Whole Blood: ____ Packed Cells: ____		
Platelets: ____ Plasma: ____	15" ____ BP: ____	
Fibrinogen: ____ Gamulin D: ____	TPR	
Checked by: ____ RN	Completion ____ BP: ____	Patient tolerated:

____ RN	CLINICAL SYMPTOMS OF REACTION	If reaction, was Reaction Procedure followed? Yes No
Started by: ____	Low back pain Yes No	
	Chest discomfort Yes No	
Solution used: ____	Chilling Yes No	1. Urine specimen Yes No
	Drop in BP Yes No	
Amount: ____	Flushing of face Yes No	2. Blood samples drawn Yes No
	Distended neck veins Yes No	
Needle size: ____	Headache Yes No	3. Blood samples to Blood Bank Yes No
	Dizziness Yes No	
Type: ____	Respiratory discomfort Yes No	
Filter: New Yes No Changed Yes No	Nausea-vomiting Yes No	4. Transfusion: continued discontinued
	Urticarial Eruptions Yes No	
Location: ____	Urine output adequate Yes No	
Rate of flow: ____	Pt. observed by: ____	5. Antihistamine antipyretic therapy Yes No
	M.D. notified:	

BALLARD COMMUNITY HOSPITAL
SEATTLE, WASHINGTON

BLOOD RECORD

Figure 57–3 The blood record documented by the nurse.

Date and Time	AMOUNT SOLUTION ADDITIVES (number consecutively)	Rate and Regulator	Added By	Needle Type Started	Size Site By:	Tubing Chng. By:	Site Care and Observations	Solu' Time	DC'd Amount Absorb.	SHIFT TOTALS Time	SHIFT TOTALS Total
Date: 7/27/94 Time: 0200	WB #MH70529	25 gtts/min	(PJ)	Vital signs: Initiation:		97^8	-64-18 110/70	1100	500 cc	6-2	500
				10 Minutes:		98^4	-66-18 114/78				
Date: Time:				Completion:		98^8	-68-16 116/78				
				Reaction: Yes ☐ No ☒							
Date: Time:											
Date: Time:											
Date: Time:											
Date: Time:											
Date: Time:											
Date: Time:											

Identify Initials with Signature:	4.	8.
1. PJ P. Jones RN	5.	9.
2.	6.	10.
3.	7.	11.

ADDRESSOGRAPH:

Bertha Johnson F-54
537-34-1409
Dr. James Gusher

CODE: "*" = see Nurses Narrative

THE SWEDISH HOSPITAL MEDICAL CENTER
SEATTLE, WASHINGTON

N-1547 Nursing Rev. 6/80 FC/TSHMC

Figure 57–4 Recording blood administration on a parenteral therapy record.

saline, remove the tape securing the intravenous tubing, clamp the tubing on the IV that is running, remove the tubing from the needle and cap it with the sterile needle and cover, remove the sterile cap from the blood tubing and connect it to the needle hub, open the clamp on the tubing, and check for patency).

9. Adjust the flow rate to administer the platelets as rapidly as possible, *because they must be administered within 4 hours of pooling at the blood bank* (20–30 minutes for 6 units). Pressure cuffs or pumps should not be used with platelets *because the cells are easily damaged.*

10. Follow steps 19–27 of the procedure for administering whole blood and packed red cells (tape the tubing in place; monitor vital signs 5 and 15 minutes after the blood product is started; check periodically for the rate of infusion and symptoms of reaction; if a transfusion reaction occurs, stop the platelets, keep the IV open with normal saline, recheck the vital signs, notify the physician for further orders; on completion of the transfusion, resume the IV, discontinue the IV, or apply a heparin lock, as ordered; monitor vital signs; discard the blood administration set; place the blood bag in a plastic bag and return it to the facility blood bank; remove gloves and wash your hands).

Evaluation

11. Evaluate, using the following criteria:
    a. Correct blood product at correct rate.
    b. TPR within normal limits and patient free of other signs of reaction.
    c. Patient comfortable.

Documentation

12. Record the following:
    a. Type and amount of blood product.
    b. Blood unit identification number.
    c. Time started and completed.
    d. Vital signs before, at 5 and 15 minutes after initiation of infusion, and on completion of transfusion.
    e. Flow rate.
    f. Pertinent patient responses and clinical observations.

Albumin

Assessment

1. Check the physician's orders.

2. Check the existing IV for patency or initiate IV therapy.

Planning

3. Wash your hands *for infection control* and put on clean gloves.
4. Gather the equipment. If it is necessary to start an intravenous infusion, you will need the equipment discussed in Module 56, Starting Intravenous Infusions, step 3, in addition to the following:
    a. Albumin solution (albumin NSA)
    b. Secondary tubing
    c. Alcohol swab
    d. Tape
5. Prepare the equipment.
    a. Insert the administration set into the albumin container according to the package directions.
    b. Fill the drip chamber half full.
    c. Clear the tubing of air, and clamp.

Implementation

6. Identify the patient *to be sure you are performing the procedure for the correct patient.*
7. Explain the procedure to the patient.
8. Measure and record the patient's blood pressure.
9. Adjust the flow rate of the primary set to slow the drip, and lower the primary bag or bottle to a point below where the albumin is hanging.
10. Prepare the injection port closest to the patient, using an alcohol swab.
11. Attach the albumin tubing to the injection port, using a 19-gauge or larger needle.
12. Leave the clamp open on the primary tubing. It will not flow until the albumin infusion is complete.
13. Open the clamp on the albumin tubing.
14. Adjust the rate of the albumin as ordered by the physician. The rate should not exceed 2 ml/min *because it can increase intravascular volume rapidly, resulting in congestive heart failure or pulmonary edema.*
15. On completion of the albumin:
    a. Close the clamp on the albumin tubing.
    b. Raise the primary bag or bottle to its original position. Readjust the flow rate.
    c. Check the patient's blood pressure.
    d. Remove the albumin bottle and tubing and discard gloves.

Evaluation

16. Evaluate, using the following criteria:
    a. Albumin infused at appropriate rate.

b. Blood pressure checked before and after albumin infusion.

c. Patient comfortable.

Documentation

17. Record the following:
    a. Amount of albumin administered.
    b. Time started and finished.
    c. Patient's blood pressure before and after albumin administration.
    d. Other pertinent reactions of the patient to the procedure.

Cryoprecipitate

Assessment

1. Check the physician's orders.
2. Check the existing intravenous infusion or heparin lock for patency and needle size or initiate an intravenous infusion with a 21-gauge needle (23-gauge needle for young children and infants).

Planning

3. Wash your hands *for infection control* and put on clean gloves.
4. Gather the equipment. If it is necessary to start an intravenous infusion, you will need the equipment discussed in Module 56, Starting Intravenous Infusions, step 3. In addition you will need:
    a. Blood administration set
    b. Bottle or bag of normal saline with a secondary administration set, as facility policy indicates. Normal saline is the only IV fluid that can be mixed with cryoprecipitate.
    c. Tape
5. Obtain the cryoprecipitate from the facility's blood bank as soon as it arrives *because it must be administered within 4 hours of the time it is thawed and pooled.*
6. With another nurse, compare the patient's name and spelling, hospital number, and physician's name on the face sheet in the chart with that on the blood bank invoice. Verify the dose size by comparing the number of units ordered with the number of units listed on the cryoprecipitate bag and on the invoice.
7. You and the other nurse sign your names, titles, date, and time on blood bank invoice if all the above information checks out.
8. Prepare the equipment as follows:
    a. Turn the control on the blood tubing to the off position.

b. Open the entry port on the cryoprecipitate bag.

c. Insert the administration set into the cryoprecipitate bag.

d. Squeeze the drip chamber and release it, to allow cryoprecipitate to flow into the filter chamber. Repeat until the filter is completely covered.

e. Clear the tubing of air, and clamp.

Implementation

9. Identify the patient *to be sure you are performing the procedure for the correct patient,* checking identification band against the blood bank invoice.
10. Explain the procedure to the patient.
11. Hang the cryoprecipitate bag on the IV stand.
12. Remove the tape securing the intravenous tubing.
13. Clamp the tubing on the intravenous infusion that is running.
14. Remove the tubing from the needle and cap it with the sterile needle and cover.
15. Connect the cryoprecipitate tubing to the needle hub.
16. Open the clamp on the tubing and check for patency.
17. Adjust the flow rate. Cryoprecipitate should be administered rapidly (i.e., 10–12 units [200–250 ml] can be administered in 20–30 minutes), *because it loses its effectiveness if not administered within 4 hours of the time it is thawed and pooled.*
18. On completion of the cryoprecipitate, connect the normal saline or discontinue the intravenous infusion, as ordered.
19. Discard the blood administration set and cryoprecipitate bag.
20. Remove gloves and wash your hands.

Evaluation

21. Evaluate, using the following criteria:
    a. Cryoprecipitate infused at appropriate rate.
    b. Patient comfortable.

Documentation

22. Record the following:
    a. Amount of cryoprecipitate.
    b. Blood bank check numbers, as facility policy indicates.
    c. Time started and completed.
    d. Pertinent patient responses and clinical observations.

Home Care

Persons who have hemophilia, including children, have frequently received infusions of cryoprecipitate at home. This procedure has been done by a family care provider or sometimes by the adult patient. *Reactions rarely occur with the use of this product so that self-administration is considered safe.*

However, the administration of blood in the home setting can have much more serious consequences. The administration of blood products in the home care setting is presently being done experimentally under the guidelines of several central blood centers in the United States. Studies are underway *to determine whether more reactions occur at the time of transfusion in the home and whether a quick and appropriate response can be made should a serious reaction occur.* Blood centers strongly recommend that only specially trained and competent licensed persons administer the blood. In fact, some blood centers will not release the product unless they are assured that the person who will be administering the blood is competent in doing so. Home care administration of blood products has merits *in that it would avoid having those very ill and weak persons being cared for in the home transported to and from an acute care setting for this procedure.* As more home health nurses are available for giving care, this procedure may become more common in the home setting.

LONG-TERM CARE

Residents in the long-term care facility occasionally receive blood products. The product used is often packed red blood cells to treat serious chronic states of anemia. Older residents with chronic leukemia may receive either red blood cells or platelets. An order is needed from the physician and it is necessary for the blood product to be identified and picked up by an employee of the facility. The nurse administering the blood product must be licensed and understand the policies and procedures *for safe administration.*

It should be recognized that elderly patients have an increased risk for reactions related to transfusion. *They have body systems that are less active and more fragile than those who are younger.* Older people who require blood transfusion may also have a heightened sense of anxiety about the procedure *because they hold a lifelong view that receiving blood is a fearful and lifesaving action rather than the common treatment modality it is considered today.* Clear, calm, and supportive explanations should be given to allay any fear the resident may have.

References

American Association of Blood Banks. (1989). *Blood Transfusions, 89*(4), 486–489.

Birdsall, C., Carpenter, K., & Considine, R. (1988). How is autologous done? *American Journal of Nursing, 88*(1), 108–111.

Butler, S. (1989). Current trends in autologous transfusion. *RN, 52*(11), 44–55.

Monks, M. L. (1988). Home transfusion therapy. *Journal of Intravenous Nursing, 11*(6), 389–396.

Performance Checklist

Administering Whole Blood and Packed Red Cells	Unsat	Needs More Practice	Sat	Comments
Assessment				
1. Check physician's orders.				
2. Check existing IV or initiate IV therapy.				
Planning				
3. Wash your hands.				
4. Gather equipment. a. Blood administration set				
b. Normal saline				
c. Tape				
5. Obtain blood product from facility blood bank.				
6. With another nurse, check: a. Patient's name and spelling, hospital number, and physician's name on face sheet with blood bank invoice.				
b. Blood product type, Rh, and blood unit administration number on blood bag with blood bank invoice.				
c. Expiration date on blood bag.				
7. Sign blood bank invoice.				
8. Prepare equipment. a. If used, obtain pump.				
b. Y blood administration set				
(1) Close all clamps on Y set.				
(2) Insert one administration set spike into normal saline bag.				
(3) Open clamp closest to normal saline bag and fill drip chamber half full.				
(4) Open lower control clamp and flush air from tubing; reclamp.				
(5) Insert other spike of administration set into blood bag.				
(6) Open clamp closest to blood and squeeze filter chamber and release until filter is completely covered with blood; reclamp.				

Administering Whole Blood and Packed Red Cells *(Continued)*	Unsat	Needs More Practice	Sat	Comments
(7) Open lower control clamp and flush the tubing with blood.				
c. Primary blood administration set				
(1) Turn control on blood tubing to off.				
(2) Open entry port on blood bag.				
(3) Insert administration set into blood bag.				
(4) Squeeze and release drip chamber to allow blood to flow into drip chamber. Repeat until filter is completely covered.				
(5) Clear tubing of air, and clamp.				
Implementation				
9. Identify patient.				
10. Explain procedure to patient and list signs of a reaction.				
11. Measure and record vital signs.				
12. Hang blood bag on IV stand while wearing clean gloves.				
13. Remove tape securing IV tubing.				
14. Clamp tubing on IV running.				
15. Remove IV tubing from needle, cap with sterile needle and cover.				
16. Remove sterile cap from blood tubing and connect to needle hub.				
17. Open clamp on tubing.				
18. Calculate flow rate to run over 2–6 hours.				
19. Tape blood tubing in place.				
20. Adjust flow rate to run at TKO rate for first 15 minutes.				
21. Recheck vital signs 5 and 15 minutes later.				
22. Regulate the rate to run as calculated.				
23. Check periodically for rate of infusion and symptoms of reaction.				
24. If transfusion reaction occurs: a. Stop blood, maintaining venous access.				

Administering Whole Blood and Packed Red Cells *(Continued)*	Unsat	Needs More Practice	Sat	Comments
b. Recheck vital signs.				
c. Notify physician.				
25. On completion of transfusion: a. If IV is to be resumed:				
(1) Remove tape from blood tubing.				
(2) Clamp blood tubing and remove from needle.				
(3) Connect normal saline to flush tubing and needle or catheter.				
(4) Clamp normal saline tubing and remove from needle.				
(5) Connect previous intravenous infusion.				
(6) Release clamp on IV tubing, adjust flow rate, and secure tubing with tape.				
b. If IV is to be discontinued:				
(1) Clamp blood tubing and remove needle.				
(2) Check to make sure infusion device is intact.				
(3) Apply pressure and raise patient's arm.				
(4) Apply adhesive bandage.				
c. If heparin lock is to be applied:				
(1) Clamp blood tubing and remove from needle.				
(2) Immediately connect heparin solution-filled lock adapter.				
(3) Flush with remaining heparin solution or saline.				
(4) Secure with tape.				
26. Monitor vital signs and compare with baseline measurements.				
27. Discard blood administration set.				
28. Place blood bag in plastic bag and return to facility blood bank.				
29. Remove gloves and wash your hands.				

Administering Whole Blood and Packed Red Cells *(Continued)*	Unsat	Needs More Practice	Sat	Comments
Evaluation				
30. Evaluate, using the following criteria: a. Correct blood product at correct rate.				
b. TPR within normal limits and patient free of other signs of reaction.				
c. Patient comfortable.				
Documentation				
31. Record the following: a. Type and amount of blood product.				
b. Blood unit identification number.				
c. Time started and completed.				
d. Vital signs before, at 5 and 15 minutes after initiation of infusion, and on completion of transfusion.				
e. Flow rate.				
f. Pertinent patient responses and clinical observations.				
Administering Platelets				
Assessment				
1. Follow Checklist steps 1 and 2 for Administering Whole Blood and Packed Red Cells (check physician's orders, check existing IV for patency and needle size, or initiate an IV).				
Planning				
2. Follow Checklist steps 3–5 for Administering Whole Blood and Packed Red Cells (wash your hands, gather necessary equipment, obtain blood product from facility's blood bank).				
3. With another nurse check: a. Patient's name and spelling, hospital number, and physician's name on face sheet with blood bank invoice.				
b. Blood type of platelets with blood type of patient.				

Administering Platelets *(Continued)*	Unsat	Needs More Practice	Sat	Comments
c. Blood type and unit numbers listed on platelet pack with blood type and unit numbers on the invoice.				
4. Sign blood bank invoice.				
Implementation				
5. Put on clean gloves and follow Checklist steps 9–17 for Administering Whole Blood and Packed Red Cells (identify patient, explain procedure, measure and record vital signs, hang blood product bag and normal saline, remove tape securing IV tubing, clamp tubing on IV that is running, remove tubing from the needle and cap with sterile needle and cover, remove sterile cap from blood tubing and connect it to needle hub, open clamp on tubing, and check for patency).				
6. Adjust flow rate.				
7. Follow Checklist steps 19–27 for Administering Whole Blood and Packed Red Cells (tape blood tubing in place; monitor vital signs 5 and 15 minutes after blood product is started; check periodically for rate of infusion and symptoms of reaction; if transfusion reaction occurs, stop blood product, keep IV open with normal saline, recheck vital signs, notify physician for further orders; on completion of transfusion, resume IV, discontinue IV or apply heparin lock, as ordered; monitor vital signs; discard blood administration set; place blood product bag in plastic bag and return to facility blood bank; remove gloves and wash your hands).				
Evaluation				
8. Evaluate, using the following criteria: a. Correct blood product at correct rate.				
b. TPR within normal limits and patient free of other signs of reaction.				
c. Patient comfortable.				
Documentation				
9. Record the following: a. Type and amount of blood product.				

Administering Platelets *(Continued)*	Unsat	Needs More Practice	Sat	Comments
b. Blood unit identification number.				
c. Time started and completed.				
d. Vital signs before, at 5 and 15 minutes after initiation of infusion, and on completion of transfusion.				
e. Flow rate.				
f. Pertinent patient responses and clinical observations.				

Administering Albumin

Assessment

1. Follow Checklist steps 1 and 2 for Administering Whole Blood and Packed Red Cells (check physician's orders, check existing IV for patency and needle size, or initiate an IV).				

Planning

2. Wash your hands and put on clean gloves.				
3. Gather equipment. a. Albumin solution				
b. Secondary tubing				
c. Alcohol swab				
d. Tape				
4. Prepare equipment: a. Insert administration set into albumin container.				
b. Fill drip chamber half full.				
c. Clear tubing of air, and clamp.				

Implementation

5. Follow Checklist steps 9 and 10 for Administering Whole Blood and Packed Red Cells (identify patient, explain procedure).				
6. Measure and record blood pressure.				
7. Slow flow rate of primary bag and lower.				
8. Prepare injection port.				
9. Attach albumin tubing to injection port.				

Administering Albumin (Continued)	Unsat	Needs More Practice	Sat	Comments
10. Close clamp on primary tubing if reflux valve is not present.				
11. Open clamp on albumin tubing.				
12. Adjust rate of albumin.				
13. On completion of albumin: a. Close clamp on albumin tubing.				
b. Raise primary container and adjust flow rate.				
c. Check patient's blood pressure.				
d. Remove albumin bottle and tubing.				
14. Discard gloves and wash your hands.				
Evaluation				
15. Evaluate, using the following criteria: a. Albumin infused at appropriate rate.				
b. Blood pressure within normal limits.				
c. Patient comfortable.				
Documentation				
16. Record the following: a. Amount of albumin administered.				
b. Time started and finished.				
c. Patient's blood pressure before and after albumin administration.				
d. Other pertinent reactions of the patient to the procedure.				
Administering Cryoprecipitate				
Assessment				
1. Follow Checklist steps 1 and 2 for Administering Whole Blood and Packed Red Cells (check physician's orders, check existing IV for patency and needle size, or initiate an IV).				
Planning				
2. Wash your hands and put on clean gloves.				
3. Gather equipment. a. Blood administration set				

Administering Cyoprecipitate *(Continued)*	Unsat	Needs More Practice	Sat	Comments
b. Normal saline with secondary set				
c. Tape				
4. Obtain cryoprecipitate from facility blood bank.				
5. With another nurse, compare patient's name and spelling, hospital number, and physician's name on face sheet of chart with that on blood bank invoice.				
6. Sign blood bank invoice.				
7. Prepare equipment: a. Turn control on blood tubing to off.				
b. Open entry port on cryoprecipitate bag.				
c. Insert administration set into cryoprecipitate bag.				
d. Squeeze and release drip chamber to allow cryoprecipitate to flow into drip chamber. Repeat until filter is completely covered.				
e. Clear tubing of air and clamp.				
Implementation				
8. Follow Checklist steps 9 and 10 for Administering Whole Blood and Packed Red Cells (identify patient, explain procedure).				
9. Hang cryoprecipitate bag on IV stand.				
10. Remove tape securing IV tubing.				
11. Clamp tubing on IV running.				
12. Remove tubing from needle, cap with sterile needle and cover.				
13. Connect cryoprecipitate tubing to needle hub.				
14. Open clamp on tubing.				
15. Adjust flow rate.				
16. On completion of the cryoprecipitate, connect normal saline or discontinue IV, as ordered.				
17. Discard blood administration set and cryoprecipitate bag.				
18. Remove gloves and wash your hands.				

Administering Cryoprecipitate (Continued)	Unsat	Needs More Practice	Sat	Comments
Evaluation				
19. Evaluate, using the following criteria: a. Cryoprecipitate infused at appropriate rate.				
b. Patient comfortable.				
Documentation				
20. Record the following: a. Amount of cryoprecipitate.				
b. Blood bank check numbers as facility policy indicates.				
c. Time started and completed.				
d. Pertinent patient responses and clinical observations.				

Quiz

Short-Answer Questions

1. What are the five methods used in blood transfusion?

   a. _____

   b. _____

   c. _____

   d. _____

   e. _____

2. Why are more autologous transfusions now being administered?

   _____

   _____

   _____

   _____

   _____

3. What tests are done on autologous blood as compared with the tests done on nonautologous blood?

   _____

   _____

4. List three reasons for administering blood and blood products.

   a. _____

   b. _____

   c. _____

5. List two advantages of component therapy.

   a. _____

   b. _____

6. List the two indications for the administration of whole blood.

   a. _____

   b. _____

7. Name the four main blood groups in the ABO system of typing.

   a. _____

   b. _____

   c. _____

   d. _____

8. List four potential complications of transfusion.

   a. _____

   b. _____

   c. _____

   d. _____

9. List four signs and symptoms of a hemolytic reaction.

   a. _____

   b. _____

   c. _____

   d. _____

10. List three actions you would take in the event of a mild allergic reaction.

    a. _____

    b. _____

    c. _____

11. How can air embolus be prevented? _____

    _____

12. Why is dextrose in water *not* used with blood and blood products?

    _____

13. What five items should be checked before a unit of blood is administered?

    a. _____

    b. _____

    c. _____

    d. _____

    e. _____

Module 58
Parenteral Nutrition

Module Contents

Rationale for the Use of This Skill
Total Parenteral Nutrition
Partial Parenteral Nutrition
Complications of Parenteral Nutrition
Solutions Used for Parenteral Nutrition
General Procedure for Administering
     Parenteral Nutrition
    Assessment
    Planning
    Implementation
    Evaluation
    Documentation

Procedure for Administering Fat Emulsions
    (Lipids)
Procedure for Administering Partial
    Parenteral Nutrition
Discontinuing Parenteral Nutrition
Long-Term Care
Home Care

Prerequisites

Successful completion of the following modules:

VOLUME 1

Module 1 An Approach to Nursing Skills
Module 2 Basic Infection Control
Module 3 Safety
Module 5 General Assessment Overview
Module 6 Documentation
Module 13 Inspection, Palpation, Auscultation, and Percussion
Module 15 Intake and Output
Module 16 Temperature, Pulse, and Respiration
Module 17 Blood Pressure

VOLUME 2

Module 35 Sterile Technique
Module 53 Preparing and Maintaining Intravenous Infusions
Module 54 Administering Intravenous Medications
Module 55 Caring for Central Intravenous Catheters

Overall Objective

To safely administer parenteral nutrition through an existing intravenous line or a central venous catheter.

Specific Learning Objectives

	Facts and Principles	Apply Facts and Principles	Demonstrate Ability	Evaluate Performance
1. *Types of parenteral nutrition*	Know the two types of parenteral nutrition.	Given a situation, state rationale for the type of parenteral nutrition in use.	In the clinical setting, identify patients receiving the two types of parenteral nutrition.	Verify your knowledge with instructor.
2. *Equipment*	List the various items of equipment used to administer parenteral nutrition.	Given a physician's order list the equipment needed to give parenteral nutrition.	In the clinical setting, gather the equipment needed for the ordered parenteral nutrition.	Validate your choice of equipment with your instructor.
3. *Administering parenteral nutrition*	List steps in administering parenteral nutrition.	Given a specific situation, identify the steps necessary in the administration procedure.	In the clinical setting, correctly administer parenteral nutrition.	Evaluate performance with your instructor.
4. *Administering lipids (fat emulsions)*	List steps in administering lipids.	Given a specific situation, identify the steps necessary in the administration of lipids.	In the clinical setting, correctly administer lipids.	Evaluate performance with your instructor.
5. *Potential complications*	Name the complications that can occur with parenteral nutrition.	Given a patient situation, state appropriate assessment and preventive actions.	In the clinical setting, make appropriate assessments and take any action needed to prevent complications.	Evaluate own performance with instructor.

Learning Activities

1. Review the Specific Learning Objectives.
2. Read the section on nutrition and intravenous infusions in Ellis and Nowlis, *Nursing: A Human Needs Approach,* or comparable material in another textbook.
3. Look up the module vocabulary terms in the Glossary.
4. Read through the module and mentally practice the procedures.
5. In the practice setting:
   a. Examine the parenteral nutrition equipment. Identify the following:
      (1) A simulated order for parenteral nutrition
      (2) A practice parenteral nutrition bag
      (3) An infusion pump
      (4) Pump tubing with a filter
      (5) Pull-tapes used for connections
   b. After checking the order against the printed contents of the bag, practice setting up the parenteral nutrition bag using the tubing. Insert the tubing correctly into the pump.
   c. Using a waste basket to catch the flow, set the flow rate and operate the pump.
6. In the practice setting:
   a. Examine the fat emulsion equipment. Identify the following:
      (1) A simulated order for fat emulsion
      (2) A practice fat emulsion bottle
      (3) A microdrip, vented, unfiltered tubing
      (4) A 20- or 21-gauge sterile needle.
   b. After checking the order against the bottle label, practice setting up the lipids using the tubing.
   c. Insert the needle into the primary parenteral nutrition tubing.
   d. Using the roller clamp, regulate the flow rate, practicing a rate of 8 drops over 15 seconds and 3–4 drops over 15 seconds.
7. Practice documenting the parenteral nutrition on an intravenous record form.
8. In the clinical setting, when your instructor approves your practice performance, administer both total and partial parenteral nutrition. Also, seek out the opportunity to administer fat emulsions (lipids).

Vocabulary

amino acids	hyperalimentation	lumen
cycling	hyperglycemia	parenteral
dextrose	hypertonic	positive nitrogen
fat emulsions	infusion pump	balance
finger stick	lipids	test dose

Parenteral Nutrition

Rationale for the Use of This Skill

More and more individuals are receiving parenteral nutrition in the hospital, in the long-term care setting, and in the home. This has occurred because of the improvements in central venous lines, the availability of intravenous nutritional solutions, and the increasing number of people with long-term illnesses that interfere with normal nutrition. The complexity of the procedure and the potential for complications demand a high level of nursing skill.[1]

TOTAL PARENTERAL NUTRITION

For most patients, parenteral nutrition is total in that all nutrients needed by the body are supplied by accessing a central line and infusing a specially formulated solution into the central circulation. For position of a central line and other details, see Module 55, Caring for Central Intravenous Catheters. The nutrients supplied by total parenteral nutrition include dextrose, protein, electrolytes, amino acids, and vitamins. These substances are mixed with sterile water into a hypertonic solution. The maximum dextrose concentration for total parenteral nutrition solutions is 35%. Several terms are used for this therapy—hyperalimentation (sometimes referred to as "hyperal") and the initials TPN which stand for "total parenteral nutrition." Some patients also receive fats or lipids in a separate solution which is infused by "piggybacking" it into the hyperalimentation line. For guidelines on this procedure, see Module 54, Administering Intravenous Medications. Patients receiving total parenteral nutrition are usually *those who cannot eat over a long period of time due to major trauma, pathology of the intestinal tract, or long-term illness such as cancer, AIDS, or renal failure.* Other patients appropriate for total parenteral nutrition are those who cannot eat normally, preventing them from taking in a sufficient amount of nutrients. These persons may have been maintained on peripheral intravenous fluids for a number of days.

Most hospitals have a medical policy that a patient should not be sustained on peripheral intravenous solutions alone for more than a few days. Depending on the policy, this may be 3–5 days. The policy requires that after the designated period of time, an alternate method must be provided *for nutritional re-*

[1] You will note that rationale for action is emphasized throughout the module by the use of italics.

quirements. Although peripheral intravenous solutions provide water, calories, and some electrolytes, *prolonged use leads to protein depletion and malnutrition* (Cerrato, 1986). Because of this, these persons are candidates for placement of a central line and the initiation of parenteral nutrition.

PARTIAL PARENTERAL NUTRITION

Some persons who are unable to eat properly for an extended period of time and are nutritionally depleted may receive partial parenteral nutrition as a *temporary adjunct to their nutritional status.* These patients are able to eat some of their diet but not enough to be nutritionally healthy. In partial parenteral nutrition, the solution is infused through a peripheral intravenous line. This route is not recommended for any length of time *due to the irritating properties of the solution on the veins.* The dextrose concentration should not exceed 10%.

COMPLICATIONS OF PARENTERAL NUTRITION

There are potential complications with either total or partial parenteral nutrition. One of these is inflammation and sepsis of the catheter insertion site. It is not true, as once thought, that the administration of these solutions with lipids, in particular, increases the risk for developing sepsis of the central catheter. (Young, Alexeyeff, Russell, & Thomas, 1988). However, the catheter site should be carefully assessed by the nurse each time parenteral nutrition is administered and any signs of inflammation or infection reported.

Another common complication is hyperglycemia. *The solutions contain large amounts of dextrose which, in some persons, may cause increased amounts of glucose in the blood.* If hyperglycemia is allowed to continue, the patient may become dehydrated and confused and experience a decreasing level of consciousness. These persons are assessed for the presence of hyperglycemia on a continuing basis. This is done by obtaining either fractional urine samples or blood collected and monitored for glucose (see Module 20, Performing Common Laboratory Tests). If hyperglycemia becomes a problem, the physician may order that a small amount of insulin be added to the solution or given subcutaneously.

During the early phases of parenteral nutrition, fluid and electrolyte imbalances can also occur. The

INITIATION OF TPN – ADULT

☐ 1. STANDARD CENTRAL VENOUS FULL-STRENGTH TPN SOLUTION
D50W 500ml (850 Calories) + Amino Acids 10% 500ml (50 Grams Protein)
Final Concentration = Dextrose 25% & Amino Acids 5%

NaCl	30 mEq	Reg. Insulin _0_ u.
KCl	25 mEq	Multivitamins (MVI) 1 pack (10ml) daily
KPhos	15 mEq	Multitrace Elements (MTE) 1ml daily
CaGluc	8 mEq	Vitamin C 500mg daily
MgSO4	8 mEq (except BMT = 16 mEq)	Vitamin K 10mg weekly (Sundays)

2. RATE: TO INFUSE AT _____ ml/hr TO PROVIDE A TOTAL OF _____ liter(s)/day.

☑ 3. NON-STANDARD CENTRAL OR PERIPHERAL FORMULA (Note: Non-standard TPN material and labor costs are higher than for the standardized solution above.)

SPECIFY: A) solution type, strength and amount   B) additives and amounts

D10W _____ ml   Amino Acid 8.5% _____ ml   NaCl _7_ mEq   Reg Insulin _∅_
D20W _____ ml   Amino Acid 10% _500_ ml   NaAcet _40_ mEq   Multivitamins (MVI) _1_
D40W _____ ml   Hepatamine 8% _____ ml   KCl _40_ mEq   Multitrace Elements (MTE) _1_
D50W _500_ ml   KPhos _20_ mEq   Vitamin C _500_
D70W _____ ml   CaGluc _8_ mEq   Vitamin K _____
        MgSO4 _16_ mEq   Other _____

C) FINAL Concentration Dextrose _25_ % & Amino Acids _5_ %

4. RATE: TO INFUSE AT _40_ ml/hr TO PROVIDE _1_ liter(s)/day.

☑ 5. INTRAVENOUS FAT EMULSION

_✓_ 10% (1.1 calories/ml) _50_ ml/hr over _10_ hours (minimum 4 - 6 hours)
_____ 20% (2.0 calories/ml) _____ ml/hr over _____ hours (minimum 8 - 10 hours)

6. Non-BMT and Non-ICU Patients: Begin fat infusion after TPN (Hyperal) Screen is drawn and before 0600.

7. Infuse initial dose slowly. 10%: begin at 60ml/hr × 30 min.; 20%: begin at 30ml/hr × 30 min.
(Note: some patients may react adversely to subsequent exposures.)

The following orders are standard for all non-bone marrow transplant patients. Delete only if crossed out by physician.

PRE-TPN ORDERS

8. Central venous catheter placement verification: (circle one)
ⓐ CXR asap for placement needed
b. Catheter tip location: _____ ; may begin TPN infusion.

9. Baseline Lab: ZINC, COPPER, TRIGLYCERIDES, TPN (Hyperal) SCREEN I (CBC w/diff, Protime, Ca, PO4, Mg, GOT, Bilirubin, Lytes, BUN, Glucose, Albumin, Prealbumin)

TPN INITIATION AND MAINTENANCE ORDERS

⑩ Initiate TPN Nursing Protocol.

⑪ Nutritional Assessment – notify Unit Dietitian.

12. TPN LAB:
Lab Draw Times: ICU Patients – draw TPN labs in AM; Non-ICU Patients – draw TPN labs in the evenings before 1900

✓ Daily × 1st 3 Days: lytes & glucose (already included in Monday & Thursday labs)

✓ Mondays: TRIGLYCERIDES, if IV fat administered.
TPN (Hyperal) SCREEN I (includes CBC w/diff, Protime, Ca, PO4, Mg, GOT, Bilirubin, Lytes, BUN, Glucose, Albumin, Prealbumin)

✓ Thursdays: TPN (Hyperal) SCREEN II (includes CBC, Lytes, Glucose, Ca, PO4, Mg)

✓ Chemstick: Q 8 hrs × 1st 48 hours. Thereafter, urine fxs Q 8 hrs on fresh specimen – Chemstick for trace or greater.
Chemstick Results: Chemstick > 240 notify MD if no sliding scale ordered
Chemstick > 400 notify MD & obtain stat glucose
Chemstick for S/S hypoglycemia: < 60 notify MD & obtain stat glucose

⑬ Daily Weight; Strict I&O

Date _7/15/95_ MD Signature _A. Bryant, M.D._

SWEDISH HOSPITAL MEDICAL CENTER
Seattle, Washington

PH-390 Rev. 4/90 FC/SHMC SN-5650

Figure 58–1 The order form that is filled out by the physician.

nurse is responsible for scheduling the periodic laboratory tests, which are ordered by the physician *to detect any potential fluid or electrolyte problems. Changes are then made in the solution in order to correct any imbalance.*

Because patients on total parenteral nutrition lack adequate amounts of vitamins K and B_{12}, bleeding tendencies and anemias can occur. This is prevented through the weekly addition of these vitamins to the parenteral solution.

SOLUTIONS USED FOR PARENTERAL NUTRITION

The solutions prepared for parenteral nutrition follow a standard for the facility with individualized adaptations for the specific needs of the patient. Figure

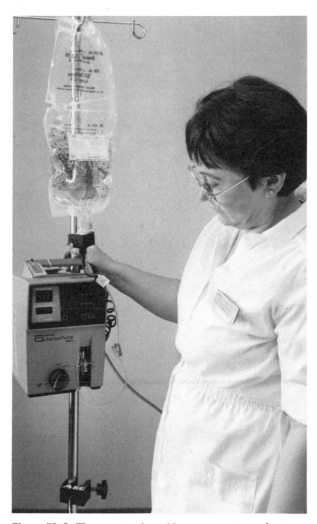

Figure 58–2 The parenteral nutrition components are kept separated until just before infusing.

58–1 shows a sample form listing the contents of routine parenteral nutrition solutions. The formula is ordered by the physician who may consult with the pharmacist, nutritionist, or nurse specialist. These nurses specialize in the care of patients receiving parenteral nutrition therapy and teach the procedure to the patient and the family when appropriate. The solutions are prepared under sterile conditions in the pharmacy of the facility. The dextrose is kept separate from the protein solution because of their instability. This is done by either mixing them just before administration or using a two-part plastic bag as seen in Figure 58–2. The lower portion contains the dextrose solution while the upper compartment contains the protein solution. The usual ratio used is 25% dextrose solution to 5% protein solution. Standard electrolytes are added to each bag or bottle. These are allowed to mix just prior to being transported to the nursing unit. Multivitamins are added daily. Trace elements and vitamins K and B_{12} are added weekly.

Lipid emulsions are usually referred to as "lipids" and are delivered to the nursing unit in a glass container and appear as a white milky solution. The concentration of fatty acids contained in these solutions is ordered by the physician at either 10% which provides 1.1 calorie/ml or 20% which provides 2.0 calories/ml. Only the lesser 10% emulsion is given by peripheral route.

GENERAL PROCEDURE FOR ADMINISTERING PARENTERAL NUTRITION

The following guidelines are those for initiating parenteral nutrition to the patient for the first time.

Assessment

1. It is important to have certain information concerning the patient who is to receive parenteral nutrition. The following are essential:
   a. The patient's diagnosis. The diagnosis *may indicate whether the patient will be on long-term or short-term therapy. It may also tell you of any particular complications for which the patient may be at risk.* For example, if the patient is a diabetic, close monitoring of the glucose component of the solution may be of added importance.
   b. The patient's age and condition. *If the patient is of advanced age and in precarious health, the impact of parenteral nutrition therapy on other systems of the body may be*

much greater than if the patient is younger and in relatively stable health.

   c. Height and usual weight. *This information gives you baseline data so that you can monitor the patient's fluid and nutritional status on an ongoing basis.*

   d. Intake and output. All patients on parenteral nutrition are placed on intake and output measurement *in order to assess daily nutritional and fluid status.*

   e. Allergies. A report of any previous allergies is important. Some patients have allergic reactions to tape or iodine-based solutions that are often used to prepare and maintain the central line insertion site. Other patients may have allergies to components of the solutions. *Reactions can often be avoided if known allergies are reported before starting the therapy.*

   f. The patient's usual vital signs. *By knowing this, you will be much more likely to detect fluctuations in vital function and detect complications before they become severe.* Patients receiving this therapy are placed on vital signs every 4 hours.

   g. Knowledge of procedure. *Some patients become very involved with their therapy and are helpful in the monitoring process. Other patients find it stressful to become involved and choose not to actively participate.*

   h. Mental status. *The ability to both understand the procedure and participate and help in its implementation may be affected* if the patient's level of awareness is decreased or if mental status is impaired.

2. Assess the patient's unit to determine which items of equipment are already in the room and what needs to be obtained.

Planning

3. Wash your hands *for infection control.*

4. Check the physician's order:

   a. Solution to be given.

   b. Length of infusion time.

5. Take the parenteral nutrition solution out of the refrigerator *so that it can warm to room temperature.*

6. Gather the equipment: infusion pump, filtered tubing, an alcohol swab, tape for connections, and clean gloves. Use an infusion pump that is volume controlled. (See Module 53, Preparing and Maintaining Intravenous Infusions regarding volume-controlled infusion pumps.)

Parenteral nutrition is always infused by pump in order *to ensure that an exact amount of solution is given over a prescribed period of time.* Use filtered tubing. *The filter on the tubing prevents any particulates from entering the system.* Check the policy of your institution and note the time and date on either a tubing sticker or in a space provided on the intravenous record *so that the tubing will be changed if the time of infusion exceeds 24 hours.* New tubing is used with each bag of solution or changed after 24 hours *to decrease chances of infection.* Tubing changes are more frequent when giving parenteral nutrition than when giving regular intravenous solutions *because the high glucose content and protein component can promote bacterial growth.*

7. Explain the procedure and rationale to the patient and family if they are present. Answer any questions.

Implementation

8. Check the bag for the date of expiration, any cloudiness, or other imperfections. Compare the written contents of the solution on the bag against the order card *for accuracy.* Note that multivitamins are added to one bottle or bag every 24 hours. The solution with the multivitamins can be identified by its yellow color. Figure 58–3 is an example of an order card.

9. Depending on the type of solution bottle or bag being used, pull off the rubber or plastic cover, insert the spike of the tubing into the port.

10. Flush the tubing with solution, following the directions for the specific infusion pump being used.

11. Maintain infection control at all times, covering the distal end of the tubing with the sterile cap before carrying it with the pump to the bedside.

12. Hang the bag on the hook of the stand that holds the infusion pump.

13. Identify the patient.

14. Inspect the central line site for signs of inflammation or infection.

15. The tubing will go directly into the central line catheter. Put on clean gloves to protect yourself from contact with blood. Clamp the central line, remove the heparin lock cap and firmly attach the parenteral solution tubing. Infusing the solution directly into the catheter

HA ORDERS

DATE: _____

Dextrose ___*25*___ %   Amino Acids ___*5*___ %
Rate ___*1*___ L/Day   _____ cc/hr
Volume _____

NaCl _____	mEq/ *30*	Date ord. _____
Na Acetate _____	mEq/ ____	Date ord. _____
K Cl _____	mEq/ *25*	Date ord. _____
K Phos _____	mEq/ *15*	Date ord. _____
K Acetate _____	mEq/ ____	Date ord. _____
Ca Gluc _____	mEq/ ____	Date ord. _____
Mg SO₄ _____	mEq/ *8*	Date ord. _____
		Date ord. _____
		Date ord. _____
Reg. Insulin *0* u/ _____		Date ord. _____

Reg. Insulin *0* u/ _____   Date ord. _____
MVI _____ *10* ml/Day
Trace Minerals *1* ml/Day
Vit. K _____ *10* mg/wk   *(Sun.)*
Vit. C _____ *500* mg/Day

Lipids ___*20*___ % ___*500*___ cc/Day
Rate: *50* cc/hr

Maintenance IV rate: _____ cc/hr
Maximum IV rate: _____ cc/hr

NU-1192 Nursing Rev. 2/89 FC/SHMC

Figure 58–3 A medication card used by the nurse to check the contents of the parenteral nutrition bag.

and not through a needle *decreases chances for infection.* Some central lines have more than one port so you will have to verify which is being used for parenteral nutrition.

16. Place a pull-tape on the connection for safety (see Module 54, Administering Intravenous Medications).

17. For the first hour of infusing every bottle or bag, the solution is given at a rate not greater than 50–85 ml/h in order to avoid fluctuations in blood glucose. Then, the rate is adjusted to the ordered infusion time.

Persons receiving parenteral nutrition may also be "cycled." This means that for the first few days, the solution may be given over a 24-hour period and the time is then gradually decreased to 12 hours. In this manner, the rate of administration is gradually increased until the patient is receiving the optimum calories and nutrients for each 24-hour period. This is called "cycling up."

When it has been determined that the parenteral nutrition is to be discontinued, a similar procedure is used in reverse. The length of time that the solution is infused is

increased so that the person is getting less solution. This is called "cycling down." Cycling *allows the body to adjust to the rate of flow of the solutions.* Figure 58–4 is an example of a cycling form. Check the specific policy of your facility and the physician's orders.

18. Within 4 hours after beginning parenteral nutrition, check the patient's vital signs and urine and blood glucose levels.

Evaluation

19. Evaluate using the following criteria:
    a. Correct functioning of the equipment.
    b. Patient's vital signs remain stable with no rise in temperature.
    c. No evidence of either hypoglycemia or hyperglycemia when testing urine or blood.
    d. No untoward reactions such as nausea, vomiting, or diarrhea.
    e. Patient demonstrates desired weight gain.

Documentation

20. These fluids are usually documented as you would intravenous solutions (Figure 58–5). Any untoward reactions are recorded on the nursing progress notes.

PROCEDURE FOR ADMINISTERING FAT EMULSIONS (LIPIDS)

To administer fat emulsions along with parenteral nutrition, follow Assessment steps 1 and 2 and Planning steps 3–7 for total parenteral nutrition.

Implementation

8. Check the order against the label on the lipid glass bottle.
9. Select macrodrip, unfiltered, vented intravenous, or pump tubing if a pump is used.
10. Remove the metal covering around the top of the bottle without touching the sterile, black cap beneath.
11. Insert the spike of the tubing into the port of the bottle.
12. Flush the tubing as you would when administering intravenous fluids. Replace the sterile cover over the end of the tubing to maintain sterility.
13. Secure an alcohol swab, a sterile needle, size 20 or 21. Carry the lipids with tubing attached to the bedside.
14. Hang lipids bottle on same stand as hyperalimentation bag.

(text continues on p. 561)

DATE	TIME	PHYSICIAN'S ORDERS	NOTED BY
		TPN CYCLING ORDERS FOR NON-BMT PATIENTS	
12/26/94	1000	(1.) CYCLE SCHEDULE	

(Final goal: _2_ liters at night over _12_ hours)

	DATE	START TIME	BAG #	LITERS	RATE	HOURS
DAY 1	12/26	1900	5	1	110	10
DAY 2	12/27	0500	6	1	110	10
DAY 3	12/27	1900	7	1.5	135	16
DAY 4	12/28	1900	8	1.5	155	14
DAY 5	12/29	1900	9	1.5	185	12

2. TAPERING:

Start infusion at 50 ml/hour for 1/2 hour.

End infusion at 50 ml/hour for 1/2 hour.

3. Infuse _500_ ml intravenous Fat Emulsion 10%/20%

every _day_. Infuse over _4-6_ hours.

Begin when TPN started.

4. Heparin Lock catheter when TPN completed.

5. DC all sliding scale insulin coverage.

DC previous chemstick orders.

DC urine fractionals.

6. Obtain chemsticks each day of Cycle Schedule:

a. 2 Hours after TPN initiated

b. 1/2 hour after TPN completed

c. Notify Dr. _Norman_ if chemstick results are

>240 or <60.

7. DC chemsticks when Cycle Schedule is completed if chemstick results are

within normal limits.

DATE _12/26_ RPh/RN SIGNATURE _Nancy Alkins, RN._

PHYSICIAN SIGNATURE _N. Norman_

A DRUG EQUIVALENT MAY BE DISPENSED UNLESS CHECKED ☐

SIGNATURE IS REQUIRED FOLLOWING ENTRY OF EACH ORDER

SWEDISH HOSPITAL MEDICAL CENTER
Seattle, WA

PH-122 Rev. 6/90 FC/SHMC

Figure 58–4 A "cycling" form used by the physician to prescribe the rate of flow.

Date and Time	TUBING CHANGE: MACRO SET	MICRO SET	PUMP SET	BLOOD SET	DEVICE: PUMP	CONTR-OLLER	Initials	AMOUNT-SOLUTION-ADDITIVES (number consecutively)	Rate	SHIFT TOTALS: Time	Total	Solu' DC'd: Time	Amount Absorb.
Date: 8/1/94 Time: 2100	✓			✓	✓		V.P.	#1 1 unit RBC's O Pos. Vital Signs: Initiation: 98^7-88-18 116/84	80 ml.				
Date: Time:								10 Minutes 98^4-84-18 122/84 Completion: 98^8-88-20 126/82 Reaction: *Yes ☐ No ☒		06	250		250
Date: 9/2/94 Time: 0100	✓				✓		MM	#2 1 unit RBC's O Pos. Vital Signs: Initiation: 99-84-20 120/80	80 ml.				
Date: Time:								10 Minutes 98^4-88-20 124/84 Completion: 98^6-84-18 124/84 Reaction: *Yes ☐ No ☒		06	250		250
Date: Time:													
Date: Time:													
Date: Time:													
Date: Time:													
Date: Time:													

Identify Initials with Signature:

1. Vicky Paulson, R.N.	4.	7.
2. Mary Marcus, R.N.	5.	8.
3.	6.	9.

ADDRESSOGRAPH:

Cynthia Grant F-40
539-26-4967
Dr. John Torres

CODE: * see Nurses Progress Notes

SWEDISH HOSPITAL MEDICAL CENTER
SEATTLE, WASHINGTON

NU-1547 Nursing Rev. 10/86 FC/SHMC SN-6111

Figure 58–5 A form used by the nurse to document parenteral nutrition.

15. Put the needle on the tubing.
16. Choosing a port below the infusion pump and the filter, clean with an alcohol swab and insert the needle. The lipid solution is run below the filter so that its viscosity will not obstruct the flow by being trapped in the filter.
17. Secure with tape if a needle lock device is not used.
18. Using the roller clamp, manually time the lipids which will infuse with the parenteral nutrition solution.
19. If this is the first time a patient has received lipids, a test dose is given which means the lipids are started at a very slow rate. For example, if the equipment delivers 15 gtt/ml:
   a. 10% at 1 ml/min for 15 minutes, then the remainder over 4 hours (8 drops over 15 seconds).
   b. 20% at 0.5 ml/min for 15 minutes, then the remainder over 8–10 hours (3–4 drops over 15 seconds).
   Untoward reactions to lipid infusion include changes in vital signs, dyspnea, dizziness, chest and eye pain, nausea and vomiting, and a metallic taste in the mouth.

PROCEDURE FOR ADMINISTERING PARTIAL PARENTERAL NUTRITION

To administer partial parenteral nutrition through an existing intravenous line, follow the guidelines outlined for administration of total parenteral nutrition with the following adaptation:
1. Put on clean gloves for protection.
2. Discontinue other intravenous fluids or remove the heparin lock device if the port is not being used.
3. Insert the sterile end of the parenteral nutrition tubing directly into the needle hub. Place a pull-tape over the connection.
4. If lipids are ordered, administer them following the directions above.

DISCONTINUING PARENTERAL NUTRITION

The fat emulsions may be completely infused before the parenteral nutrition solution is infused. If this occurs, discontinue the lipids as you would other piggyback solutions. When the parenteral nutrition solution is completely infused, again discontinue the

therapy as you would do with other intravenous fluids. Reinstate previous fluids using a new, sterile needle if the fluids have not expired. If no other intravenous fluids are ordered, replace the heparin lock (see Module 53, Preparing and Maintaining Intravenous Infusions).

LONG-TERM CARE

Many long-term care settings accept residents who are receiving parenteral nutrition. In some agencies, the solutions are prepared and delivered by a commercial medical supply company. In others with a complete pharmacy department, the solutions may be prepared within the facility. Regardless of where

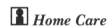 *Home Care*

Parenteral nutrition may be needed for an extended period of time after a patient is discharged. Nurses within the hospital teach the procedure to patients and their care providers. The teaching is well planned and directions in written form as well as demonstrations are given. The care provider finally gives the nutritional support to the patient within the hospital environment before taking the person home. It is important that they feel comfortable and confident before attempting the procedure alone in the home.

The general procedure is the same as that used in the hospital or long-term care facility. In urban areas, the solutions and equipment are purchased from one of a number of commercial companies. These companies usually make deliveries to the home at least twice weekly. They also act as a resource to the family *if any difficulties arise after the hospital nurse or nutritionist makes an initial visit to the home.* In nonurban areas, the family may have to make special arrangements regarding where and how to obtain the solution and equipment for the procedure.

The solutions are prepared as ordered by the physician and the family member is taught to add vitamins or insulin, if needed, at specific designated times.

the solutions are prepared, the general procedure for assessing the patient and administering and monitoring parenteral nutrition must be conscientiously followed *in order to ensure safety.* Your involvement as part of the nursing staff is to be knowledgeable and competent in administering parenteral nutrition to residents.

References

Cerrato, P. L. (1986). Will IV feeding endanger your patient? *RN, 49*(12), 59–61.

Young, J. P., Alexeyeff, M., Russell, D. M., & Thomas, R. (1988). Catheter sepsis during parenteral nutrition: The safety of long-term OpSite dressings. *Journal of Parenteral and Enteral Nutrition, 12*(4), 365–371.

Performance Checklist

General Procedure for Administering Parenteral Nutrition	Unsat	Needs More Practice	Sat	Comments
Assessment				
1. Gather the following assessment information as appropriate: a. Diagnosis				
b. Age and physical condition				
c. Height and usual weight				
d. Intake and output				
e. Allergies				
f. Usual vital signs				
g. Knowledge of procedure				
h. Mental status				
2. Assess the patient's unit regarding equipment needed.				
Planning				
3. Wash your hands.				
4. Check order, including solution and time for infusion.				
5. Take solution out of refrigerator to warm.				
6. Gather equipment: infusion pump, filtered pump tubing, alcohol swab, tape, and clean gloves.				
7. Explain procedure and rationale to patient.				
Implementation				
8. Check bag for imperfections and content orders.				
9. Pull off rubber or plastic cover and spike bag with tubing.				
10. Flush tubing with solution.				
11. Cover distal end of tubing with sterile cap and carry to bedside.				
12. Hang bag on stand holding pump.				

General Procedure for Administering Parenteral Nutrition *(Continued)*	Unsat	Needs More Practice	Sat	Comments
13. Identify the patient.				
14. Inspect central line for signs of inflammation or infection.				
15. Put on clean gloves and connect directly into central line catheter.				
16. Place a pull-tape on connection.				
17. Open all clamps and begin infusion rate at 50–85 ml/h or as ordered.				
18. Check urine or blood glucose level within 4 hours.				

Evaluation

	Unsat	Needs More Practice	Sat	Comments
19. Evaluate: a. Correct functioning of equipment.				
b. Patient's vital signs are stable, no evidence of rise in temperature.				
c. No evidence of hypoglycemia or hyperglycemia.				
d. No other untoward reactions.				
e. Patient demonstrates desired weight gain.				

Documentation

	Unsat	Needs More Practice	Sat	Comments
20. Document according to the policy of your facility.				

Procedure for Administering Fat Emulsions (Lipids)

Assessment

	Unsat	Needs More Practice	Sat	Comments
1. Assess as in Checklist steps 1 and 2 of procedure for giving total parenteral nutrition (gather baseline information, assess unit for equipment).				

Planning

	Unsat	Needs More Practice	Sat	Comments
3. Plan as in Checklist steps 3–7 of procedure for giving total parenteral nutrition (wash hands, check order, warm solution, gather equipment, explain procedure to patient).				

Procedure for Administering Fat Emulsions (Lipids) *(Continued)*	Unsat	Needs More Practice	Sat	Comments
Implementation				
8. Check the order against label on bottle.				
9. Select macrodrip, unfiltered, vented tubing.				
10. Remove metal cover without touching sterile, black rubber cap beneath.				
11. Insert tubing spike into port of bottle.				
12. Flush tubing as you would for intravenous fluids.				
13. Gather an alcohol swab, 20- or 21-gauge needle, and carry lipids and tubing to bedside.				
14. Hang lipid bottle on stand.				
15. Put needle on end of tubing.				
16. Insert needle into a port on hyperalimentation tubing which is below infusion pump and filter.				
17. Secure with tape.				
18. Time lipids as ordered.				
19. If test dose, give as follows: a. 10% at 1 ml/min for 15 minutes, then over 4 hours (8 gtt/15 sec).				
b. 20% at 0.5 ml/min for 15 minutes, then over 8–10 hours (3–4 gtt/15 sec).				
Evaluation				
20. Evaluate the patient for any of the following untoward reactions: changes in vital signs, dyspnea, dizziness, chest and eye pain, nausea and vomiting, metallic taste in mouth.				
Documentation				
21. Document according to the policy of your facility.				

Procedure for Administering Partial Parenteral Nutrition

	Unsat	Needs More Practice	Sat	Comments
1. Put on clean gloves.				

Procedure for Administering Partial Parenteral Nutrition *(Continued)*	Unsat	Needs More Practice	Sat	Comments
2. Discontinue other intravenous fluids or remove heparin lock device.				
3. Insert sterile end of tubing directly into needle hub. Place pull-tape over connection.				
4. Administer lipids, if ordered, following the previous directions.				

Quiz

Short-Answer Questions

1. The nutrients supplied by total parenteral nutrition are _____

   _____

2. Total parenteral nutrition is appropriate for which type of patients? _____

3. Partial parenteral nutrition is appropriate for which type of patients? _____

4. An infusion pump is always used to infuse the parenteral nutrition
   solution because _____

   _____

5. The solution is given directly into the central line catheter and not
   through a needle to decrease the risk of _____

6. Peripheral parenteral nutrition is usually only given for a limited period
   of time because _____

   _____

7. A common complication of parenteral nutrition is _____

8. This complication can be detected early by performing

   _____

9. Lipids may be given along with parenteral nutrition in order to supply
   the patient with _____

10. Lipids are available in which two concentrations? _____

11. How are the test doses for giving 10% lipid solutions administered?

    a. _____

    b. _____

Module 59

Giving Epidural Medications

Module Contents

Rationale for the Use of This Skill
Nursing Diagnoses and Potential
    Complications
Types of Epidural Catheters
Catheter Identification
Epidural Catheter Exit Site Care
Procedure for Administering a Medication
    Through an Epidural Catheter
    Assessment
    Planning
    Implementation
    Evaluation
    Documentation

Procedure for Setting Up a Continuous
    Epidural Infusion
    Assessment
    Planning
    Implementation
    Evaluation
    Documentation
Home Care

Prerequisites

1. *Successful completion of the following modules:*

VOLUME 1

Module 1   An Approach to Nursing Skills
Module 2   Basic Infection Control
Module 3   Safety
Module 5   General Assessment Overview
Module 6   Documentation

VOLUME 2

Module 35 Sterile Technique
Module 37 Wound Care
Module 49 Administering Oral Medications
Module 53 Preparing and Maintaining Intravenous Infusions
Module 54 Administering Intravenous Medications
Module 55 Caring For Central Intravenous Catheters

2. *Review the anatomy of the spinal cord and spinal canal.*

569

© 1992 by J.B. Lippincott Company

Overall Objective

To administer analgesics through an epidural catheter, maintaining safety for the patient.

Specific Learning Objectives

	Know Facts and Principles	Apply Facts and Principles	Demonstrate Ability	Evaluate Performance
1. *Purposes*	State reasons epidural catheter is used for narcotic administration.	Given an example of a patient with an epidural catheter, identify its purpose.	In the clinical setting, identify the reason a specific patient has an epidural catheter.	Evaluate with your instructor.
2. *Safety concerns*	State four safety concerns related to the administration of epidural narcotics.	Given an example of a patient, identify safety concerns present.	In the clinical setting, plan specific actions to maintain patient safety.	Evaluate with your instructor.
3. *Exit site care*	State usual procedure for exit site care.		In the practice setting, change an exit site dressing.	Evaluate with your instructor.
4. *Administering narcotics through the epidural catheter*	List supplies needed to administer narcotics through an epidural catheter by direct injection. List supplies needed to administer narcotics through an epidural catheter by continuous infusion.	Explain rationale for supplies needed. Explain rationale for supplies needed.	In the practice setting, administer a narcotic through an epidural catheter by direct injection. In the practice setting, administer a narcotic through an epidural catheter by continuous infusion.	Evaluate with your instructor. Evaluate with your instructor.

Learning Activities

1. Review the Specific Learning Objectives.
2. Look up the module vocabulary terms in the Glossary.
3. Read through the module and mentally practice the skills.
4. Review the procedures in your facility in regard to caring for epidural catheters.
5. Arrange for time to practice using an epidural catheter.
6. In the practice setting:
   a. Practice the procedures outlined in the Performance Checklist.
   b. When you have mastered these procedures, select a partner and critique each other's performance using the Performance Checklist.
   c. Arrange for your instructor to evaluate your performance.
7. In the clinical setting:
   a. Identify patients with epidural catheters in place.
   b. Arrange for an opportunity to observe care for these patients.
   c. Ask your instructor for an opportunity to carry out the specific care needed by the patient.

Vocabulary

analgesic
anesthetic
epidural
subdural

Giving Epidural Medications

Rationale for the Use of This Skill

The technology associated with providing pain relief is constantly expanding. One aspect of this technology is the administration of analgesic narcotics through an epidural catheter. Nurses caring for patients with epidural catheters must understand where the catheter is placed and how the system works in order to provide effective care and optimum pain relief.[1]

[1] You will note that rationale for action is emphasized throughout the module by the use of italics.

▶ *Nursing Diagnoses and Potential Complications*

The epidural administration of a narcotic carries hazards for patients, *so a narcotic antagonist should be available on the unit when epidural narcotics are administered.* The physician identifies the situations when the narcotic antagonist is to be used and orders the dosage.

Although one of the advantages of epidural narcotic administration is less frequent respiratory depression than with other methods of narcotic administration, Ineffective Breathing Pattern: Respiratory Depression still can occur. It is more likely if the patient is lying flat while an infusion is given *because the medication ascends along the dura.* The physician may order a narcotic antagonist for respiratory depression.

Alteration in Urinary Elimination: Retention arises *if innervation of the bladder is disturbed by the narcotic on spinal receptors.* Measure urinary output and palpate the bladder for distention. Catheterization may be needed.

Potential Complication: Hypotension may occur *because of the narcotic's action on receptor sites related to vascular responses.* Special attention to safety is necessary *because hypotension may cause dizziness.* A narcotic antagonist is only ordered if the blood pressure drop is precipitous.

Alteration in Comfort: Pruritis *that is sometimes accompanied by a rash is a fairly common adverse response to epidural narcotics.* For some individuals it is only mildly annoying and may be alleviated by lotion on the skin. For others it is extremely uncomfortable, necessitating administration of a narcotic antagonist. *As the narcotic antagonist relieves the pruritis, it also diminishes the pain relief.* Therefore, the narcotic antagonist may be given in small increments *to attempt relief of the pruritis without loss of pain control.* If that is unsuccessful, another method of pain management is necessary.

Potential Complication: Reversible Paraparesis weakness of the lower extremities may occur if a medication with a preservative or one not intended for epidural use is injected into the catheter and causes damage to nervous system tissue.

Potential Complication: Neural irritation related to particulate matter. A filter is placed on the epidural catheter *to ensure that no particulate matter, which might cause local irritation, is injected into the catheter.* The cap on the tubing is changed at regular intervals, depending on the frequency of use, *to prevent leakage from repeated puncture.* Check your facility's policy.

High Risk for Injury related to administering intravenous medications or solutions into an epidural catheter. Because the epidural catheter looks exactly like an intravenous catheter, a special safety concern is clearly identifying these two lines and not confusing them. *Medications intended for intravenous use may be neurotoxic and the dosage of narcotic given epidurally may be life-threatening when given by direct intravenous push.* In some facilities a brightly colored label specifying "epidural catheter" is placed on the epidural line next to the injection port. In other facilities the policy is that two nurses verify that the line is the epidural catheter immediately before giving any medication. We recommend that a large, very legible label be placed on the line next to any port (if there are several ports on the line use a label for each port). As a student, you may wish to always have a registered nurse identify the line with you. In all cases follow the hospital policy.

There is no danger if air enters the catheter, as there is with an intravenous line.

TYPES OF EPIDURAL CATHETERS

Epidural catheters are silicone rubber catheters that look like Hickman central intravenous catheters (see Module 55, Caring For Central Intravenous Catheters) and are used to administer a narcotic into the epidural or subarachnoid space. The catheter is placed by a physician (usually an anesthesiologist). When the catheter is used for long-term control of chronic pain, it is sutured in place and tunneled through the subcutaneous tissue to an exit site on the abdomen (Figure 59–1). When the catheter is intended for short-term use, it may not be sutured in place and may exit on the back under the insertion site dressing.

The catheter is the same type used to administer regional anesthetic for childbirth and some types of surgery. In some instances of chronic terminal pain, a low-dose anesthetic agent (such as Marcaine) is infused continuously into an epidural catheter *to provide pain relief.* When regional anesthetic agents are used in an epidural catheter, most states require that they be administered by an anesthesiologist or nurse anesthetist *because of the risk of serious complications.*

In this module we will discuss the administration of narcotic analgesics by direct injection or infusion into an epidural catheter. Although there are potential problems associated with the use of narcotics in this manner, they are not as serious as those from the use of anesthetic agents. Therefore, narcotics are commonly administered by registered nurses using the epidural route.

The major advantage of epidural administration of narcotics is that a lower total dose per day is needed to maintain adequate pain relief. This in turn allows the person to be more alert, more mobile, and less drowsy. In addition, respiratory depression is less common, as are other side effects of narcotics such as nausea, constipation, and dizziness.

CATHETER IDENTIFICATION

Because the epidural catheter looks exactly like an intravenous catheter, a special safety concern is clearly identifying these two lines and not confusing them. *Medications intended for intravenous use may be neurotoxic and the dosage of narcotic given epidurally may be life-threatening when given by direct intravenous push.* In some facilities a brightly colored label specifying "epidural catheter" is placed on the epidural line next to the injection port. In other facilities the policy is that two nurses verify that the line is the epidural catheter immediately before giving any medication. We recommend that a large, very legible label be placed on the line next to any port (if there are several ports on the line use a label for each port). As a student, you may wish to always have a registered nurse identify the line with you. In all cases follow the hospital policy.

There is no danger if air enters the catheter, as there is with an intravenous line.

EPIDURAL CATHETER EXIT SITE CARE

The temporary epidural catheter is covered with a surgical dressing after insertion, and this dressing is not usually changed. The care of the exit site for the permanent epidural catheter is usually identical to care of the exit site of a Hickman catheter. Be sure to follow the procedure outlined for your facility, or follow the general procedure for Hickman site care outlined in Module 55, Caring for Central Intravenous Catheters.

PROCEDURE FOR ADMINISTERING A MEDICATION THROUGH AN EPIDURAL CATHETER

For postoperative patients, epidural narcotics are injected intermittently into the epidural catheter. The medication gradually diffuses across the dura to contact opiate receptors in the spinal cord. *Because of this gradual diffusion,* the injections may be made every 8–12 hours. The amount used is often small, but *because it is concentrated where the receptors are located, pain relief is maintained.* The following procedure is

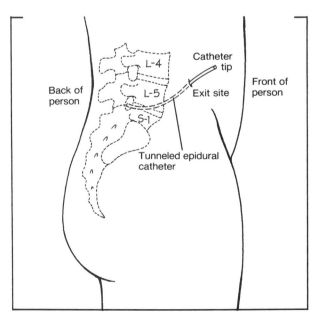

Figure 59–1 Epidural catheter for long-term use.

for the intermittent injection of narcotics into the epidural catheter.

Assessment

1. Check the physician's order for the medication.
2. Gather information on the drug to be administered.
3. Check for the type of epidural catheter in place (temporary or permanent).

Planning

4. Wash your hands *for infection control.*
5. Gather the appropriate equipment:
   a. Povidone-iodine swabs *to clean the tops of the vials and to swab the injection port. Alcohol causes pain and is toxic to nervous tissue and therefore is not used when preparing medications for epidural administration or on the injection port of an epidural catheter.*
   b. A 10- or 12-ml syringe with a 20-gauge, 1-inch needle *to administer the diluted preservative-free narcotic.* In addition, you will need a small syringe *if the narcotic comes in an undiluted form and must be drawn up and measured before dilution.*
   c. Sterile 2×2 gauze sponge

Implementation

6. Read the name of the medication from the medication record and check the label on the available medication *for your first check.*

   Use a prediluted preservative-free narcotic solution such as Duramorph, or a preservative-free narcotic and preservative-free sodium chloride for diluting it. *A large volume of fluid permits the narcotic to contact the optimum number of receptors. Preservatives used in multiple-dose vials may be toxic to nervous tissue.* Some facilities do allow narcotics with preservatives to be used in long-term epidural catheters as long as they are diluted with preservative-free saline. Be sure you follow the policy in your facility.
7. Recheck the medication record and the label on the medication after you have removed it from the drawer or shelf *for the second check.*
8. Follow your facility's procedure for recording the use of narcotics.
9. Prepare the medication, using sterile technique.
   a. If a prediluted narcotic is used, draw it up into the large syringe.
   b. If an undiluted narcotic is used:
      (1) Draw it up into the small syringe.
      (2) Draw up 10 ml of preservative-free saline into the large syringe and pull back to allow enough space for the narcotic.
      (3) Remove the needle from the large syringe and insert the needle from the small syringe into the tip of the large syringe. Inject the narcotic into the saline.
      (4) Replace the needle on the large syringe.
10. Recheck the medication record, the label on the medication container, and your syringe *for the third check.*
11. Identify the patient.
12. Explain the procedure to the patient, emphasizing what the patient will experience. The injection should not be painful.
13. Give the medication in the appropriate manner.
    a. Identify the epidural catheter.
    b. Clean the injection cap on the epidural catheter with a povidone-iodine swab.
    c. Dry the injection cap with the sterile 2×2 gauze. *Povidone-iodine may form a sticky residue if left on the cap.*
    d. Insert the needle into the cap.
    e. Aspirate. *If blood is returned, the catheter may have eroded into a blood vessel. Do not give the medication; remove the syringe and report to the physician. If more than 1 ml of clear fluid is aspirated, the catheter may have eroded into the subarachnoid space. Do not give the medication; remove the syringe and report to the physician.*
    f. Inject the medication. *You are injecting it into the epidural space, where it will be utilized gradually. It is not like an intravenous medication, which goes immediately into the circulation.* If the patient indicates discomfort, slow the injection. It may be hard to push the medication in *because the catheter is small and long.* If you are unable to inject the medication, check the tubing for kinks. If you are still unable to inject, withdraw the syringe and report.
    g. Remove the needle.
14. Dispose of the syringe and needle in the appropriate "sharps" container.

Evaluation

15. Evaluate the patient's response:
    a. Level of pain relief.
    b. The presence of any adverse effects:
       (1) Respiratory depression.
       (2) Hypotension.
       (3) Weakness or unsteady gait.

(4) Abnormal sensation in lower extremities.

(5) Lightheadedness or confusion.

(6) Sedation.

(7) Pruritus.

Documentation

16. Record the medication administered. Include name, dose, time, route, and patient's response.

A special flow sheet may be used to facilitate the documentation of pain status and assessment to identify adverse effects. See Module 54, Administering Intravenous Medications, Figure 54–3 for an example of such a flow sheet.

PROCEDURE FOR SETTING UP A CONTINUOUS EPIDURAL INFUSION

For patients with long-term pain, such as those with major trauma, a complicated recovery, or cancer, a continuous infusion of an epidural narcotic may be used *for pain management.* The continuous infusion is set up using an intravenous pump that is volume controlled *to provide the precise control of the dosage that is needed.*

Assessment

1. Check the physician's orders for the medication.
2. Gather information on the drug.
3. Check type of epidural catheter in place.
4. Take vital signs and note degree of pain *to use as a baseline for evaluation.*

Planning

5. Wash your hands *for infection control.*
6. Select the appropriate equipment. You will need a volume-controlled intravenous pump, the special pump tubing, the appropriate in-line filter if one is not already on the epidural catheter, 20-gauge 1-inch needle, povidone-iodine swabs, sterile 2 × 2 gauze sponge, tape, and labels indicating "epidural line."

Implementation

7. Read the name of the medication to be given from the medication record and compare with the infusion bag label. Be certain that it is labeled "for epidural use."
8. Recheck the medication record and label on the medication.
9. Record the use of narcotics in the manner prescribed in your facility.
10. Calculate the hourly rate of the infusion based on the ordered dosage per hour. Some

pharmacies print this information on the label, but others do not because it is confusing if the dosage is changed while the same bag is in use. As a student it is wise to have a registered nurse double-check your dosage calculation.

11. Recheck the medication record and the infusion bag label.
12. Attach the pump tubing to the medication container, set up the pump, attach the filter and needle to the line, and attach appropriate labels.
13. Identify the patient *for safety.*
14. Explain the procedure to the patient *to alleviate anxiety.*
15. Set up the infusion:
    a. Identify the epidural catheter by noting the written label.
    b. Clean the injection cap on the catheter with povidone-iodine. Do not use alcohol *because it is neurotoxic.*
    c. Dry the injection cap with a sterile 2 × 2 gauze.
    d. Attach the infusion set to the epidural catheter by inserting the needle into the injection cap.
    e. Tape the connection.
    f. Turn on the pump and set it according to the manufacturer's directions to deliver the prescribed dosage per hour.

Evaluation

16. Evaluate patient's response:
    a. Level of pain relief.
    b. Presence of adverse effects.

Documentation

17. Record on the medication record of the facility. Include name of medication, dose, time, route, and patient's response.

🏠 *Home Care*

Both intermittent and continuous epidural narcotics are used in the home setting to provide pain management to individuals with terminal pain. In these cases, family caregivers must be instructed in the techniques of epidural medication administration. In addition, they will need to learn how to care for the catheter exit site. After initial teaching in the hospital, a home care nurse is needed for ongoing assessment and support for the patient and family.

Performance Checklist

Administering a Medication Through an Epidural Catheter	Unsat	Needs More Practice	Sat	Comments
Assessment				
1. Check physician's order.				
2. Gather information on drug.				
3. Check whether temporary or permanent catheter is in place.				
Planning				
4. Wash your hands.				
5. Gather appropriate equipment. a. Povidone-iodine swabs				
b. 10–12-ml syringe with 20-gauge, 1-inch needle				
c. Sterile 2 × 2 gauze sponges				
Implementation				
6. Read name of medication from medication record and compare with medication label. a. Medication is dilute solution, or preservative-free sodium chloride is obtained for dilution.				
7. Recheck medication record and label on medication.				
8. Record use of narcotics.				
9. Prepare medication, using sterile technique. a. If prediluted, draw up into large syringe.				
b. If undiluted narcotic:				
(1) Draw narcotic into small syringe.				
(2) Draw 10 ml of preservative-free saline into large syringe and air to equal narcotic volume.				
(3) Remove needle from large syringe and insert needle of small syringe into large syringe tip. Inject narcotic into saline.				
(4) Replace needle on large syringe.				
10. Recheck medication record, label on medication container, and syringe.				

Administering a Medication Through an Epidural Catheter (Continued)	Unsat	Needs More Practice	Sat	Comments
11. Identify the patient.				
12. Explain the procedure to the patient.				
13. Give the medication. a. Identify the epidural catheter by noting written label.				
b. Clean injection cap on catheter with povidone-iodine.				
c. Dry injection cap with sterile 2×2 gauze.				
d. Insert needle into cap.				
e. Aspirate. If blood or more than 1 ml clear fluid returned, do not give medication.				
f. Inject medication.				
g. Remove the needle.				
14. Dispose of syringe and needle in "sharps" container.				
Evaluation				
15. Evaluate patient's response: a. Pain relief.				
b. Adverse effects.				
Documentation				
16. Record on medication record of facility. Include name, dose, time, route, and patient's response.				

Setting up a Continuous Epidural Infusion

Assessment

	Unsat	Needs More Practice	Sat	Comments
1. Check physician's order.				
2. Gather information on the drug.				
3. Check type of epidural catheter.				
4. Take vitals and check pain level.				
Planning				
5. Wash your hands.				

Setting up a Continuous Epidural Infusion
(Continued)

	Unsat	Needs More Practice	Sat	Comments
6. Select appropriate equipment. a. Volume-controlled pump				
b. Pump tubing				
c. In-line filter				
d. 20-gauge, 1-inch needle				
e. Povidone-iodine swab				
f. Sterile 2 × 2 gauze				
g. Tape				
h. Label indicating "epidural line"				

Implementation

	Unsat	Needs More Practice	Sat	Comments
7. Read name of medication from medication record and compare with infusion bag label. Check that it is labeled "for epidural use."				
8. Recheck the medication record and label on the infusion bag.				
9. Record use of narcotic.				
10. Calculate hourly rate of infusion.				
11. Recheck the medication record and the infusion bag label.				
12. Attach pump tubing to the medication bag, set up pump, attach needle and label to line.				
13. Identify the patient.				
14. Explain the procedure to the patient.				
15. Set up the infusion: a. Identify epidural catheter.				
b. Clean injection cap with povidone-iodine swab.				
c. Dry injection cap with 2 × 2 gauze				
d. Attach infusion set to epidural catheter.				
e. Tape the connection.				
f. Turn on and set pump.				

Setting up a Continuous Epidural Infusion (Continued)	Unsat	Needs More Practice	Sat	Comments
Evaluation				
16. Evaluate patient's responses: a. Level of pain relief.				
b. Presence of adverse effects.				
Documentation				
17. Record on medication record of facility. Include name of medication, dose, time, route, and patient's response.				

Quiz

Short-Answer Questions

1. Give two reasons epidural narcotics may be used instead of oral narcotics.

   a. _____

   b. _____

2. Identify two safety precautions related to the administration of epidural narcotics.

   a. _____

   b. _____

3. How does the exit site care differ for a temporary and for a permanent epidural catheter?

   _____

   _____

   _____

4. List four adverse responses to epidural narcotics?

   a. _____

   b. _____

   c. _____

   d. _____

5. What action would be taken if the patient experiences respiratory depression from an epidural narcotic?

   _____

   _____

   _____

6. What action is commonly taken if the patient experiences pruritis from an epidural narcotic?

   _____

   _____

   _____

Glossary

abdominal breathing Respirations in which the abdominal muscles and diaphragm are active; the abdomen moves out on inspiration and in on expiration; also called *diaphragmatic breathing*.

additive A substance that is added to a medication or intravenous solution.

adhesive A substance that causes two surfaces to stick to each other.

aeration Exchanging oxygen and carbon dioxide between the blood and inspired air in the lungs.

AIDS (Acquired Immunodeficiency Syndrome) A viral disease causing dysfunction of the immune system that can be transmitted through the blood and certain body fluids of infected persons.

air embolism A bubble of air moving within the circulatory system.

alimental Pertaining to nutritive material.

allergic reaction Reaction to a blood transfusion in which the recipient experiences an antibody reaction to allergens in the donor's blood.

allergy An abnormal body hypersensitivity to a specific antigen that is ordinarily harmless.

alveoli Air sacs of the lungs, at the termination of a bronchiole.

ambient Surrounding; encircling. Used to describe the normal air found in a room as ambient air.

ambulatory surgery Surgery done on the same day as the patient is admitted and discharged.

amino acid An organic compound containing both an amino (nitrogen) group and a carboxylic acid (carbohydrate-related) group that is the basic component of the protein molecule.

amoeba Any of various protozoans of the genus *Amoeba* and related genera, occurring in water, soil, and as internal animal parasites, characteristically having an indefinite, changeable form and moving by means of pseudopodia.

ampule A small, sterile glass container that usually holds a parenteral medication.

analgesic Any substance that relieves pain.

anastomose To surgically connect two tubular organs.

anesthesia (1) The total or partial loss of sensation. (2) The agents that are used to induce a loss of sensation.

anesthesiologist A physician with special training in the science and skill of administering anesthetic agents.

anesthetic Any agent that causes unconsciousness or insensitivity to pain.

anesthetist A nonphysician who is skilled in administering anesthetic agents.

anoxia A pathologic deficiency of oxygen.

antecubital space A depression in the contour of the inner aspect of the elbow; also called *antecubital fossa*.

anticoagulant Any substance that suppresses or counteracts coagulation, especially of the blood.

antiembolic stockings Stockings that are designed to aid the venous flow of immobilized persons or persons with circulatory impairment, or to decrease peripheral venous disorders; also called *support hose* or *TEDs*.

antimicrobial Capable of destroying or suppressing the growth of microorganisms.

antineoplastic An agent which inhibits the growth of abnormal cell tissues or neoplasms.

antiseptic Any substance that halts the

Selected definitions in this glossary are from *The American Heritage Dictionary of the English Language*, copyright © 1976 Houghton Mifflin Company. Reprinted by permission from *The American Heritage Dictionary of the English Language*.

growth of microorganisms, not necessarily by killing them.

apical pulse The heartbeat heard through a stethoscope held over the apex of the heart.

apnea The absence of respiration.

appliance Any device worn by a person to facilitate the meeting of basic needs; for example, any device worn to contain drainage from an ostomy.

armboard A firm, flat padded device that is used to straighten the arm and/or hand, to keep an intravenous infusion in place.

ascitic fluid An abnormal accumulation of serous fluid in the abdominal cavity; also called *ascites*.

aseptic Preventing contamination by microorganisms; also see *surgical asepsis*.

asepto syringe A medical instrument that is used to aspirate and instill a fluid. The tip is graduated in size so that it fits into tubings of various sizes; the rounded bulb is used to create suction to fill the barrel and pressure to expel the fluid.

asphyxiation Suffocation.

aspirate To remove gases or fluids by suction.

aspiration pneumonia An acute disease, marked by inflammation of the lungs, that is caused by inhaling substances (vomitus, mucus) into the lungs.

asymmetry Different in form or function on opposite sides of the body.

atelectasis The collapse of a group of alveoli due to blockage of the bronchiole passage by secretions.

auricle The external part of the ear; the pinna.

auscultation Listening with a stethoscope to the sounds produced by the body.

autoclave A device that establishes special conditions for sterilization by steam under high pressure.

autologous transfusion A blood transfusion of the person's own blood that was donated previously or recovered and processed during a surgical procedure.

axilla The area under the arm at the shoulder joint (the armpit).

barrel In a syringe, the cylinder that holds the fluid.

bevel On a needle, the slanting end that contains the opening.

bifurcation The point at which a structure divides or separates into two parts or branches.

bolus A measured amount of medication delivered at one time, usually into a vein or intravenous device.

bronchi The branches of the trachea that lead directly to the lungs.

bronchial Pertaining to or affecting one or more bronchi; see *bronchi*.

bronchiole The fine, thin-walled, tubular branches of a bronchus.

Broviac catheter A single-lumen intravenous catheter with an internal diameter of 1.0 mm designed to be surgically implanted into a large central vein.

buccal Pertaining to the cheeks or oral cavity.

butterfly (1) A type of tape that is used to secure two wound edges together. (2) A device that is used to start intravenous infusions; named for its plastic "wings," which are used to secure the device in place.

button A small, round, plastic device that is used to plug a tracheostomy opening.

cannula A tube that is inserted into a bodily cavity to drain fluid or to insert medication.

canthus The corner at either side of the eye that is formed by the meeting of the upper and lower eyelids. The *inner canthus* is the corner next to the nose; the *outer canthus* is the corner to the outside of the face.

capsule A soluble gelatinous sheath that encloses a dose of oral medication.

cardiac output The amount of blood pumped by the heart in a minute. It is the volume pumped in each stroke times the number of beats per minute. In the normal resting adult it is usually 2.5–3.6 L.

catheter A slender flexible tube, of metal, rubber, or plastic, that is inserted into a body channel or cavity to distend or maintain an opening; often used to drain or to instill fluids.

catheterization The process of inserting a catheter; most commonly used to refer to inserting a catheter into the bladder.

catheter-tip syringe Any syringe that has a

smooth, funnel-type tip to allow it to fit tightly into any type of tubing.

caustic Able to burn, corrode, dissolve, or otherwise eat away by chemical action.

cecostomy A surgically devised opening directly from the cecum to the abdominal wall.

cephalic vein A large superficial vein of the upper arm.

cerumen A yellowish waxy secretion of the external ear; earwax.

circulatory overload A situation in which the volume of fluid circulating in the body is more than the heart can handle adequately. It can develop if a large amount of blood or fluid is infused in a short period.

citrated blood Blood that is prevented from coagulating by the presence of citrate-phosphate-dextrose or acid-citrate-dextrose.

claustrophobia A pathologic fear of confined places.

clockwise In the same direction as the rotating hands of a clock.

collaborative problem A patient problem that the nurse must assess for, identify when present, and report to the physician for treatment.

colostomy A surgically devised opening directly from the large intestine to the abdominal wall.

combustion Burning.

compatibility A situation in which two substances can be mixed without a reaction occurring.

compatible In agreement, harmony, or congenial combination. No reaction occurs when two agents are combined.

complete blood count (CBC) A measurement that establishes the values of a variety of components of the blood, usually including red blood count, white blood count, hemoglobin, and hematocrit.

compromised host A person with a suppressed immune system, who is therefore less capable of self-protection against pathogens.

concentration of solution The amount of a specified substance in a unit amount of another substance; may be expressed as a percentage (20% solution), or as a ratio

(1:1000), or as a weight in a fluid amount (100 mg/L).

conjunctival sac The saclike inner fold of membrane on the lower eyelid.

constriction A feeling of pressure or tightness.

contaminated Having been in contact with microorganisms.

cough To expel air from the lungs suddenly and noisily.

cough reflex An involuntary nerve response that causes a cough.

counterclockwise In a direction opposite that of the movement of the hands of a clock.

cryoprecipitate A component of blood that contains Factor VIII—the factor hemophiliacs lack.

culture The growing of microorganisms in a nutrient medium.

cyanotic The presence of a bluish discoloration of the skin due to oxygen deficiency.

cycling Occurring in a pattern of regular repeated events. Used to refer to total parenteral nutrition or tube feeding schedules in which the daily intake is provided during a set number of hours followed by a number of hours with no feeding.

dead-air space The portion of the airway in which gas exchange does not take place.

debride To remove dead or necrotic tissue from the surface of a wound.

dehiscence The splitting or bursting open of a wound, usually of the abdomen.

depilatory A substance or device that is used to remove hair.

dermatologic Pertaining to the skin.

descending colostomy A colostomy performed on a portion of the descending colon.

dextrose A simple sugar found in animal and plant tissue. Also called glucose.

diaphragm (1) A muscular membranous partition that separates the abdominal and thoracic cavities and that functions in respiration. (2) On a stethoscope, the flat, drumlike head that is used most often for listening to lung and bowel sounds.

diluent A substance that is used to dilute or dissolve.

disinfect To clean or rid of pathogenic organisms.

disinfectant An agent that disinfects by destroying, neutralizing, or inhibiting the growth of pathogenic microorganisms.

diuretic A drug that increases the production of urine.

donor One who donates blood, tissue, or an organ for use in a transfusion or transplant.

dorsal recumbent position Person lies on back with knees bent.

dose A specified quantity of a therapeutic agent, prescribed to be taken at one time or at stated intervals.

double-barrel colostomy A colostomy in which there are two openings—one that leads to the proximal colon and one that leads to the distal colon.

douche A stream of water that is applied to a part or cavity of the body for cleaning or medicinal purposes; most frequently, in relation to the vagina.

droplet nuclei Microscopic particles that, when surrounded by moisture, become airborne.

dyspnea Difficulty in breathing.

edema An excessive accumulation of serous fluid in the tissues. *Dependent edema* is fluid that has accumulated in the lower areas of the body due to gravity; *periorbital edema* is fluid that has accumulated in the soft tissue around the eyes; and *pretibial edema* is fluid that has accumulated over the tibia.

embolus A moving particle in the bloodstream.

emulsify To combine two solutions that do not normally mix into one liquid, resulting in a suspension of globules.

endotracheal tube A rubber or plastic tube that is placed in the trachea for purposes of ventilation.

enteral Within the gastrointestinal tract.

enterostomal therapist A person, often a nurse, with specialized preparation in the care of individuals with ostomies and skin management problems.

epidural Outside of the dura mater that covers the brain and spinal cord.

epithelial Related to the cellular surface of the skin or mucous membrane.

erythrocyte Red blood cell.

ethmoid sinus The open cavity in the ethmoid bone that lies between the eyes and forms part of the nasal cavity.

evisceration Protrusion of a part through an incision after an operation.

excoriate To chafe or wear off the skin.

expectorate To eject from the mouth; spit.

expiration Breathing out.

explosive Pertaining to a sudden, rapid, violent release of energy.

exudate Fluid drainage from cells.

fat emulsion A form of fats in which the particles are finely disbursed so as to form a smooth fluid.

febrile reaction Reaction to a blood transfusion that occurs when the recipient is sensitive to white cells in the blood being transfused and a fever develops.

fenestrated tracheostomy tube A tracheostomy tube that allows air to pass through the larynx, allowing the individual to talk while the tracheostomy tube is in place.

fibrin An insoluble protein essential to clotting of blood.

finger stick A method used to optain a drop of blood for testing.

first-intention healing Uncomplicated wound healing that occurs when tissue is constructed between two wound surfaces that touch; also called *primary-intention healing.*

five rights A safety measure that is used to ensure the correct drug administration process. (1) The right drug is given (2) in the right dosage (3) by the right route (4) to the right patient (5) at the right time.

flowmeter A mechanical device that monitors the flow of oxygen or other gases or liquids.

fluid overload A situation in which there is more fluid in the circulatory system than it can handle; also called *circulatory overload.*

Foley catheter A rubber urethral catheter with an inflatable balloon at its end. When inflated, the balloon holds the catheter in place.

foreskin The loose fold of skin that covers the glans of the penis; the prepuce.

gag reflex A sudden involuntary spasm of the pharynx.

gatched bed A hospital bed that can be bent and raised at the knee area.

gauge A measurement of the diameter of a needle; a large number indicates a smaller diameter.

gavage Feeding by means of a tube.

Groshong catheter A central intravenous catheter that is inserted surgically and emerges from a subcutaneous tunnel on the chest. This catheter is characterized by a special tip which eliminates the need for heparin to maintain patency of the catheter.

hemodilution The dilution of blood by the presence of other fluids. Done purposefully before surgery when a patient's blood is donated and then replaced with intravenous fluids. The donated blood is returned to the patient during or after the surgical procedure as replacement for the diluted blood lost during surgery.

hemolytic reaction A reaction in which red blood cells are broken down as a result of incompatibility of the donor's red cells and the recipient's red cells.

hemophilia A hereditary, plasma-coagulation disorder principally affecting males but transmitted by females and characterized by excessive, sometimes spontaneous bleeding.

hemophiliac A person who suffers from hemophilia.

hemopneumothorax The presence of blood and air in the pleural space.

hemorrhage Bleeding; especially copious discharge of blood from the vessels.

hemothorax The presence of blood in the pleural space.

heparin trap A device filled with anticoagulant solution, used to provide ready access to a vein, making the presence of an infusing IV unnecessary.

hepatitis Inflammation of the liver, caused by infectious or toxic agents, characterized by jaundice and usually accompanied by fever and other systemic manifestations.

Hickman catheter An intravenous catheter with an internal lumen diameter of 1.6 mm designed to be surgically implanted into a large central vein. Both single- and multiple-lumen models are available.

Homan's sign Pain in the dorsal calf when the foot is firmly flexed; may be indicative of thrombophlebitis.

hub On a needle, the portion that attaches to a syringe or tubing.

human serum albumin A protein component of blood that increases the colloidal osmotic pressure of the blood.

humidifier An apparatus that increases the humidity of an enclosure.

hydrogen peroxide A colorless, strongly oxidizing liquid made of hydrogen and oxygen.

hyperalimentation Nutrition provided outside of the alimentary tract. Another term for parenteral nutrition; the introduction of nutrients into a large vein.

hypercalcemia An excessive amount of calcium in the serum; greater than 10.5 mg/dl.

hyperglycemia An excessive amount of glucose in the blood; greater than 120 mg/100 ml.

hyperkalemia An excessive amount of potassium in the blood; greater than 5 mEq/L.

hypertonic Having a higher osmotic pressure than body fluids.

hyperventilation Abnormally fast or deep respiration in which excessive quantities of air are taken in and excessive carbon dioxide is expelled, which causes buzzing in the ears, tingling of the extremities, and sometimes fainting.

hypothermia A condition in which body temperature is lower than that necessary for body processes to function adequately.

hypoventilation Abnormally slow or shallow respirations that result in inadequate air movement and thus inadequate oxygenation.

hypoxemia Inadequate oxygenation of the blood.

hypoxia An oxygen deficiency of body tissues.

ileoconduit A surgically constructed pathway for urinary drainage in which a segment of ileum is detached from the rest of the bowel, the ureters are attached to this ileal segment, and one end of the segment is closed while the other opens onto the abdomen in a single stoma; also called *ileobladder* and *ileoloop*.

ileostomy A surgically devised opening from the ileum to the abdominal wall, the drainage of which is liquid and contains some digestive enzymes.

incubate To provide conditions for growth.

inferior vena cava The large vein that returns blood to the heart from the lower body.

infiltration Leaking of fluid from an intravenous line into the tissue surrounding the vein.

inflammation Localized heat, redness, swelling, and pain as a result of irritation, injury, or infection.

inflatable cuff A plastic balloonlike device, such as the one around a tracheostomy tube, that, when filled with air, expands, producing pressure on surrounding tissues.

Infus-a-port A brand of surgically inserted subcutaneous central intravenous access port.

infusion pump A mechanical device used to control the rate and volume of fluids administered parenterally.

infusion The introduction of a solution into a vessel; commonly, the introduction of a solution into a vein.

inpatient A patient occupying a bed and receiving treatment in a hospital.

inspection A careful, critical visual examination.

inspiration The act of breathing in; inhalation.

instill To pour in drop by drop; commonly used to indicate very slow fluid introduction.

instillation The process of pouring in drop by drop; commonly used to indicate a slow process of introducing fluid.

intensive care unit (ICU) An area of a hospital set aside for the care of the critically ill.

intermittent Stopping and starting at intervals.

intermittent infusion adapter A device used to convert a regular intravenous needle into a heparin trap. (See *heparin trap.*)

intermittent infusion set A set that delivers intravenous solutions into a vein at intermittent time periods; also called *heparin lock* or *heparin trap*.

intracranial pressure The pressure existing within the cranium.

intradermal Injected into the skin layers.

intramuscular (IM) Injected into the muscle tissue.

Intrasil catheter An intravenous catheter designed to be inserted at a peripheral site on the arm and threaded through the vein until the tip rests in the right atrium.

intravenous Placed into a vein; often used to refer to the fluid being given directly into a vein.

intubation The placement of a tube into an organ or passage; often used to refer to placing an endotracheal tube into the trachea.

irrigate To wash out with water or a medicated solution.

isolation To set apart from the environment so that organisms cannot be readily transferred from one person to another.

ketone body A substance synthesized by the liver as a step in the metabolism of fats. May be present in abnormal amounts in situations such as uncontrolled diabetes mellitus.

laminar airflow hood A device that provides a controlled flow of microorganism-free air layers within a hood; used to create an environment for the sterile preparation of medications.

laparotomy A surgical incision into any part of the abdominal wall.

lateral Toward the side; away from the midline of the body.

lather A light foam that is formed by soap or detergent agitated in water.

lavage Washing, especially of a hollow organ (stomach or lower bowel) by repeated injections of water.

lesion A wound or injury in which tissue is damaged.

Levin tube A slender rubber or plastic tube that is usually used for decompression or nasogastric feedings; also called *nasogastric tube.*

lingula The projection from the lower portion of the upper lobe of the left lung.

liniment A medicinal fluid that is applied to the skin by rubbing.

lipids (fats) A term used to indicate the fat emulsion given as part of total parenteral nutrition.

liter The metric equivalent of 1.0567 quarts, equal to 1000 milliliters.

lobe A subdivision of the lung that is bounded by fissures and connective tissue.

local Of or affecting a limited part of the body; not systemic.

lotion A medicated liquid, especially one containing a substance in suspension for external application.

Luer-Lok A brand name that is commonly used to refer to a type of syringe tip that fastens securely to the needle by a twisting action.

lumen The inner, open space of a needle, tube, or vessel.

lung A spongy, saclike respiratory organ; also see *lobe* and *segment.*

maceration A process in which an area of skin softens and deteriorates following prolonged contact with moisture.

meatus The opening of the urethra onto the surface of the body.

medial Toward the midline of the body.

mediastinum An area in the center of the chest which contains the heart, great vessels, trachea, esophagus, thymus gland, and lymph nodes.

meniscus The curved, upper surface of a liquid column.

mercury A heavy poisonous liquid metal used in thermometers. Also used for weighting nasogastric tubes to facilitate passage.

microorganism An animal or plant of microscopic size, especially a bacterium or protozoan.

mucous Pertaining to mucus.

mucus The viscous suspension of mucin, water, cells, and inorganic salts that is secreted as a protective lubricant coating by glands in the mucous membranes.

nasal mucosa The mucous membrane lining of the nose.

nasogastric tube A long slender rubber or plastic tube that is introduced through the nose and esophagus into the stomach for purposes of feeding or aspiration.

nasopharynx The part of the pharynx immediately behind the nasal cavity and above the soft palate.

nebulizer A device that converts a liquid into a fine spray.

necrosis The death of living tissue.

needle A hollow, pointed device that is used to deliver medication into the tissue or to aspirate from the tissue.

noncoring needle A needle constructed so that it cuts a slit in a rubber stopper or diaphragm and does not cut out a cylindrical core.

normal flora Those microorganisms that are usually found at a site and that do not cause disease by their presence there.

NPO Nothing by mouth.

obturator Any device that closes the opening in a channel, such as a tracheostomy tube.

ocular Of or pertaining to the eye.

OD The right eye.

ointment One of the numerous, highly viscous or semisolid substances that are used on the skin as a cosmetic, an emolient, or a medicament; an unguent; a salve.

ophthalmic Of or pertaining to the eye or eyes; ocular.

oropharynx The part of the pharynx between the soft palate and the upper edge of the epiglottis.

OS The left eye.

ostomate A person who has an ostomy.

ostomy A surgically constructed opening from a body organ to the exterior of the body.

otic Of or pertaining to the ear.

OU Both eyes.

outpatient A patient who comes to the hospital, clinic, or dispensary for diagnosis and/or treatment but does not remain for ongoing care.

oxygenation Treating, combining, or infusing with oxygen.

packed red blood cells Components of blood that make up the blood product remaining after most of the plasma is removed from whole blood.

paralytic ileus Immobilization of the intestinal wall resulting in acute obstruction and distention.

parenteral Administered into the body in a

manner other than through the digestive (enteral) tract; for example, through intramuscular or intravenous injection.

parenteral fluid   Fluid given directly into tissues or blood vessels.

parietal pleura   The serous membrane that lines the walls of the thoracic cavity.

Parkinson's position   The patient is supine with the head tilted back hanging over the edge of the bed, and tilted to one side, to facilitate the administration of nose drops.

patent   Open.

pathogen   Any agent, especially a microorganism, such as a bacterium or fungus, that causes disease.

pectoralis muscles   Four muscles of the chest.

penis   The male organ of copulation and urinary excretion.

Penrose drain   A flat, soft-latex tubing; short lengths are often used to provide drainage from a surgical wound, while longer lengths are sometimes used as tourniquets.

percussion   (1) A process of striking a finger held against the body surface with a fingertip of the opposite hand and listening to the resulting sound as a part of assessment. (2) The striking of a hand on the chest wall to produce a vibration or shock that loosens secretions retained in the lungs.

perineal   Pertaining to the perineum.

perineum   The portion of the body in the pelvic area that is occupied by urogenital passages and the rectum.

peristalsis   Wavelike muscular contractions that propel contained matter along the alimentary canal.

pharynx   The section of the digestive tract that extends from the nasal cavities to the larynx, there becoming continuous with the esophagus; functions as a passageway for both food and air.

phlebitis   Inflammation of a vein.

piggyback   An intravenous infusion setup in which a second container is attached to the tubing of the primary container through a short tubing.

pinna   The flaring portion of the external ear that aids in the reception of sound waves. The auricle.

plasma   The liquid portion of the blood after red and white blood cells and platelets are removed.

platelets   Small, disk-shaped cells in the blood that adhere to any damaged surface and begin the clotting process; also called *thrombocytes*.

pleural space   A potential space formed by the visceral and parietal pleura and containing only enough lubricating fluid to allow the two surfaces to slide smoothly over each other during inhalation and exhalation.

plunger   In a syringe, the pistonlike rod that expels the fluid from the barrel.

pneumonitis   Acute inflammation of the lung.

pneumothorax   Accumulation of air or gas in the pleural cavity, occurring as a result of disease or injury or sometimes induced to collapse the lung in the treatment of tuberculosis or other lung diseases.

point   On a needle, the sharpened end.

Port-a-cath   A brand of surgically inserted subcutaneous central intravenous access port.

positive nitrogen balance   A condition in which the amount of nitrogen taken into the body is greater than the amount excreted.

postanesthesia care unit (PACU)   *see* postanesthesia recovery room.

postanesthesia recovery room (PARR)   An area of the hospital set aside for the care of the immediate postoperative patient; also called the recovery room (RR) or postanesthesia care unit (PACU).

postural hypotension   A sudden drop in blood pressure that is caused by a change in position, from lying to sitting or standing; may cause dizziness, fainting, and falling; also called *orthostatic hypertension*.

Proetz's position   The patient is supine with a pillow or other support under the shoulders, so that the head tilts straight back, to facilitate the administration of nose drops.

prongs   (1) Sharp or pointed projections. (2) A device that delivers oxygen at the nares.

prophylactic   Acting to defend against or to prevent something, especially disease.

pulmonary embolus   Obstruction of the

pulmonary artery or one of its branches by an embolus.

purulent Containing or secreting pus.

pylorus The passage connecting the stomach and the duodenum.

recipient Person receiving blood, tissue, or an organ as a transfusion or transplant.

recovery room (RR) An area of a hospital set aside for the care of the immediate postoperative patient; also called the post-anesthesia recovery room (PARR).

rectal Pertaining to the rectum.

respirator A mechanical apparatus that administers artificial respiration; a ventilator.

right atrium The chamber on the right side of the heart that receives unoxygenated blood from the body.

route In medication, a path of administration.

rubber-shod The presence of rubber tubing over the tips of hemostats or Kelly clamps to make them less traumatic.

saliva The secretion of the salivary gland, which contains mucus and digestive enzymes.

salvaged blood transfusion A transfusion using blood that is recovered and processed during a surgical procedure in order to be reinfused into the patient.

sanguineous Pertaining to or involving blood; containing blood.

sclerose To develop scarring or connective tissue. In a blood vessel, this causes the vessel to be occluded.

second-intention healing Healing that occurs through granulation beginning at the base of the wound; also called *secondary-intention healing*.

secretions Substances that are exuded from cells or blood.

segment A subdivision of a lobe of the lung.

semi-Fowler's position A supine position with the head raised 12–18 inches.

sensory deprivation A lower level of sensory input than that required by an individual for optimum functioning.

septicemia An infection in which the pathogens are circulating in the bloodstream.

serosanguineous Containing both serum and blood.

serous Containing, secreting, or resembling serum.

serum hepatitis A form of hepatitis caused by a virus transmitted primarily by blood and body fluids; also called hepatitis B.

shaft On a needle, the long narrow stem.

shock A syndrome characterized by insufficient blood and oxygen supply to the tissues; may be caused by hemorrhage, infection, trauma, and the like.

silicone A flexible material used in the manufacture of tubes and prosthetic devices.

Sims' position A side-lying position with the top leg flexed forward.

singultus Hiccup.

skin barrier An agent to protect the skin from the discharge of urine or feces.

sphenoid sinus The open area in the center of the sphenoid bone that lies at the base of the brain.

spore (1) An asexual, usually single-celled reproductive organism that is characteristic of nonflowering plants, such as fungi, mosses, and ferns. (2) A microorganism in a dormant or resting state that is especially resistant to destruction.

sputum Expectorated matter that contains secretions from the lower respiratory tract.

stab wound A small intentional wound made with a scalpel in order to introduce a trocar, tube, or drain.

sterile Free from bacteria or other microorganisms and their spores.

sterile technique A method of functioning that is designed to maintain the sterility of sterile objects.

sterilize To render sterile; also see *sterile*.

sternum A long flat bone that forms the midventral support of most of the ribs; the breastbone.

stethoscope An instrument that is used for listening to sounds produced in the body; also see *diaphragm*.

stock drugs Medications kept in a general supply, to be dispensed to individual patients.

stoma The opening on the skin of any surgically constructed passage from a body organ to the exterior of the body.

stopcock A valve that regulates a flow of liquid through a tube.

straight catheter A plain catheter without a bulb or balloon on its end.

stylet A thin metal wire or probe which fits inside a catheter or tube making it more rigid and easier to insert.

subclavian vein A vein of the upper body that lies under the clavicle.

subcutaneous (SC) Pertaining to tissue beneath the layers of the skin; sometimes called *hypodermic (H)*, a term that can also mean "injection," and is, therefore, not recommended usage.

subcutaneous catheter port A wholly implanted device for access to a central vein consisting of a flexible rubber intravenous line and a rounded metal reservoir with a rubber diaphragm which is entered through a skin puncture with a special needle.

subcutaneous emphysema Air trapped in the subcutaneous tissue that "crackles" when palpated.

subdural Immediately under the dura mater that covers the brain and spinal cord.

sublingual Beneath the tongue.

subungual Under a fingernail or toenail.

suction Withdrawing (gas or fluids) through the use of negative pressure.

superior vena cava The large vein that returns blood to the heart from the upper body and head.

suppository A solid medication that is designed to melt in a body cavity other than the mouth.

suppuration The formation or discharge of pus.

surgical asepsis The techniques that are designed to maintain the sterility of previously sterilized items and to prevent the introduction of any microorganisms into the body.

suspension A relatively coarse, noncolloidal dispersion of solid particles in a liquid.

symmetry The equal configuration of opposite sides.

syringe A medical instrument that is used to aspirate and expel fluids.

syrup A concentrated solution of sugar in water. A medicinal syrup has a drug added to the solution.

systemic Of, pertaining to, or affecting the entire body.

tablet A small flat pellet of medication that is taken orally.

TEDs A brand name that is commonly used as a synonym for antiembolic stockings; see *antiembolic stockings.*

tension pneumothorax A situation in which air gets trapped in the pleural space leading to buildup of pressure, which collapses the lung and causes mediastinal shift.

test dose A small amount of any substance that is given in order to assess for adverse reactions before regular administration is begun.

thoracentesis The insertion of a trocar into the pleural space of the chest for the removal of abnormal fluid.

thoracotomy A surgical incision of the chest wall.

three checks A safety measure that is used to ensure procuring the correct drug. The label is checked (1) before picking up the medication, (2) while holding it in the hand, and (3) after returning the container to its storage place.

thrombophlebitis Inflammation of a vein resulting from the presence of a thrombus.

thrombus A clot formed in a blood vessel.

thyroid gland A two-lobed endocrine gland that is located in front of and on either side of the trachea.

tidal volume The volume of air moved in or out during a normal breath.

tidaling Fluctuation of the water level in the long tube in the waterseal bottle.

tolerance In activity, the capacity to endure.

Toomey syringe A large-barreled syringe with a graduated tip that fits into a tubing.

topical Applied or pertaining to a local part of the body.

tortuous Having or marked by repeated turns or bends; winding; twisting.

tourniquet Any device that is used to stop temporarily the flow of blood through a large artery in a limb.

trachea A thin-walled tube of cartilaginous and membranous tissue that descends from the larynx to the bronchi, carrying air to the lungs.

tracheal ring The proximal, cartilaginous ringlike structure that surrounds the trachea.

tracheostomy A surgically devised opening into the trachea from the surface of the neck.

transfer forceps A sterile instrument with pincer or pronglike tips that is used to move sterile items from one sterile area to another.

transfer needle A double-ended needle used to transfer medication from the medication container to the fluid container prior to intravenous administration.

transverse colostomy A colostomy performed on a portion of the transverse colon.

Trendelenburg's position Position in which the head is lower than the feet, with the body on an inclined plane.

triage A process that prioritizes patients according to their condition so that the most expedient and appropriate treatment can be given to a large number of patients.

Tubex A brand name for a system of metal or plastic syringes and prefilled medication cartridges.

tympanic membrane The thin, semi-transparent, oval-shaped membrane that separates the middle ear from the inner ear; also called *eardrum*.

type To determine the type of a blood sample.

type and crossmatch A laboratory procedure used to identify whether the donor's and the recipient's blood are compatible. First, the type of blood (A, B, AB, and O and Rh factor) is determined. Then, the donor and recipient blood of the same type are mixed in order to observe for reactions.

umbilicus The navel; the site on the abdomen where the umbilical cord was attached during gestation.

unit dose A system of dispensing drugs in which each dose is packaged and labeled individually.

ureterostomy A surgically devised opening in which a ureter is brought out to drain directly through a stoma onto the abdomen.

urethra The tubular structure leading from the bladder to the surface of the body.

uvula The small, conical fleshy mass of tissue that is suspended from the center of the soft palate above the back of the tongue.

vagina The passage leading from the external genital orifice to the uterus in female mammals.

vaginal Pertaining to the vagina.

venipuncture The puncture of a vein; for example, in drawing blood or administering intravenous fluids and medication.

vesicant An agent which can cause blistering, necrosis, or the sloughing of tissues.

vial A small glass container that is sealed with a rubber stopper; may be used for single or multiple doses of a parenteral medication.

vibration A rapid, rhythmic to-and-fro motion.

visceral pleura The serous membrane that covers the outside walls of the lungs.

viscosity The degree of resistance to flow; thickness.

void The emptying of urine from the bladder through the urethra; to urinate.

waterseal drainage A chest drainage system that allows escape of air through a vent but prevents air from traveling back up the tube and into the pleural space.

wheal A small acute swelling on the skin; may be caused by intradermal injections or by insect bites and allergies.

whole blood Blood drawn from a living human being which contains all blood components and is prepared for use in transfusion.

xiphoid process Bone of the sternum at the level of the seventh rib.

Z-track A method for injecting medications that are particularly irritating or which stain the tissues; does not allow medication to track out through the needle hole.

Answers to Quizzes

Module 34 Isolation Technique

1. **a.** To protect the patient
   b. To protect the environment
2. Strict isolation
3. Enteric isolation
4. Any three of the following: private room with running water; sign on door; stand outside door for equipment; laundry hamper inside room; wastebasket lined with plastic; thermometer and blood pressure equipment
5. No special precautions are used.
6. Thoroughly wash your hands, doing a complete scrub.
7. To protect the patient from infection
8. Sensory deprivation
9. Any three of the following: give her care first; answer her call light promptly; stop and visit often; find diversions for her

Module 35 Sterile Technique

1. d
2. d
3. d
4. b
5. c
6. c
7. a
8. d
9. T
10. F
11. T
12. F
13. F
14. Any two of the following: heat-sensitive tape on outside of package; glass-tubing indicator inside pack; vacuum seal on bottle; intact seal on commercial package

Module 36 Surgical Asepsis: Scrubbing, Gowning, and Gloving

1. **a.** To remove microorganisms
   b. To remove dirt and oil
   c. To leave an antibacterial residue on the skin
2. Infection Control Committee
3. **a.** When serving as a scrub nurse in the operating room
   b. When serving as a scrub nurse in the delivery room
   c. When assisting with certain invasive diagnostic procedures
4. Because jewelry is a reservoir for bacteria
5. Because the wood may splinter and harbor microorganisms
6. It continues to inhibit the growth of microorganisms.
7. So that the water containing dirt, oil, and microorganisms drains off the elbows, keeping the hands the cleanest part
8. It lessens the possibility of contaminating the gloves while putting them on.
9. Your back is considered potentially contaminated because you cannot see what happens to it.
10. Notify the appropriate person for assistance in changing.

Module 37 Wound Care

1. **a.** Protection
   b. Absorption
   c. Application of pressure
2. **a.** To maintain sterile technique
   b. To observe and describe the wound
   c. To use appropriate dressing materials
3. **a.** Amount
   b. Color

592

    c. Consistency
    d. Odor
4. Any three of the following: edges approximated; smooth contour; minimal inflammation; minimal edema
5. Nonadherent
6. Paper tape
7. **a.** Breast surgery
    b. Hip surgery
    c. Perineal surgery
8. To protect the skin from the drainage
9. This action prevents spreading microorganisms from one site to another.
10. To debride the wound

Module 38 Ostomy Care

1. An opening from the ileum (small intestine)
2. The drainage is liquid and contains digestive enzymes, which increases the potential for skin breakdown.
3. Red and smooth without ulceration
4. **a.** Use a syringe without a needle to aspirate the urine.
    b. Use a tongue blade to gently remove feces from the stoma.
5. An ileoloop drains urine; it serves as a drainage path from the ureters. An ileostomy drains fecal material.
6. Seated on a toilet or commode
7. Approximately 1000 ml
8. 240 ml in each of three syringes, for a total of 720 ml
9. 3–5 inches
10. Approximately 15 minutes
11. Approximately 30 minutes after the patient gets up from the toilet
12. Because of the potential for urinary tract infection
13. Health teaching
Referring patient and family to community resources

Module 39 Catheterization

1. Any three of the following: fear of pain; anxiety over intrusion into body; embarrassment over lack of privacy; anxiety over relationship to reproductive system

2. There was no opportunity for the patient to express concerns or ask questions.
3. It is normal to experience some frequency; often urine will be in small amounts; minimal burning; increase fluids and call the nurse to measure the output for 24 hours.
4. b
5. c
6. c
7. c
8. a
9. a
10. c
11. b
12. d

Module 40 Administering Oxygen

1. **a.** Oxygen tent
    b. Nasal catheter
    c. Nasal cannula
    d. Oxygen mask
2. c
3. b
4. d
5. b
6. c
7. b
8. d
9. d
10. d

Module 41 Respiratory Care Procedures

1. Because persons who are immobile tend to breathe shallowly, leaving areas of the lungs unused. These areas may collapse or accumulate secretions. Deep breathing opens and expands the areas and encourages secretions to move.
2. 1:2
3. To use gravity to facilitate the movement of secretions from the lungs to an area where they can be coughed up and expectorated
4. **a.** Sitting upright
    b. Leaning 45° to right
    c. Leaning 45° to left
    d. Leaning 45° forward
    e. Leaning 30°–45° backward

5. All positions are lying head down at a 30°–45° angle:
   a. Lying on right side, shoulders at a 90° angle to bed
   b. Lying on right side, shoulders at a 45° angle to bed
   c. Lying flat on back
   d. Lying on abdomen
6. To loosen secretions so they will drain
7. To encourage deep breathing by giving immediate feedback on performance

Module 42 Oral and Nasopharyngeal Suctioning

1. a. To allay fears
   b. To elicit cooperation
2. Because pathogens can travel down the moist, continuous respiratory tract
3. To remove amniotic fluid and mucus that accumulate in the back of the throat and interfere with breathing
4. To obtain adequate suction, or pull
5. Lateral position facing you
6. a. To promote drainage of secretions
   b. To prevent aspiration
7. 15 seconds
8. Three times
9. When the oxygen level of the patient is critical
10. When the infant is suspected of having an infection

Module 43 Tracheostomy Care and Suctioning

1. c
2. b
3. a
4. d
5. c
6. c
7. a
8. d

Module 44 Caring for Patients with Chest Tubes

1. a. To remove air
   b. To remove fluid

c. To restore the normal negative intrapleural pressure
2. Air in the pleural space
3. Anteriorly through the second intercostal space
4. Air rises.
5. a. Promotes drainage because of gravity
   b. Prevents backflow of bottle contents into pleural space
6. Controls amount of suction applied to the chest tube
7. a. Airtight system except for vent in waterseal bottle
   b. Vent open
   c. Waterseal in operation
8. Tension pneumothorax
9. Anxiety and pain
10. a. The lung is expanded.
    b. No air has entered the pleural space.

Module 45 Nasogastric Intubation

1. Any three of the following: feeding; instilling medications; irrigating the stomach; gastric suction
2. So as not to damage the mucosa on insertion
3. Nausea; gagging
4. c
5. b
6. c
7. d
8. b

Module 46 Preoperative Care

1. Elective surgery is planned; emergency surgery is urgent.
2. Your care must fit the specific time frame but will include the essentials of care.
3. a. Deep-breathing and coughing
   b. Moving in bed and getting in and out of bed
   c. Leg exercises
4. To empty the contents of the stomach, thereby preventing vomiting and possibly aspiration
5. a. To remove dirt, oil, and microorganisms from the skin
   b. To prevent the growth of remaining microorganisms

   c. To leave the skin undamaged and unirritated
6. Because studies have shown a reduced infection rate over earlier preoperative shaves
7. **a.** It is more comfortable for the patient.
   b. There is less chance of nicks and cuts.
8. **a.** To establish a baseline
   b. To detect whether the patient is febrile, which might indicate infection
9. **a.** Removing colored nail polish
   b. Removing makeup
   c. Removing dentures
10. **a.** To notify them in case of emergency
    b. To tell them when the surgery is completed
11. b
12. d
13. a
14. c

Module 47   *Postoperative Care*

1. **a.** Tissues
   b. Emesis basin
   c. Equipment for taking vital signs (thermometer, stethoscope, sphygmomanometer, blood pressure cuff)
   d. IV stand
2. Any six of the following: time of arrival on unit; responsiveness; vital signs; skin condition; dressing; presence of IV; presence of bladder catheter; presence of other drainage tubes; safety and comfort
3. **a.** Is the catheter unclamped?
   b. Is the catheter connected to the appropriate drainage container?
   c. Is the catheter freely draining?
   d. What are the amount and characteristics of the urine?
4. 2:30 PM. Received from PARR. Drowsy, but answers to name call. T–97°; P–78; R–20, deep and easy; and BP–128/88. Skin warm and dry. Dressing clean, dry, and intact. P. Johnson, RN
5. Any seven of the following: operation performed; postoperative diagnosis; anesthetic agents used; estimated blood loss; blood and/or fluid replacement in surgery and PARR; type and location of drains; vital signs when patient left

PARR; medications administered in PARR; output; physician's orders
6. Any three of the following: localized pain; heat and swelling in lower extremities; positive Homan's sign
7. All of the following: encourage early ambulation; encourage fluids; administer stool softeners per physician's orders
8. Any two of the following: encourage early ambulation; encourage patient's participation; keep patient and unit tidy; listen; do patient teaching
6. Temperature (heat) in area
   Swelling
   Homan's sign (positive with thrombophlebitis)
7. Ambulation
   Encouraging fluids
   Give ordered stool softener
8. Any three of the following:
   Help person focus on the improvements seen
   Teach expected course of recovery
   Encourage use of support persons
   Encourage participation in care
9. Place flat with legs elevated
   Report status to surgeon
   Be prepared to administer prescribed: IV fluids, blood, medications
10. Alteration in Urinary Elimination: Retention
    Alteration in Bowel Elimination: Constipation
11. Decreases the incidence of postoperative complications
    Patients feel less stress.
12. Statements regarding anxiety and feelings of "nervous"
    Rapid pulse and respiration

Module 48   *Irrigations: Bladder, Catheter, Ear, Eye, Nasogastric Tube, Vaginal, Wound*

1. **a.** Cleaning
   b. Instilling medications
2. To instill medication
3. One of the following: eye, wound; bladder; catheter
4. One of the following: ear, nasogastric tube; vagina
5. **a.** Too high temperature
   b. Too great pressure

c. Incorrect solution concentration
6. That the drainage or outflow tubing not be blocked or clamped while fluid is being introduced
7. When the tympanic membrane is not intact
8. The fluid will tend to drain out too quickly and not come in contact with all vaginal surfaces.
9. To prevent the spread of microorganisms from one eye to the other
10. For seriously contaminated, traumatic wounds
11. Eye irrigations to remove dust particles and secretions, ear irrigations to remove buildup of ear wax, and catheter irrigations to keep catheter patent to decrease risk of infection.
12. The antiseptic powders used may cause irritation in some susceptible females.

Module 49   *Administering Oral Medications*

1. a. Stock supply
   b. Individual patient supply
2. a. As it is taken off the shelf
   b. Before opening
   c. Before it is replaced
3. a. Right drug
   b. Right dose
   c. Right route
   d. Right patient
   e. Right time
4. a. Identification band
   b. Ask to state name
5. gr 1/60
6. 30 ml
7. 15 or 16 min
8. 1 ʒ
9. 300 mg
10. 2 teaspoons
11. d
12. c
13. b

Module 50   *Administering Topical Medications*

1. a
2. c
3. b

4. Because of the danger of aspiration pneumonia with oil-based solutions
5. Ethmoidal and sphenoidal sinuses
6. Any three of the following: to protect, to soften, to soothe, to provide relief from itching
7. a. Dorsal recumbent position with knees flexed
   b. Sims' position
8. 20 minutes
9. Beyond the internal sphincter
10. To help the patient relax

Module 51   *Giving Injections*

1. a. Glass or Luer-Lok
   b. Disposable plastic
   c. Prefilled
   d. Cartridge
2. There are 100 units of insulin in 1 ml.
3. Length, gauge
4. a. Vials
   b. Ampules
5. Vial
6. Any three of the following: almost complete absorption; more rapid absorption; gastric disturbances do not affect the medication; patient does not have to be conscious or rational
7. 25-gauge, ⅝-inch needle
8. a. Upper arms
   b. Anterior aspect of thighs
   c. Lower abdominal wall
9. Intramuscular route
10. 22-gauge, 1½-inch needle
11. a. Upper iliac crest
    b. Inner crease of the buttocks
    c. Outer lateral edge of the body
    d. Lower (inferior) gluteal fold
12. Any three of the following: no large nerves or blood vessels; cleaner; less fatty; several positions can be used; better for small children because gluteal muscle is not well developed until after a child walks
13. a. Small muscle, so not capable of absorbing large amounts of medication
    b. Danger of injury to the radial nerve
14. The plunger is pulled back (aspiration).
15. To see whether the needle has penetrated a blood vessel

16. a
17. b

Module 52 Administering Medications to Infants and Children

1. 25.88 mg
2. 192,000 units
3. Four or 5 years of age
4. Dosages are small, so an error that is numerically small may have profound effects.
5. To enable the parent to maintain the role of comforter and protector
6. The choice of *not* taking a medication is an unacceptable action and should not be offered to a child.
7. A tuberculin (1 ml) syringe
8. **a.** 1600 mg/24 h
   b. 400 mg/dose
9. **a.** Preference of the child
   b. Nature of the medication
   c. Taste of the medication
   d. Diet prescribed for the child
10. **a.** The infant might not take it all and you would be unable to determine dosage given.
    b. The infant might reject the bottle.

Module 53 Preparing and Maintaining Intravenous Infusions

1. Microdrip set
2. Secondary administration set
3. No contaminated air can enter the container and come in contact with the sterile fluid.
4. Obtain another container and return the cloudy one to the source.
5. **a.** Hang it so the fluid level is higher.
   b. Put the second container on an extension hanger to make it lower than the first.
6. **a.** 31 gtt/min
   b. 24 gtt/min
   c. 33 gtt/min
   d. 33 gtt/min
7. Container every 24 hours, tubing every 48–72 hours
8. Too much fluid over a short period of time will simply be excreted *or* will cause

fluid overload; too little fluid may not meet the body's needs for fluid.
9. **a.** Direct pressure on the site
   b. Raising the patient's arm above the head
10. **a.** Clot over the needle lumen
    b. Clogged filter
    c. Lumen of the needle against the vein wall
    d. Kinking or pressure on the tubing
    e. Arm position
11. **a.** Pain
    b. Redness
    c. Swelling
    d. Warmth
12. **a.** Pallor
    b. Swelling
    c. Coolness
    d. Pain
    e. Diminished IV flow
13. **a.** Review entire system.
    b. Check container.
    c. Check drip chamber.
    d. Check tubing.
    e. Check IV site.
    f. Check extremity if armboard is in use.

Module 54 Administering Intravenous Medications

1. Because ports are made of self-sealing rubber. If a needle were inserted into plastic, the system would leak.
2. Slowly (approximately 1 ml/min), because it will be less irritating
3. To prevent the patient from receiving an inaccurate dosage of a lighter or heavier additive rather than the primary solution
4. Visual and chemical
5. A drug text or the manufacturer's literature
6. To provide access to the circulatory system without having to do repeated venipuncture
7. So that the pump mechanism will deliver the drug at the desired rate
8. To keep blood from coagulating in the lock
9. 50–100, depending on the drug manufacturer's directions

Module 55 *Caring for Central Intravenous Catheters*

1. **a.** To permit the infusion of solutions that would be too irritating to peripheral veins
   b. When peripheral veins have been used extensively or are otherwise unsuitable for intravenous lines
2. **a.** Infection
   b. Air embolism
3. **a.** To allow for assessment of the entry site
   b. To thoroughly cleanse the area and remove debris
   c. To apply antiseptic or antimicrobial ointment to decrease future growth of organisms
   d. To replace potentially contaminated dressings with sterile ones
4. Acetone increases the incidence of local skin irritation without decreasing the incidence of infection.
5. To provide a chemical and mechanical barrier to microbes
6. Because it might easily be mistaken for a peripheral IV. This could have serious consequences.
7. To prevent air embolus
8. The Hickman catheter has an internal diameter of 1.6 mm and can be used for drawing blood and administering nutrients, fluids, and medications. The Broviac catheter has an internal diameter of 1.0 mm and cannot be used for drawing blood but can be used for all infusions.
9. Repeated punctures of the cap with needles large enough to draw blood will damage the cap, leading to leakage.
10. To prevent air from entering and causing an air embolism
11. A noncoring needle (sometimes called a Huber needle)
12. Iodophor-iodine solution

Module 56 *Starting Intravenous Infusions*

1. **a.** May imply serious illness
   b. Pain
   c. Immobility
2. Any two of the following: to maintain daily fluid requirements; to replace past losses; to provide large amount of fluid rapidly; to provide medication
3. **a.** Short-beveled needle
   b. Butterfly
   c. Intravenous catheter inside a needle
   d. Intravenous catheter over a needle
4. **a.** Scalp
   b. Less chance of dislocation because less movement in that area
5. **a.** Applying a tourniquet
   b. Hand pumping
   c. Keeping arm in dependent position
   d. Applying warm, moist heat
6. Tincture of iodine; 70% alcohol
7. Date; time; type of device; catheter gauge; initials

Module 57 *Administering Blood and Blood Products*

1. **a.** Blood donated by an unrelated donor.
   b. Blood donated by a related donor.
   c. Blood donated by the recipient before elective surgery.
   d. Blood obtained before surgery and replaced with blood expanders until blood is needed and reinfused.
   e. Blood salvaged during surgery, filtered and reinfused.
2. Increasing fear of the transmission of certain diseases.
3. The same tests are performed on autologous blood and blood from an unrelated donor.
4. **a.** Restoration of circulating blood volume
   b. Replacement of clotting factors
   c. Improvement of oxygen-carrying capacity
5. **a.** Makes it possible to serve more needs with fewer donations
   b. Decreases the risk of complications
6. **a.** To increase oxygen-carrying capacity
   b. To increase circulating blood volume
7. **a.** A
   b. B
   c. AB
   d. O
8. Any four of the following: hemolytic, febrile, allergic, transmission of disease, circulatory overload, hypothermia, hyperkalemia, hypocalcemia, air embolus

9. Any four of the following: flank pain, dark urine, chest constriction, tachypnea, fever, chills, apprehension
10. a. Slow transfusion.
    b. Notify physician.
    c. Give antihistamine as ordered.
11. By covering the blood filter completely with blood before infusing
12. Because it may hemolyze the red cells it contacts
13. a. Recipient's name and spelling
    b. Recipient's hospital number as on face sheet of patient record
    c. Blood product type and Rh
    d. Blood unit identification number
    e. Expiration date on blood bag

Module 58 *Parenteral Nutrition*

1. Dextrose, protein, electrolytes, amino acids, vitamins, and calories
2. Patients who cannot eat for long periods of time or those who have sustained major trauma, pathology of the intestinal tract, or long-term illness
3. Patients who only need a temporary adjunct to their nutritional status
4. The rate of infusion must be controlled accurately.
5. Infection
6. Of irritation of the veins

7. Hyperglycemia
8. Fractional urine or blood specimens
9. Fat emulsions
10. 10% and 20%
11. If 10%, 1 ml/minute for 15 minutes
12. If 20%, .5 ml/minute for 15 minutes

Module 59 *Giving Epidural Medications*

1. a. To decrease the side effects and allow the patient to be more alert
   b. To allow lower doses of narcotics to be used
2. Identification of the catheter and observation for adverse reactions
3. Permanent catheter is dressed in the same way as an indwelling central intravenous catheter.
   Temporary catheter has an occulsive dressing that is not changed until the catheter is removed.
4. Any four of the following: respiratory depression, urinary retention, hypotension, pruritis, reversible paraparesis
5. Administer the ordered narcotic antagonist.
6. An antihistamine is given. If that is not successful, a narcotic antagonist is given in small incremental doses.

Index

Page numbers followed by f *indicate illustrations;* t *following a page number indicates tabular material;* g *following a page number indicates a glossary entry.*

603